W9-AQM-832

Drugs, Society, & Human Behavior

PSB 3442
Oct
UNIVERSITY BOOKSTORE
1 $30.95

Drugs, Society, & Human Behavior

OAKLEY RAY, Ph.D.

Professor, Departments of Psychology and Psychiatry,
Associate Professor, Department of Pharmacology,
Vanderbilt University and Vanderbilt University School of Medicine,
Nashville, Tennessee

CHARLES KSIR, Ph.D.

Professor, Department of Psychology
University of Wyoming
Laramie, Wyoming

FIFTH EDITION
with 119 illustrations

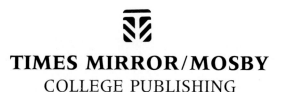

TIMES MIRROR/MOSBY
COLLEGE PUBLISHING

ST. LOUIS • TORONTO • BOSTON   1990

Acquisitions Editor: Pat Coryell
Developmental Editor: Vicki Van Ry
Project Manager: Carol Wiseman
Production Editor: Pat Joiner
Editing and Production: Editing, Design & Production, Inc.
Designer: Rey Umali

Cover photography: © G. Robert Bishop, 1989

Fifth Edition

Copyright © 1990 by Times Mirror/Mosby College Publishing

A division of The C.V. Mosby Company
11830 Westline Industrial Drive
St. Louis, Missouri 63146

All rights reserved. No part of this publication may be reproduced, stored in a retrieval system, or transmitted, in any form or by any means, electronic, mechanical, photocopying, recording, or otherwise, without prior permission from the publisher.

Previous editions copyrighted 1972, 1978, 1983, 1987

Printed in the United States of America

Library of Congress Cataloging in Publication Data

Ray, Oakley Stern.
    Drugs, society & human behavior/Oakley Ray, Charles Ksir—5th
  ed.
      p. cm.
    Includes bibliographical references.
    ISBN 0-8016-5048-8
    1. Psychotropic drugs.   2.   Drug abuse.
3. Neuropsychopharmacology.   I. Ksir Charles. II. Title.
III. Title: Drugs, society, and human behavior.
RM315.R37 1990
615'.1—dc20   89-20238
                              CIP

GW/D/D 9 8 7 6 5 4 3

Contents

Preface

The first edition of *Drugs, Society, & Human Behavior* was published in 1972, in a time of intense curiosity about psychoactive drugs and little understanding of how they worked and how they related to society. People were then most curious about LSD, marijuana, and amphetamine. This text provided students with factual, unbiased information about those and other drugs in a way that could be understood without a background in biology or chemistry. There was a need for such information, and *Drugs, Society, & Human Behavior* met that need for thousands of students. However, perhaps the greater benefit was provided by the historical and social context in which the drugs were presented. Students learned that human psychoactive drug use is not a new nor isolated phenomenon, but rather a feature of every human society. They learned that alcohol, coffee, and cigarettes were drugs, too, and learned to compare their actions, effects, and social roles with those of the illicit drugs.

RECENT DEVELOPMENTS

Times have changed since the early 1970s. People are now more interested in learning about "crack," "crank," and "ecstasy" than about amphetamine and LSD. Moreover, the general level of social understanding has changed. Given the history of our society since the 1960s, it is no longer possible to view widespread use of illicit drugs as new. After years of public discussion of drug use most of us have been forced to realize that "drugs" are not just used by some isolated, immoral subculture that can be suppressed through zealous law enforcement. Also, thanks partly to *Drugs, Society, & Human Behavior* and to other texts like it, more people now accept the notion that "nondrug" drugs (alcohol, tobacco, and coffee) have potentially damaging effects and are in fact drugs that are comparable to other psychoactive substances.

The rate of progress in the neurosciences was remarkable during the 1970s and 1980s, leading to new levels of understanding of the actions and effects of psychoactive drugs. It is particularly satisfying that many students who first became interested in psychopharmacology by taking a course based on *Drugs, Society, & Human Behavior* are now themselves scientists, physicians, or clinical psychologists engaging in research on the behavioral, biological, and social causes of drug dependence.

THE FIFTH EDITION

This new edition builds upon the many strengths of the fourth edition. Throughout the text, photographs, charts, and tables have been added or updated. Sections of each chapter have been rewritten to provide more recent information on self-reported drug use, medical emergencies, illicit drug supplies, and other drug-related statistics. The 1988 federal Anti-Drug legislation provided major new approaches to controlling illicit drugs.

The sections on mental disorders and on substance abuse and dependence were revised as needed to reflect the 1987 revision of the Diagnostic and Statistical Manual of the American Psychiatric Association (DSM-III-R). In addition, an alcoholism self-test is provided, as well as more information about the twelve steps of Alcoholics Anonymous.

For many of the major drug types, recent knowledge about mechanisms, toxicity, or medical uses has been added. These include new research on how alcohol works at the level of the neuron, new data on toxic effects caused by marijuana, and recent results of studies on the use of aspirin to prevent heart attacks.

One chapter, dealing with drugs and athletics, has been added. In keeping with the tradition of this text, the use of drugs by athletes is viewed first in a historical context. An effort is made to present a factual, unbiased account of the effects of stimulants, steroids, and other performance-enhancing agents, and of urine testing and other attempts to control abuses of these drugs by athletes.

It is our hope that this updated and expanded text will continue to serve the needs of both teachers and students by providing a basis for understanding drugs and drug use from pharmacological, psychological, and social perspectives.

LEARNING AIDS

1. *Objectives* are provided as an aid at the beginning of each chapter to alert the student to what he or she will be learning in that chapter.
2. A *summary* is provided at the end of each chapter to reinforce the major themes in the chapter and to provide an overall perspective.
3. *Key terms* are indicated in boldface so that

important concepts are pointed out to the student for study.
4. A *glossary* of all the key terms is found at the end of the book so that a definition can be found readily.
5. *"Your turn"* boxed items provide suggested exercises that involve the students directly in the material covered in each chapter.
6. *Issue* boxes in each chapter point to current concerns or controversies related to that chapter. This is a unique feature intended to enhance the relevance and currency of the text material for the student.
7. *Tables, charts, diagrams, and photographs* are used extensively throughout the text to increase interest, help explain key concepts, and focus attention on major ideas.
8. *Checklist for knowledge and interest.* This useful checklist allows the student to assess his or her level of knowledge and interest in each of the major topics covered in the text. Instructors may use a compilation of this checklist to design the course around student interests and needs.
9. *Appendices.* Appendix A provides a list of drug names, allowing for quick reference to determine the different types of drugs and a cross-reference to brand and generic names. Appendix B contains a list of drug information organizations and resources, including addresses and "hotlines" the student can contact for additional information.
10. *New four-color insert* displays different forms of illegal and over-the-counter drugs. This will help students to identify different drugs as they are reading about them!

SUPPLEMENTARY MATERIALS

1. Instructor's Manual

Prepared by Raymond Goldberg, Ph.D., of the State University of New York at Cortland, this comprehensive, unique Instructor's Manual includes the following practical features:

- A Testbank of more than 1000 examination questions, including multiple choice, true/false, matching, and essay questions
- Chapter overviews
- Chapter outlines with teaching suggestions, key terms and relevant transparency masters noted in margins
- Student activities, exercises, and assignments, which assist the student in evaluating his or her own values regarding drug use and abuse
- Related issues, including current topics for class discussion
- Current resources lists, including annotated readings, films, journals, etc.
- Transparency masters of the most important and useful illustrations found in the text, as well as some additional illustrations which are not included in the text

2. **Computerized Test Bank (Diploma II)**

   This software provides a unique combination of user-friendly aids and enables the instructor to select, edit, delete, or add questions and construct and print tests and answer keys. The Gradebook segment features computerized record-keeping, and class, test, or individual grade analysis displayed on bar charts. The Proctor segment allows instructors to set up student tutorials, using items from the Test Bank or specially written tests. The computerized Test Bank package is compatible with the IBM, Apple IIc, and Apple IIe microcomputers.

Acknowledgments

We would like to express our appreciation to the following instructors who reviewed the fourth edition and helped lay the groundwork for the improvements and changes that were needed in the fifth edition:

Pat McGarry
Texas Tech University

Rustem Medora
University of Montana

Helen Mountain
Lakewood Community College

Debbie Portch
Montana State University

Stephen Roberts
University of Toledo

I am very fortunate to have the opportunity to collaborate with Dr. Ray, and he has been most generous and supportive. Sandy and Amy continue to provide reasons for working and enjoying life. I would like to thank John Wilkinson, Sally Patton, Sue Rardin, and Max Rardin for pointing out important references or bringing news items to my attention.

Charles Ksir

Chapter 1

Drug Use: An Overview

OBJECTIVES

After reading this chapter, you should be able to:

Analyze a discussion, article, or presentation about a drug problem by seeing how well it answers a list of six questions.

State four general principles about psychoactive drugs and understand how each of these principles relates to the effects of the drug.

Describe four pharmacological revolutions that have altered our thinking about drugs and how each influenced our thinking.

Discuss the cultural changes that have occurred in the United States since World War II and how those changes relate to drug use.

Describe at least two methods for gathering information about drug use, and point out some advantages and disadvantages of each method.

Cite the approximate percentages of high school seniors and young adults reporting current use of alcohol, tobacco, marijuana, and cocaine, and describe in general terms any recent trends in those figures.

Name several psychosocial variables that have been found to be correlated with marijuana use among adolescents, and know which are the most highly correlated.

The interaction between drugs and behavior can be approached from two overall perspectives. Certain drugs, the ones we call **psychoactive,** produce profound effects on behavior. So part of what a book on this topic should do is to describe the effects of these drugs *on* behavior, and later chapters will do that in some detail. Another perspective, however, views drug taking *as* behavior. The psychologist sees drug-taking behaviors as interesting examples of human behavior that are influenced by many psychological, social, and cultural variables. In the first section of this text we focus on drug taking as behavior that can be studied in the same way that other behaviors such as aggression, learning, or human sexuality may be studied.

WHAT ARE WE TALKING ABOUT?
Talking about Drug Use

Phrases such as "drug use" or "drug and alcohol abuse" are heard almost daily on television or in discussions of social problems. But what do these phrases mean? Before you can meaningfully evaluate the extent of such a problem or propose possible solutions, it helps to define what you're talking about. In other words, it helps to be more specific about just what the problem is. Most of us don't really view drug use as the problem, if that includes your Aunt Margie taking two aspi-

1

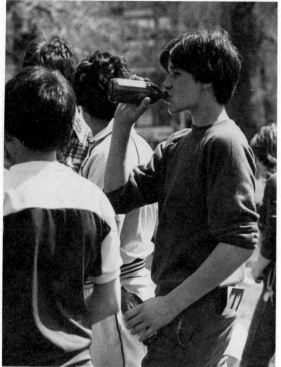

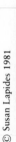

© Susan Lapides 1981

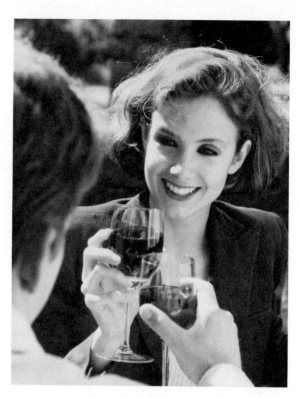

Our concern about the use of a substance often depends on who is using it.

rins when she has a headache. What we really mean is that use of certain drugs by certain people or in certain situations constitutes problems with which our society must deal.

Journalism students are told that an informative news story must answer who, what, when, where, why, and how. Let's see how answering those same questions plus one more can assist us in analyzing drug use as behavior.

Who is taking the drug? Obviously, we are more concerned about a 15-year-old girl drinking a beer than we are about a 21-year-old woman doing the same thing. We worry more about a 10-year-old boy chewing tobacco than we do about a 40-year-old man chewing it (unless we happen to be riding right behind him when he spits out the window). And, although we don't like anyone taking heroin, we undoubtedly get more upset when we hear about the girl next door becoming an addict.

What drug are they taking? This should be an obvious question, but often it is overlooked. One common example is a statement that some high percentage of students are "drug users." We don't know if there has been an epidemic of PCP abuse or a flood of heroin addiction or if the drug referred to is alcohol (more likely). If someone begins to talk about a serious "drug problem" at the local high school, the first question should be "what drug?"

When and where is the drug being used? The situation in which the drug use occurs often makes all the difference. The clearest example is the drinking of alcohol; if it is confined to appropriate times and places most people accept drinking as normal behavior. When an individual begins to drink on the job, at school, or in the morning, we have evidence that indicates a potential drinking problem. Even subcultures that accept the use of illegal drugs may distinguish between acceptable

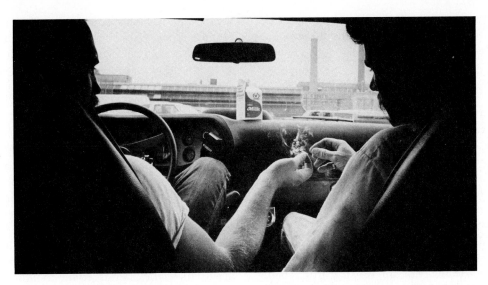

Drug use may be seen as more or less of a problem depending on when and where it occurs. How sharp will these guys be after their lunch break?

and unacceptable situations; some college-age groups might accept marijuana smoking at a party, but not just before going to a calculus class!

Why a person takes a drug or does anything else is a tough kind of question to answer. Nevertheless, we can see that it is important in some cases. If a person takes a **narcotic** drug because she just wrecked her knee while skiing and the drug was prescribed by her physician, most of us see no problem. If, on the other hand, she took that narcotic just because she likes the way it makes her feel, then we should begin to worry about her developing a dependency. One of the ways a psychologist can try to answer "why" questions is to look for consistency in the situations in which the behavior occurs (when and where). If a person drinks only when with other people who are drinking, we may suspect social motives; if a person often drinks when alone, we may suspect the person is trying to forget personal problems by drinking.

How the drug is taken can often be critical. South American Indians who chew coca leaves absorb cocaine slowly over a long period of time. The same total amount of cocaine "snorted" into the nose produces a more rapid, more intense ef-

fect of shorter duration and probably leads to much stronger dependence. Smoking cocaine in the form of "crack" produces an even more rapid, intense, and brief effect, and dependence occurs very quickly.

How much drug is being used? This isn't one of the standard journalism questions, but it is important when describing drug use. Often the difference between what one considers normal use and what one considers abuse of, for example, alcohol or a prescription drug, comes down to how much a person takes.

The importance of these questions for specifying drug use can be emphasized with one more example. It has been said many times in recent years that by the time America's young people graduate from high school, "the majority of them will have used drugs." Strictly speaking, that statement is true, as we will see later in this chapter. However, by asking some of our questions we also will be able to learn that the only drug other than alcohol used by even half of them is marijuana, and most of them have only experimented with it and are not current or regular users. The statement could be turned around and still be true: The vast majority of America's high school seniors are not current users of any illicit drug, and most of them have never experimented with any illicit substance other than marijuana.

Some Principles to Keep in Mind

Now that we've seen how helpful it can be to be specific when talking about drug use, let's look for some organizing principles.

Are there any general statements that can be made about psychoactive drugs—those compounds that alter consciousness and affect mood? In fact, there are four basic principles that seem to apply to all these drugs.

First, *drugs*, per se, *are not good or bad*. There are no "bad drugs." When drug abuse is talked about, it is the behavior, the way the drug is being used, that is being referred to. This statement sounds controversial and has angered some prominent political figures and drug educators. It therefore requires some defense. From the point of view of a pharmacologist, it is difficult to view the drug, the chemical substance itself, as somehow possessing evil intent. It sits there in its bottle and does nothing until we put it into a living system. From the perspective of a psychologist who treats drug addicts, it is difficult to imagine what good there might be in heroin or cocaine. However, heroin is a perfectly good painkiller, as effective as morphine, and it is used medically in many countries. Cocaine is a good local anesthetic and still is used for some medical procedures even in the United States. If nothing else, both drugs are useful to the scientist trying to understand the

---

Some terms that won't be defined—and why

Some terms that are commonly used in discussing drugs and drug use are difficult to define accurately, partly because they are so widely used. Let's start with the word *drug*. One definition that has been offered is "any substance, natural or artificial, that by its chemical nature alters structure or function in the living organism." Clearly antibiotics and alcohol fit this definition, but unfortunately one could also argue that food, oxygen, and water would fit. We should realize that in the context of a pharmacist discussing an order with a drug supplier the word drug may mean one thing and in the context of a policeman discussing problems at the local junior high it might mean something very different. One way to deal with this confusion would be to select an arbitrary definition appropriate for the material covered in this book and then stick to it. But what would be the purpose of such a definition? One purpose would be to help us answer a question, such as "is alcohol really a drug or not?"

In some contexts, such as a wine sauce to put on chicken, the alcohol probably would not be viewed as a drug. For the purposes of this book on psychoactive drugs, alcoholic beverages clearly deserve to be considered as drugs, along with cocaine and marijuana. Therefore our arbitrary definition should be such that the answer would be, "Yes, alcohol is a drug," but that answer isn't very informative unless we know the context in which the definition of drug was established.

Drug abuse is a term that has been used in many different ways in many different settings, and proposed definitions seem to immediately reflect the values of the definer. Some would consider any use of an illegal drug to be abuse, but many people who have tried marijuana on occasion would argue that they didn't abuse it. Other definitions of abuse rely on the notion of actual or potential harm. The problem is, the use of almost any drug, even under the orders of a physician, has at least some potential for harm. Again, we could set some definition and then use it to answer "is that behavior drug abuse or just drug use?" There would seem to be more useful ways of evaluating an example of behavior than putting it into one or the other side of this particular two-chambered box.

Drug addiction won't be defined either, but for different reasons. The concept of addiction has undergone some changes over the past 20 years, and a full discussion of this issue is included in Chapter 2.

Those interested in exploring these terms in depth are referred to the *Guide to Drug Abuse Research Terminology*, published in 1982 by the National Institute on Drug Abuse (NIDA). They spend a total of 2½ pages on these three terms and don't provide a simple definition for any of them either.

biology of addiction. Each of these drugs can also produce bad effects when people use them in particular ways and under particular circumstances. In the cases of heroin and cocaine, our society has balanced the perception of the risks of bad consequences against the potential benefits and decided that we should severely restrict the availability of these substances. It is wrong, though, to place all the blame for these bad consequences on the drugs themselves and to conclude that they are simply "bad" drugs.

A second basic, and often forgotten, fact about psychoactive drugs is that *every drug has multiple effects.* Although a user may focus on a single aspect of a drug's effect, we do not yet have compounds that alter only one aspect of consciousness. That a drug usually has many *different* effects on the individual using it might be expected from the fact that most drugs act at many different places in the brain.

This brings us to a third principle about psychoactive drug effects. *The effects of a drug depend on the amount the individual has taken.* This relationship between dose and effect works in two ways. By increasing the dose, there is usually an accentuation of effects noticed at lower drug levels. Also, and frequently this is a more important relationship, at different dose levels there is often a change in the kind of effect, an alteration in the quality of the experience. Varying doses,

then, can change not only the magnitude but also the character of the drug effect. Do certain dose levels constitute an abuse of a drug while other dose levels do not?

The fourth item of general relevance about psychoactive compounds is that *their effect, in part, depends on the individual's history and expectations.* Since these drugs act to alter consciousness and thought processes, the effect they have on an individual depends on what was there initially. The attitude an individual has can have a major effect on his or her perception of the drug experience. The fact that some people can experience a *real* high when smoking oregano and dry oak tree leaves—thinking it's good marijuana—should come as no surprise to anyone who has arrived late at a swinging cocktail party and been turned on after one martini rather than the usual two or three. It is not possible, then, to talk about many of the effects of these drugs independent of the user's attitude and the setting.

If there is one point about which every student of the drugs agrees, it is that there is no such thing as the drug experience per se—no experience which the drugs, as it were, merely secrete. Every experience is a mix of three ingredients: drug, set (the psychological makeup of the individual) and setting (the social and physical environment in which it is taken).[1,p.158]

There is, in addition, one fact about human conduct that we should keep in mind throughout this book: in spite of good, logical evidence telling us we "should" avoid certain things, we all do some of them anyway. We know that we shouldn't eat that second piece of pie or have that third drink on an empty stomach. Cool-headed logic tells us so. We would be hard pressed to find good, sensible reasons why we should smoke cigarettes, drive faster than 55 miles per hour, go skydiving, sleep late when we have work to do, flirt with someone and risk a good relationship with someone else, or use cocaine. Whether one labels these behaviors sinful or just stupid, they don't seem to be designed to maximize our health or longevity.

But humans do not live by logic alone; they

Your turn: in the news

Scan some recent newspapers or magazines for articles about drug or alcohol problems. Using the journalism questions (who, what, when, where, why, how, and how much?), evaluate the information contained in one or two of the articles. Be careful! The article may tell "who" said something and "what" was said without indicating "who" is supposed to be using the drug and "what" drug is being used. How complete were these articles in answering your questions? Did you find it easier or harder than you expected to find articles on drug problems by just scanning current issues?

are social animals who like to impress each other, and they are pleasure-seeking animals as well. These factors help to explain why people do some of the things they shouldn't, including drugs.

HOW DID WE GET HERE?
Have Things Really Changed?

Drug use is not new. As we shall see in later chapters, humans have been using alcohol and plant-derived drugs for thousands of years—as far as we know, since *Homo sapiens* first appeared on the planet. What recorded history we have indicates that some of these drugs were used not just for their presumed therapeutic effects, but also for recreational purposes. In some of the highly developed ancient cultures, psychoactive plants played important economic and religious roles. There is evidence that people have always over-used, misused, or abused these substances.

Although drugs appear to have always coexisted with humans, they certainly play a much different role in modern society than they did even 100 years ago. Major events have occurred in pharmacology and medicine that have produced revolutionary changes in the way we view drugs. In addition, recent cultural revolutions have influenced our attitudes and behavior regarding drugs and drug use.

Pharmacological Revolutions

One hundred years ago, most Americans had a very different view of drugs and their effects than we have today. There were only a few drugs that had powerful effects, and these were not very selective. For example, morphine is a powerful pain reliever, no matter whether the pain is caused by injury, infection, surgery, or cancer. The idea that a drug could be a specific treatment for a specific disease was only a dream. As a consequence, most people had limited faith in the power of drugs and were cautious about using them. Our modern attitudes about drugs are based to a great extent on several important advances in pharmacology.

The first revolution is the one that brought the major communicable diseases well under control. The use of **vaccines,** which began with Pasteur, Jenner, and Koch in the nineteenth century, certainly has had a major impact on our society. The deadly disease smallpox has been entirely eliminated, and other serious diseases are virtually a thing of the past; diphtheria, polio, and whooping cough are unheard of except when we refer to the vaccines for them. Measles, mumps, and tetanus also are preventable now through the development of specific vaccines. These advances helped to convince the public that medicine is capable of producing drugs with very powerful and very selective beneficial effects.

The second pharmacological revolution resulted from the introduction of **antibiotics:** "sulfa" drugs, penicillin, and then others. Proven effective first during World War II, they continue to save lives daily. These drugs not only can cure such previously dreaded diseases as syphilis and pneumonia; they can prevent or be used to treat infections resulting from injury or surgery, thus saving both lives and limbs. This revolution helped give us faith in drugs as real cures for serious illnesses. We now expect that when we get sick we will go to a physician who will prescribe a drug that will make us better.

The first two revolutions may be too pervasive and too close-to-home for most of us to appreciate their importance. This is not the case with the third pharmacological revolution—the development of **psychopharmacology** that began in the 1950s (Chapter 13). The most important single event was the introduction of the antipsychotic drugs for the treatment of schizophrenia and other major psychotic disorders. These drugs freed thousands of patients from long-term hospitalization and have helped to restructure our society's approach to mental illness on several levels. One important, but little-studied, effect on our culture came about because these drugs have their primary effect on mental processes. We came to accept the notion that drugs could have powerful and selective effects on our mind, our emotions, and our perceptions. Has modern medicine provided keys to the understanding of these long-hidden processes?

Perhaps the psychopharmacological revolution of the 1950s helped to set the stage for the "psychedelic" experimentation of the 1960s.

The fourth pharmacological revolution, the development of the oral contraceptive, contributed to the sexual revolution that was beginning to occur in the 1950s and has not yet resolved into stability. It is probably true that the opportunity for young, unmarried women to engage in sex without fear of pregnancy contributed to a greater sexual freedom in the 1960s and 1970s. That a married woman could be relatively certain for the first time of having even several years of her life uninterrupted by pregnancy made it possible for her to commit to more education and to developing her career. Perhaps those social changes were ready to happen without "the pill," but we all began to think in terms of scheduling pregnancies when they were most convenient. In fact, this convenience factor may be one of the most pervasive and subtle influences of the oral contraceptive on our society's view of drugs. For the first time, powerful chemicals clearly labeled as drugs were being used not to prevent or treat disease, but by healthy people because of their social convenience. Does this contribute to our perception of drugs as providers of gratification without worry?

Cultural Change

The present comes so quickly now that it's difficult to remember the past. When the rate of change in a society is slow, certain truths are self-evident and affect everyone's behavior. With moderate cultural movement the future is predictable. It is easy to feel secure extrapolating from where we are to where we will be in 10 to 20 to 50 years. With a predictable future you can make plans, follow through with them, and expect them to work out. As a guide to what you should plan for and educate for, you look to the past and see where society has been. With a slow rate of social change, your personal and society's history are important in planning for the future.

It's hard to keep track of all the social revolutions that have occurred since World War II. There were so many, and they came so fast, they seem to meld together. America bounded out of the war with a belief in the future that was untarnished by minor setbacks, such as an Iron Curtain, the Korean War, and an economic recession here and there. Everything seemed to be moving up after the depression of the 1930s and the war of the 1940s. This was the time to make it big, to make up for not having, for sacrificing.

The bright-eyed boys and girls who applauded the American flag when it appeared in the movies during the world war grew up, got married, and moved to the suburbs. These were the men in the gray flannel suits, and they *knew* progress was the most important product—their own progress. They knew where they were headed. They were after goodies. The formula was simple: hard work leads to advancement, which leads to more goodies, which. . . . Hard work and time, take aim and GO! Two cars, one acre, and zero crabgrass! This *was* the good life—and their kids would have it even better! When the harvest is good and the barns are full, even the tight people loosen up. It was Fat City! The children of the late 1950s grew up with everything. Honesty in history so all would know that the heroes of old had clay feet. Television so you could learn that there were better lives and that people would work hard to make you happy.

The guys in the button-down collars did it. They got what they wanted, and some that they didn't ask for. The world was no longer predictable; there were no more heroes. But the organization men of the 1950s and 1960s had made an affluent society. This was an important determiner of the Aquarian and hang-loose ethics of the 1960s and 1970s. Because it was possible to live adequately with very little work (and if you've always had everything, it seems easier to give it up than if you never had it) and because there was little training for achievement, the Protestant Ethic fast disappeared. This belief in self-restraint, drive, and hard work as the way to get ahead and be happy was gone for many people. Why work hard to have leisure time to enjoy life when you can work less, have more leisure time, and still survive?

I'll tell you what I think of hard work and conformity and your system. You tell me and teach me to think for myself. You stress the rights of the individual. So what if I mess around, my television tells me "nice people do get VD." Look at you, dad. What did all that hard work get you? A crummy house in suburbia—big deal. I want to do my own thing—be myself. I'm not sure who I am—but I know I'm not what you think I am. I'm a person, a unique individual, and I'm going to find me.

When you reject the hardworking 1950s, you appear in the "live and let live" 1960s. Being, not having, was a basic component of the youth philosophy. You can *be* only if you've experienced—yourself, the environment, the world around you. Individualism in clothes, actions, and thoughts were all components of the Aquarian philosophy. Give to others as Aquarius the water-bearer gives; but first know yourself, be yourself, and experience yourself, through drugs if necessary.

To reject the Aquarian age you have to tighten your belt and aim for something, and that's what we started to do in the late 1970s. The reaction began slowly—the shift to conservatism began, and economic growth slowed. The expansion of individual liberties and civil rights faltered and bogged down. The slowing was, in part, to digest the big changes that society had swallowed since the late 1950s.

Even as the slowdown developed in the early 1980s, the mood of the country changed. A mid-1981 poll found that 46% of Americans were optimistic about the future and believed that life would be even better in 5 years.[2] A study of above-average high school students in late 1981 found a 20% to 30% increase in conservatism compared to 1 or 2 years earlier.[3]

Everywhere you look, the action-reaction has occurred. The traditional religions and God of our forefathers shifted to social psychology and ecumenicalism, where they were saying that the differences they used to teach really weren't all that important. As the rock on which the churches stood was rapidly eroded, a new fundamentalistic,

charismatic, pentecostal, full-gospel revival exploded on the scene. From God to god-is-dead to *God!* in 20 years.

Universities used to be hallowed halls covered with slow-growing ivy and filled with pipe-smoking, deep-thinking scholars. College students in the 1950s were studied and described as "politically disinterested, apathetic, and conservative."[4] The students changed, the universities changed; federal money and a young faculty made many colleges active and activist. Marijuana replaced the ivy, joints replaced the pipes, and 12 credits "just for the experience of being" pushed deep thoughts to the background. The faculty aged, money grew tight, the students changed again—and so did the colleges. The faculty increased the number of required courses and became more concerned with uniform educational standards than with the students' individual experiences. And many of the students seemed only to care about the value of their degree in terms of starting salary.

If the 1970s were the decade of the "hippie," then the 1980s have been proclaimed the decade of the "yuppie": the young, upwardly mobile professional. The ideal yuppie appears to be someone who has a very nice (well-paying) job, wears very nice clothes, drives a very nice car, and lives in a very nice apartment. If married or unmarried, the ideal yuppie has a meaningful relationship with a very nice member of the opposite sex who also has a very nice job, very nice clothes, and so on.

The stereotyped 1980s person is more interested in personal health than previous generations; running shoes, jazzercise, Nautilus centers, and home exercise equipment have burst upon us. You would expect that these health-conscious individuals would use fewer drugs and they may: light beers, low-alcohol beverages, and decaffeinated coffee and soft drinks have grown rapidly in popularity. Average consumption of alcohol and cigarettes has declined along with drops in per capita intake of sugar and red meat.[5] But this yuppie stereotype also likes to indulge the upwardly mobile tendencies: we are very status conscious.

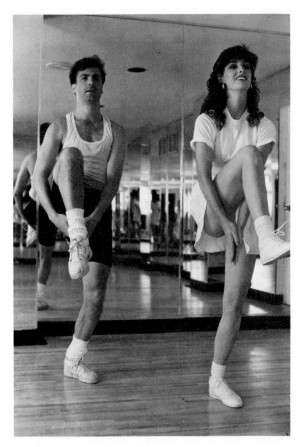

The stereotypical "yuppie" of the 1980s could be found working out at a local health club.

We may drink Perrier water when we're thirsty, but when we do want some calories, designer chocolates and imported cheese are called for. It is ironic that expensive imported beers are also selling well, even though more alcoholic and caloric than their domestic counterparts.[5]

So we seem capable of turning off our concern over health for a little self-indulgence, if what we're indulging in is chic and expensive. In that context, what was the major new drug of abuse for this generation? Until recently, considered by many to be relatively safe and nonaddicting? Expensive, supposedly glamorous, used by film and TV stars and sports figures? "Coke" is it! (And it's not the kind in the red and white cans.)

DRUGS AND DRUG USE TODAY
Extent of Drug Use

In trying to get an overall picture of drug use in today's society, we run into an issue that will be with us repeatedly throughout: getting accurate information. Measuring the use of, let us say, cocaine, in the United States is not possible to do with a high degree of accuracy. We don't really know how much is imported and sold because most of it is illegal. We don't really know how many cocaine users there are in the country because we have no good way of counting them. For some things, such as prescription drugs, tobacco, or alcohol, we have a wealth of information and can make much better estimates of per-capita use. Even there, however, our information may not be complete (home-brewed beer would not be counted, for example, and prescription drugs may be bought and then left unused in the medicine cabinet).

Let us look at some of the kinds of information that we do have. A large number of survey **questionnaire** studies have been conducted in junior highs, high schools, and colleges, partly because this is one of the easiest ways to get a lot of information with a minimum of fuss. The researcher enters a room full of people with free time and pencils or pens, who are used to doing pretty much what they're told to do in that situation and who can be assumed to be able to read and write. Questionnaires are handed to the students, asking them to report on their own drug use, and most of them do fill them out.

There are a couple of drawbacks to this type of research. The first is that you can only use this technique on the students who are in classrooms. We can't get this information from the people who have already graduated from high school and didn't go to college or from the high-school dropout. Imagine being sent to conduct such a questionnaire survey at meetings of all the Hell's Angels motorcycle gangs!

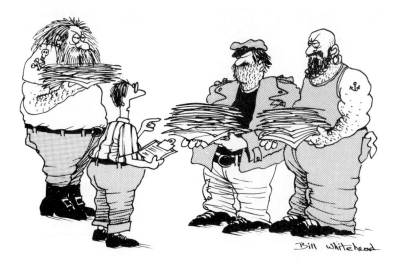

"Now, if you'll please answer these questions about your personal drug use. . . ."

A second limitation is that we must assume that most of the self-reports are done honestly. In most cases we have no way of checking to see if Johnny really did smoke marijuana last week, as he claimed on the questionnaire. Nevertheless, if every effort is made to encourage honesty (including assurances of anonymity), we expect that this factor is minimized. To the extent that tendencies to overreport or underreport drug use are relatively constant from one year to the next, we can use such results to reflect trends in drug use over time and to compare relative reported use of various drugs. Table 1-1 presents recent data from one of the best and most complete research programs of this type.[6] Data are collected each year from over 15,000 high school seniors in schools across the United States, so that nationwide trends can be assessed. We are presenting three numbers for each drug: the percent of students who have *ever* used the drug, the smaller percent who report having used it within the past *30 days,* and the still smaller percent who report *daily* use for the past 30 days. Note that almost all of these seniors have tried alcohol at some time in their lives and a large fraction have tried cigarettes. Just under half have tried marijuana, and for the rest of the drugs listed most students report never having

Table 1-1			
Percentage of high school seniors reporting use of eleven types of drugs (Class of 1988)			
Drug	**Ever used**	**Used in last 30 days**	**Used daily in last 30 days**
Marijuana/hashish	47	18	2.7
Inhalants	17	3	0.2
Hallucinogens	9	2	0.0
Cocaine	12	3	0.2
Heroin	1	0	0.0
Other opiates	9	2	0.1
Stimulants	20	5	0.3
Sedatives	8	1	0.1
Tranquilizers	9	2	0.0
Alcohol	92	64	4.2
Cigarettes	66	29	18.1

tried them. Also note that daily use of any of these drugs other than cigarettes can be considered somewhat rare. Fig. 1-1 shows trends from 1975-1988 in the reported use within the past *30 days* for several of the drugs. From this we can see the large and stable number of seniors drinking al-

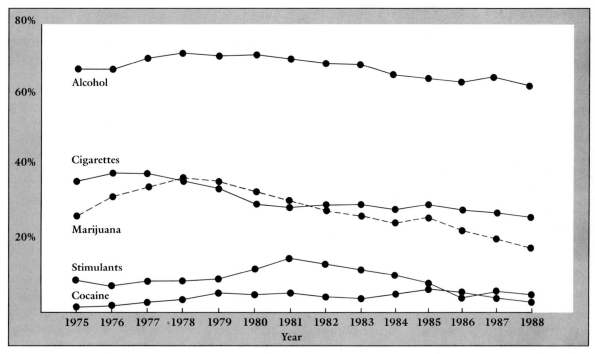

Figure 1-1. Trends in reported drug use in last 30 days for high school seniors.

cohol over these years, compared to the lower and decreasing number currently smoking marijuana. Reported current use of cocaine reached a peak in 1985, then dropped in the next three years to pre-1980 levels. Although not seen in the data presented here, it should be noted that there are fairly large regional differences in reported cocaine use, with more people in the West and Northeast reporting such use. Also, reported cocaine use is much higher in large cities than in rural areas. Regional and population density differences are not as great for the other drugs.

Another way to get broad-based self-report information is with house-to-house surveys. With proper sampling techniques these studies can estimate the drug use in most of the population, not just among students. This technique is much more time consuming and expensive, there is a greater rate of refusal to participate, and we must suspect that individuals engaged in illegal drug use would be reluctant to reveal that fact to a stranger on

their doorstep. Table 1-2 presents recent data from the National Survey on Drug Abuse,[7] obtained from over 5000 randomly selected individuals in carefully sampled households across the country. Data are shown only for reported use *ever* and in the past *30 days*. Note that data are presented for three age groups: 12 to 17, 18 to 25, and 26 and older. It should come as no surprise that the overall numbers are fairly similar to those obtained from high school seniors. Fig. 1-2 shows trends in the *30-day* figures since 1974. Again, we see evidence for a drop in marijuana use since 1979 and for a slight drop in cocaine use following the large increase in 1979.

Correlates of Drug Use

Once we know that a drug is used by some percentage of a group of people, the next logical step is to ask about the characteristics of those who use the drug as compared with those who don't.

Table 1-2

Percentage reporting use of nine types of drugs

Drug	Age 12-17 ever/last month	Age 18-25 ever/last month	Age 26+ ever/last month
Marijuana/ hashish	24/12	60/22	27/6
Hallucinogens	3/1	11/2	6/0
Cocaine	5/2	28/8	10/2
Heroin	0/0	1/0	1/0
Stimulants	6/2	17/4	8/1
Sedatives	4/1	11/2	5/1
Tranquilizers	5/1	12/2	7/1
Alcohol	56/31	93/71	89/61
Cigarettes	45/15	76/37	80/33

Often the same questionnaires that ask each person which drugs they have used also include several questions about the person completing the questionnaire. The researchers may then send their computers "prospecting" through the data to see if certain personal characteristics might be correlated with drug use. An important point to remember about these studies is that they rarely reveal much about either very unusual or very common types or amounts of drug use. For example, if we sent a computer combing through the data from 1000 questionnaires looking for characteristics correlated with heroin use, we'd fail to get an answer because only one or two people in that sample might report heroin use, and you can't correlate much based on one or two people. Likewise, it would be difficult to characterize the people who have "ever tried" alcohol, because that group usually represents over 90% of the sample.

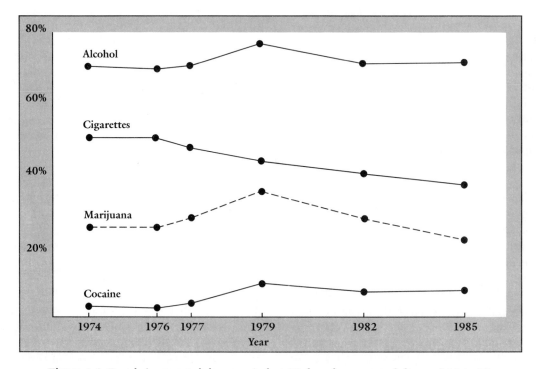

Figure 1-2. Trends in reported drug use in last 30 days for young adults aged 18 to 25.

Much of the research on correlates of drug use has used marijuana smoking as an indicator, partly because marijuana use has been a matter of some concern and partly because enough people have tried it so that meaningful correlations can be done. Other researchers focus on early drinking or on amount of drinking, and others have developed composite "drug use" scores based on use of alcohol and marijuana and experimentation with other substances. When studies of this type have been done on high school populations, the first couple of variables that always show some relationship to drug use are age and sex. It should be obvious that as these students get older they will have had more opportunities not only to experiment with more substances, but to initiate regular use of some of them. Gender differences are interesting, in that males are about twice as likely as females to be current marijuana smokers or to drink heavily, and males generally show somewhat greater use of all illicit drugs.[8] The one reversal is with cigarette smoking, which is more common among high school girls than boys (Chapter 10).

You may be surprised at some of the factors that generally do *not* correlate well with alcohol or drug use. One of these is the **socioeconomic status (SES)** of the family. Whether reporting on illicit drug use or level of drinking, most studies find little correlation to the parents' field of employment (professional, clerical, or blue-collar, for example). These results surprise some people who think it's the kids with all the money who use drugs and other people who believe that it's the poor kids who use drugs. In fact, most of these studies do not gather enough data on the most economically disadvantaged youth, and when those groups are studied there is a higher rate of drug use.[9] So, very low SES does play a role in drug and alcohol use, but for the vast majority of the population, SES is not a significant factor. Another surprise for most people is the consistent finding that **personality problems** are such poor predictors of drug use. In spite of the fact that many theories of drug use assume that people use alcohol or drugs because of low self-esteem,

depression, or anxiety, study after study has found that measures of these characteristics are only weakly correlated with drug use. People often report that they drink or use drugs when they're depressed or anxious, but they are probably referring to a temporary *state* of depression or anxiety, as opposed to a long-term personality *trait*.[9] Self-esteem apparently has complicated relationships to drug use, because there is evidence that young people sometimes enhance their self-esteem by becoming involved with a drug- or alcohol-using group.[10] Also, please remember that here we're trying to understand the overall range of drug or alcohol use as found in the population at large, as opposed to looking selectively at that small fraction of people who are addicts or alcoholics.

These studies are also fairly consistent in finding a collection of psychosocial factors that are related to drug use. Those students who are religious, attend school regularly and get good grades, have good relationships with their parents, and do not break the law are the students who report the least drinking and drug use. At the other end of the scale, the picture is that of general **nonconformity** to society, and drug use is one part of that overall picture. This doesn't account for every instance of drug use, but it is the most consistent overall finding. The nonconforming individual often has closer associations with peers than with his or her parents, and the peers are also likely to be nonconforming. In other words, drug-using youngsters are often part of a **deviant subculture.** Some researchers have begun to think in terms of **risk factors,** that is, indicators that a child or adolescent has become or is becoming a member of such a deviant subculture. The idea is that no one of these factors is critical, but the more risk factors one has, the more likely one is to be a drug user. An example of this kind of research is given in Table 1-3, which describes the significant risk factors derived from a group of about 3000 California students in 7th, 9th, and 11th grades, and Table 1-4, which shows how drug use was related to the number of risk factors.[11] Those with the most risk factors were much

---

Table 1-3

Risk factors for substance abuse in a group of California junior high and high school students

Risk factor and description	Correlation* with composite substance abuse score
Early alcohol intoxication: Intoxication at 12 years of age or younger (23% of respondents)	0.41
Perceived adult drug use: Number of adults you know who have used alcohol at least weekly, pills at least weekly, cannabis, or cocaine. Score of 2 or more (30% of respondents)	0.47
Perceived peer approval of drug use: What would your friends think about someone who gets "loaded" on drugs or alcohol? Score of 3 or 4 on 4-point scale (30% of respondents)	0.56
Perceived parent approval of drug use: Two 5-point scales on parent's attitude toward marijuana and alcohol use by the student. Average score of 2 or greater (25%)	0.28
Absent from school: Self-reported absences for reasons other than illness 5 or more times per year (16%)	0.33
Poor academic achievement: Self-reported D or F average (7%)	0.15
Distrust of teacher drug knowledge: (12%)	0.25
Distrust of parent drug knowledge: (11%)	0.25
Low educational aspirations: How much schooling do you plan to complete? Less than a college degree (28%)	0.27
Little religious commitment: How religious are you? Not religious at all (23%)	0.13
Emotional distress: How much were you bothered by each of seven problems during the past month? Each rated on a 5-point scale, average score of 2.1 or more (29%)	0.16
Dissatisfaction with life: Level of satisfaction with eight life areas, each on a 5-point scale. Average of 3 or less (26%)	0.15

*Correlation of 0.0 means no relationship, correlation of 1.0 means perfect predictability.

Table 1-4

Number of risk factors by abuse of five substances during the past 6 months

Risk factors	Percent reported abusing*					Abusing at least one substance
	Cigarettes	Alcohol	Cannabis	Cocaine	Hard drugs	
0	1	0	0	0	0	1
1	2	1	0	0	0	3
2	5	1	2	0	1	8
3	11	2	2	1	1	13
4	15	3	11	2	5	25
5	29	7	18	5	7	41
6	34	13	28	6	10	47
7 or more	56	18	40	7	18	71

*Abuse of cigarettes, alcohol, or cannabis was defined as at least daily use, whereas abuse of cocaine and hard drugs was defined as at least weekly use.

more likely to smoke cigarettes, drink alcohol daily, smoke marijuana daily, and use cocaine and other hard drugs. Please notice that even with seven risk factors, less than half the students smoked marijuana daily, and only 7% used cocaine. But among those with no risk factors there was no reported cocaine use and no regular marijuana use.

The other side of this picture is that the same individuals who are at risk for drug abuse are also at risk for other deviant behaviors; fighting, stealing, vandalism, and early sexual activity are correlated with drug use and heavier alcohol use. Therefore, the pattern of deviance-prone activity may have both a variety of causes and a variety of behavioral expressions, one of which is drug use.

Antecedents of Drug Use

Finding characteristics that tend to be associated with drug use doesn't help us to understand causal relationships very well. For example, do adolescents first become involved with a deviant peer group and then use drugs, or do they first use drugs and then begin to hang around with others who do the same? Does drug use cause them to become poor students and to fight and steal? In order to answer such questions it is necessary to interview the same individuals at different times, usually separated by a year or more, and look for the characteristics that predict later initiation of drug use. A few scientists have been able to follow the same group of young people at annual intervals for several years in what is known as a **longitudinal** study, and those results have been quite informative.

To answer our first question about the deviant peer group, the research results are consistent in reporting that other indicators of deviant behavior generally appear before drug use. For example, children often will be getting poor grades or getting into trouble for fighting or stealing before they first experiment with alcohol, cigarettes, or other substances.[12] This is important, because it means that in most cases the conduct problems and grade

problems are not caused by drug use. We may not know what the ultimate causes of all these behaviors are, but it is both too simple and obviously illogical to conclude that all the problems these kids have are a consequence of their using drugs, because the drug use more often than not comes later.

Gateway substances. One very important study done in the 1970s[13] pointed out that there was a typical sequence of involvement with drugs. Most of the high school students in this group started their drug involvement with beer or wine. The second stage involved either hard liquor or cigarettes or both, the third stage was marijuana use, and only after going through those stages did people try other illicit substances. Not everyone followed the same pattern, but it is interesting that only 1% of the students began their substance use with marijuana or some other illicit drug. It is as though they first had to go through the "gateway" of using alcohol and in many cases cigarettes. Let's keep our logic in order here: most of the illicit drug users had probably eaten hamburgers before they smoked marijuana, too. The point is that students who had not used beer or wine at the beginning of the study were much less likely to be marijuana smokers at the end of the study than the students who had used these substances. Cigarette smokers were about twice as likely as nonsmokers to move on to smoking marijuana. There is evidence that the gateway function of cigarettes continues to be important: In the senior class of 1985, those who were daily smokers of a pack or more of cigarettes were about 10 times as likely as nonsmokers to have used cocaine and about six times as likely to have smoked marijuana.[8]

One possible interpretation of the gateway phenomenon is that young people are exposed to alcohol and tobacco and that these substances themselves somehow make the person more likely to go on to use other drugs. Because the majority of people who use these gateway substances do not go on to become cocaine users or regular smokers of marijuana, we should be cautious about jumping to that conclusion. What seems more likely is that early alcohol use and cigarette smoking are common indicators of the general deviance-prone pattern of behavior that also includes an increased likelihood of smoking marijuana. For example, in the senior class of 1985, a student with a D average was about 10 times as likely as a student with an A average to be a pack-a-day smoker.[8] Because beer and cigarettes are more widely available to a deviance-prone young person than marijuana or cocaine, it is logical that beer and cigarettes would most often be tried first. The socially conforming students are less likely to try even these relatively available substances until they are older and less likely ever to try the illicit substances. Let's ask the question another way: What if we managed to develop a prevention program that stopped all young people from smoking cigarettes? Would that cut down on marijuana smoking? Most of us think it might, because people who don't want to suck tobacco smoke into their lungs probably won't want to inhale marijuana smoke either. Would such a program keep people from getting D averages or getting into trouble of other kinds? Probably not. In other words, we should not think of the use of gateway substances as the *cause* of later illicit drug use, but instead as an early indicator of the basic pattern of deviant behavior resulting from a variety of psychosocial risk factors.

Parent and peer influences. It is generally true that adolescents are more influenced by their peers about their immediate lifestyle and more influenced by their parents when it comes to long-term goals and plans.[14] Also, in early adolescence, parent influences are relatively strong, and as adolescence progresses peer influences become stronger. There is evidence from longitudinal research that both peers and parents influence adolescent drug-use behavior, but in general peer influences are more important. We can imagine situations in which peer and parent influences are in the same direction: a family that encourages school performance and long-term goals or a young person who does well in school and regularly attends religious services and is therefore surrounded by other young people who do well in school and hold similar values. Alternatively,

we may have an environment in which one or more parents is an alcoholic, other drugs are used openly, success in school is not valued or encouraged, the family lives in a neighborhood with many such families, and many of the other young people have the same problems. More commonly, we think of a model in which the parents oppose drug or alcohol use but the peer group encourages such behavior, and there is a conflict. Two recent longitudinal studies have tried to examine these influences over time. Although the results are complex, some of the major points can be summarized. As in previous research, the best predictors of drug use were peer variables. In one of the studies, having peers with antisocial attitudes was the strongest predictor of drug use.[12] In the other study, having peers who used marijuana was the best predictor of marijuana use.[14] The use of alcohol by parents did have an impact on alcohol use, but it is not clear whether this is because of direct "modeling" effects. For example, in one study it appeared that adolescents whose parents drank were more likely to have friends who drank, and the drinking pattern of friends was a big influence.[14] In the other study it was argued that heavy drinking by the parent might interfere with parent *monitoring* of the child's activities, and poor parent monitoring was found to be a major factor in allowing the child to associate with a deviant peer group.[12]

What advice for parents can we draw from all this research? First, encourage and reinforce the value of school and school achievement and of long-term life goals. It may or may not help to point out the incompatibility of drug abuse with that achievement and those long-term goals. Second, be on the alert for school practices such as remedial "tracks" or after-school detention that might frequently group your child with deviance-prone peers. Third, realize that you do have some influence on the types of peers your child associates with, particularly during childhood and early adolescence. Your child may associate with children who behave the way your family behaves, so it might pay to examine your own behavior. You can encourage or provide support for after-school activities that will bring your child into contact with positive peer groups. Monitoring involves knowing what your child is doing and with whom as well as showing interest in school activities and accomplishments. This advice certainly comes with no guarantee of success, but it is based on consistent research findings.

Why Do They Do It?

It doesn't seem to most of us to be necessary to find explanations for normative behavior; we don't often ask why someone takes a prescription pain killer following surgery. Our task is to try to explain the drug-taking behavior that frightens and infuriates—the illegal, excessive (abusive?) drug use.

The research on correlates and antecedents points to a variety of personal and social variables that influence our drug taking, and many psychological and sociological theorists have proposed models for explaining illegal or excessive drug use. We have seen evidence for one common reason why some people begin to take certain illegal drugs: usually young people and more often male than female, they have chosen to identify with a deviant subculture. These groups frequently engage in a variety of behaviors not condoned by the larger society. Within that group, the use of a particular drug may not be deviant at

all, but may in fact be expected. Occasionally the use of a particular drug becomes such a fad among a large number of youth groups that it seems to be a nationwide problem. However, within any given community there will still be groups of people of the same age who don't use the drug.

This isn't a book on adolescent psychology, but it is worth noting that rebellious behavior among young people serves important functions not only for the developing individual but also for the evolving society. Adolescents seem to enjoy impressing people, including their parents, which is a hard thing for them to do. An adolescent who

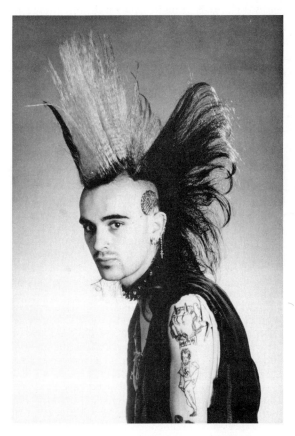

Young people sometimes do things so outrageous that their elders can't help but be impressed. Some of the more dangerous forms of drug use may serve this same purpose.

Your turn: cocaine in your town

Assume that you have just been appointed to a community-based committee that is looking into drug problems. You have been asked to find out what you can about the extent of cocaine use in the community and report back to the group in a month. Make a list of potential sources of information and the type of information each might provide. If you could get all the information on your list, how close do you think you could come to making an estimate of how many current cocaine users there are in your community? Do you think it would be above or below the national average?

is unable to gain respect from people or who is frustrated in his efforts to "go his own way" may engage in some particularly dangerous or disgusting behavior as a way of demanding that people be impressed.

One source of excessive drug use may be found within the drugs themselves. Many of these drugs seem to be capable of reinforcing the behavior that gets the drug into the system. What that means is that, everything else being equal, each time you take the drug you increase slightly the probability that you will take it again. Thus, with many psychoactive drugs there is a constant tendency to increase the frequency or amount of use. Some drugs appear to be so reinforcing that this process occurs relatively rapidly in a large percentage of those who use them, for example, intravenous heroin or cocaine. For other drugs, such as alcohol, the process seems to be much slower. In many people, social factors, other reinforcers, or other activities prevent the increase from occurring at all. For some, however, the drug-taking behavior

does increase and consumes an increasing share of their lives. These are the addicts and alcoholics we sometimes pity and sometimes fear, but almost never respect.

Most drug users are seeking an altered state of consciousness, a different perception of the world than is provided by normal day-to-day activities. It is impossible to separate this altered state from the reinforcing effect in most cases, because the altered state may be the psychological reflection of the reinforcing state. Many of the high school students in the nationwide surveys report that they take drugs "to see what it's like," or "to get high," or "because of boredom."[15] In other words, they are looking for a change, for something new and different in their lives. This aspect of drug use was particularly clear during the 1960s and 1970s when LSD and other perception-altering drugs were popular. We don't always recognize the altered states produced by other substances, but they do exist. A male drinking alcohol may have just a bit more of a perception that he's a tough

---

Issue: why do high school students use drugs and alcohol?

The annual survey of the drug-using habits of high school students has also made an attempt to get at the reasons for their drug and alcohol use. They did this by surveying the literature on motivations for substance use and then by adding some of their own reasons, and allowing the students to mark those reasons that they felt motivated their own use of each type of substance. To assume that these are the *real* motivations, we have to assume that the students are consciously aware of their motives and that they report them honestly. Although we have no way of knowing if those assumptions are valid, the answers do give us an interesting look at which motives seem to account for drug or alcohol use.

In a 1986 article, the scientists who have been conducting the national survey presented the data on reasons for use from a variety of perspectives.[16] If all substances are combined (remember that this will be heavily weighted toward alcohol, marijuana, and tobacco cigarettes), 65% said they used a substance

"to have a good time with my friends." This most common reason would be classed as a social motive and reflects the fact that drug use is most often a social behavior. The next most common reason (54% agreement) was "to experiment, to see what it's like." This reflects the fact that these are young people who may have used these substances only once or a few times. After this (20% to 40% agreement) come some motives that seem more personal, reflecting a desire to alter one's own feelings: "to feel good or get high," "to relax or relieve tension," "because of boredom, nothing else to do," "to get away from my problems or troubles," and "because of anger or frustration." While this sort of use of alcohol or another substance is sometimes seen as beneficial to the user over the short run, there is the danger that anytime things don't go the way you want or you don't feel just exactly the way you want, you will turn to a drug. That, of course, leads to trouble.

guy, that the world is his oyster, that he is well liked. A cocaine user may get the seductive feeling that everything is great and that she is doing a great job (even if she isn't). Many drug-abuse prevention programs have focused on efforts to show young people how to feel good about themselves and how to look for excitement in their lives without the use of drugs.

Summary

Drug use is such an emotional topic in our society that we sometimes forget that it is a form of behavior that has many things in common with other behaviors, and many of the same kinds of controlling variables. There is also a tendency to lump all drug use into a single category. Before making any headway in explaining or understanding drug use, we must be careful to specify exactly what we're talking about: who is using the drug, what drug, and so forth. We should also keep in mind that any individual drug may have various effects, depending on who has taken it and how much has been taken.

Drug use and problems caused by drug use are probably as old as mankind. Nevertheless, the types of drugs that are most commonly used do change, as do our attitudes about those drugs. Because of several important advances in pharmacology, our society has come to view drug use as an effective and convenient way to influence our minds. The drugs that we use recreationally seem to reflect the needs of society at a given point in time. Changes in American society since the 1950s have influenced fashion in many areas, and recreational drug use is no exception.

There are many ways of attempting to measure the extent of use of various licit and illicit drugs. The greatest amount of information probably comes from large-scale nationwide surveys done in high schools or households. Through these surveys we can monitor changes in the reported frequency of use of a given substance.

Attempts to find other variables that correlate with or predict illicit drug use have indicated that drug use is greater among those who are more rebellious and who engage in other deviant (for high school) behaviors, such as heavy drinking.

Attempts to explain why some people use certain drugs or use them in a deviant way usually focus on what the drugs do for the individual. Psychoactive drugs can be behaviorally reinforcing, they can produce altered states of consciousness, and they can help an individual make a social statement about what group he or she belongs to and what groups he or she disdains.

REFERENCES

1. Smith H: Do drugs have religious import? In Solomon D, editor: LSD: the consciousness-expanding drug, New York, 1964, GP Putnam's Sons.
2. Clymer A: Poll indicates turn toward optimism on nation's future, New York Times, July 1, 1981, p A1.
3. Conservatism is found in top teen students, New York Times, December 3, 1981, p C11.
4. Suchman EA: The "hang-loose" ethic and the spirit of drug use, Journal of Health and Social Behavior 9:146-155, 1968.
5. Sherman SP: America's new abstinence, Fortune, p 20-23, March 18, 1985.
6. Johnston LD: Summary of 1988 Drug Study Result, Press release from the Institute for Social Research, University of Michigan, February 28, 1989.
7. National Institute on Drug Abuse: National household survey on drug abuse: main findings 1985, DHHS Publication No (ADM)88-1586, Washington, DC, 1988, US Government Printing Office.
8. Johnston LD, O'Malley PM, and Bachman JG: National trends in drug use and related factors among American high school students and young adults, 1975-1986, DHHS Publication No (ADM)87-1535, Washington, DC, 1987, US Government Printing Office.
9. Oetting ER and Beauvais F: Common elements in youth drug abuse: peer clusters and other psychosocial factors. In Peele S, editor: Visions of addiction, Lexington, Mass, 1988, DC Heath and Company.
10. Stein JA, Newcomb MD, and Bentler PM: Personality and drug use: reciprocal effects across four years. Personality and Individual Differences 8:419-430, 1987.
11. Newcomb MD, Maddahian E, Skager R and others: Substance abuse and psychosocial risk factors among teenagers: associations with sex, age, ethnicity, and type of school, American Journal of Drug and Alcohol Abuse 13:413-433, 1987.

12. Dishion TJ, Patterson GR, and Reid JR: Parent and peer factors associated with drug sampling in early adolescence: implications for treatment. In Rahdert ER and Grabowski J, editors: Adolescent drug abuse: analyses of treatment research, NIDA Research Monograph 77, Washington, DC, 1988, US Government Printing Office.

13. Kandel D and Faust R: Sequence and stages in patterns of adolescent drug use, Archives of General Psychiatry 32:923-932, 1975.

14. Kandel DB and Andrews K: Processes of adolescent socialization by parents and peers, The International Journal of the Addictions 22:319-342, 1987.

15. Johnston LD and O'Malley PM: Why do the nation's students use drugs and alcohol? Self-reported reasons from nine national surveys, The Journal of Drug Issues 16:29-66, 1986.

Chapter 2

Drug Use as a Social Problem

OBJECTIVES

After reading this chapter, you should be able to:

Explain what is meant by *laissez faire* and "victimless crimes," and give three general motivations for societal regulations on drug use.

Define four categories of toxicity and give an example of each.

Describe the DAWN system and the two basic types of information it collects.

Define each of the following terms: tolerance, physical dependence, and psychological dependence.

Describe the changes that have taken place in our views of the term *addiction* and why.

Give a few brief factual statements about whether heroin addicts become criminals as a result of their addiction.

Discuss the ways in which alcohol contributes to *violent* crime.

Drugs are widely used, some legally and some illegally. If you hear someone talking about the drug problem, the reference is probably to those situations in which groups or individuals are using drugs in such a way as to attract the disapproval of the rest of society (in other words, the type of deviant or excessive drug use described at the end of Chapter 1). One possible way to look at the "drug problem" is as a social conflict between drug-using or drug-selling individuals and the majority social group.

LAISSEZ-FAIRE

In the America of the 1800s, the federal government had virtually no laws governing drug sales and use. The idea seemed to be that if the seller wanted to sell it and the buyer wanted to buy it, let them do it—**laissez-faire** in French. This is a term that has been used to characterize the general nature of the U.S. government of that era. Some current thinkers have advocated a return toward that attitude.[1] After all, buying and selling marijuana or cocaine can be called, like prostitution, a "victimless" crime. Both parties get what they want from the transaction, and neither party complains. Since that is often true, the only way society through its enforcement agencies can make many arrests for these crimes is to go looking for trouble, by pretending to be either buyer or seller. Instead why not just look the other way?

In fact, state and federal laws controlling drug sales were passed because it was believed that there were victims in some of these transactions. Three main concerns aroused public interest: (1) Some drug sellers were considered to be endangering the public health and victimizing individuals because they were selling dangerous, *toxic* chemicals often without labeling them or putting appropriate warnings on them; (2) some sellers were seen as victimizing individuals and endangering their health by selling them *habit-forming* drugs, again often without appropriate labels or warnings; and (3) the drug user came to be seen as a threat to public safety—the attitude became widespread that drug-crazed individuals would

freely engage in horrible, violent *crimes*. In Chapter 3 we will look at the roots of these concerns and how our current legal structures grew from them. For now, let's look at each issue and develop some ground rules for the discussion of toxicity, addiction, and drug-induced criminality.

TOXICITY
Categories of Toxicity

The word **toxic** refers to something that is poisonous, deadly, or dangerous. We will use the term to refer to those effects of drugs that interfere with normal functioning in such a way as to produce dangerous or potentially dangerous consequences. Seen in this way, for example, alcohol could be toxic in high doses because it suppresses respiration—this may be dangerous if one stops

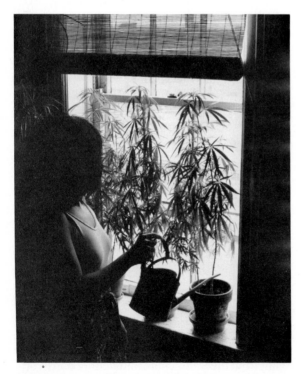

Should this woman be allowed to grow marijuana for her own private consumption?

> **Your turn: marijuana laws**
>
> A hypothetical case: An adult, well educated and fully informed about the effects of marijuana (she just finished this course), obtains marijuana seeds, plants them in her own back yard, harvests the crop, and smokes the marijuana in the privacy of her own home. By growing, possessing, and using the marijuana she has no doubt violated several state and federal statutes.
>
> The hypothetical situation was described in such a way that most of us probably don't feel too threatened by this behavior. How do you react to those who advocate changing our marijuana laws to allow for personal growing and use of marijuana?
>
> If such behavior were to be allowed, think about some of the other things that would have to be resolved: Where would a person obtain seeds? Should anyone be able to sell or transfer seeds to anyone else without restriction? Suppose the grower and private user were to smoke marijuana all day on the front porch while chatting with the neighborhood kids—should this kind of example be allowed? What if the private grower wanted to share some of her marijuana with a friend who came over? Or to send some home with the friend? Or to sell some to the friend? Think about how you would set up the laws to make them as fair as possible.

breathing long enough to induce brain damage or death. But we can also consider alcohol to be toxic if it causes a person to be so disoriented that otherwise normal situations become dangerous, for example, driving a car or swimming. This latter is an example of something we refer to as **behavioral toxicity.** We will make a somewhat arbitrary distinction, then, between behavioral toxicity and "physiological" toxicity—perhaps taking advantage of the widely assumed mind-body distinction that is more convenient than it is real. The only reason for making this distinction is that it helps to remind us of some important kinds of toxicity, which are sometimes overlooked in these discussions.

Another arbitrary distinction that we will make for the purpose of discussion will be the **acute** vs **chronic** distinction. Most of the time when people use the word acute, it is to mean sharp or intense. In medicine, an acute condition is one that comes on suddenly, as opposed to a chronic or long-lasting condition. When talking about drug effects, we can think of the acute effects as those that result from a single administration of a drug or are a direct result of the actual presence of the drug in the system at the time. For example, taking an overdose of heroin can lead to acute toxicity. By contrast, the chronic effects of a drug would be those that result from long-term exposure and may be present whether or not the substance is actually in the system at a given point

in time. For example, smoking cigarettes may eventually lead to various types of lung disorders. If one has emphysema from years of smoking, that condition is there when you wake up in the morning and when you go to bed at night, and whether you've smoked a cigarette 5 minutes ago or 5 days ago doesn't make much difference.

Using these definitions, Table 2-1 can help give us an overall picture of the possible toxic consequences of a given type of drug. However, knowing what is *possible* is different from knowing what is *likely*. How can we get an idea of which drugs are most likely to produce adverse drug reactions?

Drug Abuse Warning Network

In an effort to monitor the toxicity of drugs other than alcohol, the federal government set up the Drug Abuse Warning Network **(DAWN).** This system collects data on drug-related crises from over 800 hospital emergency rooms in metropolitan areas around the country. If an individual comes to the emergency room with any sort of problem and if in the *patient's* opinion the problem is related to the use of some drug, then that drug is counted as having been "mentioned" in connection with a medical emergency. Note that this incident could arise because a person swallowed a bottle of sleeping pills that might cause death or it might arise because someone smoked part of a marijuana joint and then suffered a panic reaction:

Table 2-1		
Examples of four types of drug-induced toxicity		
	Acute	**Chronic**
Behavioral	"Intoxication" from alcohol, marijuana, or other drugs that impair behavior and increase danger to the individual	Personality changes reported to occur in alcoholics and suspected by some to occur in marijuana users (the amotivational syndrome)
Physiological	Usually result from taking too much of a drug, as in overdose	Heart disease, lung cancer, and so on related to smoking; liver damage resulting from chronic alcohol exposure

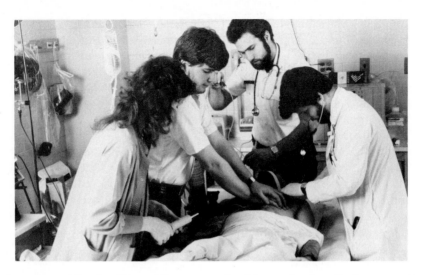

The Drug Abuse Warning Network keeps records of drug-related medical emergencies.

rapid, shallow breathing; tightness in the chest; and being very frightened. In the latter case, if the person had not gone to the emergency room probably no lasting harm would have occurred, but each incident counts as one mention anyway. You can imagine that doing the record-keeping in any other way would require many subjective judgments on the part of the emergency room physicians: Was it really a serious medical emergency? Was that drug really responsible? This would probably result in systematic differences from one hospital or one city to another.

If a person actually dies and a drug is involved in some way, then the medical examiner (coroner) is expected to report in a consistent way to the DAWN system, and these drug-related deaths form a second set of statistics (with, of course, smaller numbers of mentions).

Before looking at some of the DAWN results, it is important for us to remember a couple of important facts. First, alcohol is not counted if it is the only drug mentioned, but it is counted in the category "alcohol-in-combination" if it is mentioned along with other drugs. Second, more than one drug may be mentioned per incident, and each drug will be counted as a separate "mention."

Now let's look at Table 2-2, listing the most frequently mentioned drugs in the recent DAWN reports.[2] Probably the most obvious thing is that alcohol-in-combination is near the top in both lists, a place it has held for several years. In fact, if alcohol were counted alone and treated similarly to other drugs in the system, it would so overwhelm both sets of data that all the other drugs would appear to be unimportant beside it. This would seem to indicate that alcohol is a pretty toxic substance. It is, but let us also remember that most adult Americans drink alcohol on a fairly regular basis, whereas only a small number of people use heroin or morphine, a category of drugs that has also consistently been near the top of both DAWN lists. The DAWN system does not correct for frequency of use, but rather gives us an idea of the total impact of a substance on medical emergencies or drug-related deaths.

Diazepam (Valium), which is a sedative, is among the most widely prescribed drugs in the United States and has also been near the top of both tables for several years. It consistently shows up higher on the emergency room reports than on the coroner's reports. One reason for this may be that diazepam is frequently used in suicide attempts, most of which do not succeed. Aspirin,

Table 2-2

Drug mentions in the DAWN system for 1987

Emergency rooms			Medical examiners		
Drug name	Number of mentions	Percent of total episodes	Drug name	Number of mentions	Percent of total episodes
1 Cocaine	46,331	31.57	1 Alcohol-in-combination 2/	1,730	36.98
2 Alcohol-in-combination 1/	40,644	27.69	2 Cocaine	1,696	36.25
3 Heroin/morphine 1/	18,566	12.65	3 Heroin/morphine 2/	1,572	33.60
4 Marijuana/hashish 1/	10,083	6.87	4 Codeine	590	12.61
5 PCP/PCP combinations	9,545	6.50	5 Quinine	403	8.61
6 Diazepam 1/	7,277	4.96	6 Diazepam 2/	312	6.67
7 Acetaminophen	6,469	4.41	7 Amitriptyline	299	6.39
8 Aspirin	5,688	3.88	8 PCP/PCP combinations	249	5.32
9 Alprazolam	3,835	2.61	9 D-Propoxyphene	241	5.15
10 Ibuprofen	3,612	2.46	10 Acetaminophen	230	4.92
			11 Marijuana/hashish	146	3.12

which is also frequently used in this way, shows a similar pattern.

The importance of drug combinations, particularly combinations with alcohol, in contributing to these numbers cannot be overstressed. For example, it has been argued that diazepam almost never kills by itself, but that virtually all diazepam-related deaths are actually a result of diazepam plus alcohol.[3] Also, in a study of heroin overdose deaths in Washington, D.C., most of those dying with heroin in their blood also had significant levels of alcohol.[4]

How Dangerous Is It?

Now that we have seen how complex the interpretation of these tables can become, let's see if we can use the information they present to ask some questions about the relative danger to a person of taking one drug vs another. We have seen that the DAWN data do not correct for incidence of use. Let's do something foolhardy and use the data presented in Table 1-2, Chapter 1, obtained from home surveys, as a rough estimate of the relative proportions of use of these drugs in our

society. Please note that the populations studied are not the same, and there are a large number of other reasons why we would not want to use this approach to make fine distinctions among drugs. But we can see that marijuana, which was reported to be in current use by about 20% of the young adults, was mentioned in about 3% of drug-related deaths, mostly in combination with cocaine, alcohol, or heroin. Less than 1% of young adults reported using heroin, but it accounts for a large fraction of drug-related deaths. From this we can draw the obvious conclusion, even from imperfect data, that heroin is many more times lethal than marijuana.

Cocaine, which was reported in current use by many fewer people than marijuana, was mentioned in many more drug-related deaths than marijuana. And, although cocaine was used by many more people than used heroin, it was named about equally often in drug-related deaths. We can conclude from this that cocaine use is probably more toxic than marijuana use and less toxic than heroin use. Please keep in mind, however, that the amount taken and how a drug is taken can greatly influence toxicity. Heroin was

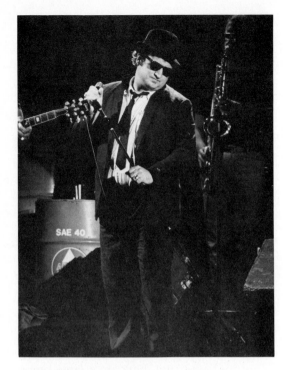

Comedian John Belushi died after injecting a combination of cocaine and heroin.

once sold in small doses in tablet form. If it were still available in that form as a prescription drug, many more people would be taking it but almost none of those would die from it, and our estimates of heroin's relative toxicity would drop drastically. Cocaine is often "snorted" into the nose, whereas heroin is often injected intravenously. A rat experiment indicated that rats allowed to self-inject as much cocaine as they wanted intravenously were more likely to die than rats allowed to self-inject as much heroin as they wanted,[5] so it may be that if the two drugs were both taken intravenously by all human users, cocaine would cause more deaths than heroin.

We cannot tell precisely from the DAWN data how many total deaths are related to the use of cocaine or heroin, because not all coroners are included in the system. Data are gathered from metropolitan areas that include about a third of the U.S. population, but they are areas that have

higher-than-average use of illicit drugs. A rough estimate of the total annual number of deaths related to cocaine, for example, might be twice the reported DAWN figure, or about 3000 per year. The total for all illicit drugs, including cocaine, heroin, marijuana, and PCP, might be approximately 6000 or 7000. In a country in which over two million people die each year, this is a relatively minor cause of death, a fact that is surprising to many people. For comparison, it is estimated that alcohol is responsible for about 100,000 deaths annually (Chapter 9) and over 350,000 annual deaths are attributed to cigarette smoking (Chapter 10). Of course many more people use those substances, and in terms of *relative* danger of toxicity, heroin and cocaine are probably as bad as or worse than alcohol or cigarettes. However, in looking at the *overall* impact of these drug-related deaths on American society, if you were about to conclude that politicians and the news media have been paying a disproportionate amount of attention to cocaine-related and heroin-related toxicity, you would be right.

AIDS

There is a great deal of concern about the spread of acquired immune deficiency syndrome (AIDS) among drug abusers. The human immunodeficiency virus (HIV) is a blood-borne agent capable of spreading the disease among addicts who share needles. The insidious thing about HIV is that one can be infected for a year or two with no overt symptoms, and during that time the disease can be spread to others. Both AIDS and hepatitis-B, another blood-borne disease, have been responsible for hundreds of deaths among intravenous drug abusers. In New York City, at least half the intravenous drug users are thought to be infected with HIV.[6] Because AIDS also can be transmitted sexually, the public at large is at some risk, especially considering that many female drug addicts earn money through prostitution.

It is important to point out that this is a type of drug-associated toxicity that is not due to the action of the drug itself, but is incidental to the sharing of needles, no matter which drug is injected. While the initial spread in New York City was among heroin users, it has been pointed out that intravenous cocaine users give themselves more frequent injections and therefore might be at greater risk.[7] In a sense, the spread through needle sharing is due less to the drug addiction itself than to laws designed to prevent addiction, in particular the laws restricting the sale of hypodermic equipment, which New York City has enforced for decades. In Liverpool, England, an aggressive campaign of providing clean syringes and needles has prevented the spread of HIV among the needle-using addicts, whereas in Edinburgh, Scotland, no such program was established and HIV infections are found in a large proportion of addicts.[8] Some U.S. cities, including Boulder, Colorado, are now experimenting with needle-exchange programs, but in most cities this idea has been rejected so far. Instead, some areas have established education programs aimed at getting addicts to clean their syringes with household bleach or alcohol, and to get them to use condoms to prevent the spread of AIDS through sexual contact.

DRUG ADDICTION
Problems of Definition

Another of the concerns expressed by those urging passage of drug controls in the early 1900s was for the victims of drug addiction. Those who unknowingly or carelessly took these habit-forming drugs stood at risk of becoming enslaved by them. The unscrupulous sellers of these drugs were thus assured a steady market for them, while the addicts were forced to continue to endanger their own health and perhaps to undermine their own mental and moral strength. That is one major reason that the habit-forming drugs, such as cocaine and the opiates, were singled out for special taxation and record keeping in 1914.

There have been many definitions offered over the years for the term *drug addiction,* and this term has been so widely used and discussed that it has passed into that group of terms that elude precise definition (see box on p. 4). But the concepts that have been included within various definitions of

and discussions of drug addiction are important to this book, so they bear some examination. Discussions of addiction usually include some mixture of three more definable concepts: **tolerance, physical dependence,** and **psychological dependence.**

Tolerance

Tolerance refers to a phenomenon seen with most drugs in which repeated exposure to the same dose of the drug results in a diminishing effect. There are many ways in which this diminished effect can occur, and some examples will be given in Chapter 6. For now, it is enough for us to think of the body as developing ways to compensate for the unbalancing actions of these drugs. In many cases, as the individual experiences less and less of a desired effect, it is possible to increase the dose of the drug so as to counteract the tolerance. Since tolerance usually also develops to the dangerous effects of these drugs, some regular drug users may eventually build up to taking much more of the drug than it would take to kill a nontolerant individual.

Physical Dependence

Suppose a person has begun to take a drug and a tolerance has developed. The person increases the amount of drug taken and continues to take these higher doses so regularly that his system is continuously exposed to the drug for days or weeks. With some drugs, if the person stops taking it abruptly, as the drug level in the system drops a set of symptoms begin to appear. For example, as the level of heroin drops in a heroin addict, his nose may run and he may begin to experience chills and fever, diarrhea, and so on. When we have a drug that produces a consistent set of these symptoms in different individuals, we refer to the collection of symptoms as a **withdrawal syndrome.** The withdrawal syndrome from all narcotics is similar to the heroin withdrawal syndrome, but different from the withdrawal syndrome produced by sedatives and sleeping pills. Our model for why these withdrawal symptoms appear is that the individual's nervous system has compensated for the presence of the drug and that some of these compensating mechanisms produce an imbalance when the drug is removed. An obvious example occurs among users of narcotic drugs, which tend to slow intestinal movement and produce constipation. After many days of constant narcotic use, other mechanisms in the body tend to counteract this effect and get the intestine moving again. If the narcotic is suddenly stopped, diarrhea is one of the most reliable and dramatic withdrawal symptoms.

Because of the presumed involvement of these compensating mechanisms, the presence of a withdrawal syndrome is said to reflect physical dependence on the drug. In other words, the individual has come to depend on the presence of some amount of that drug to maintain a balance; removing the drug leads to an imbalance, which is slowly corrected over a period of a few days.

Psychological Dependence

Psychological dependence or sometimes "behavioral dependence" can also be defined or described in many ways. Some approaches to this have referred to the amount of effort an individual exerts in "drug-seeking" behavior, some to the frequency or regularity of drug taking, some to a stated craving for the drug. A major contribution of behavioral psychology has been to point out the scientific value of the concept of **reinforcement** in this context. It appears that some drugs have an ability to reinforce the behaviors that led up to the drug's presence in the system, in the same way that food pellets can reinforce lever-pressing behavior in hungry rats. Those drugs that have powerful reinforcing properties are the ones that we will consider to have a greater potential for producing psychological dependence. If a person takes a drug and the drug reinforces the drug-taking behavior, that means that if drug availability and the availability of other behaviors and other reinforcers remain relatively constant, the drug-taking behavior is likely to occur again.

The Changing Views of Addiction

Whether or not a drug is considered to be addicting may depend more on the definition of addiction than on the drug. Since the generally accepted view of addiction has shifted somewhat over the past 20 years, this has meant that some drugs once considered nonaddicting are now considered addicting. Although we don't want to imply that one view is now wrong and the other right or that everyone has changed his or her viewpoint in this time period, it is probably fair to distinguish an older and a more recent view of addiction.[9]

When experts first began studying and defining addiction, the primary data with which they worked were the experiences of people addicted to heroin or other narcotic drugs. In fact, for many years concern about drug abuse was so focused on narcotics that all illegal drugs, including marijuana and cocaine, were referred to as narcotics in federal laws. Users of true narcotics sometimes show remarkable levels of tolerance and the withdrawal symptoms may be quite dramatic, and it was these on which the experts naturally focused in their definitions of addiction. Thus, addiction was usually defined largely in terms of physical dependence.

It began to become a public issue in the 1960s that some drugs, particularly marijuana, were not really narcotics and did not produce the typical dramatic withdrawal syndromes. It became popular among the growing group of interested scientists to refer to drugs like marijuana, amphetamines, and cocaine as producing psychological dependence, whereas heroin produced a true addiction, including physical dependence. The idea seemed to be that psychological dependence was merely mental, whereas with physical dependence real bodily processes were involved, subject to physiological and biochemical analysis and possibly to improved medical treatments for addiction. Let us refer to this as the older view of addiction, the one held by most enlightened experts in the late 1960s.

At about this time a remarkable series of experiments began to appear in the scientific literature; experiments in which laboratory monkeys and rats were given intravenous **catheters** connected to motorized syringes and controlling equipment in such a way that pressing a lever would produce a single brief injection of morphine, a heroinlike narcotic. As these scientists began to publish their results and as more experiments like this were done, they pointed out some interesting facts. First, it was not necessary to select monkeys with "addictive personalities" or rats born on the wrong side of the cage—virtually every animal given the opportunity to press for morphine injections did so. Second was the degree to which results using morphine as a reinforcer could build on the vast literature of results using food or water reinforcers with animals: by requiring first 2 presses, then 5, then 10, then 30 per injection the animals could be made to display a large amount of behavior leading up to each injection. Just as with food, there was a point at which too large a response requirement would produce erratic responding or failure to respond at all. If you want maximum performance from a rat pressing a lever for food, you don't fill its cage with rat chow for each press nor do you give the rat small specks of food for each press. The same with drugs: you can draw a nice curve showing how the rate of responding first increases and then decreases as you systematically increase either the dose of drug per press or the amount of food per press. Thus, the idea spread that drugs can act as reinforcers of behavior and that this might be the basis of what had been called psychological dependence.[10] Drugs like amphetamines and cocaine could easily be used as reinforcers in these experiments, and they were known to produce strong psychological dependence in humans.

These results seemed to indicate that psychological dependence might be more important than physical dependence in narcotic addiction, and led people to examine the lives of addicts from a different perspective.[9] Stories were told of addicts who occasionally stopped taking heroin, voluntarily going through withdrawal so as to reduce their tolerance level and get back to the lower doses of drug they could more easily afford. When we examine the total daily narcotic intake of most current addicts, we see that they do not have large habits and that the agonies of withdrawal they experience are probably more like a mild case of intestinal flu. We have known for a long time that heroin addicts who go through either rapid or slow withdrawal in treatment programs have a high probability of returning to active heroin use. In other words, if all we had to worry about was addicts avoiding withdrawal symptoms, the problem would be a much smaller one that it actually is.

Psychological dependence, based on reinforcement, is apparently the real driving force behind even narcotic addiction, and tolerance and physical dependence are less important contributors to the basic problem. This is what we will refer to as the more recent view of addiction. In this text we have not gone so far as to redefine the word addiction itself in terms of psychological dependence, because that might simply lead to more confusion at this point. For now it is probably better to leave addiction undefined and to use the more specific terms as defined.

Now that we have a better understanding of some of the basic forces driving addiction, it is clear that addiction is a muddy term, in part because it doesn't describe a single process. There is no such thing as "the" basis for addiction, because addiction is just a convenient term for the fact that some people (and other animals) develop strong patterns of behavior that are motivated by drugs. However, not all people who are exposed to narcotics or to alcohol do develop such strong drug-motivated behavior patterns. We can again turn to animal experiments to give us an idea of one type of controlling variable. In the standard drug self-administration experiment, the rats or monkeys are housed in a small cage with nothing much to do except press the drug-producing lever. Under those circumstances it is easy to demonstrate that some drugs are powerful reinforcers. But what if there are other, more "natural" reinforcers available? In one series of experiments, rats were allowed to drink a morphine solution, either when they were isolated in a small cage or when

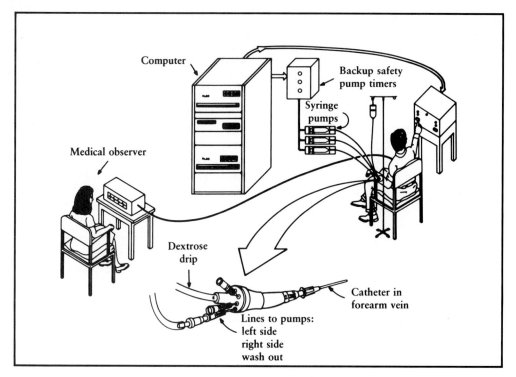

Labels in figure:
- Computer
- Backup safety pump timers
- Syringe pumps
- Medical observer
- Dextrose drip
- Catheter in forearm vein
- Lines to pumps: left side right side wash out

When humans are allowed to work for intravenous injections of small amounts of cocaine, heroin, or nicotine in a laboratory situation, they will do so.

they were living in a large, complex "Rat Park" with other rats of both sexes. The rats in Rat Park did not increase their morphine consumption very much, whereas the isolated rats did drink more and more morphine as the days went by.[11] This indicates that the reinforcing effect of a drug may have to compete with other reinforcers in most natural settings and may help to explain why many people who are exposed to addicting drugs do not become addicted.

An interesting book *The Meaning of Addiction*, examines historic views of addiction and reviews information that points to the fact that these compulsive behaviors that we call addiction, far from being easily characterized, uniform patterns of behavior, reflect much of the variety that is seen with other forms of human behavior.[12] The exact manner in which addiction does or does not appear in each individual depends on that person's history, personality, and the social and economic setting, just as with other behaviors.

The closest thing to an "official" definition of these problems comes from the American Psychiatric Association's Diagnostic and Statistical Manual (DSM III-R). This manual describes "psychoactive substance dependence," which includes tolerance and physical dependence among its criteria, and "psychoactive substance abuse," which is based principally on behavioral symptoms (see box). These definitions are meant to be applied to patterns of use once called "drug addiction" and to another controversial term, "alcoholism." In other words, the "disorders" are considered the same, whether the substance is alcohol, heroin, cocaine, tobacco, or some other psychoactive substance.

Diagnostic criteria for psychoactive substance dependence

A. At least three of the following:
  1. substance often taken in larger amounts or over a longer period than the person intended
  2. persistent desire or one or more unsuccessful efforts to cut down or control substance use
  3. a great deal of time spent in activities necessary to get the substance (e.g., theft), taking the substance (e.g., chain smoking), or recovering from its effects
  4. frequent intoxication or withdrawal symptoms when expected to fulfill major role obligations at work, school, or home (e.g., does not go to work because hung over, goes to school or work "high," intoxicated while taking care of his or her children), or when substance use is physically hazardous (e.g., drives when intoxicated)
  5. important social, occupational, or recreational activities given up or reduced because of substance use
  6. continued substance use despite knowledge of having a persistent or recurrent social, psychological, or physical problem that is caused or exacerbated by the use of the substance (e.g., keeps using heroin despite family arguments about it, cocaine-induced depression, or having an ulcer made worse by drinking)
  7. marked tolerance: need for markedly increased amounts of the substance (i.e., at least 50% increase) in order to achieve intoxication or desired effect, or markedly diminished effect with continued use of the same amount.
     NOTE: The following items may not apply to cannabis, hallucinogens, or phencyclidine (PCP):
  8. characteristic withdrawal symptoms (see specific withdrawl syndromes under Psychoactive Substance-Induced Organic Mental Disorders)
  9. substance often taken to relieve or avoid withdrawal symptoms
B. Some symptoms of the disturbance have persisted for at least one month or have occurred repeatedly over a longer period of time.

Diagnostic criteria for psychoactive substance abuse

A. A maladaptive pattern of psychoactive substance use indicated by at least one of the following:
  1. continued use despite knowledge of having a persistent or recurrent social, occupational, psychological, or physical problem that is caused or exacerbated by use of the psychoactive substance
  2. recurrent use in situations in which use is physically hazardous (e.g., driving while intoxicated)
B. Some symptoms of the disturbance have persisted for at least one month, or have occurred repeatedly over a longer period of time.
C. Never met the criteria for Psychoactive Substance Dependence for this substance.

Adapted from the Diagnostic and Statistical Manual, third edition, revised 1987 by the American Psychiatric Association.

CRIME AND VIOLENCE
Narcotic Addicts

It may seem obvious to a reader of today's newspapers or to a viewer of today's television that drugs and crime are linked. Practically daily, there are reports of killings attributed to warring gangs of crack dealers.[13] Our prisons house a large population of people convicted for drug-related crimes, and there have been recent reports that a large fraction of arrestees for nondrug felonies have positive results from urine tests for illicit substances.

The belief that there is a causal relationship between many forms of drug use and criminality probably forms the basis for many of our laws concerning drug use and drug users. The relationship between crime and illegal drug use is complex, and only recently have data-based statements become possible. Facts are necessary because political actions are taken and laws are enacted on the basis of what we believe to be true.

The basis for concern was the belief that drug use *causes* crime. The fact that drug addicts engage in robberies or that car thieves are likely to use illicit drugs does not say anything about causality. Both criminal activity and drug use could well be caused by other factors, producing both types of deviant behavior in the same individuals. There are several senses in which it might be said that drugs cause crime, but the most frightening possibility is that drug use somehow changes the individual's personality in a lasting way, making him or her into a "criminal type." For example, during the 1924 debate that led to a complete prohibition of legal heroin sales in the United States, it was asserted by a testifying physician that the use of heroin "dethrones their moral responsibility." Another physician testified that some types of individuals will have their mental equipment "permanently injured by the use of heroin, and those are the ones who will go out and commit crimes."[14] Similar beliefs are reflected in the introductory message in the 1937 film "Reefer Madness," which referred to marijuana as "The Real Public Enemy Number One!" and described its "soul-destroying" effects as follows:

"... emotional disturbances, the total inability to direct thought, the loss of all power to resist physical emotions: leading finally to acts of shocking violence ... ending often in incurable insanity."

Such verbal excesses seem quaint and comical these days, but the underlying belief that drug use changes people into criminals still can be detected in much current political rhetoric. You should remember from Chapter 1 that longitudinal research on children and adolescents has led to the conclusion that indicators of criminal or antisocial behavior usually occur before the first use of an illicit drug. As far as we know, it makes more sense to view both criminal activity and drug use as indicators of a deviance-prone pattern of behavior, both caused by exposure to multiple risk factors in the home and among peers.

A second sense in which drug use might *cause* criminal behavior is when the person is "under the influence." Do the acute effects of a drug make a person temporarily more likely to engage in criminal behavior? There is little good evidence for this with most illicit substances. In most in-

dividuals marijuana produces a state more akin to lethargy than to crazed violence (Chapter 16), and heroin tends to make its users more passive and perhaps sexually impotent (Chapter 14). Stimulants such as amphetamine and cocaine may make people paranoid and "jumpy," and this may indeed contribute to violent behavior in some cases (Chapter 7).

If there is some question as to whether the direct influence of illicit drugs is to produce a person more likely to engage in criminal or violent behavior, there is little question about one commonly used substance: alcohol.

A large number of studies indicate that alcohol is clearly linked with violent crime. In many assaultive and sexually assaultive situations alcohol is present in both assailant and victim. You may not appreciate that most homicides are among people who know each other—and alcohol use is associated with over three fifths of all murders. Of all reported assaults, 40% involve alcohol, as do one third of forcible rape and child-molestation cases.[15,16] One 1981 study of adolescents in prison for assault reported that alcohol was involved in 61% of their assaults resulting in tissue damage, and in 67% of assaults resulting in death.[17]

A longitudinal study of males born between 1944 and 1954 reported in 1976 that "those who had used alcohol were more likely to report fights as a consequence than were users of the other drugs. When only the heavy and heaviest users of alcohol were examined, some 38 percent reported fights resulting from their use of alcohol.[18, p.78]

A 1980 review of the world literature, although critical of many studies on its topic of alcohol, violence and aggression, concluded: "It is quite clear that consumption of alcohol is associated with a wide range of violent acts which include accident, suicide, sexual assault, violence within the family, felony and homicide.[19, p.114]

There is a third sense in which drug use may be said to cause crime, and that refers to crimes carried out for the purpose of obtaining money to purchase illicit drugs. It has long been noted that heroin addicts comprise a larger proportion of those arrested for robbery than of the general population. An excellent study done in Detroit has shown that the level of property crime in Detroit is in part affected by the price of heroin. When the price rises, crime rises. When the price falls, crime falls. This finding supports the general hypothesis that criminal heroin users as a class try to maintain their level of consumption in the face of price increases, and that they rely partly on property crime for the additional funds.[20]

Although most addicts are criminals first and addicts second, a 1976 survey of heroin addicts found that most reported an increase in the amount of crime, and many started committing new types of crime, after they became addicts. A 1981 report suggests just how much criminal activity increases during periods of addiction. "When addicts were not dependent on heroin, their crime rate was 84% lower than when they were regularly using the drug.[21, p.22] Reducing ad-

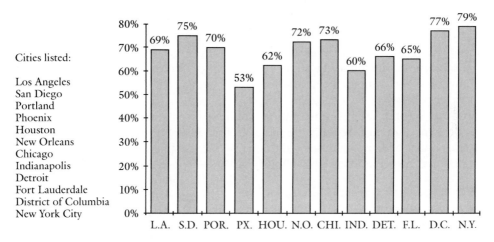

Cities listed:

Los Angeles
San Diego
Portland
Phoenix
Houston
New Orleans
Chicago
Indianapolis
Detroit
Fort Lauderdale
District of Columbia
New York City

Figure 2-1. Percentage of male arrestees testing positive for any drug, including marijuana (June-November 1987).

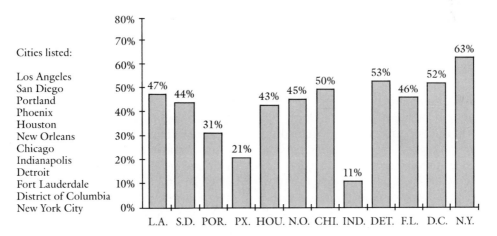

Cities listed:

Los Angeles
San Diego
Portland
Phoenix
Houston
New Orleans
Chicago
Indianapolis
Detroit
Fort Lauderdale
District of Columbia
New York City

Figure 2-2. Percentage of male arrestees testing positive for cocaine (June-November 1987).

diction will certainly result in lower crime rates.

In 1988 the U.S. Justice Department reported on their new Drug Use Forecasting project, which included a study of urine samples of more than 2000 persons arrested for serious offenses in 12 major U.S. cities.[22] Most of those tested were charged with such crimes as burglary, grand larceny, and assault, and all tests were voluntary and anonymous. Depending on the city, between 53% and 79% of the tested arrestees tested positive for some drug, including marijuana (Fig. 2-1). In New York, one-fourth of arrestees were found to have heroin in their systems. Evidence of cocaine use was found in 11% to 63% of those tested, depending on the city (Fig. 2-2). This level of drug use among those arrested for nondrug crimes is quite high; how can we account for it? First, those who adopt a deviant lifestyle may engage in both crime and drug use. Second, because most of these arrests were for crimes in which profit is the motive, the arrestees may have been burglarizing a house or stealing a car to get money to purchase drugs.

It would be remiss not to point out that the commission of crimes to obtain expensive illicit drugs is due not primarily to a pharmacological effect of the drug, but to the artificially high cost of the drugs, which results from drug controls and enforcement. Both heroin and cocaine are inexpensive substances when obtained legally from a licensed manufacturer, and it has been estimated many times that if heroin were freely available it would cost no more to be a regular heroin user than to be a regular drinker of alcohol. It is the black-market cost of these substances, combined with their addicting nature, that makes the use of cocaine or heroin consume so much money.

There is a fourth and final sense in which drug use causes crime, and that is that drug use *is* a crime. At first that may seem trivial, but there are two senses in which it is not. First, we are now making over 750,000 arrests in drug-law violations each year, and more than one-third of all federal prisoners are in jail on drug charges. Thus, drug-law violations represent one of the major *types* of crime in the United States. Second, it is

---

Your turn: are current laws fair?

There are things that people do all the time that are potentially dangerous for themselves and potentially messy and expensive for others. Driving over 55 miles per hour, driving without a seat belt, and riding a motorcycle without a helmet are examples, some of which may not be illegal where you live. In what ways are these behaviors similar to a person "snorting" cocaine or injecting heroin into his or her veins? In what ways are they different? Do you feel that the laws as they currently exist in your area are appropriate and fair in dealing with these behaviors? If it were up to you, would you outlaw some things that are now legal, legalize some things that are now controlled, or some of each?

---

likely that the relationship between drug use and other forms of deviant behavior is strengthened by the fact that drug use is a crime. It may be that some of the people who are trying to demonstrate their alienation from society choose to smoke marijuana or try heroin specifically *because* those are illegal activities. Also, if these drugs were not illegal, trying them would not be considered so socially deviant, and probably more otherwise-nondeviant types would do so. That is, of course, the major argument in favor of maintaining legal controls on these drugs.

WHY WE TRY TO REGULATE DRUGS

We can see that there are reasonable concerns about the potential toxicity, habit-forming nature, and even the criminality of some drug users. That does not mean that our current set of laws represents a rationally devised plan to counteract the most realistic of these concerns in the most effective manner. In point of fact, most legislation is passed in an atmosphere of emotionality, in response to some specific set of concerns. Often the problems have been there for a long time, but public attention and concern has been recently aroused and Congress must respond. Sometimes members of Congress or government officials play

---

Issue: smoking "crack" produces rapid dependence

In 1986, reports spread of the use of "crack," a smokable form of cocaine, in various American cities. Directors of drug abuse centers are alarmed because people who have been smoking crack for only a few weeks have developed the kind of strong dependence usually seen only in intravenous cocaine users.

The key to this strong dependence may be in the rapidity of the effect of cocaine when it is smoked. Reinforcement appears to play a major role in drug dependence, and one thing that psychologists have known for many years is that reinforcers are most effective when delivered immediately. It takes only about 8 seconds for blood to circulate from the lungs to the brain, compared to about twice that long from veins in the arm. On that basis, smoking "crack" may be even more addicting than injecting cocaine intravenously!

---

a major role in calling the attention of the public to the problem for which they offer the solution: a new law, more restrictions, and a bigger budget for some agency. This is what is known in Washington, D.C., as "starting a prairie fire." As we see in the next chapter, often the prairie fires include a lot of emotion-arousing rhetoric that borders on the irrational, and sometimes the results of the prairie fire and the ensuing legislation include some unexpected and undesirable outcomes.

Summary

American society has changed from one that tolerated a wide variety of individual drug use to one that attempts strict control over some types of drugs. This has occurred in response to social concerns about drug toxicity, dependence potential, and drug-induced crime and violence.

Toxicity may refer either to physiological poisoning or to dangerous disruption of behavior. Also, we may distinguish acute toxicity resulting from the presence of too much of a drug from chronic toxicity, which results from long-term exposure to a drug.

Addiction is difficult to define because it means different things to different people in different contexts. We may define some of its components more precisely: tolerance, physical dependence, and psychological dependence. Recent views of addiction tend to place more emphasis on psychological dependence than on physical dependence.

The idea that narcotic drugs or marijuana can produce violent criminality in their users is an old and largely discredited idea. Narcotic addicts seem to engage in crimes mainly to obtain money, not because they are made more criminal by the drugs they take. One drug that is widely accepted as contributing to crimes and violence is alcohol.

We can see that the laws that have been developed to control drug use have a legitimate social purpose, which is to protect the society from the dangers caused by some types of drug use. Whether these dangers have always been viewed rationally and whether the laws have had the intended results can be better judged after we have learned more about the drugs and the history of their regulation.

REFERENCES

1. Nadelman E: The case for legalization, Public Interest 92:3, 1988.
2. National Institute on Drug Abuse: Data from the Drug Abuse Warning Network, Annual Data 1987, DHHS Publication No (ADM)88-1584, Washington, DC, 1988, US Government Printing Office.
3. Rosenblatt S and Dodson R: Beyond Valium, New York, 1981, GP Putnam's Sons.
4. Ruttenber AJ and Luke JL: Heroin-related deaths: new epidemiologic insights, Science 226:14-20, 1984.
5. Bozarth MA and Wise RA: Toxicity associated with long-term intravenous heroin and cocaine self-administration in the rat, JAMA 254:81-83, 1985.

6. Booth W: AIDS and drug abuse: no quick fix, Science 239:717, 1988.

7. Chaisson RE and others: Cocaine use and HIV infection in intravenous drug users in San Francisco, JAMA, 261:561-565, 1989.

8. Parry A and others: Addicts, drugs, needles, AIDS, and crime in Liverpool, Presented at International Conference on Drug Policy Reform, Washington, DC, 1988. See also Mersey Drugs Journal (Liverpool) 2:7-20, 1988.

9. NIDA Research Issues No 26, Guide to Drug Abuse Research Terminology, DHHS Publication No (ADM) 82-1237, Washington, DC, 1982, US Government Printing Office.

10. Kelleher RT and Goldberg SR: Control of drug taking behavior by schedules of reinforcement, Pharmacological Reviews 27:291-299, 1976.

11. Alexander BK and Hadaway PF: Opiate addiction: the case for an adaptive orientation, Psychological Bulletin 92:367-381, 1982.

12. Peele S: The meaning of addiction, Lexington, Mass, 1985, DC Heath & Co.

13. Morganthau T and others: The Drug Gangs, Newsweek, March 28, 1988, p. 20-27.

14. Prohibiting the importation of opium for the manufacture of heroin, Hearing before the Committee on Ways and Means, House of Representatives. Congressional Record, April 3, 1924.

15. Tinklenberg JR: Alcohol and violence. In Alcoholism, progress in research and treatment, New York, 1973, Academic Press, Inc.

16. Alcohol and health: Fifth Special Report to the US Congress, DHHS Publication No (ADM) 84-1291, Washington, DC, 1984, US Government Printing Office.

17. Tinklenberg JR and others: Drugs and criminal assaults by adolescents: a replication study, Journal of Psychoactive Drugs 13(3):277-288, 1981.

18. O'Donnell JA and others: Young men and drugs—a nationwide survey, National Institute of Drug Abuse Research Monograph 5, February 1976.

19. Evans CM: Alcohol, violence and aggression, British Journal on Alcohol and Alcoholism 15(3):104-115, 1980.

20. Silverman LP and Spruill NL: Urban crime and the price of heroin, Journal of Urban Economics 4:80-103, 1977.

21. Ball JC and others: cited in Study stresses link between heroin dependence and incidence of crime, New York Times, March 22, 1981, p 22.

22. National Institute of Justice: Attorney general announces NIJ drug use forecasting system, NIJ Reports 208:8-9, 1988.

23. Church GJ: Thinking the unthinkable, Time, pp 12-18, May 30, 1988.

Chapter 3

Drug Regulations

OBJECTIVES

After reading this chapter, you should be able to:

Discuss the historical factors that led to the passage of the 1906 and 1914 laws that are the basis for our current federal drug regulations.

Explain how the rules governing pharmaceuticals have evolved since 1906 and what events led to major changes in those rules.

Describe the process by which a drug company works with the FDA to bring a new drug to market.

Explain how enforcement of the Harrison Act and subsequent federal laws have helped to shape our current illicit drug problem.

List the basic provisions of the current federal controlled substance regulations.

Describe the current federal approach to enforcement of our drug laws and some of its positive consequences and enormous difficulties.

Once upon a time there weren't any regulations about drug use—at least there weren't any federal government regulations. That lasted for about 2 years. In 1791 Congress passed an excise tax on whiskey, which resulted in a disagreement that historians call the Whiskey Rebellion. West of the Appalachian Mountains, where most whiskey was made, the farmers refused to pay the tax and tarred and feathered revenue officers who tried to collect it. In 1794 President George Washington called in the militia, and they occupied counties in western Pennsylvania and sent prisoners to Philadelphia for trial. The militia and the federal government carried the day. The Whiskey Rebellion was an important test for the new government because it established clearly that the federal government had the power to enforce federal laws within a state.

In Chapter 2 we saw that drug regulations are passed mainly for what is perceived to be the public good. As the story of the laws and regulations about drugs unfolds and the number of laws and regulations increases, it will become clear that most of the debate centers on the question: What is the public good? Issues of fact, morality, health, personal choice, and social order are intertwined—and sometimes confused. In a democratic society the debate is usually open, but not necessarily rational. It should surprise no one that our laws about drug use resemble a patchwork quilt reflecting the many different social changes that have occurred in this country. If we want to understand our current drug laws, we must see how they have evolved over the years in response to first one social crisis and then another.

THE BEGINNINGS
Reformism

The current federal approaches to drug regulation can be traced to two pieces of legislation passed in 1906 and 1914. Any student of American history will remember that the nation was moving out of the gilded age of **laissez-faire** capitalism into the reform era in which legislation was passed regulating business and labor practices, meat packing, and food production. We should also remember that this general movement toward improvement of our nation's moral character was to bring us in 1919 a constitutional amendment prohibiting the sale of alcoholic beverages. Republican president Theodore Roosevelt was in office from 1901-1909 and continued to be influential after that time; his role in involving the federal government in both foreign treaties and domestic regulation was crucial to the development of these early drug laws.

Problems Leading to Legislation

The trend toward reform was given direction and energy by the public discussion of several drug-related problems, and the forms taken by those first laws were a reflection of the problems that fueled their passage. **Opium smoking** among the Chinese, **morphinism,** cocaine use, and the peddlers of patent medicines were some of the factors that, when brought to the attention of the American public, helped to build the pressure for regulation.

   Opium and the Chinese. The roots of Chinese opium smoking and the history of the Opium Wars are discussed in the chapter on opiates. It is important, however, to say that in the mid-1800s many British and some American mer-chants were engaged in the lucrative sale of opium to the Chinese, and many reformers and world leaders disapproved. In 1833 the United States signed its first treaty agreeing to control international trade in opium, and in 1842 for the first time placed a regulatory tax on crude opium imported into this country. These first opium regulations were in the same spirit as existing taxes on alcohol and tobacco: only mildly regulatory, they still allowed a fairly free market in a now-regulated substance.

   The United States imported Chinese workers after the Civil War, mainly to help build the rapidly expanding railroads. The Chinese brought with them the habit of smoking opium. As always happens when a new pleasure is introduced into a society, the practice of opium smoking spread rapidly. A contemporary report in 1882 outlined the spread of opium smoking in San Francisco.

   The practice spread rapidly and quietly among this class of gamblers and prostitutes until the latter part of 1875, at which time the authorities became cognizant of the fact, and finding . . . that many women and young girls, as also young men of respectable family, were being induced to visit the dens, where they were ruined morally and otherwise, a city ordinance was passed forbidding the practice under penalty of a heavy fine or imprisonment, or both. Many arrests were made, and the punishment was prompt and thorough.[1, p.1]

This San Francisco act was the first ordinance in America forbidding opium smoking. In 1882 New York State passed a similar law aimed at opium use in New York City's expanding Chinatown.

   As more states and municipalities outlawed opium dens, the cost of black-market opium increased and many of the lower-class opium addicts took up morphine or heroin, which were readily available and inexpensive.

   An 1890 federal act permitted only American citizens to import opium or to manufacture smoking opium in the United States. Although this law is sometimes viewed as a purely racist, anti-Chinese policy, it was at least partly in response to an 1887 agreement with China that also for-

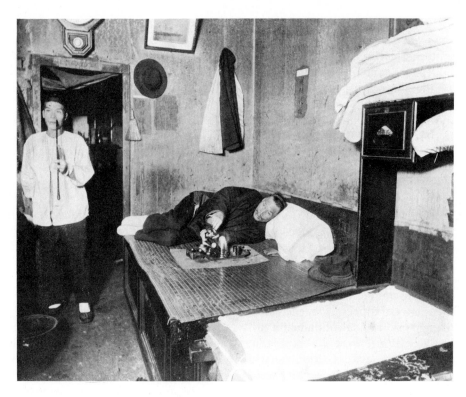

A San Francisco opium den.

bade American citizens from engaging in the Chinese opium trade.

In the early 1900s Dr. Hamilton Wright, the father of American narcotics laws, decided that the United States could gain favored trading status with China by leading international efforts to aid the Chinese in their efforts to reduce opium importation. He eventually drafted the Harrison Act of 1914 to demonstrate the willingness of the United States to control our own traffic in opium.[2]

Morphinism. The **hypodermic syringe** was introduced to the United States in 1856 and used on a large scale during the Civil War. Injecting morphine, the primary active ingredient in opium, gave near-immediate relief from pain. Morphine was used widely, and not always wisely, in the treatment of the two major afflictions in the Civil War—pain and **dysentery.** So

many soldiers became addicted to morphine that morphinism was called the "soldier's disease" or the "army disease" in the years following the war. By the turn of the century most physicians, especially those who were younger and better trained, were aware of the danger of morphine addiction and were much more conservative in their use of this drug.

Cocaine. Pure cocaine also became available at about the same time as the hypodermic needle, and physicians experimented with its many uses. It was widely touted as a cure for morphine addiction, and many physicians prescribed cocaine injections for this purpose. Within a few years it was clear that cocaine was itself habit forming and that in high enough doses a dramatic **psychotic** state occurred. By the early 1900s there was considerable medical reaction against the indiscriminate use of cocaine. The practice of "snuffing" cocaine into the nose, which was said to be popular among southern blacks, caused a great deal of concern and fear.[3, pp.197-199] Dr. Wright testified before Congress that this practice led to the raping of white women.

Patent medicines.   The broadest impact on drug use in this country came from the widespread legal distribution of **patent medicines.** Patent medicines were dispensed by traveling peddlers and were readily available at local stores for self-medication. Sales of patent medicines increased from $3.5 million in 1859 to $74 million in 1904.

Within the boundaries of the United States there was increasing conflict between the steady progress of medical science and the therapeutic claims of the patent medicine hucksters. The alcohol and/or narcotic content of the patent medicines was also a matter of concern. One medicine, Hostetter's Bitters, was 44% alcohol while another, Birney's Catarrh Cure, was 4% cocaine. In October, 1905, *Collier's* magazine culminated a prolonged attack on patent medicines with a well-documented, aggressive series, entitled "Great American Fraud."[4]

The 1906 Pure Food and Drugs Act

President Theodore Roosevelt recommended in 1905 ". . . that a law be enacted to regulate interstate commerce in misbranded and adulterated foods, drinks, and drugs."[5] The 1906 publication of Upton Sinclair's *The Jungle*, exposing the horribly unsanitary conditions in the meat packing industry, shocked Congress and America. It was the necessary straw that 5 months later, on the thirtieth of June, 1906, led to the passage of the Pure Food and Drugs Act, which prohibited the interstate commerce of adulterated or misbranded foods and drugs. This act brought the government full force into the drug marketplace, and subsequent modifications have built on it. This act defined a drug as "any substance or mixture of substances intended to be used for the cure, mitigation, or prevention of disease." Of particular importance, it developed, was the phrasing of the

law with respect to misbranding. Misbranding referred *only to the label, not to general advertising,* and covered "any statement, design, or device regarding . . . [a drug], or the ingredients or substances contained therein, which shall be false or misleading in any particular."

The act specifically referred to alcohol, morphine, opium, cocaine, heroin, *Cannabis indica* (marijuana), and several other agents. Each package was required to state how much (or what proportion) of these drugs was included in the preparation. This meant, for example, that the widely sold "cures" for morphine addiction had to indicate that they in fact contained another addicting drug.

The Harrison Act of 1914

At the request of the United States, an international conference met in The Hague in 1912 to discuss controls on the opium trade. Great Britain, which was giving up a very lucrative business, wanted morphine and cocaine included as well, because as opium was being controlled these German products were replacing it.[2, p.288] Eventually an agreement was reached in which several nations agreed to control both international trade and domestic sale and use of these substances. In response, Dr. Wright drafted a bill that was submitted by Senator Harrison of New York, titled "An Act to provide for the registration of, with collectors of internal revenue, and to impose a special tax upon all persons who produce, import, manufacture, compound, deal in, dispense, or give away opium or coca leaves, their salts, derivatives, or preparations, and for other purposes."[6] With a title like that, it's no wonder that this historic law is usually referred to as the Harrison Act!

For the first time, dealers and dispensers of the opiates and cocaine had to register annually, pay a small fee, and use special order forms provided by the Bureau of Internal Revenue. Physicians, dentists, and veterinary surgeons were named as potential lawful distributors if they registered. This was not a punitive act, penalties for violation were

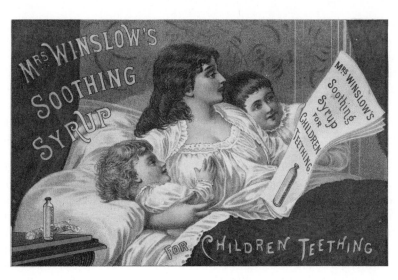

This "soothing syrup" for children contained a large amount of opium.

not severe, and the measure contained no reference to users of "narcotics."

During congressional debate there was some concern expressed about the inconvenience to physicians and pharmacists, and it is doubtful if such a law would have been passed in the United States if its purpose had been merely to meet the rather weak treaty obligations of the 1912 Hague Conference. It was not meant to replace existing laws and, in fact, specifically supported the continuing legality of the 1906 Pure Food and Drugs Act and the 1909 Opium Exclusion Act. Dr. Wright had written and lectured extensively, waging an effective public campaign for additional controls over these drugs. Probably the emotional issues added the necessary heat to make the difference: the agonies experienced by the victims of these habit-forming drugs, the racially tinged fears of Chinese opium dens, and the fear of cocaine-fueled violence among blacks.

Two Bureaus, Two Types of Regulation

By 1914 the basic federal laws had been passed that would influence our nation's drug regulations up to the current time. It may be significant that the Pure Food and Drugs Act was administered within the Department of Agriculture, whereas the Harrison Act was administered by the Treasury Department—two different federal departments administering two different laws. Many of the drugs regulated by the two laws were the same, but the political issues to which each agency responded were different. The Agriculture Department was administering a law aimed at ensuring that drugs were pure and honestly labeled, whereas the Treasury Department was trying to regulate the sale of habit-forming drugs. The approach taken by each bureau was further shaped by court decisions so that the actual effect of each law came to be something a bit different from what seems to have been intended.

REGULATING PHARMACEUTICALS

The 1906 law called for the government to regulate the purity of both foods and drugs, and evidence had been presented during the congressional debate that thousands of products in both categories were at fault. Where to begin with the task of analyzing and prosecuting? Dr. Harvey Wiley, chief chemist in the Department of Agriculture, had been a major proponent of the 1906 law and had in fact drafted most of it. He was in charge of administering the law, and he influenced the direction that its enforcement would take. His first concern was with adulterated food, so most of the initial cases dealt with food products rather than drugs.

Purity

Most large drug manufacturers made efforts to comply with the new law, although they were not given specific recommendations as to how this should be accomplished. The manufacturer of Cuforhedake Brane-Fude modified its label to show that it contained 30% alcohol and 16 grains of the active ingredient, a widely used headache remedy. The government brought the manufacturer to trial in 1908 on several grounds: the alcohol content was a bit *lower* than that claimed on the label and the label seemed to claim that the product was a "cure" and food for the brain, both misleading claims. After much arguing about different methods of describing alcohol content and about the label claims, the manufacturer was convicted by the jury, probably because of the "brane-fude" claim, and paid a fine of $700.[7, pp.3-12]

Dr. Wiley went on vigorously testing products and pursuing any that were adulterated or didn't properly list important ingredients, but he also went after many companies on the basis of their therapeutic claims. In 1911 government action against a claimed cancer cure was overturned by arguing that the ingredients were accurately labeled, and the original law had not in fact covered therapeutic claims, only claims about the nature of the ingredients. Congress rapidly passed the 1912 Sherley amendment that outlawed "false and fraudulent" therapeutic claims. Even so, it was still up to the government to prove that a claim was not only false, but that it was also fraudulent in that the manufacturer knew it to be false. In a 1922 case, the claim that "B&M External Remedy" could cure tuberculosis was ruled not to be fraudulent because its manufacturer, who had no scientific or medical training, truly believed that its ingredients (raw eggs, turpentine, ammonia, formaldehyde, and mustard and wintergreen oils) would be effective.[7, pp.88-112] This seemed to encourage the ignorant to become manufacturers of medicines!

From the beginning, the Food and Drug Administration **(FDA)** had adopted the approach of encouraging voluntary cooperation, which they could obtain from most of the manufacturers through educational and corrective actions rather than through punitive, forced compliance. As more and more cases were investigated, it became clear to the FDA officials that many of the violations of the 1906 law were unintentional and caused primarily by poor manufacturing techniques and an absence of quality control measures. The FDA began developing assay techniques for various chemicals and products and collaborated extensively with the pharmaceutical industry to improve standards. The prosperous 1920s, coupled with a friendly Republican administration and increasing scientific knowhow, resulted in many voluntary changes by the drug industry that improved manufacturing and selling practices.

In spite of these improvements, many smaller companies continued to bring forth "quack" medicines that were ineffective or even dangerous. The depression of the 1930s increased competition for business, and the Democratic Roosevelt administration took a more critical view of the pharmaceutical industry. FDA surveys in the mid-1930s showed that over 10% of the drug products studied did not meet the standards of *The United States Pharmacopeia* or *The National Formulary*. Several attempts were made during the early 1930s to enact major reforms, but concerned opposition by the manufacturers of proprietary medicines prevented this from happening.

Safety

The 1930s had seen an expansion in the use of "sulfa" drugs, which are effective antibiotics. In searching for a form that could be given as a liquid, a chemist found that **sulfanilamide** would dissolve in diethylene glycol. The new concoction looked, tasted, and smelled fine, so it was bottled and marketed in 1937. Diethylene glycol causes kidney poisoning, and within a short time 107 people died from taking "Elixir Sulfanilamide." The government seized the elixir on the grounds that a true elixir contains alcohol, and this did not—there was no legal requirement that a medicine be safe! The chemist committed suicide, the company paid the largest fine ever under the 1906 law, and the public crisis arose that led to passage of the 1938 Food, Drug, and Cosmetic Act.[7, pp.184-188]

A critical change in the 1938 law was the requirement that *before* a new drug could be marketed its manufacturer must test it for toxicity. The company was to submit a "new drug application" **(NDA)** to the FDA. This NDA was to include "full reports of investigations which have been made to show whether or not such a drug is safe for use." If the submitted paperwork was satisfactory, the application was allowed to become effective. Between 1938 and 1962 about 13,000 NDAs were submitted and about 70% were allowed to become effective.

The new drug application provision was important in two ways: First, it changed the role of the FDA from testing and challenging some of the drugs already being sold to that of a gatekeeper, which must review every new drug before it is marketed. This increased power and responsibility led to a great expansion in the size of the FDA. Second, the requirement that companies conduct research before marketing a new drug greatly reduced the likelihood of new drugs being introduced by small companies run by untrained people.

The 1938 amendments also stipulated that drug labels either give adequate directions for use or state that the drug was to be used only on the prescription of a physician. Thus federal law recognized a difference between drugs that could be sold over the counter and prescription-only drugs.

Effectiveness

In the late 1950s Senator Estes Kefauver began a series of hearings investigating high drug costs and marketing collaboration between drug companies. As the hearings progressed, manufacturers, physicians, and the FDA itself were criticized. So many new, powerful, and more complex chemicals were being introduced that it seemed more caution should be exercised at all levels. Senator Kefauver's remedial bill was introduced in 1960, but it was weakened by amendment and finally bottled up in committee. Again it took a disaster that raised public awareness and congressional concern before major reforms were implemented.

Thalidomide, a sedative and sleeping pill, was first marketed in West Germany in 1957. The drug was widely used by pregnant women because it also reduced nausea and vomiting associated with the morning sickness often experienced early in pregnancy. An American company submitted an NDA in 1960 to market thalidomide, but luckily the FDA physician in charge of the application did not approve it quickly. In 1961 and early 1962 it became clear that thalidomide had been responsible for the birth in Germany of hundreds of children with deformed limbs. The American company had released some thalidomide for clinical testing, but since its application was not approved a major disaster was avoided in the United States.[7, pp.415-418]

The 1962 Kefauver-Harris amendments added several important provisions, including the requirement that companies submit plans for and seek approval of any testing to be done with humans before the clinical trials are conducted. Another provision required advertisements for prescription drugs (mostly in medical journals) to contain a summary of information about adverse reactions to the drug.

The most important change was one requiring that every new drug has to be demonstrated to be effective for the illnesses mentioned on the label. As with the details of safety testing required by the 1938 law, this research on effectiveness was to be submitted to the FDA. Before this time, if a new drug contained harmless substances and did not make any strong claims for therapeutic effectiveness, there was no need for it to be useful at all!

The FDA was also to begin a review of the thousands of products marketed between 1938 and 1962 to determine their effectiveness. Any that were found to be ineffective were to be removed from the market. In 1966 the FDA began the process of evaluating the formulations of prescription drugs. By the end of 1974 the FDA had taken action to remove from the market 6133 drugs manufactured by 2732 companies.

Marketing a New Drug

To translate the 1962 law on the safety and effectiveness of a new drug, the FDA has established certain regular procedures and standards that must be met by the pharmaceutical house that hopes to market a prescription drug. As does the consumer of legal drugs, the pharmaceutical industry has a considerable stake in these FDA requirements. Developing a compound to the point where it can be marketed is a long and expensive procedure for the drug company, maybe costing as much as $50 to $70 million.

In an average year, researchers in the pharmaceutical industry may screen 126,000 chemical compounds for possible utilization as drugs. About 1,000 of these will prove worthy of intense investigation. Years later, if the researchers are lucky, 16 compounds may eventually make it to pharmacies.[8, p.5]

It is not only new drugs that must be evaluated by the FDA but also a new use for an established drug. A drug may prove to be effective for a group of conditions and be passed by the FDA for sale as a treatment for those conditions. If the company finds the drug is also effective for a different group of conditions, it must submit the new information to the FDA and may not advertise the drug as effective for the new conditions until permitted by the FDA. A similar situation occurs when a new form of a drug is introduced, for example, a sustained-release form; the FDA requires that it be handled as a new drug.

The FDA formally enters the picture only when a drug company is ready to study the effects of a compound in humans. At that time the company supplies to the FDA a "Notice of Claimed Investigational Exemption for a New Drug" **(IND).** This IND must include the composition of the drug, its source if a biological preparation, and complete manufacturing information. At this time the manufacturer is required to submit all information from preclinical (before human) investigations, including the effects of the drug on animals. The principal purpose of this preclinical work is to establish the safety of the compound.

As minimum evidence of safety, the animal studies must include acute, one-time administration of several dose levels of the drug to different groups of animals of at least two species. There must also be studies where the drug is given regularly to animals for a period related to the proposed use of the drug in humans. For example, a drug to be used chronically requires 2-year toxicology studies in animals. Again two species are required. The method of drug administration and the form of the drug in these studies must be the same as that proposed for human use.

In addition to these research results, the company must submit a detailed description of the proposed clinical studies of the drug in humans. Information on the physicians who will conduct the clinical studies must also be submitted so that the FDA can evaluate their competency. In addition to the credentials on the clinical investigators, the FDA requires that it receive copies of *all* information given to the investigators about the drug.

The company must also certify that the human subjects will be told they are receiving an investigational compound and that the subjects will sign a form stating that they know they are to receive such a compound and that this is acceptable to them. Finally, the company must agree to forward annually a comprehensive report and to inform the FDA immediately if any adverse reactions arise in either animals or humans receiving the investigational drug.

If the FDA authorizes the use of the drug in humans, the company can move into the first of three phases of clinical investigation.

The first phase encompasses studies with very small amounts of the drug on a limited number of healthy people—company employees, medical school personnel, prisoners and others who volunteer for such trials. At this stage, the researchers are primarily interested in learning how their drug is absorbed and excreted in healthy people, and what side effects it may trigger.[8, p.12]

There has been increasing concern about the ethics, as well as the scientific validity, of using prisoners in Phase 1 studies. Can a prisoner freely volunteer? Is a group of prisoners similar enough to those individuals who will be taking the drug therapeutically? The federal government wanted to ban all biomedical research in prisons as of 1981. A lawsuit by prisoners stopped the regulation from being implemented and drug research in prisons continues. In 1976 about 40% of Phase 1 testing was on prisoners.

Phase 2 of the human studies involves patients who have the condition the candidate drug is designed to treat. These will probably involve as many as 100 hospital patients, who are chosen because the new agent may help them. . . . If all goes well with these trials, Phase 3 will follow. It can involve thousands of patients in and out of hospitals.[8, pp.12-13]

Phase 3 is quite extensive and involves administering the drug to individuals with the disease or symptom for which the drug is intended. If the compound proves effective in Phase 3, the FDA balances its possible dangers against the benefits for the patient before releasing it for sale to the public.

There is one big, continually debated issue surrounding the FDA "drug approval" system: Why does it take so long? This issue hits the media headlines frequently as the "drug lag"—the length of time between the drug's submission to the FDA for approval and its approval for marketing.

The issue is not just one of concern for the individual who is sick. Pharmaceutical manufacturers have only a 17-year patent on a new drug. They usually patent the chemical as soon as there is some evidence that it may be marketable. The

manufacturers claim that by the time a drug is cleared for marketing, they have only about 7 years left on the patent—not long enough to reclaim costs and make a decent profit. The manufacturers have pushed for a 7-year patent extension to compensate for the FDA's slow approval process.

A survey in 1984 showed that most Americans support tough drug-testing laws in spite of the marketing delays.[9] In 1985 the FDA did set up new regulations designed to speed up the marketing of new drugs, and there was an increase in the number of new drugs allowed on the market over the next couple of years. By the end of the 1980s, about 20 new drugs per year were being approved. In one specific area, the push for new drugs to treat AIDS, the FDA is not only streamlining procedures, but is providing direct aid to the makers of potential new products to speed them through the review process.[10]

Changes to the Food, Drug, and Cosmetic Act since 1962 have been relatively minor. For example, the Prescription Drug Marketing Act of 1987 tightened the procedures whereby drug company salespeople could provide free samples to physicians, after Congress had heard testimony about widespread diversion of samples and sloppy handling and record keeping.[11] Also, because counterfeit and adulterated drugs had found their way into the U.S. market from abroad as shipments of "American goods returned," new regulations were added covering the transfer and reimportation of drugs. Both these provisions require more records and more paperwork in general and carry the potential for more bureaucratic oversight.

NARCOTICS, DANGEROUS DRUGS, AND CONTROLLED SUBSTANCES

Although the Harrison Act controlled opiates, which are **narcotics,** and cocaine, which is not, the enforcement effort focused so much on the narcotics that the term *narcotic* came to mean illegal drug to many people. Reference is even made to the Harrison Narcotics Act, although that was not its title. Later federal laws classified cocaine and then marijuana as narcotics, and the section of the Treasury Department responsible for enforcing federal drug laws was called the Bureau of Narcotics. This overextension of the word has been corrected to some extent, and those changes that have occurred in the laws and terminology once again reflect a series of public crises.

After the Harrison Act

In 1914 it was estimated that about 200,000 Americans—1 in 400—were addicted to opium or its derivatives. One way to administer the new law would have been to allow a continued legal supply of opiates to those individuals through registered physicians and to focus enforcement efforts on the smugglers and remaining opium dens. After all, the Harrison Act stated that an unregistered person could purchase and possess any of the taxed drugs if they had been prescribed or administered by a physician "in the course of his professional practice and for legitimate medical purposes." Early enforcement efforts focused on smugglers and did not result in a large number of arrests. However, one very important arrest was to have later repercussions. It seems that a Dr. Webb was taking telephone orders for narcotics, including some from people he had never seen in person. Evidence was presented that this physician would prescribe whatever amount the caller requested. He was arrested, convicted, and appealed the conviction all the way to the U.S. Supreme Court, which in 1919 upheld his conviction on the grounds that his activity did not constitute a proper "prescription" in the course of the professional practice of medicine. Although they had arrested several smugglers and a few other scoundrels who tried to take advantage of their professional positions to deal in large amounts of narcotics, the Treasury Department did not make a large number of arrests. Many addicts received narcotics quietly through their private physicians, and in most large cities there were public clinics that dispensed morphine to addicts who could not afford private care.

It is ironic that the single most important piece of legislation that has shaped the federal government's approach to drug addiction wasn't a narcotics law at all, but rather the Eighteenth Amendment prohibiting alcohol. That law was also to be enforced by the Treasury Department, and a separate Prohibition unit was established in 1919. The Narcotics Division was placed within that unit, and Colonel Levi G. Nutt was appointed the first director, with 170 agents at his disposal.[2,p.231] Although the Harrison Act itself had not changed, the people enforcing it had. Just as with alcohol, these people believed that the cure for narcotic addiction was to prevent the addict from having access to the drug, in other words, narcotic "prohibition," at least for addicts. The new enforcers interpreted the Webb case to mean that any prescription of a habit-forming drug to an addict was not a "legitimate medical purpose," and they began to charge many physicians under the Harrison Act. They seemed to be right on target when in 1922 the Supreme Court upheld the conviction of another physician, Dr. Behrman, who used the defense that his prescriptions were not given to maintain addiction, but as part of a cure program. This defense was not allowed in his case, because evidence was presented that one patient had received the equivalent of 3000 "ordinary doses."[6,p.780]

Since even cure programs were not exempt, the Internal Revenue Service (IRS) moved to close down municipal narcotics clinics in over 30 cities from coast to coast. In the period from 1919 to 1929, the Narcotics Bureau arrested about 75,000 people, including 25,000 physicians and druggists.[2,p.231] The American Medical Association, which was concerned with the reputation of the medical profession, supported tight narcotic controls. Reputable physicians were not to prescribe narcotics to addicts. Narcotic addiction was increasingly viewed as a police, rather than a medical, problem. Since there was no legal way for an addict to continue his habit, the addict was forced to look for his drugs in the illegal market. Thus, this new method of enforcing the Harrison Act resulted in the growth of an illicit drug trade that charged users up to 50 times more than the legal retail drug price.

Partly in response to this growing illicit market, Congress passed the Jones-Miller Act of 1922, which more than doubled the maximum penalties for dealing in illegally imported narcotics to $5000 and 10-years' imprisonment. This act was the first to mislabel cocaine as a narcotic, and it established the Federal Narcotics Control Board, to initiate an active program against dealers. Included also was the stipulation that the mere possession of illegally obtained narcotics was sufficient basis for conviction, thus officially making the addict himself a criminal. Because illegal narcotics were so expensive, many addicts came to prefer the most potent type available, heroin. In 1924 another act entirely prohibited importing opium for the manufacture of heroin. Already by this time several important trends had been set: addicts were criminals at odds with the regulatory agency, the growth of the illicit market was responded to with greater penalties and more aggressive enforcement, and there was a focus on attempting to eliminate a substance (heroin) as though the drug itself were the problem. In the 1925 Linder case the Supreme Court declared that it could be legal for a physician to prescribe narcotics for an addict if it was part of a curing program and did not transcend "the limits of that professional conduct with which Congress never intended to interfere."[6,p.780] However, the damage had been done, and most physicians would have nothing to do with addicts.

By 1928 individuals sentenced for drug violations made up one-third of the total population in federal prisons, a statistic which we have managed to match again in the late 1980s. Even though the 1920s was the period of alcohol prohibition, twice as many people were imprisoned for narcotics violations as for liquor violations.[12] In 1929 Congress viewed this enormous expenditure for narcotics offenders as indicating that something was wrong, and decided that addicts should be cured rather than repeatedly jailed. They voted to establish two narcotic farms for the treatment of persons addicted to habit-forming drugs (including marijuana and peyote) who had

been convicted of violating a federal law. The farm in Lexington, Kentucky opened in 1935 and generally held about 1000 patients, two-thirds of whom were prisoners.

Answering the call for new approaches to addiction, and in response to the end of Prohibition and to charges of corruption in the previous Narcotics Division, in 1930 Congress took several actions that culminated in the formation of a separate Bureau of Narcotics in the Treasury Department. Harry Anslinger became the first commissioner of that Bureau in 1932, and took office with the pledge to stop arresting so many addicts and instead to go after the big dealers. Mr. Anslinger became the first "drug czar," although he wasn't called that at the time. To some extent he followed the lead of J. Edgar Hoover, Director of the Federal Bureau of Investigation (FBI). Each

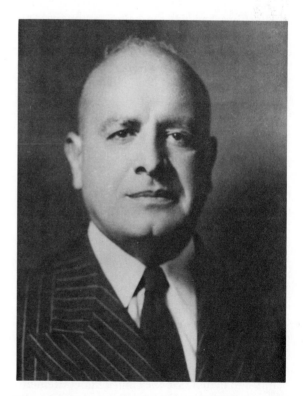

Harry Anslinger became the first commissioner of the Bureau of Narcotics in 1932.

of these men was regularly reappointed by each new president, and each built up a position of considerable power and influence. Mr. Anslinger had almost total control of federal efforts in narcotics education, prevention, treatment, and enforcement for over 30 years, from 1932 to 1962. No federal or state narcotics law was passed without his influencing it, and he also represented U.S. narcotics interests to international organizations, including the United Nations. He was tough-minded in the area of drug abuse and always opposed any form of "ambulatory" narcotic treatment (outside a secure hospital environment).

The end of Prohibition, combined with depression-era cutbacks, had reduced the manpower available for enforcement, but not for long. After some newspaper reports that linked marijuana smoking with crime, Anslinger adopted this new threat and began writing, speaking, testifying, and making films depicting the evils of marijuana. This succeeded in bringing public attention to the fight his bureau was waging against drugs and also resulted in 1937 in the passage of the Marijuana Tax Act. This essentially brought marijuana under the same type of legal control as cocaine and the narcotics, in that one was supposed to register and pay a tax to legally import, buy, or sell marijuana. From 1937 until 1971, marijuana was referred to in federal laws as a narcotic.

World War II caused a decrease in the importation of both legal and illegal drugs. With the end of the war and the resumption of easy international travel, the illegal narcotic trade resumed and increased every year, in spite of the 1951 Boggs Amendment to the Harrison Act that established mandatory minimum sentences for narcotic offenses. Testimony before a subcommittee of the Senate Judiciary Committee in 1955 stated that drug addiction was responsible for 50% of crime in urban areas and 25% of all reported crimes. The subcommittee also reported that drug addiction was one of the ways Communist China planned to demoralize the United States. Remember that this was the height of the McCarthy era, during which a mere hint by Senator Joseph McCarthy that someone consorted with "known communists" was enough to ruin that person's career, and the FBI was putting most of its resources into the effort to locate communist conspirators. It may not be important, but one of those interesting little nasty bits of history has recently come out. It seems that Anslinger and FBI Director Hoover were aware that Senator McCarthy, in addition to his widely known alcoholism, was addicted to morphine. Anslinger arranged for McCarthy to obtain a regular supply of his drug from a Washington, D.C., pharmacy without interference from narcotics officers.[2,pp.283-284] With both crime and communism to combat, Congress passed the 1956 Narcotic Drug Control Act, with the toughest penalties yet. Under this law any offense except first-offense possession had to result in a jail term, and no suspension, probation, or parole was allowed. Anyone caught selling heroin to a person under 18 could receive the death penalty. Anslinger commented on that particular provision by saying, "I'd like to throw the switch myself on drug peddlers who sell their poisons to minors."[13]

Drug Abuse Control Amendments of 1965

The early 1960s saw not only an increase in illegal drug use but also a shift in the type of drug being used illegally. The trend was for the new drug users to be better educated and to emphasize primarily drugs that alter mood and consciousness, such as amphetamines, barbiturates, and hallucinogens. Some hospitals in large cities reported that up to 15% of their emergency room calls involved individuals with adverse reactions to these drugs. Although amphetamines and barbiturates were legal prescription drugs, it was felt that they should be under the same type of controls as narcotics. The 1965 Drug Abuse Control Amendments referred to these as dangerous drugs and also included hallucinogens such as LSD. Recognizing that new illicit drugs were arriving on the scene and that it was impractical to pass new legislation for each one, the bill provided that the

FDA could recommend to the Secretary of Health, Education, and Welfare that a new drug be controlled if it has a potential for abuse because of its stimulant or depressant or hallucinogenic effects. The Bureau of Narcotics later became the Bureau of Narcotics and Dangerous Drugs, and it was to carry out this enforcement. Thus the 1960s saw a number of major changes for this agency. Mr. Anslinger had retired, they had new classes of drugs to control, and they were facing widespread disregard of the drug laws by large numbers of young people who were not all members of the underprivileged and criminal classes.

Comprehensive Drug Abuse Prevention and Control Act of 1970

The Comprehensive Drug Abuse Prevention and Control Act of 1970, usually referred to as the **Controlled Substance Act of 1970,** almost lived up to its title. It was comprehensive, since it repealed and replaced or updated all previous laws concerned with both the narcotic and dangerous drugs. The law specifically stated that the drugs controlled by the act are under federal jurisdiction regardless of involvement in interstate commerce. The law did not eliminate state regulations; it just made clear that federal enforcement and prosecution is possible in any illegal activity involving controlled drugs.

The law dealt with prevention and treatment of drug abuse by appropriating funds for expanding the role of community mental health centers and Public Health Service hospitals in the treatment of those who misuse drugs. It authorized the development of educational material and drug education workshops for professional workers as well as for the public schools.

The special status of marijuana and marijuana users was evident throughout the law. Of particular note is the fact that the law established a *Commission on Marijuana and Drug Abuse.* The Commission was instructed to complete a comprehensive summary on the medical, legal, and sociocultural aspects of marijuana and marijuana use and to submit a final report with "recom-

mendations for legislative and administrative actions" within 2 years.

The control aspects of the bill were the most debated portions, and several basic philosophical, ethical, and legal issues were resolved (!) by the law. First is that this was a law to control drugs directly rather than through excise taxes. Enforcement authority was moved to the Department of Justice from the Treasury Department. A second major issue was the separation of enforcement of the law from the scientific evaluation of the drugs considered for control. The Attorney General is responsible for the administration of the control aspects of the law, but the Secretary of Health and Human Services (HHS) now makes the final decision on which drugs should be controlled. This separation of enforcement from the scientific and medical decision of what should be controlled was a major victory for those arguing for a sane drug law.

The Secretary of HHS has delegated to the FDA primary responsibility in determining whether a drug should be controlled. The FDA must consider the following factors:

1. Scientific evidence of its pharmacological effect, if known
2. The state of current scientific knowledge regarding the drug or other substance
3. What, if any, risk there is to the public health
4. Its psychic or physiological dependence liability
5. Whether the substance is an immediate precursor of a substance already controlled under this title

After specifically excluding "distilled spirits, wine, malt beverages, or tobacco" the law established five schedules of drugs that must be updated and published regularly. Table 3-1 summarizes the characteristics and penalties for illegally selling drugs in each of the five schedules. Remember that many prescription drugs are not included in these schedules, usually because they are not psychoactive, for example, antibiotics.

Several different aspects of control are contained in this law. This law reformulated some of

Table 3-1

Summary of drug schedules and penalties for violation of the Comprehensive Drug Abuse Prevention and Control Act

Sched-ule	Potential for abuse	Medical use	Produc-tion con-trolled	Examples	Maximum penalties for illegal	
					Manufacturing distribution	Possession
I	High	None	Yes	Heroin, marijuana, THC (tetrahydrocan-nabinol), LSD, mes-caline Some morphine salts, methaqualone	**Schedules I and II** Narcotics— 1st offense 15 yr/$25,000/3yr* 2nd and more offenses 30 yr/$50,000/6 yr	
II	High	Yes	Yes	Morphine, cocaine, methadone, opium, codeine, secobarbital, amobarbital, pento-barbital, meperidine, amphetamine, meth-amphetamine	Nonnarcotics— 1st offense 5 yr/$15,000/2 yr 2nd offense 10 yr/$30,000/4 yr	1st offense 1 yr/$5,000 2nd offense 2 yr/$10,000
III	Some, less than drugs in I and II	Yes	No	Nonamphetamine-type stimulants; some bar-biturates, some nar-cotic preparations, paregoric, phencycli-dine	1st offense 5 yr/$15,000/2 yr 2nd offense 10 yr/$30,000/4 yr	For first offense probation may be given
IV	Low, less than drugs in III	Yes	No	Barbital, chloral hy-drate, meprobam-ate, phenobarbital, propoxyphene, diaz-epam, chlordiaz-epoxide, certain nonamphetamine stimulants not listed in previous schedules	1st offense 3 yr/$10,000/1 yr 2nd offense 6 yr/$20,000/2 yr	Penalties for possession are the same for all schedules
V	Low, less than drugs in IV	Yes	No	Compounds, mixtures, and preparations with very low amounts of nar-cotics; dilute codeine and opium com-pounds	1st offense 1 yr/$5,000/none 2nd offense 2 yr/$10,000/none	

*Maximum prison sentence/maximum fine/mandatory probation period after release from prison.

the restrictions on drug prescriptions found in earlier acts. No prescription for a Schedule II compound can be refilled, but in an emergency a Schedule II drug can be dispensed on an oral prescription. Prescriptions for substances in Schedules III, IV, and V cannot be refilled more than five times and not at all more than 6 months after written. The label of a drug in Schedule II, III, or IV must contain this warning: CAUTION: FEDERAL LAW PROHIBITS THE TRANSFER OF THIS DRUG TO ANY PERSON OTHER THAN THE PATIENT FOR WHOM IT WAS PRESCRIBED.

The penalties for simply possessing a drug are more lenient than before and do not depend on the schedule. Therefore, an individual is theoretically guilty of the same crime whether he or she has a Darvon tablet prescribed for another person or a bag of heroin. A first offense of illegal possession of a controlled drug or "distributing a small amount of marijuana for no remuneration . . ." can be punished by a year's imprisonment and/or a fine of $5000. In lieu of this the court can place the individual on probation for up to 1 year. If there is no violation of the conditions of probation the charge is dismissed, the conviction erased from the individual's record, and, for every legal purpose, the conviction never existed.

While the individual user is less likely to serve a long prison sentence under this law, more severe penalties are prescribed for anyone over 18 who distributes a controlled substance to anyone under 21 or to those who are involved with other people in dealing in controlled substances. The idea seemed to be to focus more on the dealers, especially the organized dealers, and less on the individual user. Some have suggested that this was a result of the drug scene moving into white suburbia. "Since sons and daughters of prominent persons—including senators—started getting busted for crimes previously associated with lower-class blacks, compassion for marijuana criminals was sure to arise."[14]

It was clear before this 1970 law that many more prescription amphetamines were being manufactured than were being sold legally, so restrictions were placed on the amount of Schedule I and Schedule II drugs that could be made (since Schedule I drugs have no legal medical use, only very small amounts are legally made for research purposes).

Although terms such as *narcotic* and *dangerous drug* were generally replaced by the term *controlled substance,* there remains one problem of terminology. The penalties for distribution of Schedule I and II narcotics are higher than for distribution of Schedule I and II nonnarcotics. This, of course, requires a legal definition of the term narcotic. While pharmacologically this term should be used only for opiates such as heroin and morphine, it was previously applied to cocaine and then to marijuana. Enough people had argued in court in the 1960s that marijuana was not a narcotic that the 1970 law did not list it as one. But cocaine, which at the time was not widely used, remained on the list and is still legally a narcotic. Since there is no rational basis for higher penalties based on the narcotic vs nonnarcotic distinction, perhaps someday this problem can be corrected.

The 1988 Omnibus Drug Act made some interesting additions and adjustments to the controlled substances act.[15] There were many components to this new law, involving the registration of airplanes, money laundering, firearms sales to felons, and chemicals used to manufacture drugs. One part allowed for the death penalty for anyone who murders someone or orders the killing of someone in conjunction with a drug-related felony. Major sections of the law funded treatment and education programs as well. The most noteworthy changes were a toughening of approaches toward drug users, aimed at reducing the *demand* for drugs (as opposed to putting all federal efforts into reducing the *supply* of drugs). Before this law there were few penalties and little federal interest in convicting users for possessing small (personal-use) amounts of controlled substances. Under the new law, here are some of the unpleasant possibilities if you are convicted of possession:

- A civil fine of up to $10,000
- Forfeiture of the car, boat, or plane conveying the substance
- Loss of all federal benefits, including student

loans and grants, for up to 1 year after a first offense and up to 5 years after a second offense

The 1988 law also would also remove from public housing the entire family of anyone who engaged in criminal activity, including drug-related activity, on or near public-housing premises.

In order to better coordinate all these federal efforts, the law established the "cabinet-level" position of Director of National Drug Control Policy (popularly referred to as a "drug czar"). The first person appointed to this new office by President Bush was William Bennett, former Secretary of Education. He is ordered by the legislation to prepare a national drug-control strategy and an annual consolidated drug-control budget for all federal agencies involved, to advise the National Security Council, and to report directly to the president.

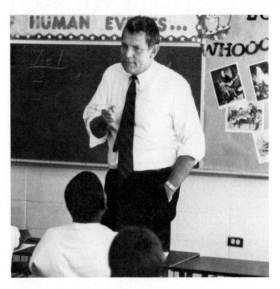

William Bennett was the first person appointed Director of National Drug Control Policy.

Drug enforcement

The current efforts at enforcing federal drug laws can be examined by asking ourselves three questions: What exactly are we doing? How much is it costing us? How effective is it?

In 1982, President Reagan announced a renewed and reorganized effort to combat drug trafficking and organized crime. What made this approach different from previous renewed efforts was its scope and degree of involvement of many federal agencies. The country was divided into 13 task force areas. The task forces were to work within their areas in cooperation with state and local authorities, and were to use the resources of the Drug Enforcement Administration **(DEA),** the FBI, the IRS, Alcohol, Tobacco and Firearms Bureau, Immigration and Naturalization, U.S. Marshals, U.S. Customs Service, and the Coast Guard. A special budget allocation of $127 million was used to hire some 1000 agents and 200 attorneys.[16] In some regions, Defense Department tracking and pursuit services would be added. This last item had been legalized earlier in the Reagan administration and signaled an important change in the role of the military; the idea of using our

military forces to police our population has long been abhorrent to Americans who have insisted that most police powers remain at the state and local level. Because of the success of smugglers, we now use Air Force radar and aircraft and Navy patrol boats to detect and track aircraft or boats that may be bringing in drugs. These efforts continued to expand throughout the 1980s. With more people and more agencies involved there was increasing conflict over budgets, territory, and control over combined operations. This was the major reason Congress established the "drug czar" position in the 1988 law—so that all the federal agencies could become more coordinated in their drug enforcement efforts.

International efforts aimed at reducing the drug supply have included State Department programs that provide aid to individual countries to help them with narcotics controls, usually working in conjunction with the DEA. The DEA has agents in more than 40 countries outside the United States, and they assist the local authorities in crop eradication, locating and destroying illicit laboratories, and interfering with the transportation of drugs out of those countries. It has been charged

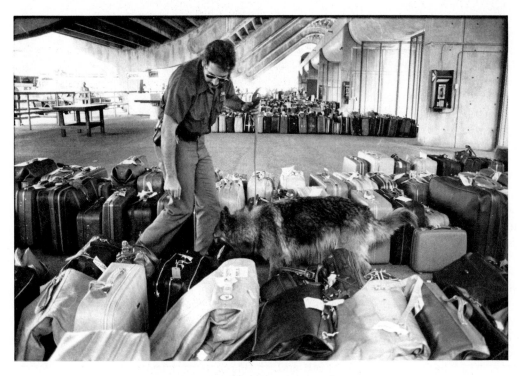

Enforcing our drug laws is a large scale enterprise.

that our previous narcotics-control aid has been used for political repression, both in Latin American and in Southeast Asia. The State Department's International Narcotics Control Program budget for 1989 had increased to over $100 million dollars to be spent in Latin America, Southeast Asia (Burma and Thailand), and Southwest Asia (mainly Pakistan). The biggest single outlays were $15 million each for Mexico, Bolivia, and Colombia. In addition, the State Department must make recommendations to the President, who must then report to Congress each year, on whether any country receiving *any* form of aid from the United States can be certified to be cooperating with antinarcotics efforts. All foreign aid is to be suspended to any country that cannot be certified to be cooperating. Other international efforts through the U.S. Agency for International Development include about $5 million for drug education projects and over $20 million for "in-

come substitution" (mostly paying farmers to switch to other, less profitable crops).[17] The 1988 law added a couple of interesting new twists, each of which sounds potentially dangerous.[15] First, the planes and helicopters that we have provided for other countries to use in their narcotics interdiction programs will now be equipped with defensive weapons, including machine guns. Second, the *Defense Department* will begin training foreign police agencies and equipping them with weapons, ammunition, and other supplies. This program will be restricted to police agencies that do not engage in a "consistent pattern of gross violations" of human rights.

Efforts within the United States have been focusing on drug trafficking organizations; there have been frequent newspaper accounts of wholesale arrests of 20 or 30 people at a time, either in various parts of the United States or in the United States and another country. Seizures of large shipments have now occurred so frequently and in such size that the large numbers no longer cause much excitement. It is interesting that once in a while the DEA seizes its own cocaine; they have been known to arrange deals with sellers in Colombia, fly the cocaine to the United States, and arrange to sell it here. The sellers and the U.S. buyers are arrested, and the DEA seizes the cocaine it brought in![18]

The international work and the organized crime crackdowns are the glamorous (and dangerous) part of it, but officials have begun to feel frustrated that they aren't making much progress in controlling the supply of drugs. At the 1988 White House Conference for a Drug-Free America, a frequent refrain was that we must move away from a focus on supply reduction and begin to put more effort into demand reduction. Partly this means more emphasis on education, but mainly it means putting more pressure on both addicts and casual users. Nancy Reagan's message to that conference was that the casual marijuana user shares the blame for the "trail of death and destruction that leads directly to his door," and "I'm saying that if you're a casual drug user, you're an accomplice to murder."[19] Armed with the 1988 laws and this attitude, we can expect to see more arrests, seizures of property, and fines for individuals possessing and using controlled substances in the 1990s.

What does all this enforcement effort cost us? Even at the federal level it is hard to determine accurately, because so many agencies are playing a part. However, it is not difficult to tell that the costs increased dramatically during the 1980s. The budget for the DEA alone more than doubled during the Reagan years, and is now over $500 million. Total federal drug enforcement costs were about $4 billion in 1988 and over $5 billion was budgeted for 1989. It is very difficult to estimate the added expenditures by state and local agencies, but most estimates are that these add up to an amount similar to the federal expenditures. Thus, a widely used figure for 1988 was $8 billion for all levels of drug enforcement,[20] and we could expect that to reach over $10 billion by the 1990s.

There are other costs, only some of which can be measured in dollars. We are paying to house a large number of prisoners: about 80,000 drug-law violators in state prisons and local jails and about 15,000 in federal prisons.[21] We should add in the cost of crimes committed to purchase drugs at black-market prices and the incalculable price of placing so many of our state and local police, DEA, FBI and other federal agents in danger of losing their lives to combat the drug trade, as some have done. A price that has been paid by many law enforcement agencies over the years is the corruption that is ever-present in drug enforcement. Because it is necessary for undercover officers to work closely with and to gain the trust of drug dealers, they must sometimes ignore an offense in hopes of gaining information about more and bigger deals in the future. They may even accept small favors from a drug dealer, and some officers have found it necessary to "use" along with the suspects. Under those circumstances, and given the amounts of money available to some drug dealers and the salaries paid to most law officers, the possibility of accepting too large a gift and ignoring too many offenses is always there, and there may be no obvious "line" between doing one's job and becoming slightly corrupted.[22] When such corruption becomes public, it can immobilize an entire police agency with mistrust, internal investigations, and changed leadership.

There are costs on the international level, also. We are put in an awkward position whenever one of our political allies becomes involved, even unwillingly, in drug trafficking. A great deal of heroin has been flowing through Pakistan, for example, and some might wonder why we haven't cut off aid to them. First, they have been trying to control heroin with our help and their limited resources but the problem is a large one.[17] From their point of view perhaps the problem is caused more by our appetite for heroin than by their need for money. Second, we cannot afford to lose them as an ally in that part of the world (they border on the Soviet Union and Iran and were an important staging area for the Afghan rebels fighting the So-

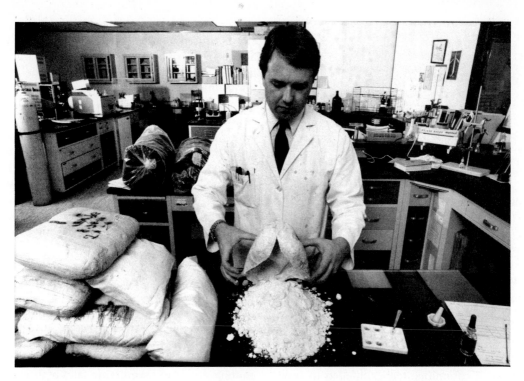

Confiscated cocaine being analyzed at a DEA laboratory in Miami.

viets with our aid). So, we must do the best we can to help them in their drug control efforts and not to offend them with too many demands. The prime ministers of both Jamaica and Haiti have complained that U.S. congressional hearings have publicly implicated them in drug trafficking, and they have demanded apologies.[23] Panama's General Noriega was actually indicted on drug-trafficking charges by a Florida grand jury. To the extent that narcotics control efforts place additional strain on our foreign policy needs in Pakistan, the Caribbean, and Latin America, this also represents a significant cost to our country.

Given this effort and these costs, are our drug enforcement efforts effective? Do they work? Critics have pointed out that despite escalating expenditures, more agents, and an increasing variety of supply-reduction efforts, the supplies of cocaine, heroin, and marijuana have not dried up. In fact, they actually may have increased. Al-

though there were record-breaking seizures of cocaine year after year, the price of cocaine did not change on the streets during the 1980s, and there seemed to be more suppliers than ever. The United States government made a decision in 1924 to make heroin completely unavailable to addicts in this country, and after more than 65 years we can say only that we have been consistent in our failure to accomplish that goal. Our efforts to eradicate illegal coca fields in South America have been described as a failure by the General Accounting Office, which pointed out that many more new acres are being planted in coca each year than are being destroyed by our program.[24] To some, the final irony of all these enforcement efforts is that they seem only to strengthen the drug-dealing organizations, which become more efficient and better armed, requiring more of our agents and more arms on our side, which means more organization, sophistication, and technology on the or-

---

Your turn: what are your rights?

Do you know what your own rights and liabilities are under the laws in your area? Suppose you are driving and a police officer stops you for driving erratically. Smelling no alcohol, she suspects some other chemical agent. Can she search your car for drugs? Just the passenger compartment or the trunk as well? Can she search the people in the car? If she finds marijuana in your car, will you be charged? What if the marijuana is found on the person of a passenger in your car? If you don't know the answer to these questions, it might be interesting to find out. You could invite a member of the police force to meet with a group of classmates to talk about this and other issues of drug enforcement. Another idea would be to interview someone from the police force regarding this issue and then write a small article for the campus newspaper.

---

ganized crime side, which means . . . . By 1988 the criticisms had reached such a level that one Congressional committee felt compelled to hold hearings on the idea of legalizing controlled substances, although the Congressmen made it clear that they were not very much interested in pursuing that course.

But the laws do work at another level. The DEA estimates that it seizes 10% to 15% of the drugs imported into the United States. In 1986, they captured over 800 pounds of heroin, 60,000 pounds of cocaine, and almost 2 million pounds of marijuana.[25] (These figures are accompanied by street values in the billions of dollars, but remember that those estimates are quite unrealistic.) Efforts to reduce opium supplies and heroin smuggling have made it difficult and expensive to do business as a major importer. Evidence of the restricted supply can be found in the high prices charged on the streets. The price is many times more than the cost of the drug itself if sold legally. It is possible that the high cost is the only thing that regulates the amount taken for some of these addicts, who might otherwise die from overdoses more often than they do. Local efforts make a difference, too. By forcing small pushers to work

out of sight, they are less able to contact purchasers and the risk is increased to both the buyer and the seller of being hurt or cheated in the transaction.[26,pp.81-83] This not only raises the cost of doing business, it probably deters some people from trying the drugs. For example, if you were curious about heroin and wanted to try some, you would have to take some money and go to a rough part of one of our larger cities. If you were "lucky enough" to find a dealer, he would not be the sort of person you would trust. The transaction would probably take place in a nonpublic place, and if you were robbed, beaten, or just sold some worthless junk, you wouldn't be in a position to call a cop!

STATE AND LOCAL REGULATIONS
Drug Laws

It is impossible to try to describe all the varied drug laws that exist in all 50 states. We should remember that most states and many local communities had laws regulating sales of drugs before the federal government got into the act in 1906. Some aspects of those old laws may still be in effect in some areas. In the area of legal sales of prescription and over-the-counter drugs, there is considerable uniformity across the states, but some details do differ. For example, in some states licensed Physician's Assistants are allowed to prescribe many types of medication, and in a few states pharmacists are now allowed to prescribe a few types of drugs that had previously required prescription by a physician or dentist.

Following the passage of the 1970 *Controlled Substances Act* at the federal level, states began to adopt the *Uniform Controlled Substances Act,* a model state law recommended by the DEA. The same set of schedules is found in these state laws, and they generally follow a similar pattern of penalties, although a given penalty may be greater in one state than in another. This model act was meant to replace all previous drug legislation in each state, but sometimes vestiges of older laws remain. For example, some states define as a special crime the smuggling of intoxicating drugs into a jail or prison. Also, many states have modified the uniform laws since they were originally passed. Several states have "decriminalized" possession of marijuana (see Chapter 16) by making it a civil offense punishable by a fine. Other states have toughened their drug laws or passed special laws to deal with specific problems, such as the growing of marijuana, the "laundering" of drug money, or the sale of kits to convert cocaine to its freebase.

Paraphernalia

In the mid-1970s a major industry grew up in the United States, selling legal items that were in some way related to the use of drugs. Sales of cigarette papers grew, while sales of loose cigarette tobacco declined. Water pipes and "bongs" (special pipes for concentrating marijuana smoke) were big items, as were decorative "roach clips," sifters, and scales. These were mainly sold in "head shops," which catered to the drug-using subculture, and in many cases were connected to record stores or other youth-oriented businesses. Although the items themselves were not illegal, their obvious relationship to illegal drug use and their visibility to young people raised concerns that drug use was being indirectly condoned and even advertised. Several communities passed ordinances aimed at controlling the sales of drug **paraphernalia,** and in 1977 Indiana passed the first statewide anti-paraphernalia law.[27] The DEA decided that it would not be a useful investment of their efforts to try to enforce a federal law on paraphernalia. In 1979 the DEA did propose, at the request of the White House, a model antiparaphernalia act that states could adopt as an amendment to the Uniform Controlled Substances Act.

Interest in drug paraphernalia seems to have reached a peak in about 1979-1980, with television and newspaper reports, congressional hearings, and much legal action. Concern was fueled by the sale of cocaine freebasing kits and other cocaine-related paraphernalia (straws, spoons, grinders, mirrors, and razors). Virtually every form of antiparaphernalia law has come under legal attack. We can best understand why by looking at the wording of a portion of the DEA's proposed model legislation, which would ban "blenders, bowls, containers, spoons, and mixing devices used, intended for use, or designed for use in compounding controlled substances."[23] Thus a spoon or a bowl might or might not be considered drug paraphernalia, depending on its "intended use." An alligator clip sold as an electronic part at Radio Shack would not be paraphernalia, but the same clip sold at Rock-n-Roll Records might be, depending on how it is displayed for sale and what the salesperson says about its use. Such laws seem vague and invite challenges in court. Because of these problems, interest in passing and enforcing paraphernalia laws has waned since the early 1980s.

Alcohol

Because alcohol has been an important part of American society since colonial times, laws regulating alcohol sales and use have a long and complex history in most states and communities. There is no more interesting exercise than comparing the drinking laws of any two of our states, much less all 50 of them. During what hours can alcohol be sold? Are sales allowed on Sunday? In Texas you can drive up to a hamburger joint and have the carhop deliver beer on a tray. Many states have drive-up windows for sales of package liquors. Either of those practices may seem horrible to a Californian but Californians can buy wine, beer, or distilled liquor in any large supermarket, a practice that would be surprising to people in most states. In Indiana, it is illegal to carry a drink from one table to another in a bar. In Utah liquor is sold only in state stores, and some restaurants contain miniature state liquor stores. Although it may seem that there is no logic to this patchwork of various laws, in every case the laws can be seen as attempts to control either the total amount of alcohol consumed or some particular drinking-related problem that at one time must have created a public outcry in that state.

One problem that has created public outcry all

Issue: the special status of dronabinol

The Controlled Substance Act lists substances under Schedules II–V based on their abuse potential. However, substances with "no medical use" all fall under Schedule I, whether they are considered to be highly addicting and dangerous (e.g., heroin) or are rarely abused and of little concern (e.g., bufotenin). The active ingredient in marijuana, delta-9 tetrahydrocannabinol (THC), has recently caused some classification headaches for the DEA. For one thing, THC does now have a medical use—treating the nausea caused by cancer chemotherapy agents. Since 1986, under the generic name dronabinol, THC has been legally marketed as a prescription drug. According to the traditional interpretation of the law, that would automatically result in rescheduling THC to Schedule II. The DEA's rather unusual response to this has been to reschedule dronabinol *when dissolved in sesame oil and sealed in gelatin capsules* as a Schedule II controlled substance. Any other preparation of THC is still Schedule I, as is marijuana itself. Of course, marijuana is also being prescribed to some people for the treatment of glaucoma, and the government is even providing "official" marijuana cigarettes for this purpose. Marijuana has also been reported to provide some relief to multiple sclerosis patients. But marijuana cigarettes are not a generally available prescription drug. These prescriptions are carried out under the guise of "research" on an investigation of a new drug (IND) application.

Reviewing all this in 1988, the DEA's administrative law judge recommended that marijuana be removed from Schedule I. According to Judge Francis L. Young, "By any measure of rational analysis, marijuana can be safely used within a supervised routine of medical care."[29] The head of the DEA has been slow to respond, and there seems to be a great deal of reluctance to appear to be "softening" the DEA's position on marijuana. This example serves to point out that even the most rational-appearing legislation is subject to political interpretation. The final decision on whether to reschedule marijuana will probably be made by the U.S. Circuit Court of Appeals.

---

over the United States in the 1980s is drunk driving. Groups like Mothers Against Drunk Driving (MADD) have lobbied city councils, local judges, and state legislators to get tough with those who drive while intoxicated. Penalties have been increased, and mandatory jail sentences or license revocation imposed in many states. In many areas laws have been passed holding bar owners or hosts liable for allowing someone to get drunk and then get behind the wheel of a car.[28] These legal efforts, combined with massive advertising campaigns, have made all Americans more aware of the dangers of drunk driving. Liquor regulation and drunk driving are discussed in more detail in Chapter 9.

Summary

In the early 1900s reformism, combined with concerns about opium smoking, morphinism, cocaine snuffing, and patent medicines containing habit-forming drugs, led to the passage of two federal laws on which our modern drug regulations are based.

The 1906 Pure Food and Drugs Act at first required only that a drug's label accurately describe what was in the drug. Later the law was amended to require that the label not contain false and fraudulent therapeutic claims. New laws were passed in 1938 and in 1962, both after public outcry over drug-related disasters. Since 1938 companies have been required to submit evidence to the Food and Drug Administration that a new drug has been tested for safety. In 1962 the safety testing requirements were strengthened and companies were also required to test the drugs for efficacy before they could be sold.

A company wishing to market a new drug must first test it on animals, then file a request to investigate the new drug in human clinical trials (IND). After a 3-phase sequence of human testing, the company can apply to have the new drug allowed on the market (NDA). Companies have been concerned about the length of time it takes to get a new drug to market, and the FDA has recently altered their procedures to allow for more rapid marketing of new drugs.

The 1914 Harrison Act regulated the sale of narcotic drugs and cocaine. Although written as a tax law, it was enforced in such a way as to prevent addicted individuals from obtaining narcotics, and thousands of physicians and pharmacists were arrested along with tens of thousands of addicts. As narcotics became more scarce and their price rose on the illicit market, this illicit market grew. Harsher penalties and increased enforcement efforts, which were the primary strategies of Commissioner of Narcotics Harry Anslinger, failed to reverse the trend. Marijuana was added to the list of narcotics in 1937, and in 1965 the dangerous drugs, such as amphetamines, barbiturates, and hallucinogens, were also brought under federal control.

The basic law that now governs our drug regulations is often called the Controlled Substances Act of 1970. Penalties for possession have been reduced, but large fines and long prison sentences are provided for repeated offenses of distributing drugs or for being involved in a drug-dealing organization.

Current federal enforcement efforts by the DEA and several other federal agencies involve thousands of federal employees and include activities in other countries, along our borders, and within the United States. This is in addition to the efforts of state and local police, who often work in cooperation with the federal officers. Each year these officers seize tons of illicit drugs and arrest thousands of people. This enforcement does limit the supply of drugs and keeps their prices high, but the high prices attract more smugglers and dealers, so that increasing amounts of cocaine are coming in each year, heroin is still available to addicts, and marijuana is still widely available. It will never be possible to "win the war" against illicit drugs. The latest approach to enforcement is to attempt to reduce the demand for drugs by putting more legal pressure on "casual users."

State and local laws reflect quite a bit of variety, but there are some consistencies. For example, most states treat prescription drugs in a consistent way, and all have adopted some form of the Uniform Controlled Substances Act regarding illicit drugs. With regard to alcohol laws there is much more variety, but recent concerns about drunk driving have led to a fairly consistent set of approaches to increase the penalties for this offense. Also, the federal government has mandated a uniform minimum 21-year-old drinking age in all states.

REFERENCES

1. Kane HH: Opium-smoking in America and China, New York, 1882, GP Putnam's Sons.
2. Latimer D and Goldberg J: Flowers in the blood: the story of opium, New York, 1981, Franklin Watts.
3. Courtwright DT: Dark paradise: opiate addiction in America before 1940, Cambridge, Massachusetts, 1982, Harvard University Press.
4. Adams SH: The great American fraud, Collier's, six segments from October 1905 to February 1906.
5. Congressional Record 40:102 (Part I), Dec 4, 1905, to January 12, 1906.
6. Terry CE and Pellens M: The opium problem, New York, 1928, Bureau of Social Hygiene.
7. Young JH: The medical messiahs: a social history of health quackery in twentieth-century America, Princeton, New Jersey, 1967, Princeton University Press.
8. A prognosis for America, Washington, DC, 1977, Pharmaceutical Manufacturers Association.
9. Majority supports tough FDA standards, Los Angeles Times, p. 18, March 28, 1984.
10. Booth W: FDA looks to speed up drug approval process, Science 241:1426, 1988.
11. Greenberg RB: The prescription drug marketing act of 1987, Am J Hosp Pharm 45:2118-2126, 1988.
12. Schmeckebier LF: The bureau of prohibition, Service Monograph No 57, Institute for Government Research, 1929, Brookings Institute. Cited in Narcotic Drug Laws and Enforcement Policies, King, Rufus: Law & Contemporary Problems 22:122, 1957.
13. US News and World Report 41:22, 1956.
14. A little less illegal, New Republic 161:11, 1969.
15. Lawrence C: In its last act, Congress clears anti-drug bill, Congressional Quarterly, Oct 29, 1988, pp 3145-3151.
16. Organized crime drug enforcement task forces: Goals and objectives, Drug Enforcement, pp 3-15, Summer 1984.
17. USAID Highlights, 5:1-4, US Agency for International Development, Washington, DC, 1988.
18. DEA flew coke cache into state, Denver Post, p 1, May 24, 1985.
19. Churchville V: First lady opens new front in drug war, attacking casual users, Washington Post, p A6, March 1, 1988.

20. Church GJ: Thinking the unthinkable, Time, pp 12-17, May 30, 1988.

21. Nadelman EA: US drug policy: a bad export, Foreign Policy, 70:83-108, 1988.

22. Eddy P, Sabogal H, and Walden S: The cocaine wars, New York, Norton, 1988.

23. Drug war earns US enemies, Denver Post, Sept 3, 1988.

24. Culhane C: US fails in South American drug war, The US Journal of Drug and Alcohol Dependence, January, 1989.

25. Statistical Abstract, U.S. Census Bureau, Washington, DC, US Government Publishing Office, 1988.

26. Kaplan J: The hardest drug: heroin and public policy, Chicago, 1983, The University of Chicago Press.

27. Community and legal responses to drug paraphernalia, DHEW Publication No (ADM)80-963, Washington, DC, 1980, US Government Printing Office.

28. Alcohol and Highway Safety 1984: A Review of the State of the Knowledge, DOT Publication No (HS)806-569, Washington, DC, 1985, US Government Printing Office.

29. Conlan MF: Top drug cop weighs use of marijuana as an Rx drug, Drug Topics, p 50, December 12, 1988.

Chapter 4

The Nervous System

OBJECTIVES

After reading this chapter, you should be able to:

Explain the need for chemical communication within the body, and know the similarities and differences between hormonal and neural communication.

Describe how neurotransmitter chemicals are released from neurons and from what parts, and understand their interaction with receptors.

Identify the major subdivisions of the nervous system and the functions of the two parts of the autonomic nervous system.

Name a few of the major structural parts of the brain and some of the chemical pathways along with the general functions served by each path or pathway.

Describe the "life cycle" of a neurotransmitter molecule and the various ways that psychoactive drugs can interact with it.

Drugs are psychoactive, for the most part, because they alter established biochemical processes in the brain. To understand how drugs influence psychological processes, it is necessary to have some knowledge of the normal functioning of the brain and other parts of the nervous system and then to see how drugs can alter those normal functions. We will not assume any background in biology or chemistry nor will we try to make neurophysiologists or biochemists of you in this chapter. It should, however, be possible to develop a good understanding of these topics at a conceptual level.

The field of neuroscience is growing and changing more rapidly than most scientific fields at this time, and there is controversy about what is important now and what people will consider to be important or fundamental in the future. However, learning certain concepts will give you a framework for understanding new information as it comes along.

CHEMICAL MESSENGERS OF THE BODY

Since the first multicellular organisms oozed about in their primordial tidal pools, some form of cell-to-cell communication has been necessary to ensure the organism's survival. Those first organisms probably needed to coordinate only a few functions, such as getting nutrients into the system, distributing them to all the cells, and then eliminating wastes. At that level of organization, perhaps one cell excreting a chemical that could act on neighboring cells was all that was necessary. As more complex organisms evolved with multicellular systems for sensation, movement, reproduction, and temperature regulation, the sophistication of these communication mechanisms increased markedly. It became necessary for many types of communication to go on simultaneously and over greater distances. Although those early organisms were at the mercy of the sea environment in which they lived, we carry our own sea water-like cellular environment around with us and must maintain that internal environment within certain limits. This process is known as **homeostasis.** This word can be loosely translated as "staying the same," and it describes the fact that many biological factors are maintained at or near certain levels. For example, most of the biochemical reactions basic to the maintenance of life are temperature dependent, in that these reactions occur optimally at temperatures near 37° Celsius (98.6° Fahrenheit). Since we cannot live at temperatures too much above or below this, our bodies have many mechanisms they can use to either raise or lower temperature: perspiration, shivering, altering blood flow to the skin, and others. Similar homeostatic mechanisms serve to regulate the acidity, water content, and sodium content of the blood, glucose concentrations, and many other critical physical and chemical factors that are important for biological functioning. To some extent these must be coordinated, since a particular homeostatic response to one factor often has an effect on another factor. In humans and other mammals, we find a variety of sophisticated systems for chemical communication within the body, presumably having evolved at different times and forming layers of communication and control that interact with one another at many levels. These chemical messengers can be divided into two broad classes: hormones and neurotransmitters.

Hormones

Hormones are chemicals that are released from specialized groups of secretory cells (often called glands) that affect other cells, which we think of as "target" cells (Fig. 4-1). For example, the male sex hormone testosterone is released from the testes into the bloodstream. It then circulates throughout the body, influencing muscular and neural development, sexual and aggressive behavior, and other functions. Another gland, the

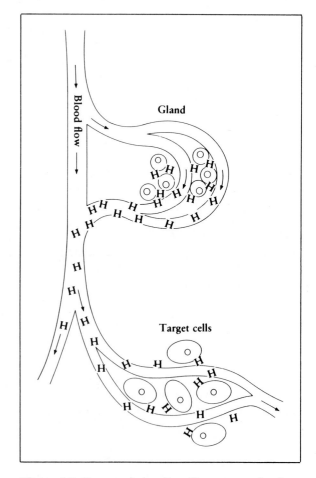

Figure 4-1. Hormonal signaling. Hormone molecules are released by secretory cells in a gland. The molecules are carried by the blood to distant target cells, where they exert their signaling effect.

pituitary (referred to as the master gland), releases several hormones that circulate through the bloodstream, each having specific effects on the appropriate target cells. In many cases these target tissues are themselves glands, and the pituitary therefore controls the release of other hormones. Some pituitary hormones have more direct actions. For example, in response to a drop in blood pressure, the pituitary releases vasopressin, which signals the kidney to release less fluid into the urine. Drinking alcohol inhibits the release of vasopressin, so the kidney releases more fluid into the urine.

You may be surprised to learn that hormones are still being discovered, including a large number since 1975. Each new discovery only helps us to appreciate more how many mechanisms are at work to coordinate our most basic biological functions.

Neurotransmitters

In the nervous system, a more discrete signaling is found (Fig. 4-2). Each cell in the nervous system (these nerve cells are called neurons) acts as a secretory cell and as a target cell. Each neuron releases one or a few specialized signalling chemicals called **neurotransmitters.** There are about 50 chemicals now believed to act as neurotransmitters, and each neuron is sensitive to one or a few of them.[1]

What makes the action of neurotransmitters more discrete than that of hormones is that they are not released into the blood, but rather into a small space, called a synapse, between two neurons. The chemical released into that synapse affects only one neuron, rather than a whole group of target cells, at once. Since only a small amount of neurotransmitter chemical is released into this small synapse, it is possible to remove it quickly once it has sent its signal. Therefore the signal is discrete in time, as well as in space. This allows the sending of detailed information from one specific place to another in the nervous system. To give some idea of scale, the synaptic space is less

than 1/10,000th of an inch across. Several thousand neurotransmitter molecules are released at once, and it takes only microseconds for these molecules to diffuse across the synapse.

Although many neurotransmitters have now been identified, we are concerned only with those few that we believe to be associated with the actions of the psychoactive drugs we are studying. Those neurotransmitters include acetylcholine, norepinephrine, dopamine, serotonin, γ-aminobutyric acid (GABA), and the endorphins.

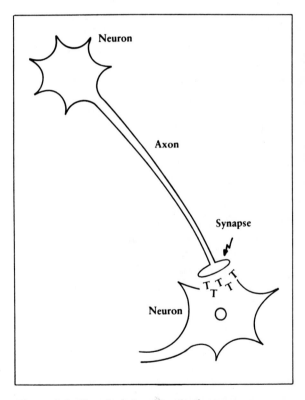

Figure 4-2. Chemical signalling in the nervous system. When an electrical signal reaches the terminal end of the axon, it causes release of neurotransmitter molecules into the synapse, a small space between the terminal and another neuron. The second neuron is affected by the transmitter molecules, which influence electrical activity in the second neuron.

Receptors

Chemical signals are useful only if the target cells are able to detect the presence of the signal molecules and then perform some action on the basis of that signal having been received. The specialized structures that perform these functions are called **receptors**—subcellular structures that are part of the target cell membrane.[2] These receptors play an important role in the actions of many of the drugs we discuss in this book, and it is therefore important for you to have a feeling for how they work in the nervous system.

As you know, chemicals may be described by their structures—the way the atoms are put together to form molecules of that chemical. Each of the neurotransmitter chemicals therefore has a unique three-dimensional structure that is characteristic of each of its molecules and different from the molecules of other neurotransmitters. The atoms often tend to make parts of the molecule electrically more positive or negative than other parts, and the locations of these electrical charges also help to make the molecule unique.

One analogy that has been used to describe the interaction between the neurotransmitter and its receptor is that of a lock and key: the neurotransmitter fits into a receptor as a key fits into a lock. That model is useful for pointing out the specificity of the interaction based on the three-dimensional structure of the neurotransmitter, but it is difficult to explain the dynamic properties of the interaction using the lock and key analogy. In fact, a given molecule may be more or less attracted to a receptor, depending on its degree of fit and the locations of electrical charges on both the molecule and the receptor. This means that molecules will vary widely in their affinity for a receptor, whereas we generally think of a key as either fitting or not fitting a lock. Fig. 4-3 shows a schematic diagram of a portion of a synapse and depicts neurotransmitter molecules being released from the terminal of one neuron and binding to receptors of another neuron. Again, remember that the structures depicted in the diagram are subcellular. The diagrams shows parts of two neurons only, and the brain contains billions of neu-

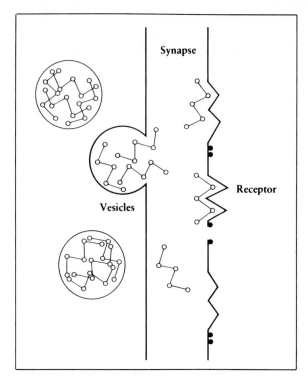

Figure 4-3. Schematic representation of the release of neurotransmitter molecules from synaptic vesicles in the axon terminal of one neuron and of the passage of those molecules across the synapse to receptors in the membrane of another neuron. A neurotransmitter molecule has bound to the center receptor and has distorted it so as to open a channel through the membrane of the second cell. This channel allows the flow of electrically charged ions through the membrane, thus altering the electrical charge on the membrane of the second cell.

rons. None of these structures is visible under a light microscope. With an electron microscope it is possible to see the synapses and vesicles and to get an idea of where the receptors are located in a membrane, but the detailed structure of a molecule or a receptor can only be inferred from indirect evidence.

In neurons, the effect of a neurotransmitter binding to its receptor is to allow an electrical current to flow through the membrane, which changes the electrical charge across the nerve

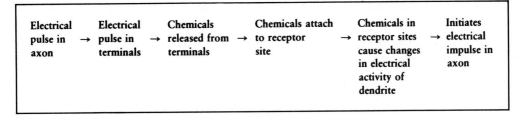

| Electrical pulse in axon | → | Electrical pulse in terminals | → | Chemicals released from terminals | → | Chemicals attach to receptor site | → | Chemicals in receptor sites cause changes in electrical activity of dendrite | → | Initiates electrical impulse in axon |

Figure 4-4. Sequence and mode of information movement in the nervous sytem.

membrane. Since neurons conduct electrical signals along their membranes, the effect of a particular type of receptor is either to *excite* this electrical activity or to *inhibit* it. Fig. 4-4 depicts information flow in the nervous system. Electrical activity along the nerve membrane conducts information from one place to another, and, once that activity arrives at the nerve terminal, it results in the release of a neurotransmitter chemical, which influences the electrical activity of the next neuron. The electrical signal traveling along the membrane is brief—the appearance of the recorded signal on an oscilloscope is so sharp that it has been called a "spike"; and if it is amplified and sent to a loudspeaker one hears only a pop as the signal travels past the recording electrode. Neurons "fire" these spikes several times a second under normal conditions, and excitatory or inhibitory influences may be seen as increasing or decreasing the firing rate of the neuron.

Whether the effect of a neurotransmitter is excitatory or inhibitory depends on the type of receptor. One of the neurotransmitters, GABA, seems to act at only inhibitory receptors. Therefore GABA is often called an inhibitory neurotransmitter. But acetylcholine probably acts at three or four different types of receptors in the brain, and its action may be either excitatory or inhibitory, depending on the receptor.

THE NERVOUS SYSTEM

Although we often speak of the nervous system, it is perhaps more appropriate to remember that there are several communication and control systems that are based on neurons and neurotransmitters. Some important distinctions among these systems will help us to understand drug actions.

Central Nervous System

The **central nervous system** (CNS) consists of the brain and spinal cord. These two structures can be seen as the central mass of nervous tissue, with sensory nerves coming in and motor nerves going out. This is where most of the integration of information, learning and memory, and coordination of activity occur. The spinal cord will be briefly discussed, although the brain will be described in detail.

Somatic System

The **somatic system** can be thought of as a group of nerves that carry sensory information into the CNS and carry motor information back out. Cranial nerves that relate to vision, hearing, taste, smell, chewing, and movements of the tongue and face are included, as well as spinal nerves carrying information from the skin and joints and controlling movements of the arms and legs. We think of this system as serving voluntary actions. For example, a decision to move your leg results in activity in large cells in the motor cortex of your brain. These cells have long axons that extend down to the spinal motor neurons. These neurons have long axons that are bundled together to form nerves, which travel out directly to the muscles. The neurotransmitter at neuromuscular junctions in the somatic system is acetylcholine, which acts on receptors that excite the muscle.

Autonomic Nervous System

The **autonomic nervous system** (ANS) controls many of the visceral, or involuntary, functions of the body, such as heart rate and blood pressure. It is important for us to understand this system, because many psychoactive drugs also have effects on the ANS.

The ANS is of interest also because it is where chemical neurotransmission was first studied. If the vagus nerve in a frog is electrically stimulated, its heart slows. If the fluid surrounding the heart is withdrawn and placed around a second frog's heart, it too will slow. This is an indication that electrical activity in the vagus nerve causes a chemical to be released onto the frog's heart muscle. When Otto von Loewi first demonstrated this phenomenon in 1921, he named the unknown chemical "vagusstoffe." We now know that this is acetylcholine. However, because of the type of receptor found in the heart, acetylcholine inhibits muscle contraction.

The ANS is further divided into **sympathetic** and **parasympathetic** branches. The inhibition of heart rate by the vagus nerve is an example of the parasympathetic branch; acetylcholine is the neurotransmitter at the end organ. In the sympathetic branch, norepinephrine is the neuro-transmitter at the end organ. Table 4-1 gives some examples of the effects of parasympathetic and sympathetic influences on various systems. Note that often, but not always, the two systems oppose each other.

Because the sympathetic system is interconnected, it tends to act more as a unit, to open the bronchi, to reduce blood supply to the skin, to increase the heart rate, and to reduce stomach motility. This has been called the "fight or flight" response and is elicited in many emotion-arousing circumstances in humans and other animals. Also, amphetamines and other diet pills, because they have a chemical structure that resembles norepinephrine, stimulate these functions in addition to their effects on the brain. Those drugs that activate the sympathetic branch are referred to as sympathomimetic drugs.

THE BRAIN
The Whole Brain

Although most of us don't think about it very often, our brain is obviously the most complex organ in our bodies and in fact represents what is still the most amazing functional system in the world. We carry around in that small package a machine capable of storing and analyzing more information than the most powerful supercomputers. It may not be as fast at repetitive calculations, but it is able to deal simultaneously with

---

Table 4-1

Sympathetic and parasympathetic effects on selected structures

Structure or function	Sympathetic reaction	Parasympathetic reaction
Pupil	Dilation	Constriction
Heart rate	Increase	Decrease
Breathing rate	Fast and shallow	Slow and deep
Stomach and intestinal glands	Inhibited	Activated
Stomach and intestinal wall	No motility	Motility
Sweat glands	Secretion	No effect
Skin blood vessels	Constriction	Dilation
Bronchi	Relaxed	Constriction

thousands of kinds of input, it can select the important from the unimportant, and it can process images in ways unmatched by the most complex video devices. We might humbly remember that it is this fantastically complex machine that we are tinkering with when we take psychoactive drugs.

The brain has a rich supply of blood from four major arteries, so that drugs circulating in the blood have rapid access to the brain. However, the capillaries in the brain are different from those in the rest of the body—the cells are tightly joined so that some molecules cannot pass freely out of the blood and into the brain. This specialization is the blood-brain barrier, and it keeps some drugs from reaching the brain. Of course, for a drug to be psychoactive, its molecules must be capable of passing the blood-brain barrier.

The brain contains billions of neurons, and each may influence or be influenced by hundreds of other neurons. If these neurons all looked alike and were connected in apparently random ways,

it would be difficult for us to begin to understand anything about the organization of brain activity and function. Therefore it would be impossible to get any understanding of psychoactive drug action by studying the brain. Luckily, the situation is not quite that bad.

Major Structures

Knowing about a few of the major brain structures makes it easier to understand some of the effects of psychoactive drugs. When looking at the brain of most mammals, and especially of a human, much of what one can see consists of **cerebral cortex,** which is a layer of tissue that covers the top and sides of the upper parts of the brain (Fig. 4-5). Some areas of the cortex are known to be involved in processing visual information, and other areas are involved in processing auditory or somatosensory information. Relatively smaller cortical areas are involved in the control of muscles (motor cortex), and large areas are referred

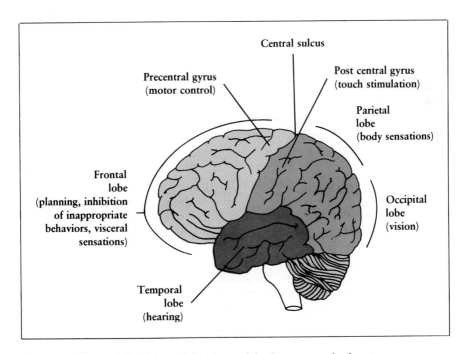

Figure 4-5. Major subdivisions of the human cerebral cortex.

to as association areas. It is often said that higher mental processes, such as reasoning, language, and fine sensory discriminations, take place in the cerebral cortex. In an alert, awake individual, arousal mechanisms keep the cerebral cortex active. When a person is asleep or under the influence of sedating drugs, the cerebral cortex is much less active, whereas other parts of the brain may be equally active whether a person is awake or asleep.

Underneath the cerebral cortex on each side of the brain and hidden from external view are the **basal ganglia.** The basal ganglia are important for the maintenance of proper muscle tone. For example, when you are standing still in a relaxed posture, your leg muscles are not totally relaxed. If they were, you would fall down in a slump. Instead, you remain standing partly because of a certain level of muscular tension, or tone, that is maintained by the output of the basal ganglia. Too much output from these structures results in muscular rigidity in the arms, legs, and facial muscles. This can occur as a side effect of some psychoactive drugs that act on the basal ganglia, or it can occur if the basal ganglia are damaged by **Parkinson's disease.**

The **hypothalamus** is a small structure near the base of the brain just above the pituitary gland. The hypothalamus is an important link between the brain and the hormonal output of this master gland and is involved in feeding, drinking, temperature regulation, and sexual behavior.

The **limbic system** consists of a number of connected structures that are involved in emotion, memory for location, and level of physical activity (Fig. 4-6). Together with the hypothalamus, the limbic system represents important mechanisms for behavioral control at a more primitive level than that of the cerebral cortex.

The **medial forebrain bundle** is sometimes considered to be part of the limbic system. This is a collection of nerve fibers that connects groups of cell bodies in the midbrain with areas of the limbic forebrain. It is interesting that rats and other animals will learn to press a lever if each lever press is followed by a brief electrical stimulation in the medial forebrain bundle. It has been proposed that drugs that have reinforcing properties activate this so-called pleasure system in the brain. Both dopamine and norepinephrine neurons are found within this bundle.

In the **brainstem** a couple of small areas of major importance are found. One area is the vomiting center. Often when the brain detects foreign substances in the blood, such as alcohol, this center is activated and vomiting results. It is easy to see the survival value of such a system to those animals, including humans, that have it. Another brainstem center regulates the rate of breathing. This respiratory center can be suppressed by various drugs, resulting in respiratory depression that may lead to death.

These structures and their functions have been understood in general terms for many years. Knowledge about such things comes partly from people who have suffered accidental brain damage and partly from experiments using animals. Since these basic structures exist in mammals other than humans and their functions and connections are basically the same, it is possible to learn a great deal about human brain function from these animal experiments.

Chemical Pathways

Recently chemical techniques have shown us another level of organization in the brain. Often, groups of cells that are found in a particular brain region will have a high probability of containing a particular neurotransmitter chemical, and axons from these cells will be found grouped together and terminating in another brain region. We now think of many psychoactive drug actions in terms of a drug's effect on one of these chemical pathways. For example, we know that cells in the basal ganglia receive input from a large number of dopamine fibers that arise in the substantia nigra in the midbrain, course together past the hypothalamus, and end in the corpus striatum (part of the basal ganglia). This **nigrostriatal** dopamine

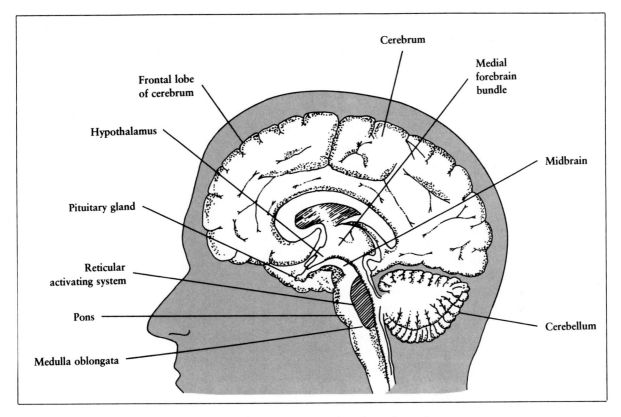

Figure 4-6. Cross-section of the brain identifying the major structures.

pathway is what is damaged in Parkinson's disease and also what is affected by the tranquilizers that produce muscular rigidity as a side effect.

Another important dopamine pathway begins in the midbrain and projects to areas in the limbic system and frontal cortex. This **mesolimbic** dopamine system, which forms part of the medial forebrain bundle, may be important for the reinforcing effects of many drugs and has also been proposed to play a role in some types of psychotic behavior.

Pathways containing acetylcholine arise from cell bodies in the *nucleus basalis* in the lower part of the basal ganglia and project to much of the cerebral cortex. In patients who have died from **Alzheimer's disease,** these cells are damaged

and the cortex contains much less acetylcholine than normal. This degenerative disease affects millions of older Americans, causing personality changes, memory loss, and generally widespread mental deterioration. Since this link with an acetylcholine pathway was only recently discovered, much research activity is currently focused on chemical means to diagnose and treat Alzheimer's disease.

Norepinephrine pathways arising from the *locus ceruleus* have numerous branches and project both up and down in the brain, influencing the level of arousal and alertness. It is perhaps through these pathways that stimulant drugs induce wakefulness. On the other hand, serotonin pathways arising from the *raphe nuclei* have been implicated in the initiation of deep sleep. The change from deep to dreaming sleep and back again seems to be controlled somewhat by the interaction of the raphe nuclei and the locus ceruleus.

DRUGS AND THE BRAIN

Drugs in the Brain

As we have seen, a drug is carried to the brain by the blood supply and, unless it is kept out by the blood-brain barrier, can diffuse out of the blood into the brain tissue itself. How does each drug know where to go once it gets into the brain? The answer is that the drug doesn't know, it goes everywhere. But because the drug molecules of LSD, for example, have their action by acting on serotonin systems, LSD affects only those brain systems that depend on serotonin. The drug molecules that are found in other parts of the brain have no particular effect of which we are aware.

Because the brain is so well supplied with blood, an equilibrium develops quickly for most drugs so that the concentration in the brain is about equal to that in the blood and the number of molecules leaving the blood is equal to the number leaving the brain to enter the blood. As the drug is removed from the blood (by the liver or kidneys) and the concentration in the blood decreases, more molecules leave the brain than enter it and the brain levels begin to decrease.

While an individual drug molecule is in the brain, we can think of it as floating around, possibly just being taken back into the blood without itself having had a specific effect. Since a large number of molecules are required to reach an overall concentration of drug sufficient to produce a drug effect, the majority of the molecules never do have a direct, specific effect.

We are currently able to explain the mechanisms by which many psychoactive drugs act on the brain. In most of these cases the drug has its effects because the molecular structure of the drug is similar to the molecular structure of one of the neurotransmitter chemicals. Because of this structural similarity, the drug molecules interact with one or more of the stages in the life cycle of that

---

Your turn: chemical causes of mental disorders

In the past you may have been only vaguely aware of the number of reports that appear in newspapers and magazines indicating a possible breakthrough in some type of mental illness. Because new brain chemicals are being discovered at a rapid rate, it is inevitable that our hopes are high for new understanding and possible new treatments for schizophrenia, depression, or other major disorders. Chapter 13 presents the current state of our understanding and treatment of these problems.

Now that you have learned some things about the brain and its neurotransmitters and hormones, you will probably pay more attention to such reports in the future. If you want to test and sharpen your understanding of this important approach to understanding human behavior, go to a library and look back over the last year's issues of a magazine, such as *Psychology Today* or *Scientific American*. A list of the brief news reports relating chemicals to mental disorders will probably include quite a few items.

---

neurotransmitter chemical. We can therefore understand some of the ways drugs can act on the brain by looking at the life cycle of a typical neurotransmitter molecule. In the next section, remember that we are going to be talking more about the neurotransmitter molecules that exist naturally in the brain than about the drug molecules that we introduce from the outside.

Life Cycle of a Neurotransmitter

The neurotransmitter molecules that are used to communicate between neurons seem to be made inside the cell from which they are to be released. This makes sense, because if they were just floating around everywhere in the brain, then the release of a tiny amount from a nerve ending wouldn't have much information value. However, the raw materials, or **precursors,** from which the neurotransmitter will be made are to be found circulating in the blood supply and generally in the brain. A cell that is going to make a particular neurotransmitter may need to bring in the right

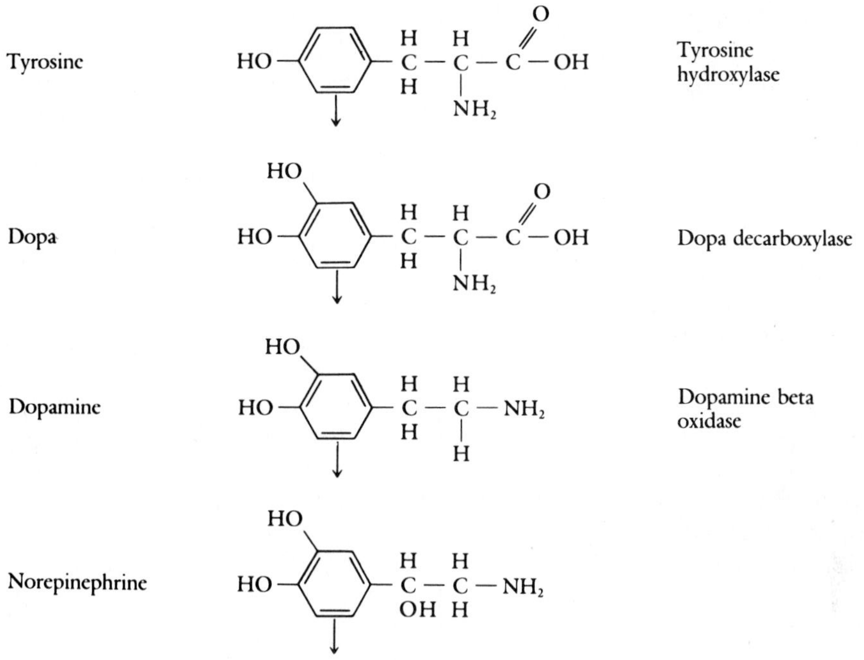

Tyrosine — [structure] — Tyrosine hydroxylase

Dopa — [structure] — Dopa decarboxylase

Dopamine — [structure] — Dopamine beta oxidase

Norepinephrine — [structure]

Figure 4-7. Steps in the synthesis of the catecholamine neurotransmitters (dopamine and norepinephrine). The precursor molecule tyrosine is acted on by the enzyme tyrosine hydroxylase, which adds an OH fragment onto the ring portion of the molecule. This new molecule is called DOPA, and it in turn is acted on by the enzyme DOPA, and it in turn is acted on by the enzyme DOPA decarboxylase to form dopamine.

precursor in a greater concentration than exists in the whole brain, and so machinery is built into that cell's membrane for active **uptake** of the precursor. In this process the cell expends energy to bring the precursor into the cell even though the concentration inside the cell is already higher than that outside the cell. Obviously, this uptake mechanism must be selective and must recognize the precursor molecules as they float by. The precursors themselves are often amino acids that are derived from proteins in the diet, and these amino acids are used in the body for many things besides making neurotransmitters. In our example diagram of the life cycle of the neurotransmitter norepinephrine (Fig. 4-7), the amino acid tyrosine is recognized by the norepinephrine neuron, which expends energy to take it in.

After the precursor molecule has been taken up into the neuron, it must be changed, through one or more chemical reactions, into the neurotransmitter molecule. This process is called **synthesis.** At each step of the set of synthetic chemical reactions, the reaction is helped along by an **enzyme.** These enzymes are themselves large molecules that recognize the precursor molecule, attach to it briefly, and hold it in such a way as to make the synthetic chemical reaction occur. Fig. 4-8 provides a schematic representation of such a synthetic enzyme in action. In our example diagram of the life cycle of the catecholamine neurotransmitters dopamine and norepinephrine (Fig. 4-7), the precursor tyrosine is acted on first by one enzyme to make DOPA and then by another enzyme to make dopamine. In some cells the process stops there as dopamine is used as the neurotransmitter. In our norepinephrine cell, a

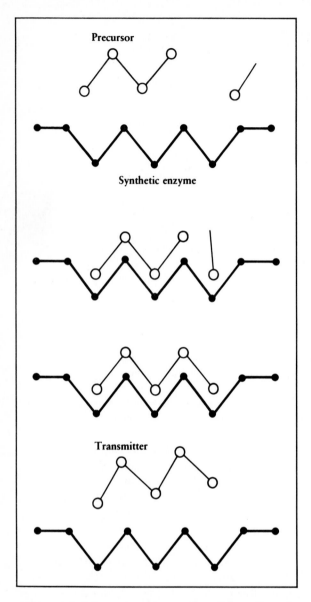

Precursor

Synthetic enzyme

Transmitter

Figure 4-8. Schematic representation of the action of a synthetic enzyme. A precursor molecule and another chemical fragment both bind to the enzyme. The fragment has a tendency to connect with the precursor, but the connection is made much more likely because of the way the enzyme lines the two parts up. After the connection is made, the new transmitter molecule separates from the enzyme.

third enzyme is present to change dopamine into norepinephrine.

After the neurotransmitter molecules have been synthesized (or perhaps as they are being synthesized), they are stored in small, round packages called *vesicles,* near the terminal from which they will be released. This storage process also consists of recognizing the transmitter molecules and concentrating them inside the vesicles.

As an electrical signal arrives at the axon terminal, some of the vesicles fuse with the cell membrane and then open, releasing several thousand neurotransmitter molecules at once. This process of neurotransmitter *release* takes place within a few thousandths of a second after the electrical signal reaches the terminal.

Once the neurotransmitter molecules are released into the small synaptic space between neurons, a particular molecule may just float around briefly, or it may be one of the ones that **bind** to the receptor on the membrane of the other neuron (Fig. 4-3). This receptor represents the most important recognition site in the entire process, and it is also one of the most important places for drugs to interact with the natural neurotransmitter. With thousands of neurotransmitter molecules floating freely in the synapse, some will come near these receptors, bind to them briefly, then float away again. In the process of binding, the neurotransmitter may distort the receptor so that a tiny passage is opened through the membrane, allowing an electrical current in the form of charged ions moving through the membrane. This opening does not last long, however, and within a few thousandths of a second the neurotransmitter molecule has left the receptor and the ion channel is closed.

The small, localized electrical current found at a single receptor might not have much effect all by itself. However, these electrical currents do spread, and, if enough receptors are activated at about the same time, then an electrical signal will be sent all the way down the axon to the terminal and a transmitter will be released there. The actual mechanisms by which this electrical current flows and moves along the membrane are too complicated to go into here. For our purposes we need only remember that electrical signals carry information within a neuron and cause the release of chemical signals that carry information between neurons. These chemical signals in turn cause electrical signals in the next neuron and so on (Fig. 4-4).

Because signalling in the nervous system occurs at a high rate, once a signal has been sent in the form of neurotransmitter release it is important to terminate that signal so that the next signal can be transmitted. Thus the thousands of neurotransmitter molecules released by a single electrical signal must be removed from the synapse. Two methods are used for this. In some cells a process of **reuptake** takes place, in which the neurotransmitter is recognized by a part of the membrane on the neuron from which is was released. The releasing neuron then expends energy to recapture its released neurotransmitter molecules. With other neurotransmitters, enzymes present in the synapse **metabolize,** or break down, the molecules (Fig. 4-9). In either case, as soon as neurotransmitter molecules are released into the synapse some of them are being removed or metabolized and never get to bind to the receptors on the other neuron. All neurotransmitter molecules may be removed in less than one hundredth of a second from the time they are released. In the case of our example neurotransmitter, norepinephrine, those molecules are rapidly taken back up into the neuron from which they were released. Once inside the neuron, most of those molecules are metabolized by an enzyme that is found in the cell.

Examples of Drug Actions

The purpose of learning about the life cycle of a typical neurotransmitter molecule is so that you can understand how foreign molecules, in the form of drugs, interact with and alter the normal machinery for synthesizing, storing, releasing, binding, reuptaking, and metabolizing those neurotransmitters.

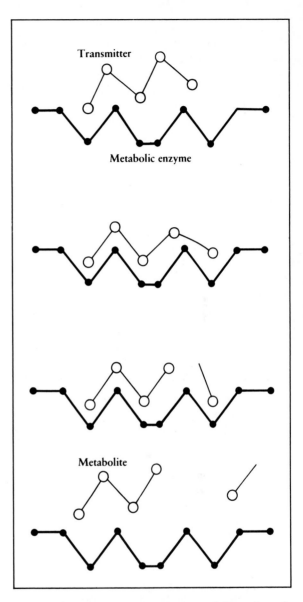

Figure 4-9. Schematic representation of the action of a metabolic enzyme. The transmitter molecule binds to the enzyme in such a way that the transmitter molecule is distorted and "pulled apart." The fragments then separate from the enzyme.

One drug that interferes with the synthesis of a neurotransmitter is methyldopa, which is used to treat high blood pressure. Methyldopa looks like DOPA, one of the chemicals produced during the synthesis of dopamine and norepinephrine. In the ANS, methyldopa is acted on by some of the enzyme molecules that normally act on DOPA. The eventual result is a false norepinephrine (methylnorepinephrine), which the neuron then stores and releases along with some regular norepinephrine molecules. However, the false norepinephrine molecules do not activate the norepinephrine receptors in the heart or the blood vessels. Since norepinephrine usually causes increases in blood pressure, the false norepinephrine molecules reduce this effect.

A great many drugs have their actions at the receptors for neurotransmitters. Because the drug molecule resembles the natural transmitter in its structure, the receptor recognizes the drug molecule. Then the drug molecule may have the same type of action as the neurotransmitter itself does on those receptors. For example, the stimulant drug amphetamine is structurally similar to norepinephrine and dopamine, and one of its effects is to mimic norepinephrine at its receptors. In other cases a drug molecule may bind to the receptor but not activate it (for instance, not distort it so as to open an ion channel). If there are enough drug molecules and they have enough of a tendency to bind to the receptor, they may prevent most of the neurotransmitter molecules from having access to a receptor. The major tranquilizers such as chlorpromazine, which are used in treating psychotic behavior, act by blocking receptors for dopamine in the brain, thus reducing the activity in those dopamine pathways.

Some drugs work by slowing the removal of a neurotransmitter from the synapse, so that the molecules stay around and continue to bind to the receptors for a longer period. The stimulant drug cocaine interferes with the reuptake of dopamine and norepinephrine, thus effectively increasing the duration and magnitude of each signal in those pathways. However, if too much neurotransmitter is left in the synapse so that the receptors are con-stantly bound to neurotransmitter molecules, information flow can cease. The most dramatic examples of this are the nerve gases, which are made up of molecules that bind irreversibly to the enzyme that normally breaks down the molecules of the neurotransmitter acetylcholine. With the enzyme thus tied up, the acetylcholine rapidly builds up in the synapse (there is no reuptake process for acetylcholine). Within minutes of exposure to a lethal dose of a nerve gas, respiration ceases and suffocation results.

CHEMICAL THEORIES OF BEHAVIOR

Drugs that affect existing biochemical processes in the brain can also affect behavior, and this has led to many attempts to explain normal (not drug-induced) variations in behavior in terms of changes in brain chemistry. For example, differences in personality between two people might be explained by a difference in the chemical makeup of their brains, or changes in an individual's reactions from one day to the next might be explained in terms of shifting tides of chemicals. The ancient Greek physician Hippocrates believed that behavior patterns reflected the relative balances of four *humors:* blood (the "hot" fluid, resulting in a sanguine or passionate nature); phlegm (the "cold" fluid, resulting in a phlegmatic or calm nature); yellow bile (the "dry" fluid, resulting in a choleric, bilious, or bad-tempered nature); and black bile (the "wet" fluid, resulting in a melancholic or gloomy nature). The Chinese made do with only two basic dispositions: *yin,* the moon, representing the cool, passive, feminine nature and *yang,* the sun, representing the warm, active, masculine nature. Thus any individual personality could be seen as a relative mixture of these two opposing forces. Unfortunately, most of the chemical-balance theories that have been proposed based on relative influences of different transmitters have not really been more sophisticated than these yin-yang or humoral notions of ancient times. Searches for differences in the amounts of norepinephrine, dopamine, serotonin, or other transmitters have not found evidence to

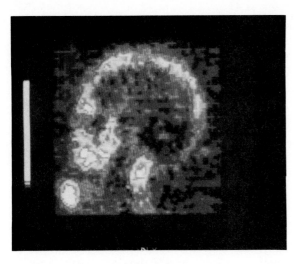

PET-scan.

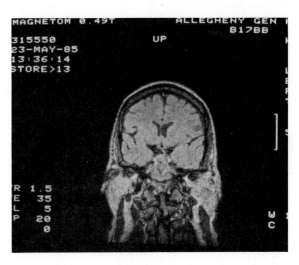

NMR scan.

relate the levels of these substances to personality differences, psychopathology, or mood swings. However, one basic idea that still seems to have a lot of merit continues to guide people's thinking about major alterations in mood, such as are seen in clinical depression. Drugs that interfere with the catecholamines (norepinephrine and dopamine) are able to bring on a depressed mood, and drugs like cocaine and amphetamines that stimulate activity in these catecholamine systems produce a temporary mood elevation. Thus the *catecholamine theory of mood* is that too little activity in these systems can cause depression and too much can cause an excited or manic state (seen with high doses of amphetamines or cocaine). Although there is clear evidence that other neurotransmitter systems also play a role in the normal modulation of mood, the catecholamine theory is able to account for many of the basic drug effects on mood.

MODERN BRAIN IMAGING TECHNIQUES

Two techniques were developed during the 1980s for obtaining chemical "maps" from the brains of living humans. These techniques offer exciting possibilities for furthering our understanding of brain chemistry, abnormal behavior, and drug effects.

One of the techniques is positron emission tomography (PET). In this technique a radioactively labeled chemical can be injected into the bloodstream, and a computerized scanning device can then map out the relative amounts of the chemical in various brain regions.[3] Since all neurons in the brain rely on blood glucose for their energy, a labeled form of glucose can be used to see which parts of the brain are most active, and these will vary depending on what the person is doing. Similarly, blood flow to a particular brain region reflects the activity there, and labeled oxygen or other gases can map regional cerebral blood flow, which also changes depending on what the person is doing. More recently, labeled drugs that bind to dopamine, serotonin, or opiate receptors have been used and it is therefore possible to "see" where the binding of those chemicals takes place in a living human brain. There is no doubt that our understanding of normal and abnormal brain function and of psychoactive drug effects will be advanced rapidly by these techniques over the next few years.

A slightly newer and more complicated tech-

Issue: Alzheimer's disease

Alzheimer's disease has been called the disease of the 1980s, becuase it was not until that decade that the widespread incidence of this disorder was recognized. This is a progressive, degenerative disease of the CNS that results in a multifaceted loss of intellectual functioning, personality changes, and eventually death. Its incidence increases dramatically in old age, and it now appears that about half of all cases of senile dementia are a result of Alzheimer's disease. For generations, we have accepted forgetfulness and mental confusion as natural consequences of growing old. Now we realize that this mental deterioration is no more natural than other diseases, and considerable efforts are being made to understand the cause of Alzheimer's disease. This may be a genetic disorder, a viral infection, some type of toxin, or some combination of those factors.

In 1986 a group of scientists from Johns Hopkins and Georgetown Universities reported that there is a selective loss of the nicotinic type of acetylcholine receptors in the brains of people who died with Alzheimer's disease.[4] There is no known relationship between smoking and Alzheimer's disease, and it is not believed that the nicotinic receptor changes are themselves the basic cellular cause of the disorder. However, the loss of those receptors might play a role in the loss of memory and other cognitive functions. Some limited improvement has already been reported in patients given treatments designed to increase acetylcholine levels in the brain. This new information—that it is one type of acetylcholine receptor that is lost—might lead to more specific drug treatments using nicotine or related chemicals.

---

nique is nuclear magnetic resonance (NMR) scanning, also called MRI (magnetic resonance imaging). Rather than using radioactive labels, the technique relies on applying a strong magnetic field and then measuring the energy released by various molecules as the field is collapsed. The signals are complex, but with the aid of computers it is possible to detect certain chemical "fingerprints" in the signals. This technique gives a high-resolution image, does not require the administration of expensive radiochemicals, and, since it can provide much information not attainable with simple x-ray studies, has been rapidly adopted by the medical community. MRI systems have been installed in most major hospitals and are in quite widespread use, considering how new the technology is.

Summary

Psychoactive drugs alter biochemical processes relating to the brain's neurotransmitters. These neurotransmitter molecules are released from neurons and act at receptors on other neurons. In addition to the effects of these drugs on the brain, they may also have effects outside the CNS, particularly on the ANS, which controls voluntary visceral functions, such as heart rate and stomach motility.

The brain can be divided into major structures based on their physical appearance, and such parts as the cerebral cortex, basal ganglia, and hypothalamus have been studied for many years. Recently it has become possible to trace pathways in the brain that use a particular neurotransmitter chemical. An understanding of the connections and functions of these chemical pathways has led to much greater understanding of the effects of many psychoactive drugs.

Molecules of a particular psychoactive drug may be found everywhere in the brain, but because that drug influences a particular neurotransmitter, it will affect only pathways that contain that transmitter. A drug may interfere with the normal precursor uptake, transmitter synthesis, storage, release, reuptake, or metabolism. In addition, many drugs have their effects by interacting directly with the receptor for the neurotransmitter, either to stimulate it or to block it. For example, cocaine interferes with the reuptake of the catecholamine neurotransmitters dopamine and norepinephrine, so that they remain in the synapse for a longer than normal time.

Athough many theories have been advanced over the years relating behavior to the balance of chemicals in the brain, it has proved quite difficult to measure these chemicals directly to test the theories, so they remain speculative. Recently developed chemical imaging techniques, such as PET and NMR, promise to reveal a great deal of information about the chemistry of the living human brain.

REFERENCES

1. Axelrod J: Neuroscience advances, Science 225:1253, 1984.
2. Snyder SH: Drug and neurotransmitter receptors in the brain, Science 224:22-31, 1984.
3. Phelps ME and Mazziotta JC: Positron emission tomography: human brain function and biochemistry, Science 228:799-809, 1985.
4. Whitehouse PJ, Martino AM, and others: Brain Research 371:146-151, 1986.

Chapter 5

Chemical Commodities

OBJECTIVES

After reading this chapter, you should be able to:

Discuss the drug marketplace and distribution patterns for both legal and illicit drugs.

Explain the difference between a brand name and a generic name.

Describe the techniques used to identify drugs.

Discuss the major issues in the current controversy over the detection of drugs in samples of body fluids.

Until now we have focused on drug-taking behavior. It is time to learn where the drugs come from, how they are named and categorized, and how they can be identified.

You're probably already aware that most of the drugs in use 50 years ago originally came from plants. Even now, most of our drugs either come from plants or are chemically derived from plant substances. Have you ever wondered why the plants of this world are such prodigious drug manufacturers? Suppose a genetic mutation occurred in a plant so that one of its normal biochemical processes was changed and a new. chemical was produced. If that new chemical had an effect on an animal's biochemistry, when the animal ate the plant the animal might become ill or die. In either case that plant would be less likely to be eaten and more likely to reproduce others of its own kind. Such a selection process must have taken place many thousands of times in various places all over the earth. Some of those plant-produced chemicals alter brain biochemistry. In controlled doses those chemicals may alter the biochemistry just enough to produce interesting or even useful effects, but in higher doses the effect is virtually always unpleasant or dangerous. Thus in most primitive cultures the people who learned about these plants and how to use them safely were important figures in their communities. Those medicine men were the forerunners of today's drug producers and sellers.

Our system for providing legal drugs for therapeutic purposes is remarkably efficient when you consider the complexities of the processes and the number of people involved. To see just how efficient it is and help you understand why drugs are such a big business, let us compare two ways of dealing with mental problems: psychotherapy and drug therapy. If a person goes to a psychiatrist who practices psychoanalysis, he expects to spend 50 minutes per session for at least several sessions, expects to be made uncomfortable during that time, and does not expect rapid improvement. On the other hand, if the psychiatrist prescribes medication, the patient might expect to have to see him for only a few minutes, and then drive to the pharmacy and pick up some pills that might begin to work right away. Even if the pills had less chance of success, most of us would prefer to try the easy way first, whether we're talking about psychotherapy or cardiac surgery as an alternative.

LEGAL DRUGS
Producers

The pharmaceutical industry is one of the largest and most profitable in the United States today. With sales well over $40 billion a year and the major companies reporting profits of about 15% based on their sales, the profits are more than double those of other American industries.[1] The pharmaceutical companies point to four factors that they believe justify their activities and profits.

1. It is a high-risk, high-cost business. Development of a new drug may cost $125 million and then not be a marketable or profitable agent.
2. Drug costs have consistently increased at a

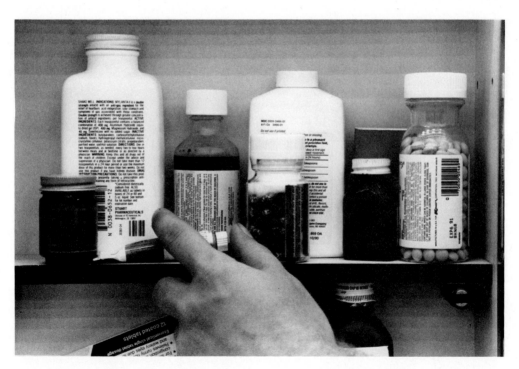

Prescription and over-the-counter drugs account for more than $40 billion a year in sales in the United States.

much lower rate than the cost of other items.

3. The industry has always invested heavily in research and development of new products—about 15% of the total sales, compared to 1.5% in other industries. (Only about 1.5% is spent by drug companies on basic research, but this is still more than other industries.)

4. Drug costs now take less of the health care dollar than at any time in recent years.

With sales in the billions of dollars, many people expect that there are zillions of drugs. Not so. Over half of all prescriptions are filled with only 200 different drugs. The 50 top-selling drugs account for almost 30% of retail sales.

There are two opposing trends underway that make it difficult to predict growth patterns. One is that as the country becomes more health conscious and health knowledgeable, life-styles change and better health habits are established. Since many of today's diseases are a result of personal decisions—such as alcohol use, cigarette smoking, and nutritional factors—and not of a germ-laden poorly sanitized environment, it is likely that the incidence of most diseases will continue to fall. Fewer diseases, less need for drugs. The opposing trend is that we're all getting older; as a nation our average age is creeping up. With advanced age there is usually more illness; the body and the mind are no longer able to withstand the slings and arrows of the world. More disease, more drug use. In 1988 12% of the population were over 65 years of age and used 30% of the prescription drugs. The average older person uses 10 prescription drugs annually, at a cost of about $300. No matter what happens, no one expects the large pharmaceutical companies to go broke.

Products from the pharmaceutical industry are grouped in two major ways. One classification dis-

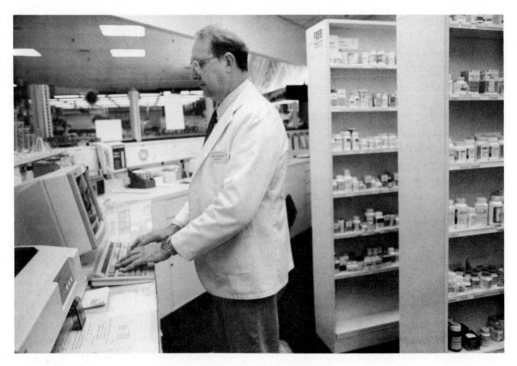

Many pharmacies now employ computers that keep track of each patient's prescriptions, point out possible drug interactions, and even help type the labels!

tinguishes ethical from proprietary products. The term *ethical* means that the products are advertised only to professionals—physicians and pharmacists—and not to consumers. *Proprietary* refers to a company that advertises its products directly to the consumer. The other classification distinguishes prescription (legend) drugs, which can be dispensed to a consumer only with a physician's approval (a written prescription), from over-the-counter (OTC) drugs. Large drug companies have both an ethical and a proprietary division. Sales of prescription drugs in the United States totaled $30 billion in 1988. OTC expenditures in the United States in the same year were $8.6 billion.

It is understandable that the big issues confronting the drug industry have to do with profits. The drug lag mentioned earlier is a major concern. An equally, perhaps even more, important problem is that of the "me too" drugs: generic products jumping on the bandwagon that a brand name drug has built and brought to speed. This issue is discussed later in the chapter.

Sellers

At 60,000 locations in the United States, 150,000 pharmacists wait patiently for you and me to bring in one of the 750 million new or 780 million refill prescriptions written yearly by one of the 550,000 physicians in this country. We're not in a big hurry since the average prescription cost in 1987 was about $15.00. The pharmacist may be mixed up in his feelings. A 1981 survey[2] showed that Americans put pharmacists a close second to clergymen in honesty and ethical practice. On the other hand, the Supreme Court Chief Justice noted that 95% of all presciptions are filled with drugs already packaged by the manufacturers and in the other 5% " . . . the pharmacist performs three tasks: (1) he finds the correct bottle, (2) he counts out the correct number of tablets or measures the right amount of liquid, and (3) he accurately transfers the doctor's dosage instructions to the container."[3]

Oh for the good old days when pharmacy was pharmacy: "the art and science of preparing from natural and synthetic sources suitable and con-venient materials for distribution and use in the treatment and prevention of disease."[4,p.1] That all started to change in 1843 when the first tablet was made; the first gelatin capsule appeared in 1863. Today's pharmacist can and should do more than count pills. If John Q. Public buys all his drugs from a single store, the pharmacist should maintain a drug profile on each customer, which he checks and adds to each time he sells a drug. He should warn his customers of possible dangerous interactions between drugs prescribed by different physicians, advise on the selection of nonprescrip-

---

Your turn: advertising prescription drugs

Although drug companies spend quite a bit of money advertising prescription drugs to physicians by purchasing advertisements in medical journals, they have not been allowed to advertise on television or in magazines or newspapers with a broader audience. In 1983 several companies were exploring the possibility of advertising directly to consumers. The American Medical Association was opposed, fearing that this process would interfere with the doctor/patient relationship. Presumably, patients would hear about a drug from such advertising and then request that their physician prescribe it for them. Consumer groups were opposed also, fearing that such advertising might lead some individuals to diagnose and treat themselves unnecessarily.

In 1985 the FDA did lift its ban on advertising, but they required that any such advertisements include all warnings and contraindications that are included in advertising to physicians. The companies have not begun wholesale direct advertising, in part because of the amount of such information that would have to be provided with each advertisement.

In your opinion, what would the effects be of widespread advertising of prescription drugs? Would the doctor/patient relationship be seriously altered? What would happen to the advertising income for medical journals? For mass-market magazines and television? Would large companies or smaller companies benefit most? Does it make sense to require a large volume of warning information with each advertisement? Would consumers buy more prescription drugs? Would their knowledge improve, leading to better choices?

tion drugs, and counsel on the proper use of prescription and nonprescription drugs. In brief, the local pharmacist should function as a knowledgeable advisor on the use of drugs and as an essential, independent monitor on prescribed drugs.

ILLEGAL PRODUCTION AND SALES

For obvious reasons, we have no accurate statistics on the production and sales of illegal drugs. However, there are government estimates of the amount of heroin, cocaine, and marijuana produced in other countries and shipped into the United States. Almost all of the heroin sold in the United States now comes from three areas of the world.[5] Southwest Asian opium is processed into heroin primarily in Afghanistan, Pakistan, and Iran (see map, Fig. 5-1). Until the mid-1980s this region probably produced just under half the U.S. heroin supply. Since that time, estimates are that

the fraction of heroin coming from Southwest Asia has declined and may have fallen below the production of Mexico. Illegal opium fields and heroin labs in Mexico accounted for a little over one-third of U.S. heroin supplies in the mid-1980s, but it appears that the figure has increased since then to perhaps over 40%. From the Golden Triangle area of Southeast Asia (Burma, Laos, and Thailand) comes most of the rest of the heroin. In the mid-1980s this represented less than 15% of the U.S. samples, but evidence indicates that this proportion has grown. A reasonable guess as of the end of the 1980s would have about 40% of our supplies coming from Southwest Asia, another 40% from Mexico, and about 20% from Southeast Asia.

Almost one-third of the available marijuana in the United States comes from Mexico, where it is grown on both small and very large farms controlled by large trafficking organizations. Almost as much marijuana is imported from Colombia,

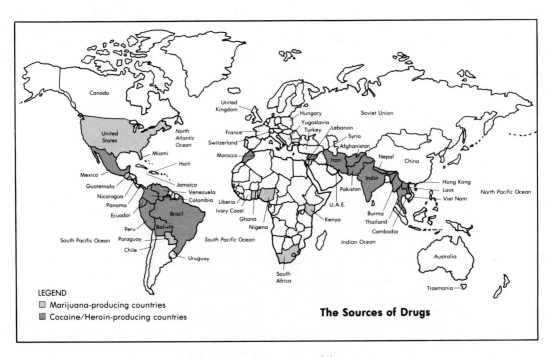

Figure 5-1. The source of drugs.

with smaller amounts coming from Jamaica, Belize, and other countries. Both the quantity and quality of "home-grown" U.S. marijuana production has been increasing, and the Drug Enforcement Administration (DEA) estimated that 19% of available marijuana in 1987 was grown in the United States.

Illegal laboratories in the United States produce a variety of synthetic drugs, including PCP, LSD, methaqualone, and especially methamphetamine ("crank"), the production of which seems to be increasing. In 1987, 682 illegal labs were seized, and 561 of them were methamphetamine labs.

The most recent boom in illegal drug sales has come from cocaine. From the late 1970s to the early 1980s, cocaine use increased dramatically in the United States. By 1985 it was estimated that over 22 million Americans had used cocaine, and perhaps over a million were at risk for continuing or increasing their use of cocaine.[6] The cocaine industry in the United States may be worth more than $50 billion a year. Miami has become the symbol of commerce in cocaine, and stories of intercepted shipments, huge profits, and gangland violence are familiar to most Americans. Houston and Los Angeles are also major sites for importation and sales, but every major American city

has become the scene of frequent cocaine dealing. In 1986 the news media began to focus on a new form of cocaine, called **crack** or **rock.** Compared to the snowlike crystals of cocaine hydrochloride, this solid form is more easily transported, divided, and sold on the streets. Since the solid form can also be heated in a water pipe and smoked, its effects are rapid, potent, and brief. For as little as $10 to $25, a small amount of crack can provide a high lasting for 20 to 30 minutes.[7]

Widespread plantings of coca fields in Peru and Bolivia in the mid-1980s pushed their production ahead of the traditional source country, Colombia. By 1987, the DEA estimated that Peru produced about 100,000 tons of coca leaf, Bolivia about 50,000 tons, and Colombia about 20,000 tons.[5] These coca leaves are processed into cocaine hydrochloride in illegal laboratories located either in Colombia, in the country of origin (Peru, Bolivia, Ecuador), or in Brazil or Argentina. Supplies of cocaine have increased and the wholesale prices have actually declined in spite of major eradication efforts. The business has come increasingly under the control of larger organizations, the biggest of which are Colombian.

The production of crack from cocaine appears to have grown rapidly from the first appearances

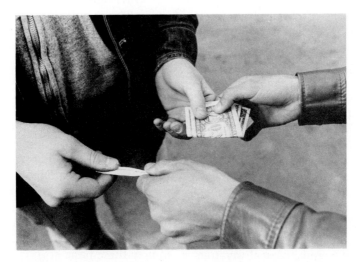

The low-level street dealer often doesn't make a great deal of money.

of this substance in the early 1980s and to have reached a peak in 1986. The process is simple, and has been carried out mostly by large numbers of small, neighborhood producers and distributors. By 1987 larger, more centralized organizations had begun to manufacture and distribute crack, sometimes in more than one city.

Heroin dealers had pioneered the use of teenagers as street dealers, because they are subject to considerably less punishment than adults. The new twist added by the cocaine business is the house or apartment with an armored door. Deals are made through a hole in the door, behind which may be a heavily armed teenager. If the police arrive, it takes a few minutes for them to get through the door, which may be enough time for the dealer to flush the cocaine down the toilet or to slip out through a back door or window.

A lot is said about the **street value** of illegal drugs. Whenever a law enforcement group confiscates an amount of illegal drug, this is invariably translated in the news release into a street value of some very impressive magnitude. You should remember that these street values are based on the estimated final sale price, not on the actual value of the amount seized. If 100 pounds of marijuana is said to have a street value of $160,000, for example, you have to assume that the marijuana is separated into individual doses, rolled into "joints," and each joint sold for a top price. This is like calculating the value of a ton of iron ore in terms of the value of the Cadillacs that could be made from it. The realities of the marketplace are quite different. There aren't that many buyers for 100 pounds of marijuana, and they're taking a big risk just handling that amount of contraband. The fewer buyers a dealer works with, the less risk, so the large dealer might, for example, sell 10 packages of 10 pounds each. If that pattern continued, the next level would involve 100 people buying 1 pound each, and finally 1600 people each buying 1 ounce. Some end-users might then roll up an ounce into individual joints, smoke some, and sell some. In reality, the final selling price of the 100 pounds would almost always total less than $160,000.

Another common theme found in stories about the illicent drug trade relates to the high profits and how easy it is to get rich quick by becoming a drug dealer. Looking at the example just given, we see that the profits are spread out over a fairly large number of people at several levels. The small dealers at the local level often make almost nothing, especially if you subtract the amounts they themselves use. The per sale profit is, of course, larger for the people who deal in larger amounts. But one does not simply walk around with 100 pounds of marijuana in one's back pocket; to deal in these larger amounts requires help in transporting, protecting, arranging deals, handling the cash, and so on, and more mouths to feed. There is no doubt that a few people do indeed make fat profits and live very well (especially considering they pay no income taxes on this cash business!). But it is a myth that anyone can get rich in a hurry just by deciding to take the chance and sell illegal drugs.

The law enforcers emphasize these large street values and the "big bucks" to remind us of how good a job they're doing and of the size and power of some of the operations they are up against. But one has to wonder if all this money talk doesn't help to glamorize the illicit drug trade and to draw susceptible individuals toward it.

It was pointed out in Chapter 3 that our efforts to regulate this illicit drug market have resulted in stronger and better organized gangs of traffickers rather than in reducing the size of the market. According to the simplest economic models, if we arrest traffickers and seize goods, the supply should be reduced. This may decrease the size of the market somewhat, but if demand does not change, the price should also increase. With most goods, except the basic necessities of life like bread and water, the demand is related to price. As price rises, the demand falls off somewhat, further shrinking the size of the market. So, any successful drug busts should result in both somewhat higher prices and somewhat fewer people using the drug. What is it about the illicit drug market that it seems to defy these basic economic principles? The answer is that these principles work fine in a *closed* economy, in which nothing new can enter the picture. But the illicit drug market is far from being a closed economy, in that as drug suppliers are arrested they are replaced by other individuals. As supplies of drugs are seized they are replaced by new supplies. In such an open economic system, the major factor regulating the size of the market is the size of the demand. What has happened to the illicit supply network can perhaps better be understood by turning away from the economic model of supply and demand and using instead the biological model of natural selection (survival of the fittest). If we look at drug suppliers as a population of predators, when we arrest some perhaps we are selectively arresting the least clever. When we frighten or shame some out of the business perhaps we are selectively eliminating the least ruthless. When we use other governments and police organizations to help us we may be selectively eliminating those suppliers who are least favored by those officials, either because they are political enemies or because they have not provided money or other favors. The remaining suppliers are the most clever, most ruthless, and have the best political connections. They wind up controlling bigger shares of the market, making greater profits, hiring and training farmers and lab workers, buying their own airplanes and airports and boats, and becoming better organized and even more profitable. This has happened over and over again, from the Mexican marijuana farms to the Colombian cocaine suppliers, and it is beginning to happen in the making of crack cocaine in our own cities.

This is not a new phenomenon. Something very similar happened with alcohol markets during prohibition. The more pressure exerted by the Treasury Department and the FBI, the more the liquor business became concentrated in the hands of a few ruthless organized crime bosses who paid bribes for local officials to look the other way, and who eliminated both their competition and the "nosy cops" with machine guns. In that case, it was decided that we would be better off to have large organizations sell us liquor who didn't use machine guns and who paid taxes and who could

be relied upon to follow certain rules—thus, alcohol prohibition was repealed.

Americans are neither morally nor politically ready to allow legal sales of heroin, marijuana, and cocaine for recreational purposes, so instead we are broadening the direction of our efforts and taking new aim at reducing the demand for illicit drugs, while continuing to put pressure on the suppliers (Chapter 3).

DRUG NAMES

Commercially available compounds have several kinds of names: **brand, generic,** and **chemical.** The *chemical name of a compound* gives a *complete chemical description of the molecule* and is derived from the rules of organic chemistry for naming any compound. Chemical names of drugs are rarely used except in a laboratory situation where biochemists or pharmacologists are developing and testing new drugs. Chemical names of drugs are given here only when the structure of a chemical is shown. There are several sets of rules for naming chemical structures. The most commonly used rules in the United States are those of *Chemical Abstracts* and those of the International Union of Pure and Applied Chemistry (IUPAC). Structures shown in this book are generally named using the *Chemical Abstracts* system, although a few have been named by IUPAC where that system's name is more common.

Much more commonly used by scientists is the simpler generic (or nonproprietary) name of a drug. Generic names are the official (that is, legal) names of drugs and are listed in the United States Pharmacopeia (USP). The generic, nonproprietary, names of chemicals are standardized by representatives of the American Medical Association, the American Pharmaceutical Association, the U.S. Pharmacopeial Convention, Inc., and the Food and Drug Administration. This group, known as the United States Adopted Name Council (USAN), has certain principles for assigning generic names to structures. Of primary importance in considering generic names are two facts: *a generic name specifies a chemical,* and *generic names are in the public domain.* The last point means they can be freely used by anyone and are not protected by trademark laws, clearly differentiating them from brand names.

The brand name of a drug specifies a particular formulation and manufacturer of a generic product. A brand name is usually quite simple and as meaningful (in terms of the indicated therapeutic use) as the company can make it. The over-the-counter compound Compōz and the prescription drug Vesprin, for example, certainly aren't stimulants. Vesprin is a tranquilizer, and the name alone almost makes you feel more relaxed, associating with it a quiet evening and vespers. Compōz, sold as a sleep aid and sedative, makes some people think of relaxation and smooth, easy experiences in life. However, brand names are controlled by the FDA, and overly suggestive ones are not approved.

BRAND-GENERIC NAME CONFLICT

When a new chemical structure, a new way of manufacturing a chemical, or a new use for a chemical is discovered, it can be patented. Patent laws in this country protect for 17 years, and, after that time, the finding is available for use by anyone. Brand names, however, are copyrighted and protected by trademark laws. These laws indefinitely restrict the use of the brand name to the original copyright holder.

For 17 years a company that has discovered and patented a product can manufacture and sell it without direct competition. If the product is a success in the marketplace, other companies will rush to discover equally effective agents with similar, but not identical, chemical structures. When the patent expires the discovery is free game for any manufacturer, and, if the drug has been a moneymaker, it is quite likely that new companies will develop the capability to produce the "same" drug. However, at this point a question arises: if the drug is chemically identical by FDA standards, is it the therapeutic equivalent?

A drug is initially released for sale by the FDA only after it has been shown to be safe and effective for the condition it is used to treat. This clearance is obtained by the original producer of the drug. The heart of the brand-generic conflict is whether it can be assumed that drugs manufactured to Food and Drug Administration standards by new companies do not have to go through the necessary preclinical and clinical trials to demonstrate safety and effectiveness.

A drug can be effective only if it is delivered to those cells where the drug acts. Almost all drugs reach the area where they are to act through the bloodstream, and any factors that influence a drug's ability to be absorbed by the bloodstream will influence its effectiveness. To separate out some of the factors involved in determining the equivalence of two drugs, three concepts have come into wide use.

The concept of *chemical equivalence* is fairly clear. Chemical equivalents are drugs that contain essentially identical amounts of the identical active ingredients in identical dosages and that thus meet present FDA physiochemical standards. *Biological equivalents* are drugs that, when administered in the same amounts, provide the same biological or physiological availability of the drug to the body tissues. The biological availability, or *bioavailability*, is usually assessed by determining the levels of the drug in the bloodstream.

Clinical equivalents are chemical equivalents that, when given in the same amounts, result in the same therapeutic effect. Thus, two drugs can be chemically equivalent but not be clinically equivalent. Whether biological equivalence is tantamount to clinical equivalence is not yet decided, but it seems probable. The primary factor involved in determining whether chemical equivalents have the same bioavailability is related to the way the drug is finally prepared for use. What would seem to be minor factors such as the hardness of the tablet of the drug and the solubility of the drug capsule become critical in determining the extent to which a drug can be absorbed into the bloodstream. If the drug does not reach the bloodstream, there is little chance it can have an effect. A study of two brands of chlorpromazine hydrochloride tablets reported the time it took for each tablet to release 60% of the active ingredient. One brand required over six times as long as the other.[8]

A case history of a brand-generic conflict involves Terramycin, the Charles Pfizer Company's brand of oxytetracycline. Terramycin was discovered by Pfizer researchers in 1949 after screening over 100,000 samples of earth (hence the name "terra") and was a highly successful antibiotic. In 1967, when the patent ran out, several companies began producing oxytetracycline, which is the generic name for Terramycin and which was the chemical equivalent according to FDA tests. Considerable money was involved, since the cost to the patient for Terramycin was about 30 cents a capsule, whereas oxytetracycline was half that price. The Pfizer Company decided to study blood levels in groups of patients receiving Terramycin or the various brands of oxytetracycline.[9]

The FDA certified the chemical composition, amount, and purity of each of the generic brands and of Terramycin, and all were equivalent. After administration of equal amounts of each drug, the blood levels of the drug in patients receiving the different brands were anything but equivalent. None of the generic brands gave blood levels (and thus "bioavailability") as high as Terramycin. The drugs produced by eight manufacturers resulted in blood levels too low to be acceptable, and the FDA called in 40 million capsules by those producers. The sales field was left to Terramycin and two generic forms of oxytetracycline that did yield adequate blood levels.

There is still no scientific resolution to the problem of therapeutic equivalence of brand name and chemically equivalent generic drugs. There are some political and economic attempts at "solving" the problem, but the plot continues to thicken. Since a patent permits manufacturing control for only 17 years, it is understandable that companies would seek other means to control the sale of the drug for a longer period of time. This is accomplished by advertising drugs under their brand names to physicians, not only through advertising in journals but also by direct contact of company representatives. According to some estimates,

pharmaceutical houses spend about $2,400 a year per physician in this area of selling.

In December 1980 the FDA decided that:

> Manufacturers will be permitted to sell generic versions of brand name drugs marketed since 1962 whose patents have expired, without repeating the costly testing done to show that the original version was safe and effective. . . .
>
> Instead of repeating studies, manufacturers need only cite studies in the literature to show that the drug is safe and effective. . . .[10,p.1]

These "paper" INDs (rather than the original research INDs) are the source of considerable debate. Consumer groups, the FDA, and the manufacturers of generics think they're the best thing since night baseball. The manufacturers of brand-name drugs are appalled and point to both administrative and scientific problems in ensuring effective, quality drugs for patients if the paper INDs are allowed to remain. They are also honest in saying that they'll lose a lot of money if things don't change. One pharmacologist said, "No amount of wishful thinking or administrative fiat can change the present state of affairs in which differences in drug bioavailability from different products are very common, and therapeutic inequivalence . . . is a potentially serious threat to patient welfare."[11,p.39] Even so, in 1980 the FDA published its first version of the *Therapeutics Equivalence List*, which is updated monthly. This list tells the pharmacists what generics they can substitute—with the FDA's approval—for a brand name drug. I'm sorry, maybe I'm more of a scientist than an administrator, but I'd like to see at least *one* study done on each different, accepted generic drug to show that there really is therapeutic equivalence—not just chemical equivalence.

In a more recent battle over licensing generics, Hoffmann-LaRoche Inc., the manufacturers of Valium (diazepam), successfully slowed the introduction of generic diazepam, but not for as long as they had hoped. Valium was the fourth best-selling prescription drug in 1984 with sales of about $240 million. Just as Valium's 17-year pa-

---

The ever-changing world of drug slang

One of the exercises in which drug agencies and drug books have engaged over the years is compiling a list of slang or street terms used for various drugs. Presumably, we should offer you a list of such terms that you could then memorize and be at home among the drug subculture, recognizing when those in the know are talking about drugs, right? Sorry, folks, but it doesn't seem to work that way.

Where do these slang terms come from? Presumably from groups of mostly young people in a relatively small, isolated subculture. Think about the names you and your friends used or now use to refer to people who are "nerds." One might begin to compile these names of animals or objects and find that the students at one school have some names that the students at another school don't have or that they change from one year to the next or that sophomores use different terms than seniors in the same school. If a particular term were used in a popular movie, it might actually be in widespread use throughout the country for a couple of years, but after that anyone who used the term would probably be one.

Something like that happens with drug slang: the name used for marijuana by a group of high school students in Los Angeles is probably different from that used by a group of college students in Dallas or a group of longshoremen in New York. And they change, so that as soon as a list is printed it is out of date.

The NIDA has compiled a list of drug slang terms taken from various sources—interesting, but perhaps not too useful for the purpose we proposed originally. Over 150 terms are listed as referring to marijuana, about 100 for heroin, and about 75 for cocaine. And some names are listed for more than one drug: "witch" and "white girl" can be found under either cocaine or heroin. One has to wonder how widely some of the terms are used: "Foo Foo Dust" for cocaine or "Red Chicken" for heroin. And even if you hear people talking about "snow," "grass," or "horse," they may very well be talking about snow, grass, or a horse.

---

tent was to expire, the company presented evidence they said indicated that even measuring blood levels to determine bioavailability was not enough. They wanted the generic manufacturers to have to conduct brain-wave recordings demonstrating the equivalence of their diazepam.[12] This would have cost the generic companies money and time. The FDA ruled against Hoffmann-LaRoche in July of 1985 and in September of that year allowed three companies to begin sales of generic diazepam.[13]

Diazepam was the seventh generic drug to be approved under the new "paper" IND procedure, and, with diazepam, nine of the ten best-selling drugs had approved generic equivalents. Generics accounted for 12% of prescription drug sales in 1988, and because several patents will be expiring it is expected that they will have 30% of the market by the mid-1990s.

CATEGORIZING DRUGS

Physicians, pharmacologists, chemists, lawyers, psychologists, and users all have drug classification schemes that best serve their own purposes. A compound such as amphetamine might be categorized as an antiappetite agent by many physicians, since it reduces food intake for a period of time. It might be classed as a phenylethylamine by a pharmacologist, since its basic structure is a phenyl ring with an ethyl group and an amine attached. The chemist wastes no time and says flat-out that amphetamine is 2-amino-1-phenylpropane. To the lawyer amphetamine may be only a drug of abuse falling in Schedule II of the federal drug law, while the psychologist may say simply that it is a stimulant. The user may call it a diet pill or an upper. The important thing to remember is that any scheme for categorizing drugs has meaning only if it serves the purpose for which the classification is being made.

The scheme presented here organizes the drugs according to their effects on the user, with first consideration given to the psychological effects. The basic outline and examples of each drug are given in Table 5-1, but it is worthwhile to point

Table 5-1

Classification of psychoactive drugs	
Type of drug	Example
Stimulant	Amphetamines, cocaine, caffeine (mild stimulant)
Depressant	Alcohol, barbiturates, other sedatives, sleeping pills, some volatile solvents, inhaled anesthetics
Narcotic	Morphine, codeine, heroin, methadone
Hallucinogen	Mescaline, LSD, PCP
Psychotherapeutic	Chlorpromazine, imipramine, lithium
Nicotine	
Marijuana	

out some of the defining characteristics of each major grouping.

At moderate doses, **stimulant drugs** produce wakefulness and a sense of energy and well-being. The more powerful stimulants, such as cocaine and amphetamines, can at high doses produce a manic state of excitement combined with paranoia and hallucinations.

If you know about the behavioral effects of alcohol, then you know about the **depressant drugs.** At low doses they appear to depress inhibitory parts of the brain, leading to disinhibition or relaxation and talkativeness that may give way to recklessness. As the dose is increased, other neural functions become depressed, leading to slowed reaction times, uncoordinated movements, and "passing out." It should be pointed out that stimulants and depressants do not have opposite effects on most functions. Although it may be possible to keep a drunk awake with stimulant drugs, he or she would still be reckless, uncoordinated, and so on. Regular use of these drugs can lead to a withdrawal syndrome characterized by restlessness, shakiness, hallucinations, and sometimes convulsions.

Narcotics are a group of analgesic (pain-kill-

ing) drugs that produce a relaxed, dreamlike state; at moderately high doses sleep is often induced. There is a clouding of consciousness without the reckless abandon, staggering, and slurred speech produced by alcohol and other depressants. Regular use of any of the narcotics can lead to a withdrawal syndrome different from that of depressants and characterized by diarrhea, cramps, chills, and profuse sweating.

The **hallucinogens** produce altered perceptions. These include unusual visual sensations and quite often changes in the perception of one's own body.

The psychotherapeutic drugs include a variety of drugs prescribed by psychiatrists and other physicians for the control of mental problems. The **antipsychotics,** such as chlorpromazine, are also called major tranquilizers. They can calm psychotic patients and over time help them to control hallucinations and illogical thoughts. The **antidepressants,** such as imipramine, help some people to recover more rapidly from seriously depressed mood states. Lithium is used to control manic episodes and to prevent mood swings in manic-depressives.

As with any system of classification, there are some things that don't seem to fit into the classes. Nicotine and marijuana are two such drugs. Nicotine is often thought of as being a mild stimulant, but it also seems to have some of the relaxant properties of a low dose of a depressant. Marijuana is often thought of as a relaxant, depressive type of drug, but it doesn't share most of the features of that class. It is sometimes listed among the hallucinogens, because it can produce altered perceptions at high doses, but that classification doesn't seem entirely appropriate for the way most people use it.

DRUG IDENTIFICATION AND DETECTION
Identification of Drugs

There are many reasons to identify exactly what drug is represented by a tablet, capsule, or plant substance. For example, the *Physician's Desk Ref-*

Issue: who must submit to drug tests?

Corporations, professional sports organizations, and government agencies are adopting urine tests to screen for illicit drugs. Some employees, unions, and civil rights organizations are opposing such testing. Why? Let's start with the fourth amendment to the Constitution of the United States:

The right of the people to be secure in their persons, houses, papers, and effects, against unreasonable searches and seizures, shall not be violated, and no warrants shall issue, but upon probable cause, supported by oath or affirmation, and particularly describing the place to be searched, and the person or things to be seized.

This limits only the powers of governments (local, state, and federal), not private employers. Urine tests are considered to fall under the "search and seizure" clause, even though Thomas Jefferson and James Madison probably never imagined that such things would exist. A conservative reading of the Fourth Amendment would say that government agencies could not test someone's urine unless they showed probable cause that that particular individual was engaged in drug use and obtained a warrant describing the individual to be tested and perhaps even the drug being tested for. The U.S. Supreme Court heard two cases in 1989, one involving railroad workers and the other customs agents. Although the Court upheld the government's testing programs in both cases, it did place restrictions on the conditions. The Federal Railway Administration will be allowed to test train crews *if they are involved in accidents*. By a narrow (5-4) vote, the practice of screening customs agents who apply for drug enforcement-related jobs will be allowed.

Conservative Justice Scalia wrote the minority opinion in this second case, and pointed out that only 5 of 3600 Customs Service employees had tested positive for drugs. Since such testing will have no real effect on drug abuse, he concluded that we are sacrificing "privacy and human dignity in symbolic opposition to drug use." Given the close decisions and the narrowly defined limits in which testing was allowed, it would seem that the federal government's plan to apply random drug tests to 400,000 federal workers will have to be scaled back considerably.[19]

With regard to private employers, Fourth Amendment protections do not apply. They must be careful not to violate civil rights laws by selectively testing certain groups, but in most cases it seems that they will be allowed to require tests. Some states do have laws that might limit a company's power to impose such tests, and other types of challenges can be brought. We can predict that many lawyers will find employment in this field over the next several years, and it will take a few years to settle the basic issues.

If you're wondering why anyone would oppose urine testing unless he or she was a drug user, it might be good to review this 1937 quote from Pastor Martin Neimoller:

In Germany they came first for Communists, and I didn't speak up because I wasn't a Communist. Then they came for the Jews, and I didn't speak up because I wasn't a Jew. Then they came for the trade unionists, and I didn't speak up because I wasn't a trade unionist. Then they came for the Catholics, and I didn't speak up because I was a Protestant. Then they came for me, and by that time no one was left to speak up. (Peter's Quotations).

---

erence (PDR) has for many years published color photographs of many of the legally manufactured pharmaceuticals.[14] In this way a physician can determine from the pills themselves what drugs a new patient has been taking and in what doses. More critically, in emergency rooms it is possible to determine what drugs a person has just taken, if some of the pills are available for viewing. During the late 1960s access to a PDR was a big deal for those who were buying and selling amphetamines and barbiturates on the streets, although the later introduction of look-alikes by unscru-

pulous street dealers made the appearance of the pills a less reliable guide. Police chemistry labs also have used the PDR as a preliminary indication of the nature of seized tablets and capsules.

Even illicit drugs can sometimes be identified by visual appearance. Sometimes the makers of illicit tablets containing amphetamines or LSD would mark them, however crudely, in a consistent way so that they would be recognized by their buyers. For example, many illicit LSD tablets were colored purple. Such visual identification is far from perfect, of course. Cocaine or heroin may also be packaged in a consistent way by dealers. Some plant materials, such as psilocybin mushrooms, peyote cactus, or coca or marijuana leaves may be fairly easy to identify visually, although again not with perfect accuracy.

If a case involving illicit drugs is to be prosecuted in court, the prosecution would usually be expected to produce the testimony of a chemist indicating that the drug had been tested and absolutely identified. The exact chemical tests performed would vary with the substance and with the laboratory doing the analyses.

Detection of Drugs in Body Fluids

The practice of using urine tests to screen individuals for drug use has become quite a fad during the 1980s. It wasn't until the 1970s that relatively inexpensive screening tests were invented that could detect a variety of abused substances or their metabolites in urine.[15] The Navy, followed by the other armed forces, was the first to employ random urine screening on a large scale. Soon to follow were people in various high-risk or high-profile positions: oilfield workers, air traffic controllers, and professional athletes. In 1986, President Reagan first declared that random urine tests should be performed on all federal employees in "sensitive" jobs.[16] He also urged companies doing business with the federal government to begin testing their employees, if they had not done so. Fuel was added to the fire by a 1987 collision between an Amtrak train and a Conrail train near Baltimore, Maryland. Sixteen people were killed, and the wreck was quickly blamed on drug use, since the Conrail engineer and brakeman had shared a marijuana joint shortly before the tragedy. The causal relationship may be argued: Warning indicators on the Conrail train were malfunctioning, and the marijuana use could be viewed as just a symptom of a general "goofing off" attitude by the railway workers. Nevertheless, the politicians and news media saw this tragedy as a clear indication of the need for random urine testing.

Private corporations, which may require urine testing before hiring a new employee and/or may periodically test employees, have two main reasons for adopting urine tests, but the bottom line in both cases is money. First, companies believe that drug-free workers will be absent less often, make fewer mistakes, have better safety records, and produce more and better work. Second, by spending a relatively few dollars on urine tests, they protect the company against negligence suits that might follow if a "stoned" employee hurt someone on the job or turned out a dangerously faulty product. By 1987 about one-third of the large companies in the United States were using urine screens, and the fraction is expected to grow in spite of legal challenges and union opposition[17] (see Issue box).

What is not widely discussed in the newspaper accounts of such testing programs is what procedures will be used, what drugs will be looked for, and how well the tests work. Most drug screening programs test urine samples, using a commercially available kit that employs a method known as EMIT (enzyme multiplied immunoassay test). This method relies on the use of antibodies that react either to the drug in question or to some metabolite (breakdown product) of the drug. A problem with this type of assay is that it is possible that some other drug or chemical might cross-react with the antibody and produce a false positive result.

Although the incidence of such false positives is fairly low, they can occur and it is best to follow up the initial screen with another more selective method, such as gas chromatography/mass spectrometry (GC/MS). This method is more specific and more sensitive, but also more expensive: A typical EMIT test can be done for about $20 per sample, but GC/MS tests cost about $100.[18] An early problem with mass screening programs was sloppy handling of the samples, allowing for false reports based on mixups. However, the labs doing this type of work have improved their handling procedures and the companies making the test kits have improved their accuracy, so that it is theoretically possible for a company or government agency to obtain very accurate information. That is not always done in practice, however. For example, several over-the-counter drug products contain ingredients such as ephedrine which are chemically similar to amphetamine, and someone taking these perfectly legal substances may show up with an EMIT test positive for amphetamine. Until recently, products containing ibuprofen could cause a positive test for marijuana. These false positives can be ruled out if another portion of the same urine sample is subjected to GC/MS, because that test can distinguish between ephedrine and amphetamine or between ibuprofen and marijuana metabolites. But the person paying for the testing has to want to spend the extra money. Sometimes people have not been hired on the basis of a single positive result on an EMIT test. In other cases, the sample may be retested using EMIT, which does not solve the problem of cross-reactivity. It would be irresponsible to take serious actions against a person, such as terminating employment, on the basis of a single positive result on an EMIT test.

These kits can detect marijuana metabolites, the cocaine metabolite *benzoylecgonine,* phencyclidine (PCP), or heroin. However, both the sensitivity and the duration over which the metabolites can be detected vary greatly among these substances. The cocaine metabolite clears within 1 or 2 days after a single use of a moderate amount, and it would probably be impossible to detect cocaine use for more than 3 or 4 days even in someone chronically using high doses. The outside limit for PCP or heroin would also probably be about 4 days. After a single use of marijuana, metabolites can be reliably detected for 5 days or more, but with chronic use of high doses, tests may be positive for 2 or 3 weeks or as long as 30 days. The point is that it is much easier for these tests to detect marijuana use for long periods of time than for them to detect other types of drug use. Combine that with the much greater frequency of use of marijuana than of these other drugs, and the odds are good that if you read that someone "flunked" a drug screen, it was probably because of marijuana metabolites.

You should also be aware that these screens

What does a drug user look like?

You've probably seen magazine advertisements or drug information that is aimed at helping you tell if someone you know and love is a drug user. Heroin addicts may have runny noses, for example, and marijuana smokers may have reddened eyes. Someone who is high on cocaine may talk in a rapid, excited fashion. The problem with most of these symptoms is that they represent drug influences that could be produced by other things, such as having a cold, seeing a sad movie, or getting excited about something. There are some signs that could be worrisome no matter what the cause, such as large sums of money disappearing for no apparent reason. Major personality changes, falling grades in school, and running around with a bunch of "losers" should cause a parent to become concerned and try to find out what is going on. But it does little good, we think, to have people trying to diagnose drug use by checking for dilated pupils or runny noses. For that reason we have chosen not to include lists of such symptoms to aid in the detection of drug use.

can detect the presence of a drug or its metabolite, but they can't tell you anything about the state of impairment of the individual. One person might show up at work Monday morning with a terrible hangover from drinking the night before, be unable to perform well on the job, and pass the drug screen easily. Another person might have smoked some marijuana on Friday night, have experienced no effect for the past day and a half, and yet fail the screen. The general idea of the screens seems to be to discourage illicit drug use more than to detect impairment of performance.

Summary

As commodities, drugs represent big business. Whether legitimate or illicit, they provide big profits for some and employment for a large number of people, some in industry, some in regulatory agencies, and some in the underworld.

The naming and classification of these drugs

are complex processes, involving considerations of scientific, political, corporate, and user perspectives. Most of the psychoactive drugs can be grouped into a fairly small number of distinct categories based mostly on their effects.

The need to identify drugs and to detect their presence in humans who have used them has led to a proliferation and refinement of chemical techniques that are increasingly specific and sensitive. What is less clear is how these techniques are to be put to use by a society concerned about the use of drugs.

REFERENCES

1. US Industrial Outlook 1989, US Department of Commerce.
2. Gallup Poll: Stat-O-Grams, Pharmacy Times, p 1, November 1981.
3. Garcha BS, editor: Is the justice blind? Pharmacists answer Burger, Drug Topics, pp 55-59, October 15, 1976.
4. Deno RA and others: The profession of pharmacy, ed 2, Philadelphia, 1966, JB Lippincott Co.
5. The supply of illicit drugs to the United States, National Narcotics Intelligence Consumers Committee. Washington, DC, US Government Printing Office, 1988.
6. Clayton RR: Cocaine use in the United States: in a blizzard or just being snowed? In Kozel NJ and Adams EH, editors: Cocaine use in America: epidemiologic and clinical perspectives, NIDA Research Monograph No 61, DHHS Publication No (ADM) 85-1414, Washington, DC, 1985, US Government Printing Office.
7. Kids and cocaine, Newsweek 107:58-65, 1986.
8. Desta B and Pernarowski M: The dissolution characteristics of two clinically different brands of chlorpromazine HCl tablets, Drug Intelligence and Clinical Pharmacy 7:408-412, 1973.
9. Biodecision Laboratories Second Annual International Symposium, Pittsburgh, September 1975.
10. HHS News: US Department of Health and Human Services, P80-59, December 8, 1980.
11. Schwartz LL: Generic drug rules: science or politics, Medical Tribune p 39, August 26, 1981.
12. Sun M: Generic Valiums clear another hurdle at FDA, Science 229:369, 1985.
13. Duke P and Waldholz M: Three drug firms get US approval to sell diazepam, The Wall Street Journal, September 5, 1985.
14. Physician's Desk Reference Oradell, NJ, annual, Medical Economics Company.
15. Employee drug screening: detection of drug use by urinalysis, DHHS Publication No (ADM) 86-1442, Washington, DC, 1986, US Government Printing Office.
16. Marshall E: Testing urine for drugs, Science 241:150-152, 1988.
17. O'Keefe AM: The case against drug testing, Psychology Today, June, 1987, pp. 35-38.
18. Drug testing: the state of the art, American Scientist 77:19-23, 1989.
19. The high court weighs drug tests, Newsweek, April 3, 1989, p 8.

Chapter 6

The Actions of Drugs

OBJECTIVES

After reading this chapter, you should be able to:

Distinguish between specific and nonspecific drug effects.

Describe dose-response relationships and how they are interpreted to reveal specific drug effects, individual differences, and multiple drug effects.

Explain how the route of administration, drug distribution, and processes of drug removal are reflected in the time course of a drug's action.

Name three possible reasons for developing tolerance, and understand how one of them relates to physical dependence.

No matter what the drug or how much of it there is, it can't have an effect until it is taken. In other words, for there to be a drug effect, we must bring the drug together with a living organism. This chapter looks at some of the ways the drug and organism interact to produce drug actions.

NONSPECIFIC FACTORS IN DRUG EFFECTS

Most of the discussion on generic and brand name drugs (see Chapter 5) involved the issue of **bioavailability:** the availability of the biologically active molecules to the cells of the body where the drug must act to have an effect. The assumption was made that the level of a drug in the circulatory system would have a high positive relationship with the effect of the drug. Drug blood level monitoring has become an important part of decision making in treatment for many drugs.

Would that life were so simple that the effect of psychoactive drugs could be predicted by their level in the blood. The psychoactive drugs appear to have their effect by altering patterns of neural functioning. Since these drugs act by altering function, it follows that the effects will in part depend on the activity that is already present. Another consideration in understanding the actions of these drugs is that they are frequently used to affect moods, feelings, and the individual's reaction to changes in environment. These kinds of changes can also be brought about by nonchemical means, and this fact must always be considered when evaluating the effects of psychoactive drugs.

The bases for the effects of a psychoactive drug are usually divided into two groups. One group consists of molecular, physiological, and biochemical changes that result from specific chemical characteristics of the drug and the cells or chemicals with which it interacts. Thus a basis for the effects of atropine in the body is the occupation of the acetylcholine receptor site by atropine. One specific effect resulting from this is the cessation of the flow of saliva and a drying of the mouth and throat. This effect will occur regardless of whether the patient believes it will happen, whether he knows he is receiving a drug, whether he likes his doctor, or whatever. The specific effects of drugs are caused by physiobiochemical actions of the drug, which depend only on the drug's reaching the site of action and a normal body chemistry.

The second group of causes for a drug's effect has only recently been widely studied and is termed **nonspecific factors,** which means merely that these effects of the drug are not based on its chemical activity. These nonspecific factors are those that reside in an individual with a unique background and a particular perception of the world. In brief, the nonspecific factors can include anything except the chemical activity of the drug and the direct effects of this activity. For example, a good "trip" or a bad trip from pure LSD seems to be dependent in part on the personality and mood of the user prior to taking the drug. In part, the kind of trip experienced depends on what the user expects to experience. The expectation is a nonspecific factor with respect to drug actions, since it influences the experienced effect of the drug but not the chemical activity of the drug.

Since the expectation of a drug effect can influence the effect that is experienced by the user or seen by an observer, most of the acceptable drug research with humans is carried out under *double-blind* conditions. In a double-blind experiment, neither the physician nor the patient knows whether the patient is receiving a drug or an inert substance — a **placebo.** When neither the patient nor his doctor knows if a drug is being used, a better evaluation can be made of the drug's specific effect on the symptoms. Another factor is necessary for a study to be considered adequately controlled. The patients should be assigned randomly to the drug and the placebo groups. A meaningful study of the effects of a drug can best be accomplished if patients are randomly assigned to groups and double-blind conditions are met.

However, even a double-blind study does not provide a pure evaluation. One investigator[1] studied the differential effects of two mild tranquilizers on anxiety in a group of patients of general practitioners. Neither the patient nor the physician knew which drug was being used, and, *prior to the start of medication,* both the physician and patient had to indicate whether they were optimistic, indifferent, or pessimistic about the outcome of treatment. After 2 months, regardless of the drug used, patients for whom the doctors were optimistic showed a 50% reduction in symptoms, whereas those patients for whom the physician had been pessimistic showed only a 20% decrease. Optimistic patients showed a 45% reduction in

---

Your turn: the placebo and you

Suppose that you have an ache in your left arm. You try aspirin, but it does no good. After living with it for several days, you go to see your physician. She examines you and can find no physical problem, but she writes out a prescription. She indicates that she thinks this drug will help you and ushers you out. You pay the receptionist $20, go to the drug store, get the prescription filled, and pay $7.50. Then you go home and take the first pill.

Now assume that your physician has decided that your problem may be psychological in origin and has prescribed a placebo, but you don't know this. Has the physician done the right thing? Do you feel that the trust you have placed in that physician was betrayed? What about the pharmacist who sold you the placebo for $7.50?

their anxiety symptoms, while the patients pessimistic about outcome showed a symptom drop of only 35%.

A nice transition from nonspecific effects of drugs and placebos to the specific effects of biologically active drugs has been developing since the late 1970s. When the term *nonspecific* is used, it just means that we don't know what factors are operating, or how they are operating, to give the effect. No one here, I hope, believes in magic or ghosts so we must agree that there are real, biophysiochemical mechanisms underlying the nonspecific and placebo effects—we just don't know what they are. However, the evidence is slowly building. There is now good reliable research that tells us some of the steps involved in the reduction of pain by placebos.

In a dental study[2] some patients receiving a placebo reported a reduction of pain. When they were given a drug whose only effect is to block the opiate receptor in the brain, pain increased (just as it would have if the pain reduction were the result of morphine rather than a placebo). It's known (see Chapter 16) that the body manufactures chemicals—**endorphins**—very similar to morphine and that these endorphins play an important role in the normal control of pain. The results of the dental study suggest that the placebo (that is, the belief that the individual was taking a drug that would reduce pain) resulted in an increase in production of endorphins and thus a decrease in pain.

However, not all placebo effects on pain are mediated by endorphins. Scientists are now investigating the possible release of other natural chemicals in response to placebos.[3]

SPECIFIC ACTIONS OF DRUGS

You might think that demonstrating specific drug actions, that is, actions that do depend on the chemical makeup of the drug, would be next to impossible with psychoactive drugs. In fact, pharmacologists have a couple of neat tricks up their sleeves: suppose you give each person the same-size capsule, but vary the number of drug molecules in the capsules (the drug dose)? If the size of the effect is related to the drug dose, this is a very good indication that the drug is having specific effects. Also, if the effect varies over time in the same way that the bioavailability of the drug molecules varies, this is an indication of the specificity of the effect of those molecules. For this reason, two basic tools of the pharmacologist are the study of dose-response relationships and time-dependent factors in drug actions.

Dose-Response Relationships

Perhaps the most fundamental concept in understanding drug actions is the dose-response curve and phenomena associated with it. In simple terms the **dose-response curve** refers to the fact that as the amount of the drug administered is varied, there may be a change in a monitored behavior. A basic point is that since the effects of a drug can be studied on many behaviors or responses, there are many different dose-response curves for the same drug.

Drug effects arise from the collective effects of many molecular interactions. The more drug molecules there are at the site of action, the more interactions there can be, and the greater their collective effects may be. A minimum number of molecular interactions is always required before the result of their collective effects can be measured. When an effect is seen, it is called a threshold response, and the dose of the drug administered is called the threshold dose.

With an increase in the amount of drug given, there is an increase in the collective effect of the molecular interactions and thus of the response being monitored. At some point molecular interactions are occurring at the most rapid rate possible; the addition of more drug does not then increase the response. This, in essence, is what a dose-response curve is. At some low dose (few drug molecules) there is an observable effect on the response system being monitored. This dose is the threshold, and, as the dose of the drug is increased, there are more molecular interactions and a greater effect on the response system. At the point where the system shows maximal response, further additions of the drug have no effect.

In some drug-response interactions, the effect of the drug is all-or-none, so that when the system does respond, it responds maximally. There may, however, be variability in the dosage at which individual organisms respond, and, as the dose increases, there is an increase in the percentage of individuals who show the response. The relationship between the change in the response system and the dose of the drug is shown in Fig. 6-1. Each of the graphs is a dose-response curve and indicates the relationship between the amount of drug administered and a particular measure of the response being monitored. Three different types of measures are used, and they all indicate the same basic relationship.

Previously, it was mentioned that as the drug dose increases, sometimes new response systems are affected by the drug. This fact suggests that some response systems have higher drug thresholds than others. Fig.6-2 shows a series of dose-response curves for three different effects of alcohol. As the dose increases from the low end, first a few and then more and more of the individuals show a slowing of their reaction times. If we also have a test for **ataxia** (staggering or inability to walk straight), we see that as the alcohol dose reaches the level at which most individuals are showing slowed reaction times, a few are also beginning to show ataxia. As the dose increases further, more people show ataxia and some become **comatose** (they pass out and cannot be aroused). At the highest dose indicated, all the individuals would be comatose. Note that we could draw curves for other effects of alcohol on such a figure; for example, at the high end we would begin to see some deaths from overdose and a curve for lethality could be placed to the right of the coma curve.

In the rational use of drugs, there are four questions about drug dosage that must be answered. First, what is the effective dose of the drug for a desired goal? For example, what dose of morphine is necessary to reduce pain 50%? What amount of marijuana is necessary for an individual to feel euphoric? How much aspirin will make the headache go away? The second question is, what dose of the drug will be lethal to the individual? How much of the drug is necessary to kill a person? Combining those two, what is the safety margin—how different are the effective dose and the lethal dose? Finally, at the effective dose level, what other effects, particularly adverse reactions, might develop? Leaving aside for now this last question, a discussion of the first three deals with basic concepts in understanding drug actions.

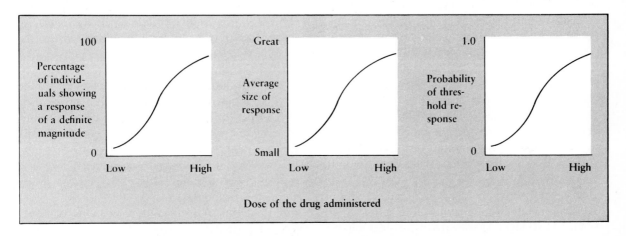

Figure 6-1. Relationships between drug dose and single-response system.

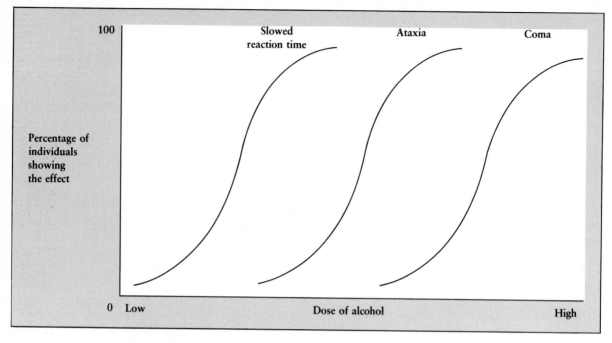

Figure 6-2. Relationship between alcohol dose and multiple responses.

In any biological system there is considerable variability; response to drugs is no different. Some individuals will be very sensitive to a drug and show the desired effect at low dose levels. Others will be quite resistant, and the desired effect of the drug will be reached only after high doses are administered. Between these sensitive and resistant individuals is usually an increasing percentage of effective responses as the dose of the drug is increased. This relationship is shown in Fig. 6-1, upper left.

The basis for this variability is partially understood and is the object of much research. Many factors about the individual contribute to drug effect variability. These include body weight, sex, and age; infants and children are usually more sensitive to drugs than adults, whereas the elderly frequently show unique responses to drugs—rate of absorption from the digestive tract, activity of the drug metabolizing enzymes in the liver, diet, and so on. Genetic factors are of considerable interest and importance in determining the rate of drug metabolism.

The **effective dose** (the dose that is effective in causing a particular effect) is abbreviated ED, and a number is attached to indicate the percentage of individuals who show the desired effects at a particular dose level. The term ED 50 means that at the indicated dose level, 50% of the people or animals showed the desired response. The ED 1 is a dose level at which the effect is observed in only 1% of the individuals, while the ED 99 is the dose at which 99% of the individuals showed the effect.

The **lethal dose,** LD, is determined in the same way; what percentage of the animals at each dose level die within a specified period of time? The *safety margin* refers to the dose difference between an acceptable level of effectiveness (ED 50? ED 90?) and the LD 1. For most psychoactive drugs there is a considerable range between the dose giving the desired effect and a lethal dose. For some experimental anticancer compounds there is a small margin of safety.

Since most of the psychoactive compounds have an LD 1 well above the ED 95 level, the

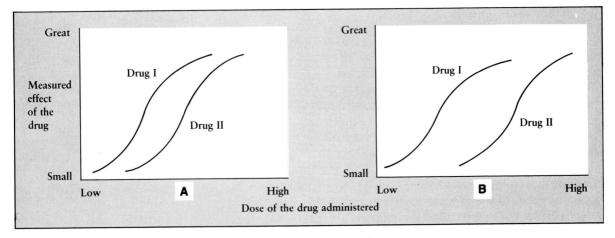

Figure 6-3. Relationship between the measured effect of two drugs at varying dose levels. In A, drug I is more potent than drug II; that is, less of drug I than of drug II is needed to obtain a given effect, but both drugs have the same maximum effect. In B, drug I is more potent, but drug II can give greater effects.

practical limitation on whether or not, or at what dose, a drug is used is the occurrence of side effects. With increasing doses there is usually an increase in the number and severity of side effects—those effects of the drug not relevant to the treatment. If the number of side effects becomes too great and the individual begins to suffer from them, the use of the drug will be discontinued or the dose lowered, even though the drug may be very effective in controlling the original symptoms. The selection of a drug for therapeutic use involves both these concepts. Drug choice should be made on the basis of specificity of action on the symptom with minimal side effects.

Potency

The **potency** of a drug is one of the most misunderstood concepts in the area of drug use. *Potency refers only to the amount of drug that must be given to obtain a particular response.* The less the amount needed to get a particular effect, the more potent the drug. Potency has nothing to do with the effectiveness of the drug. Neither is potency related to maximum effect of a drug. These relationships are indicated in Fig. 6-3. If drug A is one

half as potent as drug B, then you can get the same effect by using twice the dose of drug A as of drug B. Potency refers only to relative effective dose; the ED 50 of a potent drug is lower than the ED 50 of a less potent drug. Rarely is it true that two drugs will differ only in their potency.

Time-Dependent Factors in Drug Actions

Figure 6-4 roughly describes one type of relationship between administration of a drug and its effect over time. Between points *A* and *B* there is no observed effect, although the concentration of drug in the blood is increasing. At point *B* the threshold concentration is reached, and from *B* to *C* the observed drug effect increases as drug concentration increases. At point *C* the maximal effect of the drug is reached, but its concentration continues increasing to point *D*. Although deactivation of the drug probably begins as soon as the drug enters the body, from *A* to *D* the rate of absorption is greater than the rate of deactivation. Beginning at point *D* the deactivation proceeds more rapidly than absorption, and the concentration of the drug decreases. When the amount of

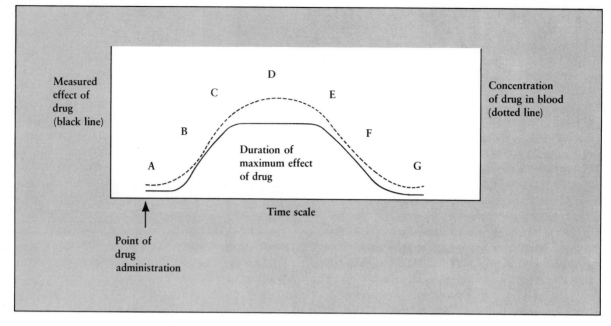

Figure 6-4. Possible relationship between drug concentration in body and measured effect of the drug.

drug in the body reaches *E*, the maximal effect is over. The action diminishes from *E* to *F*, at which point the level of the drug is below the threshold for effect, although there is still drug in the body up to point *G*.

It should be clear that if the relationship described in Fig. 6-4 is true for a particular drug, then increasing the dose of the drug will not increase the magnitude of its effect. Aspirin is probably the most misused drug in this respect — if two are good, four should be better, and six will really stop this headache. No way! When the maximum possible therapeutic effect has been reached, increasing the dose *may* prolong the effect, but such an increase primarily serves to add to the number of side effects. If a high dose is used originally, there may be some shortening of the time of onset (the amount of time between taking the drug and the experiencing of effects), but in the case of aspirin there will also be an increase in gastric irritation.

A different type of relationship between a drug and its effect is presented in Fig. 6-5, *A*. In this case the effect of the drug parallels the concentration of the drug in the body. In Fig. 6-4 the situation was shown in which a drug's maximum effect was in some way limited — perhaps all available receptor sites were occupied, or perhaps the system on which the drug was acting had reached its limit for change. Alcohol is one of the drugs in which as the concentration in the blood increases, the effects on the central nervous system increase. And with alcohol the drug effect can continue to increase until loss of consciousness or death occurs.

Alcohol is also a good example of the relationship shown in Fig. 6-5, *B*. This graph shows how drugs can have a cumulative effect so that, with repeated doses of a drug, you get increasing effects. Usually **cumulative effects** occur when a second dose is given before the first dose has been deactivated. Similar to cumulative effects are those called **additive,** which refers to the fact that different drugs can act on the same system. Even though low doses may be taken of each drug,

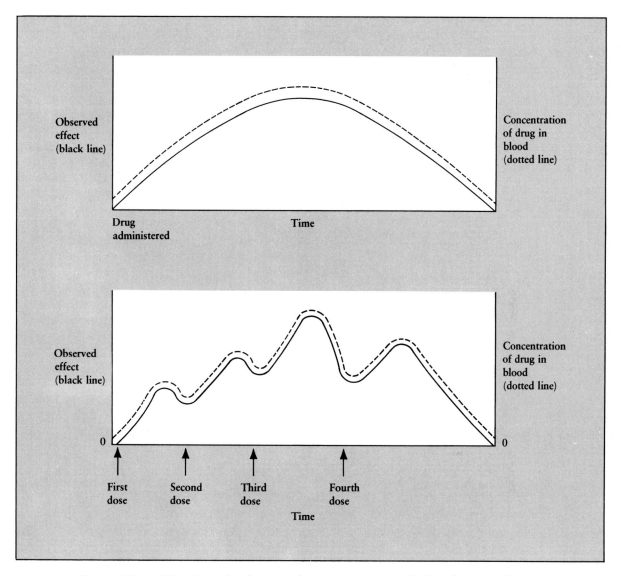

Figure 6-5. Possible relationship between drug concentration in body and measured effect of the drug.

together the effect may be the same as a high dose of a single drug. Alcohol and Valium are drugs that show additive effects—sometimes their combined depressant effects are lethal.

One of the important changes in manufacturing drugs is the development of time-release preparations. These compounds are prepared so that following oral use the active ingredient is released into the body over a 6- to 10-hour period. With a preparation of this type a large amount of the drug is initially made available for absorption, and then smaller amounts are released continuously for a long period. The initial amount of the drug is expected to be adequate to obtain the response desired and the gradual release thereafter is designed to maintain the same effective dose of the drug even though the drug is being continually deactivated. In terms of Fig. 6-4, a time-release preparation would aim at eliminating the unnecessarily high drug level at *C-D-E* while lengthening the *C-E* time interval. Unfortunately, up to this time there is no way to manufacture orally active drug products so that drugs can be retained in the gut and reliably released over more than 8 to 10 hours.

GETTING THE DRUG TO THE BRAIN

Tracing the path of drug molecules from their entry into the body to their site of action will sketch some of the factors that must then be detailed. Even though oral intake may be the simplest way to "take a drug," absorption from the gastrointestinal tract is the most complicated way to enter the bloodstream. Here the drug must first be taken up (absorbed), either by diffusion or by an active transport system, into cells lining the gastrointestinal tract. To be absorbed, the drug must have certain characteristics. It must be in solution, be lipid soluble, and be in a suitably high concentration. Not all drugs can fulfill these requirements.

Ease of movement of a drug across cell membranes is important in determining its activity. Since cell membranes have a substantial amount of lipid, drugs that are lipid soluble readily enter cells and move through capillary walls. Lipid solubility can be fairly well predicted from the chemical structure of the compound; one of the crucial factors is the degree of its ionization. As ionization goes up, lipid solubility goes down. Water solubility is increased with ionization, and this acts to keep the drug outside of cells. Because of this, ionized, water-soluble drugs, if absorbed at all, will remain extracellular, be *poorly* metabolized, and be readily filtered out by the kidneys and excreted. Physiologically active drugs and hormones that are not lipid soluble need a special transport system to cross cell membranes.

To move into the bloodstream clearly requires a series of complex steps in most cases. When a drug is delivered by injection directly into a vein, then it is in the circulation. When an intramuscular or subcutaneous injection is used, the drug enters the bloodstream by diffusion from one intercellular space where it was deposited. If taken orally, a drug must diffuse into capillaries from cells lining the stomach and intestines. Such movement occurs for some agents that move from an area of higher concentration into one of lower concentration. Other compounds cannot so easily cross the cell membrane, and an active transport system, which requires energy, is necessary.

Only three primary drug delivery methods are used with humans: oral, injection, and inhalation. **Inhalation** is used with volatile anesthetics and is also the drug delivery system used for smoking nicotine, marijuana, or crack cocaine. It is a very efficient way to deliver some drugs. Onset of drug effects is quite rapid because the capillary walls are very accessible in the lungs, and the drug thus enters the blood quickly. For psychoactive drugs, inhalation can produce more rapid effects than even intravenous administration. This is because of the patterns of blood circulation in the body. The blood leaving the lungs moves fairly directly to the brain, taking only 5 to 8 seconds to do so. By contrast, blood from the veins in the arm must return to the heart, then be pumped through the lungs before moving on to the brain, and this takes 10 to 15 seconds. Aerosol dispensers have been used to deliver some drugs via the lungs, but three considerations make inhalation of limited value. First, the material must not be irritating to the mucous membranes and lungs. Second, control of dose is more difficult than with the other drug delivery systems. Last, and perhaps the prime advantage for some drugs and disadvantage for others, there is no depot of drug in the body. This means that the drug must be given as long as the effect is desired, and also that when drug administration is stopped, the effect rapidly decreases.

Injection

Chemicals can be delivered with the hypodermic syringe directly into the bloodstream, deposited in a muscle mass, or under the upper layers of skin. With the **intravenous (IV) injection,** the drug starts in the bloodstream and does not have to be absorbed first, so the onset of action is faster than with any other means of injection. Another advantage is that very irritating material can be injected this way, since blood vessel walls are relatively insensitive. A major advantage frequently is that the material injected, the bolus, can deliver a high concentration of the drug to the brain tissues. The major disadvantage to IV injections is that the vein wall loses some of its strength and elasticity in the area round the injection site. If there are many injections into a small segment of a vein, as with an addict who must inject where he can see, the wall of that vein eventually collapses, and blood no longer moves through it, necessitating the use of another injection site.

Subcutaneous and intramuscular injections have similar characteristics, except that absorption is more rapid from intramuscular injection. Muscles have a better blood supply, and thus more area over which absorption can occur, than the underlying layers of the skin. Absorption is most rapid when the injection is into the deltoid muscle of the arm and least rapid when the injection is in the buttock. Intermediate between these two areas in speed of drug absorption is injection into the thigh. The rate of absorption can be varied in both subcutaneous and intramuscular injections by adding a vasodilator or vasoconstrictor to increase or decrease the area of absorption. When slow absorption is desired, a less soluble salt of the drug is frequently put in a suspension rather than a solution. Since only material in solution can be absorbed, the suspended material has to first go into solution. An additional factor influencing the rate of absorption is that movement into the blood depends on the concentration of the drug. As more drug enters the bloodstream, the concentration outside decreases, and so does the rate of absorption. One disadvantage to subcutaneous injection is that if the material injected is extremely irritating to the tissue, the skin around the site of injection may die and be shed. This method of injection is not very common in medical practice but has long been the kind of injection used by beginning narcotic users. Colloquially this is called "skin popping."

There is less chance of irritation if the injection is **intramuscular** because of the better blood supply and faster absorption. Another advantage is that larger volumes of material can be deposited in a muscle than can be injected subcutaneously.

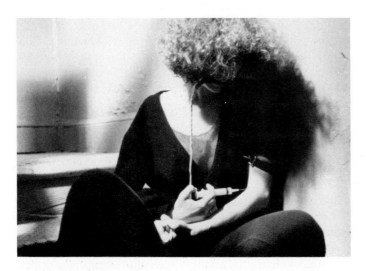

For many heroin users, the preferred route of administration is by intravenous injection.

Most of the "shots" given by a physician are intramuscular injections, and anyone who has had a series of tetanus shots may question the fact that this is one of the less irritating ways of injecting a drug.

Oral Administration

Most drugs begin their grand adventure in the body by entering through the mouth. Taking biologically active agents orally is unquestionably the oldest route of administration and probably the easiest. It is not necessarily the most effective, since a chemical in the digestive tract has to withstand the actions of the acid of the stomach and the digestive enzymes and not be deactivated by food before it is absorbed. As long as the drug remains in the digestive tract, it can be considered to be outside the body. The process of drug absorption from the stomach and intestines is a special area in and of itself.

A good example of the dangers in the gut for a drug is that which develops with tetracycline. This antibiotic readily combines with calcium and aluminum ions to form a compound that is poorly absorbed. If tetracycline is taken with milk (calcium ions) or with antacids (aluminum ions), blood levels will never be as high as if it were taken in the absence of these or similar agents.

Many factors compete in getting the drug through the cells lining the wall of the gastrointestinal tract on into the capillaries in the area. If taken in capsule or tablet form, the drug must first dissolve and, as a liquid, mix in the contents of the stomach and intestines. However, since as concentration goes down so does rate of absorption, the drug will be less rapidly absorbed when it is diluted by other material in the stomach.

Drugs are frequently prepared as salts, and they are weak electrolytes, since this ionization increases their water solubility, which is necessary for the compound to spread throughout the stomach. Once distributed, though, absorption is primarily of the nonionized form of the drug. If organic molecules are too strongly ionized, they will be poorly absorbed and pass through the intestines

to be excreted in the feces. Lipid-soluble and very small water-soluble molecules are readily absorbed into capillaries and go into the general circulation. There is very little drug absorption during the first 5 minutes, even on an empty stomach, but by 30 minutes most has been absorbed. After 6 to 8 hours, essentially all the drug will have been absorbed.

Once in the bloodstream the dangers of entering through the oral route are not over. The veins from the gut go first to the liver. If the drug is the type that is rapidly taken up and metabolized by the liver, very little may get into the general circulation. A drug may thus be ineffective by the oral route but very effective if given by injection.

The brain has a high lipid content and thus is a target organ for drugs with high lipid solubility. Drugs that act on the central nervous system are usually active when given orally because the lipid solubility of these agents increases their absorption from the gastrointestinal tract. Similarly, because of the high lipid solubility and low water solubility, these agents are usually not excreted but are reabsorbed in the kidneys and thus show cumulative effects.

As with all generalizations, there are exceptions. If a lipid-soluble drug is taken with a fatty meal, the drug will to some extent be taken up and remain in the food. Since fat is only slowly digested and the drug released, the rate of drug absorption is slowed. A slow absorption rate could possibly lower the drug concentration in the blood to an ineffective level.

Other Routes

Topical application of a drug to the skin is not widely used, because most drugs are not absorbed well through the skin. However, for some drugs this can be a method of providing a slow, steady absorption over many hours. For example, a skin patch that results in slow absorption of nicotine over an entire day has been tested. This patch has been found to help prevent relapse in people who have quit smoking. Application to mucous membranes may result in more rapid absorption than through the skin, because these membranes are moist and have a rich blood supply. Both rectal and vaginal suppositories take advantage of these characteristics, although suppositories are used only rarely. The mucous membranes of the nose are used by most cocaine users, who "snort" or "sniff" cocaine powder into the nose where it dissolves and is absorbed through the membranes.

Transport in Blood

When a drug enters the bloodstream, usually its molecules will attach to one of the protein molecules in the blood, albumin being the most common protein involved. The degree to which there is binding of drug molecules to plasma proteins is important in determining drug effects. As long as there is a protein-drug complex, the drug is inactive and also cannot leave the blood. In this condition, the drug is protected from inactivation by enzymes.

An equilibrium is established between the free (unbound) drug and the protein-bound forms of the drug in the bloodstream. As the unbound drug moves across capillary walls to sites of action, there is a release of protein-bound drug in order to maintain the bound-free equilibrium. Considerable variation exists among drugs in the affinity that the drug molecules have for establishing a bond with plasma proteins. Alcohol has a low affinity and thus exists in the bloodstream primarily as the unbound form. The salicylate ion has a high affinity, and about 80% is bound to blood proteins. Acetylsalicylic acid (aspirin), in contrast, has a low affinity. Differences in blood protein binding are reflected in their effects. Acetylsalicylic acid has a more rapid onset of action but a shorter duration than the salicylates.

Since differences exist in the affinity of drugs for the plasma proteins, one might expect that drugs with high affinity would displace drugs with weak protein bonds. And they do. This fact is important because it forms the basis for one kind of drug interaction. When a high-affinity drug is added to a situation where there is a weak-affinity drug already largely bound to the plasma proteins, the weak-affinity drug is displaced and will exist primarily as the unbound form. The increase in the unbound drug concentration helps move the drug out of the bloodstream to the sites of action faster and may be an important influence on the effect the drug has. At the very least, there will be a shortening of the duration of action.

Taking into consideration that only the free drug can leave the circulatory system, the same rules apply for leaving the bloodstream and entering cells as for leaving the stomach and moving into blood. Small, lipid-soluble, nonionized molecules diffuse through these cell membranes very easily, whereas larger lipid-insoluble, ionized molecules move more slowly, if at all, without an active transport system.

Blood-Brain Barrier

The brain is very different from the other parts of the body in terms of the ability of drugs to leave the blood and move to sites of action. A barrier acts to keep certain classes of compounds in the blood and away from brain neurons and glial cells. Thus some drugs act only on neurons outside the central nervous system, that is, those in the peripheral nervous system, whereas others may affect all neurons.

The blood-brain barrier is not well developed in infants; it reaches complete development only after 1 or 2 years of age in humans. Although the nature of this barrier is not well understood, several factors are known to contribute to the blood-brain barrier. One is the makeup of the capillaries in the brain. They are different from other capillaries in the body, since they contain no pores at all. Even small, water-soluble molecules cannot leave the capillaries in the brain; only lipid-soluble substances can pass the lipid capillary wall.

If a substance can move through the capillary wall, another barrier unique to the brain is met. About 85% of the capillaries are completely covered with glial cells; there is little extracellular space next to the blood vessel walls. With no pores and close contact between capillary walls and glial cells, almost certainly an active transport system is needed to move chemicals in and out of the brain. In fact, known transport systems exist for some naturally occurring agents.

A final note on the mystery of the blood-brain barrier is that cerebral trauma can disrupt the barrier and permit agents to enter that normally would be excluded. Concussion or cerebral infections frequently cause enough trauma to impair the effectiveness of this screen, which normally permits only selected chemicals to enter the brain.

Possible Mechanisms of Drug Actions

Many different types of actions will be suggested as ways in which drugs can affect physiochemical processes, neuron functioning, and ultimately thoughts, feelings, and other behaviors. It is possible for drugs to affect all neurons, but many exert actions only on certain presynaptic or postsynaptic processes in some neurons or only on presynaptic neurons. Since the action of a drug is usually quite specific—that is, it affects one phase of the information-processing systems—it is unusual to find a drug that has more than one of the actions to be discussed.

Effects on all neurons. Chemicals that have an effect on all neurons must do it by influencing some characteristic common to all neurons. One general characteristic of all neurons is the cell membrane. It is semipermeable, meaning that some agents can readily move in and out of the cell, but other chemicals are held inside or kept out under normal conditions. The semipermeable characteristic of the cell membrane is essential for the maintenance of an electric potential across the membrane. It is on this membrane that some drugs seem to act and, by influencing the permeability, alter the electrical characteristics of the neuron. Some drugs do affect the transport systems involved in maintaining the neuron, but usually the effect is a more general one.

Most of the general anesthetics have their effects on the central nervous system by a general influence on the cell membrane. Note that the agents which act in this way are depressants and that there are no drugs that increase the cell's activity level by affecting general membrane char-

acteristics. The classical view of alcohol's action on the nervous system is that it has effects similar to the general anesthetics through an influence on the neural membrane. However, recent evidence suggests that alcohol may have more specific postsynaptic effects.

Postsynaptic effects. Remember from Chapter 4 that the brain's natural neurotransmitters are released from one neuron, cross a small space called a *synapse,* and interact with receptors on the surface of another neuron. The neuron releasing the neurotransmitter at this synapse is call the *presynaptic* neuron, and the neuron that is acted on by the neurotransmitter is called the *postsynaptic* neuron. Psychoactive drugs may interact with these natural chemicals at various stages. Those drug actions that alter the synthesis, storage, or release of neurotransmitters are classified as presynaptic, because they act on the releasing (presynaptic) neuron. Drugs that act at the neurotransmitter receptors are said to have a postsynaptic effect, because the receptors are found on the postsynaptic neuron. By using a drug that operates only by mimicking or blocking one kind of neurotransmitter, a much greater precision of action occurs than when using a compound that acts on all neuron membranes.

Drugs that act postsynaptically can make contact with the electrical system only through the receptor itself or the enzymes that deactivate the neurotransmitters. When a drug acts at the receptor, it can have one of two possible effects. It may mimic the normal transmitter and thus cause either an increase or a decrease in the excitability of the postsynaptic neuron similar to that produced by the normal transmitter. Carbachol, which mimics the action of acetylcholine at many places in the nervous system, is a good example. It activates cholinergic fibers, but, unlike acetylcholine, it is not readily deactivated by cholinesterase. As a result, it continues to have its effect on the receptor for a longer period of time than would acetylcholine. Nicotine, at different types of receptors also mimics the action of acetycholine but initially activates and then depresses activity of the postsynaptic neuron.

Some drugs act as the postsynaptic receptor by

occupying the site but are unable to influence the electrical characteristics of the neuron. These agents are called "blockers," since by occupying the site, they prevent the normal neurotransmitters from having an effect postsynaptically. Atropine and scopolamine are well-known compounds that can occupy some cholinergic receptors and thus prevent acetylcholine from having an effect. These drugs act on both the central and the peripheral nervous systems, but if a methyl group is added to their chemical structure to form methylatropine and methylscopolamine, the effects are restricted to the peripheral nervous system. The addition of a methyl group prevents the chemical from crossing the blood-brain barrier and provides a valuable tool for research. By comparing the effects of atropine and methylatropine, important clues can be obtained to indicate which actions of the drug are mediated by the central and which by the peripheral nervous systems.

In cholinergic systems the enzyme responsible for deactivating acetylcholine is located postsynaptically. Any drug that prevents this deactivating enzyme, cholinesterase, from acting increases the duration of effect that acetylcholine can have. Cholinesterase inhibitors, then, prolong the effect of acetylcholine, which is released under normal physiological stimulation. Some drugs are short-acting, reversible inhibitors (such as physostigmine), whereas others (such as diisopropylfluorophosphate, DFP), because of the nature of their effect, are called "nonreversible" and may alter cholinesterase functioning for days.

Thus drugs acting postsynaptically can have major effects on the information-processing system. Emphasis here has been on the cholinergic system, since alteration of function in the adrenergic system is most readily accomplished presynaptically. It is quite difficult to do this with the cholinergic system.

Presynaptic effects. Drugs affect synaptic processes by acting on the presynaptic neuron in several major ways. One of these, blocking the release of the neurotransmitter, is of importance only in the peripheral nervous system and will not be discussed. The other ways of altering the effectiveness of the neurotransmitter are concerned with modifications of its synthesis, storage, uptake, and deactivation processes.

Synthesis of the endogenous neurotransmitters can be blocked by inhibiting one or more of the enzyme systems involved in the synthesis of the transmitter. Preventing or slowing new synthesis results in a depletion of the transmitter under normal functioning and thus a cessation, or at least an impairment, of synaptic transmission. Interestingly, one of the important enzymes involved in the synthesis of noradrenaline plays a similar role in building serotonin, so that inhibition of that enzyme causes a decrease in the level of both these neurotransmitters.

Some drugs effectively decrease the synthesis of the normal transmitters because they are better substrates for the synthesizing enzymes than the endogenous material. The synthesizing enzymes thus act on these drugs rather than on the normal substrate. Because the manufacturing system is not disrupted, complex molecules are built and stored in synaptic vesicles. Since these are not the same as the normal transmitters but are released in the same way as the real transmitters, these synthesized compounds are called *false transmitters*. The false transmitters are usually only moderately, if at all, effective in activating the receptor postsynaptically, so information processing is disrupted by their presence.

When a transmitter is manufactured, it must be stored in a vesicle to prevent its deactivation. Some drugs, such as reserpine, prevent the transmitter from being taken up into vesicles. The transmitter is then open to deactivation by the deactivating enzymes, but, more importantly, the vesicles are unable to collect and release the transmitter when the neuron fires. Obviously, without transmitter release, the synapse will cease to function normally.

An important distinction must be made between the cholinergic and the adrenergic systems of neurotransmission. The cholinergic system is relatively straightforward. Acetylcholine is synthesized presynaptically, bound in vesicles, released, bound to the postsynaptic receptor site (thereby changing the electrical characteristics of the dendrite), and deactivated postsynaptically. In adrenergic neurons there are a few differences. First, two classes of noradrenaline are accumulated presynaptically: a functional store, released in neural firing, and a bound (reserve) form of noradrenaline that is not used in synaptic functioning.

A second difference is that after the transmitter molecule has had its effect at the receptor, it is not usually deactivated but instead is released into the synaptic gap, where it is taken up by the presynaptic neuron and stored again in the vesicles of the functional pool of transmitter substance. Some clinically important drugs impair this reuptake, thereby increasing the noradrenaline level at the receptor. Cocaine and imipramine are drugs that have their primary action in this way.

Two enzymes are important in the breakdown of the adrenergic transmitters. One of these enzymes, monoamine oxidase (MAO), is also important for the deactivation of serotonin, so use of an MAO inhibitor results in an increase in brain levels of both noradrenaline, and serotonin. The increase in noradrenaline, however, is not an increase in the transmitter used in neurotransmission (the functional form) but rather an increase in the reserve form. Therefore there is no increase in the activity of the adrenergic transmitters after administration of an MAO inhibitor.

There are available inhibitors of the second deactivating enzyme, catechol-O-methyl transferase (COMT), but these have not been used clinically because COMT is relatively unimportant in deactivating noradrenaline. This COMT system seems to function both pre- and postsynaptically, although the postsynaptic site seems to be of primary importance.

A final presynaptic mechanism of drug action causes a continuous slow release of newly synthesized noradrenaline. Amphetamine, a stimulant, has this effect. This action (along with a second action of amphetamine, blocking noradrenaline reuptake) increases the activity of the adrenergic system and forms the biochemical basis for amphetamine's behavioral and experienced effects.

Summary of Drug Actions

Psychoactive drugs have their central effects only by changing the effectiveness and sensitivity of neurons and thus their information-processing characteristics. There are many ways in which this can be accomplished, however, and a brief survey of these methods gives only a hint of the total complexity. Some drugs act on cell membranes. Those compounds are usually nonspecific depressants, since they act similarly on all neurons. (Unique are the opiates, which have their effect through the special opiate receptor.) By interfering with synthesis, storage, release, or reuptake of a neurotransmitter or its combination with receptors, the efficiency of the synapse is modified and information transmission changed. By mimicking the transmitter at the receptor or preventing its normal deactivation, the postsynaptic neuron is changed electrically more than under normal conditions, and integrated functioning is also then impaired.

DRUG DEACTIVATION

Before a drug can cease to have an effect, one of two things must happen to it. It may be removed unchanged from the body, or it may be chemically changed so that it no longer has the same effect on the body and then is excreted from the body. Few drugs are eliminated unchanged from the body, although this is true of the volatile anesthetics. They are eliminated in the same way they enter the body—through the lungs. Alcohol, if taken in large amounts, may be partially eliminated unchanged through the lungs or sweat glands. Some drugs are excreted unchanged in the urine because they are filtered out, but not reabsorbed, in the kidneys. Even drugs that are primarily deactivated biochemically in the body are occasionally found unchanged in the urine.

Most drugs, though, are metabolized in some way in the body and the end products excreted in the urine. Drug metabolism aims primarily at two ends: inactivation of the agent and increasing the water solubility so that it can be excreted by way of the kidneys. Ionized, nonlipid-soluble substances are filtered out of the blood plasma in the kidneys and, instead of being reabsorbed, pass on into the urine for excretion. In part, the rate of excretion of ionizable substances depends on the pH of the urine, and this reflects to some extent an individual's diet.

Drug metabolism is not an incidental part of the study of drugs and drug actions. Since a drug continues to act until it is changed or excreted, the duration and intensity of a drug's action are determined to a great extent by the speed of its metabolism. Most drug metabolism is accomplished by special detoxification enzymes in the liver. The liver is *the* organ of drug metabolism; anything that interferes with the normal functioning of the liver will impair the drug-metabolizing capability of the body.

The enzymes in the liver that metabolize drugs are quite different from the enzymes in the body. These **liver microsomal enzymes** are unique in that they can use oxygen directly for metabolism, whereas most enzymes cannot. Another peculiar quality is that they are also specific for foreign compounds. They do not act on normally occuring chemicals (except steroids), but the reason for this specificity is still not clear. Interestingly, although these microsomal enzymes are specific for foreign chemicals, they are relatively nonspecific within that group of compounds. Therefore, they metabolize a number of very different drugs.

The activity of these microsomal enzymes can be affected by drugs. Over 200 drugs have been shown to increase the activity of these drug-metabolizing enzymes; meprobamate, phenobarbital, and DDT all have this effect in common. When the enzymes are stimulated, drug metabolism speeds up, and the duration of action of the drugs in the body is decreased. Some drug interactions may occur so that one drug may inhibit the metabolism of a second and thus increase the second's effects. Alcohol given after meprobamate decreases meprobamate's metabolism, thereby increasing the effects of meprobamate (perhaps sedation).

Some drugs are deactivated at their site of action and, in fact, some are altered in the process of having an action. Furthermore, some drugs are not active in the form in which they are administered but become quite active after they have been altered by the metabolizing process. Marijuana may be one example of this situation in that the metabolite is just as active as the original compound.

MECHANISMS OF TOLERANCE AND PHYSICAL DEPENDENCE

You should remember that the phenomena of tolerance and physical dependence have historically been associated with drug addiction. **Tolerance** refers to a situation in which repeated administration of the same dose of a drug results in gradually diminishing effects. Some effects of a drug may show tolerance, whereas others do not, since a drug may have multiple effects that may occur by different mechanisms. There are at least three different mechanisms by which a reduced drug response can come about.

Behavioral tolerance is the state in which an individual learns to compensate for an effect of the drug. In this type of tolerance the drug may continue to have the same chemical effect but with fewer behavioral responses. The drug user has learned to counteract or diminish the behavioral effects. Behavioral tolerance is a factor in the greater resistance of some alcoholics to the intoxicating effects of alcohol.

Tolerance can also develop because the drug is deactivated and/or excreted more rapidly on repeated administration. This is **drug disposition tolerance.** At least two mechanisms may be involved in this tolerance. Most drugs are deactivated by special enzymes in the liver. Some drugs, including alcohol, act to increase the number and activity of these enzymes. The greater the activity of the enzymes, the more rapidly drugs are deactivated. To maintain the same effect, more drug is needed, since the duration of action is briefer. But additional amounts of the drug increase the activity of the enzymes even further, and the circle continues. Some drugs are excreted unchanged in the urine. The rate at which excretion occurs varies with the acidity of the urine, as in the classic case of amphetamine. Here, too, intake of the drug is responsible for increasing the rate at which the drug is excreted, which requires even more drug intake to offset the more rapid loss—and so it goes. With a normal diet and moderate amphetamine intake, the urine stays slightly alkaline, so very little amphetamine is excreted unchanged. As the use of amphetamine increases and food intake goes down, the urine becomes more acid, and amphetamine is excreted more rapidly. More amphetamine is used, less food is eaten, the urine becomes more acid, and so on. Amphetamine is excreted 20 times as rapidly in urine with a pH of 5 as compared to a pH of 8.

Pharmacodynamic tolerance refers to the adjustment of the nervous tissue to the drug. Acting homeostatically, the nervous tissue counters the effect of the drug. As the drug is metabolized, additional drug is required, more is needed than originally, since now the drug must not only alter the normal activities of the nervous tissue but also the compensatory mechanisms used to counter the original effect of the drug. Ever-increasing amounts of the drug are thus necessary to maintain the status quo.

An understanding of one mechanism of physical dependency and the withdrawal symptoms provides a better understanding of this form of tolerance. Tolerance can occur with either stimulant or depressant drugs. When pharmacodynamic tolerance develops to a compound, it is accompanied by physical dependence on the drug. Physical dependence is said to have occurred when stopping the administration of the drug results in withdrawal symptoms. The actual symptoms observed vary from drug to drug but are based on the drug-induced changes in the activity of the cells involved.

The mechanisms underlying physical dependence are not well understood. One simple, and certainly incomplete, explanation is that when a depressant drug is administered, it sometimes has its effects by slowing the metabolic processes of cells. To offset this decrease in metabolic activity, the cells initiate processes that return cellular ac-

---

Issue: animal toxicity tests

There has been increasing interest in the welfare of laboratory animals, and this has resulted in improved standards for housing, veterinary care, and so on. Some animal welfare groups have suggested that many types of animal research should be stopped altogether, because the experiments are claimed to be either unnecessary or even misleading. The use of the LD50 test by drug companies in which the researchers estimate the dose of a drug required to kill half the animals (usually mice) has been a particular target. The groups have claimed that these tests are outmoded and that toxicity could be predicted from computer models or work on isolated cell cultures.

A pamphlet published by People for the Ethical Treatment of Animals (PETA), one of the most emotional animal rights groups, claims on the one hand that the laboratory animals are sensitive beings with "distinct personalities. Just like you and me..." but on the other hand that toxicity tests on animals are not relevant to humans. A specific case cited by PETA was thalidomide testing (see Chapter 3), which they claim "passed animal safety tests with flying colors" and later caused thousands of human deformities. Some critical points in that argument were, however, omitted. Thalidomide caused birth defects when taken during pregnancy. Otherwise, its human toxicity was quite low. Thalidomide was *not* tested on pregnant animals. If it had been, the birth defects would have been detected. And because of thalidomide, the laws were changed over 20 years ago to *require* that drugs to be used by humans during pregnancy first undergo testing in pregnant animals.

Admittedly, giving drugs to pregnant animals just to see if they produce birth defects or spontaneous abortions sounds cruel. Would you volunteer to be the first living animal to take a new drug whose toxicity had been estimated by a computer? Which pregnant humans should be the first?

---

tivity to normal even though the drug continues to have a depressant effect on the metabolism. Under this condition, to continue to affect the output of the cells, the amount of drug must be increased, since it now must depress not only the normal activity but also the compensation that homeostatic mechanisms brought into play. The necessary increase in drug dose to obtain the same effect is pharmacodynamic tolerance.

When administration of the drug is abruptly stopped, its depressant effect on cellular mechanisms disappears over a period of hours as the drug is deactivated. The compensatory mechanisms that were initiated in an attempt to maintain normal cellular functioning continue to act. Without the drug-induced depression to counteract them, the compensatory systems increase the activity of the cells above normal, and this cellular hyperactivity and hypersensitivity cause the withdrawal symptoms. Homeostatic processes again come into action, and, as the compensatory systems decrease their activity, the withdrawal symptoms subside.

Summary

Psychological processes can easily be influenced by nonspecific effects of drug administration and these placebo effects are themselves an interesting subject for research. One method of demonstrating that a drug has effects that are specifically related to its chemical makeup is to vary the dose of the drug and see if the response varies. The study of dose-response relationships also reveals interesting facts about individual variation and multiple drug effects.

That the effects of drugs also vary with time has important consequences for dosage scheduling. The time course of the effect of a drug can be examined in terms of the processes involved in getting the drug into the bloodstream, the mechanisms by which the drugs act when they reach the brain, and the processes involved in deactivating the drug and eliminating it from the system. Once those processes are understood, they aid us in understanding the several forms of drug tolerance and in understanding physical dependence.

REFERENCES

1. Wheatley D: Effects of doctors' and patients' attitudes and other factors on response to drugs. In Rickels K, editor: Nonspecific factors in drug therapy, Springfield, Il, 1968, Charles C Thomas, Publisher.
2. Fields HL and Levine JD: Biology of placebo analgesia, American Journal of Medicine 70(4):745, 1981.

Chapter 7

Stimulants

OBJECTIVES

After reading this chapter, you should be able to:

Discuss the history of the origin and early uses of both amphetamine and cocaine.

Describe the history and current status of illicit use of these drugs.

Explain how these drugs work in the brain and how their chemical structure relates to their mechanism of action.

State the previous and current medical uses of cocaine and amphetamine.

Discuss the potential for addiction and the possible toxic reactions to each of these drugs.

Stimulants are the drugs that can keep you going, both mentally and physically, when you should be tired. There have been lots of claims about the other things these drugs can do for (and to) people. Do they really make you smarter, faster, or stronger? Can they sober you up? Improve your sex life? Are they addicting?

We can divide the stimulants somewhat arbitrarily into three groups: the mild stimulants with caffeine-like actions are discussed in Chapter 11, and this chapter will cover **amphetamine** and **cocaine.** These two powerful stimulants produce effects virtually unknown to man until just over 100 years ago. Since the widespread introduction of cocaine into western Europe and the United States in the last century, there has always been a fair-sized minority of individuals committed to the regular recreational use of the stimulants, but neither cocaine nor amphetamine has ever achieved widespread social acceptance as a recreational drug. Although amphetamines have been available for only about 50 years, they enjoyed considerable medical use for several decades and a great deal is known about their pharmacology and their varied psychological effects. For that reason they will serve as our model for the stimulants.

AMPHETAMINES

History

Development and early uses. For centuries the Chinese have made a medicinal tea from herbs they call *ma huang,* which we classify in the genus Ephedra. The active ingredient in these herbs is called **ephedrine,** and it is used to dilate the bronchial passages in asthma patients. Bronchial dilation can be achieved by stimulating the sympathetic branch of the autonomic nervous system and that is exactly what ephedrine does (it is referred to as a **sympathomimetic** drug). Of course, this drug also has other effects related to its sympathetic nervous system stimulation, such as elevating the blood pressure. The story of the amphetamines starts with the search for a substitute for ephedrine. In the late 1920s researchers synthesized and studied the effects of the amphetamine salts and received the patent for them in 1932. The amphetamines came to be widely used and spawned a number of related drugs with similar properties as other companies vied for the stimulant dollar.

All major effects of amphetamine were discovered in the 1930s, although some of the uses developed later. Quite early it was shown that amphetamine was a potent dilator of the bronchial tubes and could be efficiently delivered through inhalation. To capitalize on this effect of amphetamine, the Benzedrine (brand name) inhaler was introduced as an over-the-counter product in 1932. Some of the early work with amphetamine showed that the drug would awaken anesthetized dogs. As one writer put it, amphetamine is the drug that won't let sleeping dogs lie!

Amphetamine, a CNS stimulant, seemed to be effective for the treatment of **narcolepsy** in 1935. Narcolepsy is a condition in which the individual spontaneously falls asleep, five, ten, fifty times a day (even outside the classroom). Amphetamine enables these patients to remain awake and function almost normally. In 1938, however, two narcolepsy patients treated with amphetamine developed acute paranoid psychotic reactions. The paranoid reaction to amphetamine has reappeared regularly and has been studied (as will be seen later).

In 1937 amphetamine became available as a prescription tablet, and a report appeared in the literature suggesting that amphetamine, a stimulant, was effective in reducing activity in hyperactive children. Two years later, in 1939, notice was taken of a report by amphetamine-treated narcolepsy patients that they were not hungry when taking the drug. This appetite-depressant effect became the major clinical use of amphetamine.

In 1939 amphetamine went to war. There were many reports that Germany was using stimulants to increase the efficiency of their soldiers. A 1944 report in the *Air Surgeon's Bulletin* titled "Benzedrine Alert"[1] stated that "this drug is the most satisfactory of any available in temporarily postponing sleep when desire to sleep endangers the security of a mission." Some studies were reported, including one in which

one hundred Marines were kept active continuously for sixty hours in range firing, a twenty-five mile forced march, a field problem, calisthenics, close-order drill, games, fatigue detail and bivouac alerts. Fifty men received seven 10-milligram tablets of benzedrine at six hour intervals following the first day's activity. Meanwhile, the other fifty were given placebo (milk sugar) tablets. None knew what he was receiving. Participating officers concluded that the benzedrine definitely "pepped up" the subjects, improved their morale, reduced sleepiness and increased confidence in shooting ability. . . . It was observed that men receiving benzedrine tended to lead the march, tolerate their sore feet and blisters more cheerfully, and remain wide awake during "breaks," whereas members of the control group had to be shaken to keep them from sleeping.[1]

Although the blisters may have been in a different place, it was the same desire for increased alertness that resulted in the order in 1969 to astronaut Gordon Cooper to take an amphetamine prior to his manual control of reentry of his space capsule.

These alerting characteristics had already been well noted by truck drivers and college students. A group of psychology students at the University of Minnesota began experimenting with various drugs in 1937 and found that amphetamine was ideal for "cramming." No real concern over nonmedical use of amphetamine developed until after World War II. A 1946 article, " On a Bender with Benzedrine," appeared in a popular national magazine. It made explicit just how one could get his amphetamine without a prescription.

> After I bought an inhaler, Hal worked off the perforated cap and pulled out the medicated paper, folded accordion-wise. . . . "Like this—" Hal took the innocent looking scrap of paper he had torn away and held it between thumb and finger. He alternately dunked and squeezed this paper into his glass of beer.[2]

Some of the medical and psychiatric problems that occurred when the contents of the Benzedrine inhaler were used were discussed in a 1947 report[3] in the *Journal of the American Medical Association* titled "Oral Use of Stimulants Obtained from Inhalers." Since each inhaler contained 250 mg of amphetamine, a considerable dose could be obtained if taken all at once. Of 15 army prisoners using inhaler amphetamine, hallucinations and the feeling that others were talking about them were observed in four. It was not until 1959 that the FDA banned the use of amphetamine in inhalers.

Abuse in other countries. The problems of the misuse of the amphetamines in the United States were actually minor compared to those experienced in some other countries. During World War II, amphetamines were widely used in Japan to maintain production on the home front and to keep the fighting men going. To reduce large stockpiles of methamphetamine after the war, the drug was sold without prescription, and the drug companies advertised them for "elimination of drowsiness and repletion of the spirit." As a result, "drug abuse grew as furiously as a storm."[4, p.138] Medical problems developed, and in 1948 stricter controls on amphetamine were put into force. Although they were tightened each year, the problem increased, and in 1954 the Japanese Pharmacists Association estimated that 1.5 million people (about 2% of the population) were abusing the amphetamines. In that year the penal provisions were strengthened and treatment facilities

expanded, and a year later, 1955, production was tightly controlled. A massive public education program in 1954 to 1955 completed the triad of treatment, education, and penalties. Although the Japanese government claimed to have "eliminated" the amphetamine abuse problem before 1960, there is evidence that a small number of people continued to abuse amphetamine. There were smaller "epidemics" of methamphetamine use in the 1970s and 1980s.[5]

In 1944 in Sweden, because such a large number of people were using oral amphetamines, prescriptions became tightly controlled. This resulted in a large drop in amphetamine sales and a decrease in the total number of individuals using the amphetamines. But those who were heavy abusers would not be denied, so there arose a black market in amphetamines and an amphetamine subculture similar to our American heroin subculture. To get the most value out of their expensive black-market amphetamine, some Swedes began injecting it intravenously. In addition, many began abusing other prescription amphetamine-like drugs, particularly phenmetrazine. In 1959 Sweden put tighter controls on phenmetrazine, and throughout the 1960s tried to stem the tide of smuggled amphetamines, phenmetrazine, and other stimulants coming from other countries. In 1965 they tried providing narcotics and stimulants to a small number of their users, but the plan was considered a failure and was dropped after 2 years. In 1968 Sweden banned virtually all prescriptions for amphetamines and related stimulants. The black market, of course, continued to flourish.[6]

The "speed scene" in the United States. In the United States, most of the misuse of amphetamines until the 1960s was through the legally manufactured and legally purchased oral preparation. In 1963 the AMA Council on Drugs stated "At this time, compulsive abuse of the amphetamines is a small problem. . . ."[7] But at exactly this time, trouble was brewing in California.

It is difficult to pinpoint exactly when intravenous IV abuse of the amphetamines began in the United States, but it was probably among users of intravenous heroin and cocaine. In the 1920s and 1930s, when IV use of those drugs was spreading among the drug subculture, the combination of heroin and cocaine injected together was known as the "speedball," presumably because the cocaine rush or flash occurs rapidly after injection, thus speeding up the high. So, on the streets, one name for cocaine was "speed." When the amphetamines became so widely available after World War II, some of these enterprising individuals discovered that they could get an effect similar to that of cocaine if they injected amphetamine along with the heroin. Thus slowly and out of the awareness of most Americans, the amphetamines came to be known as **speed** by that small drug underground that used IV mixtures of heroin and other drugs. By the 1960s amphetamines became so widely available at such a low price that more IV drug users were using them, either in combination with heroin or alone. Although they were prescription drugs, it was not difficult to obtain a prescription to treat depression or obesity.

The most desired drug on the streets was methamphetamine, which was available in liquid form in ampules for injection. Hospital emergency rooms sometimes used this drug to stimulate respiration in patients suffering from overdoses of sleeping pills (no longer considered an appropriate treatment), and physicians also used injectable amphetamines intramuscularly to treat obesity. In the San Francisco Bay area, reports appeared in the early 1960s of apparently unscrupulous "fat doctors" who had large numbers of patients coming in regularly for no treatment other than an injection of methamphetamine.

Because some of the local heroin addicts would inject amphetamines alone when they could not obtain heroin, some physicians also felt that methamphetamine could serve as a legal substitute for heroin and thus be a form of treatment. In those days amphetamines were not considered to be addicting, so these physicians were quite free with their prescriptions.[6] Reports of those abuses led to legislation, including federal regulation of amphetamines within the new concept of dangerous drugs in the 1965 law. Unfortunately, all the publicity associated with these revelations and the ensuing legislation fell on the ears of young people whose identity as a generation was defined largely by experimentation with drugs their parents and government told them were dangerous. To the Haight-Ashbury district of San Francisco came the flower children, to sit in Golden Gate Park, smoke marijuana, take LSD, and discuss peace, love, and the brotherhood of man. They moved in next door to the old, established drug subculture in which IV drug use was endemic. That mixture resulted in the speed scene and young people who became dependent on IV amphetamines. Although in historical perspective the speed scene of the late 1960s was relatively short-lived and only a few people were directly involved, it was the focus of a great deal of national concern, and it helped to change the way the medical profession and the society at large viewed these drugs that had been so widely used.

As amphetamine use began to be considered abuse, physicians prescribed less and less of the drugs. Their new legal status as dangerous drugs put restrictions on prescriptions and refills, and in the 1970s there were limits placed on the total amount of these drugs that could be manufactured. Thus, within less than a decade, amphetamines went from widely used and accepted pharmaceuticals to less widely used, tightly restricted drugs associated in the public mind with drug abuse.

As controls tightened on legally manufactured amphetamines, there were at least three reactions that continue to affect the current drug scene. One reaction was that a market began to develop for so-called "look-alike" pills, which are legal, milder stimulants (usually caffeine) packaged in tablets and capsules that are virtually identical in color, shape, and markings to prescription amphetamines. Later the makers of look-alikes began to expand the variety of shapes and sizes to attract a wider market. Because these pills contain legally available, over-the-counter ingredients, their sellers could not be prosecuted. By the early 1980s these products were so popular that the odds were good that if someone bought "speed" pills from a street dealer they were actually getting look-alikes. The national high school survey had to apply a correction factor to their data to account for these look-alikes and get a more accurate measure of actual amphetamine use. The FDA began to crack down on manufacturers and distributors of pills containing large amounts of caffeine or mixtures of caffeine and other legal stimulants, and states passed regulations making it illegal to distribute any substance that is misrepresented to be a controlled substance.

Another reaction to limited amphetamine availability was an increase in the number of illicit laboratories making methamphetamine, which acquired the name "crank." Although both the process for making methamphetamine and the name "crank" have been around on the streets since the 1960s, by the late 1980s the increasing number of confiscations by authorities led some to wonder if this would be the next drug "fad."[8]

The reduced availability of legally manufactured amphetamines had one more important effect. As the price went up and the quality of the available speed became more questionable, the drug subculture began, slowly and without fanfare, to rekindle its interest in a more "natural," reportedly less dangerous stimulant—cocaine. By 1970, federal agents in Miami reported "the traffic in cocaine is growing by leaps and bounds."[6] And as we now know, they hadn't seen anything yet.

Basic Pharmacology and Mechanism of Action

Chemical structures. Take a couple of minutes to look at Fig. 7-1. We're not trying to make medicinal chemists out of anyone, but we want you to see some similarities in the structures of amphetamines and related drugs. First, note the similarity between the molecular structures of the catecholamine neurotransmitters (dopamine and norepinephrine) and the basic amphetamine molecule. It does appear that amphetamine produces its effects because it is recognized as one of these catecholamines at many sites in both the central

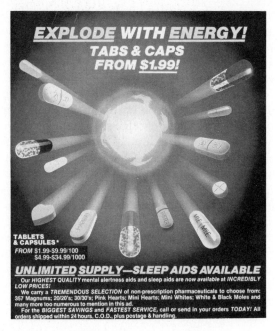

These tablets and capsules contain caffeine, ephedrine, or PPA, but many look like prescription amphetamine products. They are sometimes resold on the street as speed by unscrupulous individuals.

and the peripheral nervous systems. The amphetamine molecule has both "left-handed" and "right-handed" forms (*l* and *d* forms). The original Benzedrine was an equal mixture of both forms. The *d* form is several times more potent in its CNS effects, however, and in 1945 *d*-amphetamine was first marketed as Dexedrine for use as an appetite suppressant. Next, look at the methamphetamine molecule, which simply has a methyl group added to the basic amphetamine structure. This methyl group seems to make the molecule cross the blood-brain barrier more readily and thus further increases the CNS potency. (If more of the molecules get into the brain, then fewer total molecules have to be given.)

We're not through with the molecules yet! Next, look at the structures for ephedrine, the old Chinese remedy that is still used to treat asthma, and for phenylpropanolamine (PPA). PPA is an ingredient in all over-the-counter (OTC) weight

Dopamine

Norepinephrine

Amphetamine

Methamphetamine

Ephedrine

Phenylpropanolamine

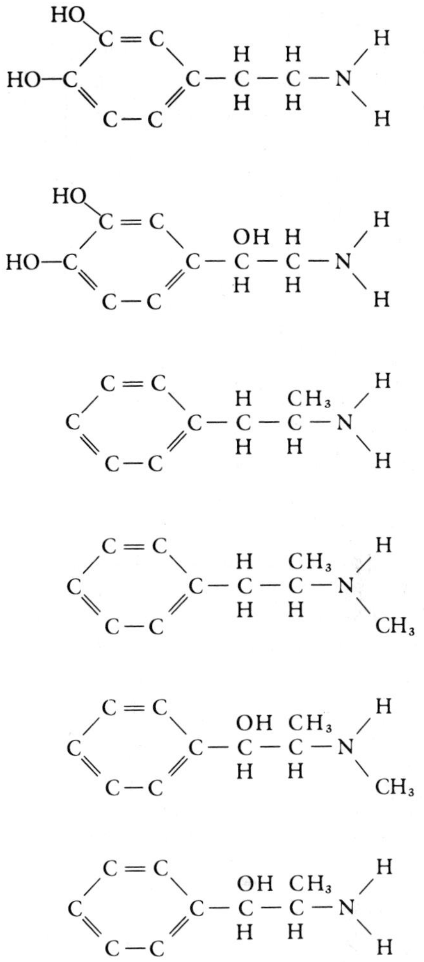

Figure 7-1. Molecular structures of stimulants.

control preparations (see Chapter 12) and in many of the look-alikes mentioned earlier. Both of these molecules have a structural addition that makes them not cross the blood-brain barrier as well, and therefore they produce peripheral effects without as much CNS effectiveness.

Effects on catecholamine systems. The stimulant types of amphetamine have at least two effects on catecholamine (dopamine and norepinephrine) synapses. The presynaptic storage mechanism recognizes and tries to store amphetamine molecules, which results in the leakage of catecholamines into the synapse, where they can interact with the receptor. Second and probably less important, is the ability of amphetamine molecules to occupy the reuptake mechanism so that catecholamines released into the synapse are not taken back up as readily and therefore stay longer in the synapse. Both of these mechanisms produce increased stimulation of the dopamine and norepinephrine receptors.

Exactly which of amphetamine's effects are related to which neurotransmitter is controversial, but current theories can be summarized. Stimulation of the norepinephrine neurons arising from the locus ceruleus would produce the alerting and antifatigue effects, and stimulation of the meso-limbic dopamine pathway would produce euphoria and increased motor activity. Higher doses would activate the nigrostriatal dopamine pathway to produce stereotyped, repetitive movements. Too much activity in the mesolimbic system could be responsible for the paranoid psychotic reaction seen with very high doses.

Absorption and elimination. Amphetamines may be taken by a variety of routes. When taken orally, the peak effects are found 2 to 3 hours after ingestion. The half-life is 10 to 12 hours, so that a fairly stable blood level can be achieved with oral administration at 4- to 6-hour intervals, and virtually complete elimination of the drug would occur within 2 days after the last dose. With IV injection, peak effects are much more rapid. With higher doses a tachyphylaxis (rapid tolerance) may be seen. Since amphetamine produces its effects largely by displacing the catecholamine transmitters from their storage sites, with large doses the catecholamines may be sufficiently depleted so that another dose within a few hours may not be able to displace as much catecholamine and a reduced effect will be obtained.

Beneficial Uses

Previous medical uses. During the 1950s and early 1960s, amphetamines were prescribed for depression and feelings of fatigue. If we look at an individual's mood as potentially ranging from very depressed, up through sadness into a normal range, and then into euphoria and finally an excited, manic area (Fig. 7-2), we can better understand amphetamine's effects on mood. Note that the person who is seriously depressed is not just sad; he or she feels helpless and hopeless with no energy and may think of suicide or of death in general. Amphetamines are capable of temporarily moving the mood up the scale, so that a depressed person may, for a few hours, move into a normal range. The problem is that when the

drug wears off, that person doesn't stay "up." The mood drops, often below the predrug level. To keep the mood up, one needs to keep taking amphetamine. Amphetamine does reduce appetite and interfere with sleep, two problems that many depressed people already have. Some physicians prescribed sleeping pills for nighttime. In any case, these patients often went for a daily "ride" on an emotional roller coaster, waking up depressed and taking a pill to get going in the morning, and either coming off the drug or taking a "downer" at night. As we shall see in Chapter 15, other treatments are now used for depression and amphetamines are not recommended.

Probably the most common medical use for the amphetamines through the mid-1960s was weight control. It is clear that amphetamine can reduce food intake and body weight. This is obvious in people of normal or below-average weight who take the drug for other reasons and especially obvious in those who have built up to taking large doses. Studies on rats show without doubt that amphetamine reduces food intake and body weight compared to rats given placebo. With one third of Americans overweight, there is a vast market for a pill that would help us lose weight. For years, the common medical response was some form of amphetamine or related sympathomimetic stimulant. Physicians dispensed prescriptions for pills and some gave injections, and some people did lose some weight. But in the 1960s when people began to view the amphetamines with greater concern, it was also clear that some people who had begun taking small doses for weight control had developed large dependencies and many people who took these stimulants regularly were still overweight. People began to weigh the costs vs the benefits and eventually reached some new conclusions.

To understand the role of these drugs in weight control, let's imagine a typical experiment to test the value of amphetamine in treating obesity. Patients are selected for the study who meet some criterion for overweight. All are brought to a hospital or clinic where they are weighed, interviewed, given physical exams, and given a diet to

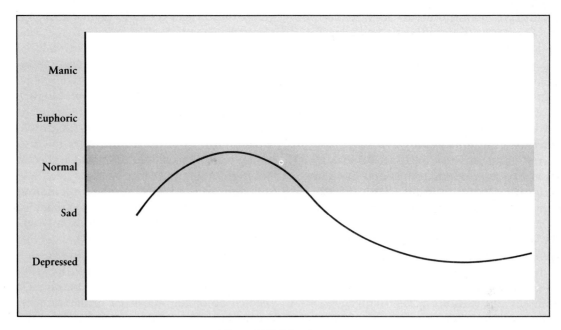

Figure 7-2. Mood ranges.

follow. Half are given amphetamine and half a placebo in a double-blind design. Each week the patients return to the hospital where they are interviewed, weighed, and given their supply of drug for the next week. After 2 months the drug code is broken and the amount of weight loss in each group is calculated. This type of study virtually always finds that both groups lose weight, mostly in the first 2 or 3 weeks. After that, the weight loss is much slower. This initial weight loss by both groups probably is a result of beginning a new diet and being involved in a medical study in which they know they will be weighed each week. Over the first 2 or 3 weeks the amphetamine group will lose a little more weight than the placebo group. The difference between the two groups after 2 or 3 weeks might be about 2 or 3 pounds, which is statistically significant but probably not medically significant. The interesting thing is that as the study goes on, the gap doesn't widen, but stays about the same. In other words, the amphetamine effect is real but small and limited in duration in such studies. Even with mod-

erate dose increases, 4 to 6 weeks seems to be the limit before tolerance occurs to this effect. Increasing to high doses might produce some further effect, but these experiments don't allow that and it would be foolhardy as a treatment approach. The use of amphetamines for weight reduction came under attack from various sources, and the FDA in 1970 restricted the legal use of amphetamines to three types of conditions: narcolepsy, hyperkinetic behavior, and short-term weight reduction programs.[9]

Current medical uses. Although the NAS/NRC again recommended in 1972 that the prescription antiappetite drugs, including amphetamine, should stay on the market, they insisted that "the clinically trivial contribution of these drugs to the overall weight reduction is properly emphasized."[10] In 1989, preparations of *d*-amphetamine and methamphetamine were still available by prescription for short-term weight loss, as were the other sympathomimetics diethylpropion, phentermine, phenmetrazine, phendimetrazine, and some related but slightly different drugs, fenfluramine and mazindol. The package insert for each of these drugs includes the following FDA mandated statements: "The natural history of obesity is measured in years, whereas most studies cited are restricted to a few weeks duration; thus, the total impact of drug induced weight loss over that of diet alone must be considered clinically limited. . . .(Drug name) is indicated in the management of exogenous obesity as a short-term (a few weeks) adjunct in a regimen of weight reduction based on caloric restriction. The limited usefulness of agents of this class. . . must be weighed against possible risk factors inherent in their use. . . ."[11]

So, although the companies have succeeded in keeping these drugs on the market and in allowing the prescribing physician to decide what constitutes a "few weeks," the perspective of the medical community has been drastically changed regarding these drugs. Prescriptions for amphetamines dropped from 24.5 million in the peak year of 1965 to 3.3 million by 1978. However, sales of the OTC sympathomimetic phenylpropanolamine for weight reduction have increased dramatically. This drug is discussed in Chapter 12.

Narcolepsy. Narcolepsy is a sleep disorder in which individuals do not sleep normally at night and in the daytime experience uncontrollable episodes of muscular weakness and falling asleep. Although there has been increased interest in sleep disorders in general and sleep disorder clinics are now associated with almost every major medical center in the United States, the best available treatment still seems to be to keep the patient awake during the day with amphetamine or methylphenidate, a related stimulant. There is no doubt that some individuals who receive stimulants from a general practitioner under the diagnosis of narcolepsy are actually suffering from some other sleep disorder or from depression, which often includes disruptions of normal sleep patterns. Accurate diagnosis of narcolepsy requires checking in to a sleep disorder clinic for some sleep recordings of an electroencephalogram (EEG). However, for these recordings to be ac-

curate, the programs usually require a 2 to 3 week drug-free period.

Hyperactive children. Even though it has been more than 50 years since the first report that amphetamine could reduce activity levels in hyperactive children, and even though hundreds of thousands of children are currently being treated with stimulant drugs for this problem, we still have controversy over the nature of the disorder being treated, we still don't understand what the drugs are doing to reduce hyperactivity, and we still don't have a widely accepted solution to the apparent paradox: what's a "stimulant" drug doing producing what appears to be a "calming" effect?

The disorder itself was referred to as childhood hyperactivity for many years, and the children who received that label were the ones who seemed absolutely incapable of sitting still and paying attention in class. Many of these children had normal or even above average IQ scores, yet were failing to learn. During the 1960s it was proposed that lead toxicity or early oxygen deprivation might be the cause of a small amount of brain damage. Pointing out that many of these children exhibit "soft" neurological signs (impairments in coordination or other tests that are not localizable to a particular brain area), the term "minimal brain dysfunction" (MBD) became popular. By 1980 there was a feeling that there had been too much focus on activity levels, and that the basic disorder was a deficit in attention, which usually but not always was accompanied by hyperactivity. Thus, the **Diagnostic and Statistical Manual** of the American Psychiatric Association used the term "attention deficit disorder." However, the latest revision of that manual, the 1987 **DSM-III-R** recognizes the strong relationship between attention deficit and hyperactive behavior by using the term "attention-deficit hyperactivity disorder" (ADHD).[12] The criteria used to diagnose this disorder are listed in the shaded box.

The cause (or causes) of the disorder is not known. One idea that attracted a lot of attention suggested that it was the additives in the foods we

Diagnostic criteria for attention-deficit hyperactivity disorder

---

Diagnostic criteria for attention-deficit hyperactivity disorder

Note: Consider a criterion met only if the behavior is considerably more frequent than that of most people of the same mental age.

A. A disturbance of at least six months during which at least eight of the following are present:

  (1) often fidgets with hands or feet or squirms in seat (in adolescents, may be limited to subjective feelings of restlessness)

  (2) has difficulty remaining seated when required to do so

  (3) is easily distracted by extraneous stimuli

  (4) has difficulty awaiting turn in games or group situations

  (5) often blurts out answers to questions before they have been completed

  (6) has difficulty following through on instructions from others (not due to oppositional behavior or failure of comprehension), e.g., fails to finish chores

  (7) has difficulty sustaining attention in tasks or play activities

  (8) often shifts from one uncompleted activity to another

  (9) has difficulty playing quietly

  (10) often talks excessively

  (11) often interrupts or intrudes on others, e.g., butts into other children's games

  (12) often does not seem to listen to what is being said to him or her

  (13) often loses things necessary to tasks or activities at school or at home (e.g., toys, pencils, books, assignments)

  (14) often engages in physically dangerous activities without considering possible consequences (not for the purpose of thrill-seeking), e.g., runs into street without looking

Note: The above items are listed in descending order of discriminating power based on data from a national field trial of the DSM-III-R criteria for Disruptive Behavior Disorders.

B. Onset before the age of seven.

C. Does not meet the criteria for a Pervasive Developmental Disorder.

---

eat that were the basis for ADHD with hyperactivity. Many studies were done and in 1982 a blue ribbon panel handed down the verdict on diets without food additives: ". . . there is no firm evidence that the diets work. Claims that the diets produce dramatic effects simply did not hold up in well-designed clinical trials."[13,p.958]

Some hyperactive children have histories of difficult births or contracting encephalitis when very young. Some reports indicate a higher incidence of abnormal EEGs in these children than in nonADHD children. There are as many children, however, who do not show abnormal EEGs or medical histories, so the importance of these factors is not clear. There is also no evidence that a large percentage are mentally retarded, although school achievement is usually quite poor. Some believe[14] that these ADHD children suffer only from a maturational lag: they are exhibiting behavior that is typical of children several years younger.

It is interesting that the disorder is at least three times more common in boys than in girls, though that fact hasn't helped us to understand its cause. Also, in many cases the problems seem to be reduced once the child reaches puberty. It was once thought that this was an absolute developmental change, but now we recognize that as many as one third of the children continue to have hyperactivity problems even into adulthood, and there are arguments as to whether the disorder fades in the other children or just changes its character to something such as antisocial personality disorder.[12]

Regardless of the cause, there is clear evidence of the beneficial effect of both amphetamine and methylphenidate (Ritalin). Methylphenidate is now considered the drug of choice for treating ADHD. It is a milder stimulant than amphetamine, with a potency between the amphetamines and caffeine. Why either type of stimulant drug should work is still not known. One theory that has been around for years is worth considering, even if it is has been difficult to test experimentally: assume that the ADHD child is receiving inadequate sensory input to the CNS, and his noisiness, rocking movements, running, and crashing into things are an effort to obtain sensory stimulation. The stimulant drugs may arouse the CNS partly by allowing sensory information more direct access to the thalamus and cerebral cortex. Thus, children treated with stimulants could better attend to environmental stimuli and would have less need for hyperactivity and noisiness. While this theory is plausible, please understand that there are other theories and that none has yet been widely accepted.

One of the more disturbing side effects of stimulant therapy is a suppression of height and weight increases during drug treatment.[14] Amphetamine has the greater effect compared to equally effective but higher daily doses of methylphenidate. Amphetamine reduced the average growth to 70% to 80% of normal, whereas methylphenidate reduced growth to 80% to 90% of normal. In children in whom drug treatment was stopped over the summer vacation, there was a rebound and a growth spurt of 15% to 68% greater than the growth rate shown by nondrug-using children. The indications are that this accelerated rate of growth diminishes after 2 to 3 months.

The seemingly indiscriminate but medically prescribed use of stimulant drugs to influence the behavior of school-age children has evoked much social protest and commentary. After widespread publicity about the use of amphetamines for this purpose in the late 1960s, coinciding with public reaction against amphetamine use, there was a decline in stimulant prescriptions for children and a switch to methylphenidate. During the 1970s and 1980s there has apparently been a steady increase in the proportion of school children receiving stimulant medication for hyperactivity, and it is now estimated that over 750,000 public school children are currently receiving such treatment in the United States. What is not clear is whether this increase represents more awareness of the disorder and its proper treatment or whether more children are being given the medication inappropriately.[15,16] It should be empha-

sized that whenever drug therapy is used, it should be only one component of an effective treatment program.

Other claimed benefits. In the 1960s there were a number of studies that seemed to show rats learned faster and performed better if they were given amphetamine or some other stimulant. Abbott Laboratories obtained a patent for the stimulant they named Cylert, which they were testing as a "smart pill." A great deal of animal and human research has since been done on the role of stimulants in improving mental performance, and it is now possible to summarize the ideas that have come from that work. One way to represent the effects of stimulants can be seen in Fig. 7-3, which schematically relates degree of mental performance to the arousal level of the CNS. At low levels of arousal, such as when the individual is sleepy, performance suffers. Increasing the arousal level into the normal range with a stimulant could then improve performance. At the very high end of the arousal scale the person is so maniacal or so involved in repetitive, stereotyped behavior that performance suffers, even on the simplest of tasks. In the region of the graph labeled "excited," it can be seen that some simple tasks may be improved above normal levels, but complex or difficult tasks are disrupted because of difficulty in concentrating, controlling attention, and making careful decisions. It has been suggested, for example, that a professional quarterback might benefit from a low dose of amphetamine to give him the energy to get through the game and to keep him alert, whereas a defensive tackle would benefit from a larger dose, not just because they tend to be larger people but because the "manic high" resulting from the higher dose would give them a sort of mindless intensity that could be useful to them but disruptive of the quarterback's decision-making ability.[17]

From the schematic we can see that anyone trying to improve his or her mental performance level with amphetamines or other stimulants is taking a chance. Depending on the type of task, predrug performance level, and dose, one might obtain improvement or disruption. A small dose

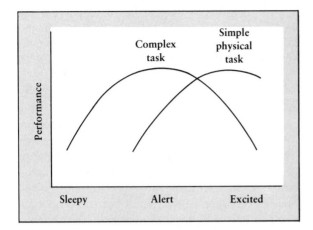

Figure 7-3. Effects of stimulants on performance.

could be beneficial to a tired person driving alone at night on a deserted interstate highway, but would probably only add to the confusion of a school bus driver trying to negotiate a Los Angeles freeway interchange at 7:30 AM with a load of noisy students. As for the students themselves, a small dose of a stimulant might help keep one awake to study when he or she should be sleeping, but a larger dose? There's an ancient piece of college folklore (at least 20 years old) that probably never really happened but has the ring of possible truth to it. It involves a student who stayed awake for days studying with the help of amphetamines, went into a final exam "wired up," wrote feverishly and eloquently for 2 hours, and only later when he received an "F" saw that he had written the entire answer on one line, using it over and over so that it was solid black and the rest of the paper was blank.

Athletics

An excellent review of the literature on amphetamine and athletic performance[18] confirmed what an earlier extensive laboratory study had indicated[19]; that under some conditions the use of amphetamine at an appropriate dose can produce slight improvements in athletic performance. The effects are so small as to be meaningless for most

athletes, but at the highest levels of competition even a one or two percent improvement can mean the difference between winning a medal or coming in sixth. The temptation has been strong for athletes to use amphetamines and other stimulants to enhance their performances, and this topic is discussed in more detail in Chapter 19.

Causes for Concern

Dependence potential. For years experts argued about whether the amphetamines were truly "addicting." As we saw in Chapter 2, for many years most experts in this field equated addiction with physical dependence. Since amphetamine withdrawal didn't produce the kinds of obvious physical symptoms seen with heroin or barbiturate withdrawal, most people decided that amphetamine did not produce physical dependence. Yet there is evidence that repeated use of high doses of amphetamine produces a consistent set of withdrawal symptoms: several hours after the last dose the user "crashes," mood and energy level drop dramatically, and the user may then sleep for 24 or more hours. On awakening, the user is in a depressed mood that may last for days. During this time the individual feels helpless, worthless, and as though they could "just sit there and die." Talk of death is common during this period. Of course, taking amphetamine again seems the most rapid way to overcome this mood and get high again.

It has been known for years that amphetamines could be habit forming, that is, produce psychological dependence. Until a few years ago that was not considered to be too important. Amphetamine was even considered by some to be a so-called soft drug. It was available by prescription, it produced only psychological dependence, and most users did not develop even psychological dependence. The idea seemed to be that while it could be habit forming in some individuals, its potential for abuse was limited. Now we realize that important factors, such as dose and route of administration, were not being taken into account. Small doses (5 or 10 mg) taken orally by people acting under their physician's orders for some purpose other than achieving a high rarely resulted in dependence. A larger dose injected intravenously for the purpose of getting high results in very rapid development of strong psychological dependence. Taken in this way, amphetamine is as addicting as any drug we know. Animal studies reveal that rats or monkeys will quickly learn to press a lever that produces intravenous injections of amphetamine. If required to do so an animal will press hundreds of times for a single injection.[20]

Toxicity potential. During the period of amphetamine intoxication with above-normal doses, what dangers are caused by the altered behavior patterns? As we have seen, even at moderately high oral doses there may be impairments in complex discrimination or decision making. At higher doses there is a tendency to be easily panicked and to become suspicious to the point of paranoia. Because of this, the "speed freak" is a very unreliable person. Stores from the Haight-Ashbury "speed scene" point out that these people were often unable to remain calm enough to pass a faked prescription, but would panic and run out of the pharmacy. Of greater concern was the reported hostility and violence associated with amphetamine use.

Amphetamine, and other stimulants to some extent, has two effects that suggest a relationship to violent behavior. Even low doses increase activity level, and, as the dose increases, there is an increase in feelings of power and capability. Large doses used chronically or an abrupt increase in the amount of amphetamine used frequently causes a paranoid, psychotic reaction. This latter behavior is primarily associated with the injection of amphetamine—speed freaks.

One authority has stated:

From all evidence, amphetamines do tend to set up conditions in which violent behavior is more likely to occur than would be the case had the individual not used it. Suspiciousness and hyperactivity may combine to induce precipitous and unwarranted assaultive behavior. Under the influence of amphetamines, lability of mood is common, the user abruptly shifting from warmly congenial to furiously hostile moods for the most trivial of reasons.[21,p.16]

There were multiple reports of the association of amphetamine use and violence and aggression in the late 1960s and early 1970s. In almost every case large amounts of amphetamines were used, which resulted in suspicious ideas and hostile behavior. This type of emotional arousal can easily explode into violence and homicide if the appropriate conditions are met. Users of large amounts of amphetamine (especially if taken by injection) are good people to stay away from.

One study[22] of 13 amphetamine abusers who committed murder while under the influence of amphetamine reported that seven were paranoid at the time of the killing, three were impulsive, and two panicked during a robbery. This triad of paranoid ideas, impulsive behavior, and hypersensitivity is directly related to the pharmacological actions of the amphetamines, no matter what the personality of the user is in the absence of the drug.

A review of the world literature on amphetamine use and crime and/or violence de-emphasized the large-dose users and the resulting paranoia predisposing to hostility and violence. It was then possible for the author to generalize and conclude, truthfully, that "the use of amphetamine per se is not particularly conducive to violence."[23] There is clear evidence, though, that high doses of amphetamine result in paranoid suspiciousness, and that, coupled with hyperactivity and hypersensitivity, makes aggressive behavior very probable.

Whereas the amount of demonstrated violence because of amphetamine use cannot compare to that resulting from alcohol use, it is still a matter of concern, especially when the two are combined. Stimulants and alcohol do not counteract one another in most behavioral effects, and in the case of violence they combine to form an especially explosive mixture.

The development of a paranoid psychosis has been long known to be one of the effects of sustained cocaine use. The first amphetamine psychosis was described in 1938, but little attention was given this syndrome until the late 1950s. There have been many suggestions as to the reason for the psychosis: that heavy methamphetamine users have schizoid personalities or that the psychosis is really caused by sleep deprivation, particularly dream-sleep deprivation. The question of the basis for the amphetamine psychosis was resolved by the demonstration that it could be elicited in the laboratory in individuals who clearly were not prepsychotic and who did not experience great sleep deprivation. It seems, then, that the paranoid psychosis following high dose intravenous use of amphetamine is primarily the result of the drug and not the personality predisposition of the user.

The amphetamine psychosis has been studied many times, both in and out of the laboratory. One researcher[24] commented about his results:

The psychosis was the facsimile of the disorder observed during drug abuse—a schizophrenic-like state of paranoia in a setting of clear consciousness accompanied by auditory or visual hallucinations, or both, but without thought disorder . . . in some cases the onset of the psychosis was sudden and occurred within one hour of commencing the intravenous injection. . . .

There is evidence that the paranoid psychosis results from dopaminergic stimulation, probably in the mesolimbic system.

There is another behavior induced by high doses of amphetamine: compulsive and repetitive actions. The behavior may be acceptable (the individual may compulsively clean a room over and over) or it may be bizarre (one student spent a night counting cornflakes). There is a precedent for this stereotyped behavior in animal studies using high doses of amphetamine; it probably results from an effect of amphetamine on dopaminergic systems in the basal ganglia.

In some cases in which paranoid psychoses have been produced by amphetamines, the paranoid thinking and loss of touch with reality have been slow to return to normal, persisting for days or even weeks after the drug has left the system. There is no good evidence for more long-lasting behavioral disruption. At one time there was concern that high doses of amphetamines would push the blood pressure so high that small strokes would occur and cause some slight brain damage, which would of course be cumulative for repeated high-dose users. However, no direct human evidence was obtained indicating this to be a problem. More recently, it has been demonstrated in rats that high doses of methamphetamine result in the production in the brain of a chemical that selectively destroys catecholamine neurons.[25] The possible long-term behavioral consequences for humans could be great from such damage, but as of yet we have no evidence that this occurs in human amphetamine users.

Patterns of amphetamine abuse. A major reason for concern over the number of people using prescription amphetamines in the 1960s was the possibility of beginning to take them under a physician's orders and then escalating the dose into oral abuse. Many individuals occasionally took 5 to 20 mg of amphetamines orally to allay fatigue, elevate mood while doing an unpleasant task, produce prolonged wakefulness, help recover from a hangover, or to "get high." In this pattern, the individual obtains amphetamine pills from the doctor for weight control, but takes the pills three to four times a day for the stimulation and euphoria produced by the drug. A strong psychological dependence on the pills may develop, and the person may feel that it is not possible to get along without them. If the daily amphetamines are stopped, withdrawal depression occurs.

These days there are many fewer people using prescription amphetamines, but there is a fair-sized market in oral doses of illicit speed. Although many purchasers may have in mind an occasional small dose to help them stay awake, it is probably the case that most oral users are out to "get a buzz"—to get high. This is more dangerous, because to get an obvious effect in a hurry, there is a tendency to start with higher doses. And if a little will get you feeling good, then a lot will get you feeling great, right? But remember that after the party's over the user may feel depressed and turn to the drug again. And *there's no such thing as a drug that makes you feel great and isn't addicting.* In 1989 there were reports from Hawaii of a new drug called "ice." This is a smokable form of methamphetamine, and, if it receives enough publicity, we may experience a new wave of amphetamine abuse and dependence.

There are still some people using amphetamines intravenously. Intravenous amphetamine use may begin with only (!) 30 mg. In a long run (speed binge) of 3 or 4 days with injections occurring every 2 or 3 hours, tolerance develops rapidly, and 500 to 1000 mg may be injected at one time. The peripheral effects show greater tolerance than those of the CNS, so only moderate cardiovascular effects may occur even with high doses that still yield the euphoria. The effects of single and repeated doses have been well described:

> After the intravenous user injects the drug in sufficient quantity he experiences a "flash or rush" which he describes as orgasmic in nature. After this initial experience he usually becomes euphoric, with an increase in motor and speech activity. The individual may stay hyperactive for many hours with no signs of fatigue. . . .
>
> The action phase of the "speed binge" is in effect repeated injection of the drug from one to ten times per day. With each "hit," the individual experiences the desired "flash" which the user often describes as a "full-body orgasm." Between "hits" the user is euphoric, hyperactive and hyperexcitable. This action phase of stimulation may last for several days in which the individual does not sleep and rarely eats.
>
> For a variety of reasons this action phase terminates, however. The user may stop voluntarily because of fatigue, he may become confused, paranoid or panic-stricken and stop "shooting," or he may simply run out of drug.

Even if the user doesn't run out of drug he is destined to "**crash**"; tolerance to these high doses builds up rapidly and after a few days of high doses it appears that new catecholamines cannot be synthesized fast enough. Since the amphetamine effect depends on the availability of dopamine and norepinephrine, the drug will eventually lose its effect. The emotional distress of this "crash" and its associated depression are so great that users have a hard time describing how bad it is. So after a couple of days' rest they climb back on the roller coaster. . . .

COCAINE

The drug that replaced amphetamine as the recreational stimulant drug of the 1980s is a drug that was around before amphetamine was invented: cocaine.

History

The coca plant.   A grave in Peru dating from about 500 AD contains an early record of use of **coca** leaves. Included along with other necessities for the afterlife were several bags of the leaves. Use of coca in this way gives no hint of the extent of cultivation or general use of the leaf at the time, but it certainly must have produced "exaltation of spirit, freedom from fatigue, and a sense of well being,"[26,p.12] even as it does today. By 1000 AD the coca shrub was extensively cultivated in Peru; today approximately 50 million kg of coca leaves are produced each year. Less than 5 million kg are exported for legal use or consumed by the 2 million Peruvians who live in the highlands. Simple and inexpensive processing of 500 kg of coca leaves yields 1 kg of cocaine.

Growing coca is illegal in Bolivia and Colombia, and no new plantings have been authorized by the government of Peru since 1964. The terrain of the Andes in Bolivia and Peru is poorly suited for growing almost everything. *Erythroxylon coca,* however, seems to thrive at elevations of 2000 to 8000 feet on the Amazon slope of the mountains, where there is over 100 inches of rain annually. The shrub is pruned to prevent it from reaching the normal height of 6 to 8 feet, so that the picking, which is done three or four times a year, is easier to accomplish. The shrubs are grown in small, 2- to 3-acre patches called *cocals,* some of which are known to have been under cultivation for over 800 years.

Before the sixteenth-century invasion by Pizarro, the Incas had built a well-developed civilization in Peru. The coca leaf was an important part of the culture, and, although earlier use was primarily in religious ceremonies, it was treated as money by the time the conquistadors arrived. The Spanish adopted this custom and paid coca leaves to the native laborers for mining and transporting gold and silver.

The mountain natives at that time, as today, chewed coca leaves almost continually, keeping a ball of them tucked in their cheek as they went about their business. The habit was so common that distances were measured by how far one could travel before it became necessary to stop and replenish the leaves. Even then, the leaf was recognized as increasing strength and endurance while decreasing the need for food. Early European chroniclers of the Inca civilization recorded and reported on the unique qualities of this plant, but it never interested Europeans until the last half of the nineteenth century. At that time the coca leaf contributed to the economic well-being and fame of three individuals. They, in turn, brought the Peruvian shrub to the notice of the world.

One of these men was Angelo Mariani, a French chemist. His contribution was to introduce the coca leaf indirectly to the general public. Mariani imported tons of coca leaves and used an extract from them in many products. The quid of leaves was gone, but you could suck on a coca lozenge, drink coca tea, or obtain the coca leaf extract in any of a large number of products. It was Mariani's coca wine, though, that made him rich and famous. Assuredly, it had to be the coca leaf extract in the wine that prompted the pope to present a medal of appreciation to Mariani. Not only the pope but royalty and the man in the street benefited from the Andean plant. For them, as it had for the Incas for 1000 years and was to do for Americans who drank Coca-Cola (Chapter 11), the extract of the coca leaf lifted their spirits,

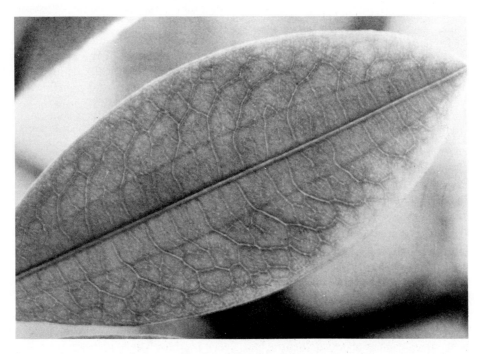

The coca leaf is somewhat distinctive because of the bilateral veins running parallel to the leaf's center.

freed them from fatigue, and gave them a general good feeling.

Early uses of cocaine. Coca leaves contain, besides the oils that give them flavor, the active chemical cocaine (up to almost 2%). Cocaine was isolated before 1860, but there is still debate over who did it first and exactly when. An available supply of pure cocaine and the newly developed hypodermic syringe improved the drug delivery system, and in the 1880s two famous physicians began to experiment with it. In the United States, Dr. W.S. Halsted, who was later referred to as "the father of modern surgery," experimented with the ability of cocaine to produce local anesthesia and to block sensation from a large area if the drug was injected near a nerve trunk. And in Vienna, a young medical doctor named Sigmund Freud studied the drug's psychological effects:

In 1884 Sigmund Freud wrote his fiancée that he had been experimenting with "a magical drug". After dazzling success in treatment of a case of gastric catarrh he continues "If it goes well I will write an essay on it and I expect it will win its place in therapeutics by the side of morphium, and superior to it. . . . I take very small doses of it regularly against depression and against indigestion, and with the most brilliant success." He urged his fiancée, his sisters, his colleagues, and his friends to try it . . . extolled the drug as a safe exhilarant which he himself used and recommended as a treatment for morphine addiction. For emphasis he stated, in italics, that "Inebriate asylums can be entirely dispensed with". . . .[27,p.17]

In an 1885 lecture before a group of psychiatrists, Freud commented on the use of cocaine as a stimulant, saying, "On the whole it must be said that the value of cocaine in psychiatric practice remains to be demonstrated, and it will probably be worthwhile to make a thorough trial as soon as the currently exorbitant price of the drug becomes more reasonable." The first of the consumer advocates!

Freud was more convinced about another use of the drug, however, and in the same lecture said:

We can speak more definitely about another use of cocaine by the psychiatrist. It was first discovered in America that cocaine is capable of alleviating the serious withdrawal symptoms observed in subjects who are abstaining from morphine and of suppressing their craving for morphine. . . . On the basis of my experiences with the effects of cocaine, I have no hesitation in recommending the administration of cocaine for such withdrawal cures in subcutaneous injections of 0.03-0.05 g per dose, without any fear of increasing the dose. On several occasions, I have even seen cocaine quickly eliminate the manifestations of intolerance that appeared after a rather large dose of morphine, as if it had a specific ability to counteract morphine.[28]

Even great men make mistakes. The realities of life were harshly brought home to Freud when he used cocaine to treat a close friend, Fleischl, to remove his addiction to morphine. Increasingly larger doses were needed, and "Freud spent one frightful night nursing Fleischl through an episode of cocaine psychosis and thereafter was bitterly against drugs. . . ."[29,p.17]

Even before Freud became aware of the problems with cocaine, Louis Lewin had attacked his proposal to use cocaine to cure morphine addiction and referred to Freud as "Joseph, the dream interpreter"!

The psychological effects of cocaine, both the initial stimulation and the later depression, were well appreciated by 1890, as indicated in a piece of fiction written in that year by Arthur Conan Doyle:

Sherlock Holmes took his bottle from the corner of the mantelpiece, and his hypodermic syringe from its neat morocco case. With his long, white nervous fingers, he adjusted the delicate needle and rolled back his left shirtcuff. For some little time his eyes rested thoughtfully upon the sinewy forearm and wrist, all dotted and scarred with innumerable puncture-marks. Finally, he thrust the sharp point home, pressed down the tiny piston, and sank back into the velvet-lined armchair with a long sigh of satisfaction.

Three times a day for many months I had witnessed this performance, but custom had not reconciled my mind to it. . . .

"Which is it today," I asked, "Morphine or cocaine?"

He raised his eyes languidly from the old black-letter volume which he had opened.

"It is cocaine," he said, "a seven-per-cent solution. Would you care to try it?"

"No, indeed," I answered brusquely. "My constitution has not got over the Afghan campaign yet. I cannot afford to throw any extra strain upon it."

He smiled at my vehemence. "Perhaps you are right, Watson," he said. "I suppose that its influence is physically a bad one. I find it, however, so transcendently stimulating and clarifying to the mind that its secondary action is a matter of small moment."

"But consider!" I said earnestly. "Count the cost! Your brain may, as you say, be roused and excited, but it is a pathological and morbid process which involves increased tissue-change and may at least leave a permanent weakness. You know, too, what a black reaction comes upon you. Surely the game is hardly worth the candle. Why should you, for a mere passing pleasure, risk the loss of those great powers with which you have been endowed? Remember that I speak not only as one comrade to another but as a medical man to one for whose constitution he is to some extent answerable."

He did not seem offended. On the contrary, he put his finger-tips together, and leaned his elbows on the arms of his chair, like one who has a relish for conversation.

"My mind," he said, "rebels at stagnation. Give me problems, give me work, give me the most abstruse cryptogram, or the most intricate analysis, and I am in my own proper atmosphere. I can dispense then with artificial stimulants. But I abhor the dull routine of existence. I crave for mental exaltation."[30,pp.91-92]

Although physicians were well aware of the dangers of using cocaine regularly, nonmedical as well as quasimedical use of cocaine was widespread in the United States around the turn of the century. It was one of the secret ingredients in many patent medicines and elixirs but was also openly advertised as having beneficial effects. The Parke-Davis Pharmaceutical Company noted in 1885 that cocaine "can supply the place of food, make the coward brave, and silent eloquent . . . " and called it a "wonder drug."[31]

Legal controls on cocaine. With so much going for cocaine, and its availability in a large number of products for drinking, snorting, or injection, it may seem strange that between 1887 and 1914, 46 states passed laws to regulate the use and distribution of cocaine. One author provided extensive documentation and concluded:

All the elements needed to insure cocaine's outlaw status were present by the first years of the twentieth century: it had become widely used as a pleasure drug, and doctors warned of the dangers attendant on indiscriminate sale and use; it had become identified with despised or poorly regarded groups—blacks, lower-class whites, and criminals; it had not been long enough established in the culture to insure its survival; and it had not, though used by them, become identified with the elite, thus losing what little chance it had of weathering the storm of criticism.[32]

Cocaine was included in all sorts of nerve tonics, patent medicines, and home remedies, often without being mentioned on the label, until the 1906 Pure Food and Drugs Act was passed. As we saw in Chapter 3, for various political reasons coca and cocaine were included along with opium and its derivatives in the Harrison Act of 1914, which taxed its importation and sale. During the Prohibition era of the 1920s, when the Harrison Act was used by federal Treasury agents as a tool to suppress drug addiction, cocaine became less available and more expensive. Not that it went away: cocaine was sometimes mixed with heroin and injected intravenously (the combination was called a "speedball"), and some of the carefree and wealthy young people of the era dabbled in its use. "Cocaine Lil," a song written in the 1920s, included the line, "Lil went to a 'snow' party one cold night, and the way she sniffed was sure a fright." Cole Porter's "I Get a Kick out of You" in 1934 originally contained the verse:

> I get no kick from cocaine
> I'm sure that if
> I took even one sniff
> It would bore me terrifically too
> But I get a kick out of you.

With the introduction in the 1930s of inexpensive and easily available amphetamine, the use of cocaine declined among both occasional recreational users and serious drug addicts. Little concern was given to cocaine until, at the end of the 1960s when amphetamines became harder to obtain, cocaine use again began to increase. In 1970 it was reported that federal agents were becoming

New Life, New Vigor

Experienced by all who have had occasion to use

VIN MARIANI

This Popular French Tonic-Stimulant is Invariably Agreeable and Efficacious,

STRENGTHENS, REFRESHES, RESTORES
THE VITAL FORCES,

When overworked, and for body or mental fatigue, nothing equals " VIN MARIANI " for immediate and lasting beneficial effect.

This assertion is based on

WRITTEN ENDORSEMENTS

from over 7,000 eminent Physicians and continued use over 30 years, in Hospitals, Public and Religious Institutions everywhere.

AT DRUGGISTS AND GROCERS.

For Illustrated Book with Portraits and Autographs of Celebrities, address:

Mariani & Co., New York.

The tonic in this 1893 advertisement was made from 2 ounces of coca leaves soaked in 18 ounces of red wine. Although the cocaine content of the leaves varied, a typical glass probably contained less than 100 mg (1/10 g) of cocaine.

concerned; the amount of cocaine seized by U.S. Customs agents had increased from about 50 pounds in 1967 to almost 200 pounds in 1969.[6] Yearly seizures increased throughout the 1970s and 1980s, and in 1984 customs agents seized over 50,000 pounds of cocaine in Miami and Ft. Lauderdale, Florida alone!

Basic Pharmacology

Chemical characteristics. In the process of making illicit cocaine, the coca leaves are mixed with an organic solvent, such as kerosene or gasoline. After thorough soaking, mixing, and mashing, the excess liquid is filtered out to form a substance known as **coca paste.**[33] In South America this paste is often mixed with tobacco and smoked, but that practice has not caught on in the United States, perhaps because the lingering solvent gives the smoke a unique flavor. The paste can be made into cocaine hydrochloride, a salt that is stable and mixes easily in water. Some U.S. users who want to smoke the cocaine convert it into **freebase** by extracting it into a volatile organic solvent, such as ether. The freebase can be smoked, but putting fire and ether fumes together can be an enlightening experience, since ether is so explosive. The popularity of this form of freebasing began to decline with the discovery that cocaine freebase could be made by mixing cocaine with baking soda and water. When a piece of this cocaine **crack** or **rock** is heated, cocaine vapors are produced and may be inhaled.

The chemical structure of cocaine is shown in Fig. 7-4. Notice that it is much more complex than the structure of amphetamine and that it doesn't bear any obvious resemblance to dopamine or norepinephrine. In fact, the structure of cocaine doesn't give us much help at all in understanding how the drug works on the brain, which is still something of a mystery.

Mechanism of action. The more we learn about cocaine's effects on brain biochemistry, the more complex its actions seem. For many years it was believed that the primary CNS effects of cocaine resulted from its interfering with the reuptake of norepinephrine, thus prolonging the effect of each packet of norepinephrine released from a neuron. However, other drugs that also block the reuptake of norepinephrine, such as the antidepressant drugs, do not result in stimulation of the CNS. Cocaine also blocks the reuptake of dopamine and seotonin, and it alters the metabolism of serotonin. Cocaine does appear to attach to

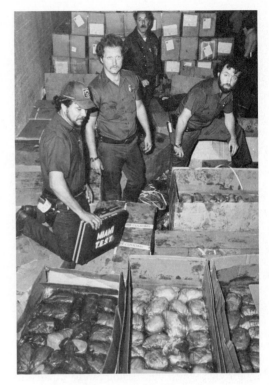

Figure 7-4. Cocaine.

specific sites in the brain, and many of these sites may be located on serotonin neurons.[34]

Absorption and elimination.   People can, and do, use cocaine in many ways. Chewing and sucking the leaves allows the cocaine to be absorbed slowly through the mucous membranes. This results in a slower onset and much lower blood levels than are usually obtained by the most common recreational method of "snorting" or sniffing. In snorting the attempt is to get the very fine cocaine hydrochloride powder high into the nasal passages—right on the nasal mucosa. From there it is absorbed quite rapidly and, through circulatory mechanisms that are not completely understood, reaches the brain rather quickly.

The intravenous use of cocaine delivers a very high concentration to the brain, producing a rapid, powerful, and brief effect. For that reason, IV cocaine has been a favorite among compulsive users, many of whom switched from intranasal to IV use. However, another method that produces effects even faster has become the preferred route by most compulsive users—the smoking of crack. Because the lungs provide a large surface area for absorption, and blood circulation from the lungs to the brain is quite rapid, smoking crack produces more rapid and profound dependence than even IV use.

The cocaine molecules are metabolized by enzymes in the blood and the liver, and the activity of these enzymes is variable from one person to another. In any case, cocaine itself is rapidly removed, with a half-life of about 1 hour. The major metabolites, which are the basis of urine screening tests, have a longer half-life of about 8 hours.[35]

U.S. customs agents in Miami with an intercepted shipment of cocaine.

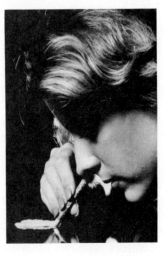

The most common method of cocaine use is snorting it into the nose.

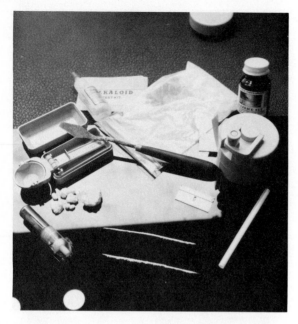

Cocaine paraphernalia includes a small balance for weighing, a test kit, a razor blade and grinder for preparing the "lines" of cocaine powder, and a plastic straw through which the cocaine can be inhaled into the nose.

Beneficial Uses

Local anesthesia. The local anesthetic properties of cocaine, that is, the ability to numb the area to which it is applied, were discovered in 1860 soon after its isolation from coca leaves. It was not until 1884 that this characteristic was used medically; the early applications were in eye surgery and dentistry. The use of cocaine spread rapidly, since it apparently was a safe and effective drug. The potential for misuse soon became clear, and a search began for synthetic agents with similar anesthetic characteristics but little or no potential for misuse. This work was rewarded in 1905 with the discovery of procaine (Novocaine), which is still widely used.

Local anesthetics probably block pain by preventing the generation and conduction of nerve impulses. They seem to act quite specifically on the nerve membrane. By disrupting the membrane processes necessary for the initiation and generation of electrical impulses, impulse conduction and information processing are stopped. Many drugs have been synthesized since 1905 that have local anesthetic properties similar to those of cocaine but have little or no ability to produce CNS stimulation. Those drugs have largely replaced cocaine for medical use. However, because cocaine is absorbed so well into mucous membranes, it remains in use for surgery in the nasal, laryngeal, and esophageal regions.

Other claimed benefits. Because cocaine produces a feeling of increased energy and well-being, it has an important status among modern achievers who self-prescribe it frequently to overcome fatigue. It seems that many athletes and entertainers feel that they cannot consistently perform at their peak without the assistance of cocaine, and this has resulted in widespread cocaine use among these groups. It should be remembered that cocaine has not been used medically for its CNS effects for many years because its effects are brief, there is a subsequent period of depressed mood, attempts to maintain the euphoria lead to rapid tolerance and acceleration of the dose, and high doses result in unpleasant restlessness, paranoia, and other side effects. Thus whereas the drug can provide a brief sense of increased energy, the long-term consequences are frequently disruptive.

Causes for Concern

Dependence potential. There is no doubt that cocaine produces powerful psychological dependence in some users, particularly among those who inject it or inhale the vapors of cocaine base. This phenomenon is backed up by a large number of animal experiments demonstrating that rats or monkeys will rapidly learn to press levers that lead to cocaine injections and that these animals will continue to respond even when large numbers of presses are required for each injection.[36] Thus it appears that cocaine can be a powerfully reinforcing drug: take it and it will make you want to take it again.

Throughout the 1970s the importance of this

dependence potential went unrecognized, partly because cocaine was expensive and in short supply and largely because the only common method of using cocaine during this time was snorting it. The 1980s saw the introduction of freebasing and recently the more stable form of smokable cocaine known as "crack" or "rock." As large numbers of people began to smoke cocaine in the mid-1980s, the powerful dependence potential of this form of use became clear for the first time.

Since at one time addiction was linked to the presence of tolerance and physical dependence, there have been a number of experiments that asked whether these occur with repeated cocaine use. Experiments in which animals were given cocaine each day often found increased, rather than decreased, behavioral effects. After prolonged daily cocaine administrations there were no obvious withdrawal signs, and so many scientists concluded that cocaine produced no tolerance or physical dependence and was therefore not an addicting drug. Experience with amphetamine led to a different way of looking at this issue: cocaine is a short-acting drug. Repeated administrations within a single day do demonstrate a rapid tolerance (tachyphylaxis), just as is seen with amphetamine. As cocaine wears off, there is a dysphoric reaction (the cocaine blues). If cocaine use has been prolonged and high doses have been used, the withdrawal period produces a powerful sense of psychological depression (profound anguish), as is seen with amphetamine. Although this withdrawal syndrome is seen by many as a psychological symptom, since it occurs consistently after repeated exposure to cocaine and can be reversed by readministering cocaine, it does fit our definition of physical dependence. Thus it is now clear that both tolerance and physical dependence are possible with cocaine (Table 7-1).[37]

Toxicity potential.   There is no evidence that occasional use of small amounts of cocaine is a threat to the individual's health. Regularly snorting cocaine, and particularly cocaine that has been "cut" with other things, may irritate the nasal septum, leading to a chronically inflamed, runny nose. The major concerns seem to be the

---

Your turn: cocaine and friendship

Imagine you have a good friend who has been using cocaine off and on for a year. However, in the past couple of months it seems the use has become more and more frequent. You have had to stop lending your friend money because it never gets paid back. When you hinted that the cocaine use might be getting out of hand there was no response. When you tried direct confrontation, you got angry denial that there was any problem. You are still good friends. You certainly don't want to turn your friend in to the police, but you are getting pretty worried. What do you think you should do?

Obviously there is no correct answer to this problem, but it might be interesting to discuss this hypothetical situation with a group of people who are your friends. Find out how they would want to be treated under the circumstances. How would you yourself want to be treated?

---

effects of chronic use on behavior and the acute physiological effects of overdoses.

Use of cocaine in a binge, in which the drug is taken repeatedly and at increasingly high doses, leads to a state of increasing irritability, restlessness, and paranoia. This may in severe cases result in a full-blown paranoid psychosis in which the individual loses touch with reality and experiences auditory hallucinations (threatening voices). This experience is of course disruptive and quite frightening. However, most individuals seem to recover from the psychosis as the drug leaves the system. They then have to deal with a longer-lasting period of depression.

Acute cocaine poisoning leads to profound CNS stimulation, progressing to convulsions that may lead to respiratory or cardiac arrest. This is in some ways similar to amphetamine overdose, with the exception that there is much greater individual variation in the uptake and metabolism of cocaine, so that a lethal dose is much more difficult to estimate.[38] In addition, there are very rare, severe, and unpredictable toxic reactions to cocaine and other local anesthetics in which individuals die rapidly, apparently from cardiac failure. Intra-

Table 7-1			
Dependence liability of stimulants			
Drug and route	Tolerance	Physical dependence	Probability of behavioral dependence
Amphetamines, oral	Yes, both short- and long-term	Yes, at high doses	Moderate
Amphetamines, intravenous	Yes, long-and short-term	At high doses	Very high
Cocaine, snorted	Yes	At high doses	High
Cocaine, intravenous	Yes	At high doses	Very high
Cocaine, freebase inhaled	Yes	At high doses	Very high

venous cocaine users may also experience an allergic reaction, either to the drug or to some additive in the street cocaine. The lungs fill rapidly with fluid, and death may occur.

It is clear that cocaine was the drug of abuse for the 1980s. As discussed in Chapter 1, the national household survey of 1985 reported increasing use, with about 5.8 million Americans estimated to have used cocaine in that year. The annual national high school senior survey reported in 1987 that fewer students were using cocaine, whereas the 1987 DAWN data found large increases in the number of emergency room visits and drug-related deaths associated with cocaine. The price and purity of available cocaine have not changed greatly, but indications are that during the 1980s there may have been a slight decrease in price and increase in purity of street cocaine, reflecting the vast and increasing amounts of cocaine smuggled into the United States. About 200 tons annually were flowing into the States at the end of the 1980s, and more lucrative markets were beginning to develop in Europe.[33]

Freebasing. Large numbers of people using cocaine might not cause a great deal of concern if it seems that the vast majority of users are using the drug occasionally in a nondestructive manner,

as appeared to many to be the case in the 1970s. But the 1980s brought us more than an increase in cocaine use. It was in this decade that people looking for a more rapid effect and more "bang for the buck" sought to maximize cocaine's psychological effects by converting the drug from the hydrochloride salt into the more volatile freebase so that it could be smoked. The smoking of freebase cocaine became a popular pasttime for a relatively small group of cocaine users, however, because of the incovenience of converting the freebase just before smoking it. Because the conversion to freebase involves extraction of the chemical into ether, which is highly explosive, the freebase must be thoroughly dried before smoking it.

Crack. In the mid-1980s it was discovered that mixing the cocaine base with some simple household chemicals, including baking soda, before drying it resulted in a lump of cocaine in a stable, smokable form. These small cocaine "rocks" could be prepared in small lumps or in larger ones that were then cracked to provide small pieces. When smoked, a relatively small amount of cocaine can produce a rapid and short-lived high, and the street sales of crack or rock made this experience available to anyone with

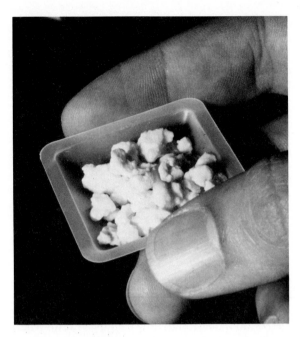

Crack—smokable cocaine—in a Miami crime lab.

$10, a butane torch or lighter, a pipe, and access to a dealer. The practice spread rapidly during 1985 and 1986, at first in the ghetto areas of large cities. Cocaine, which had come to symbolize the rich and famous, was now accessible to the poor.

Because batches of crack can be cooked up fairly easily once one has the cocaine, crack "factories" tend to be small operations, run by only a few people and supplying a fairly small number of dealers. This makes law enforcement more difficult than would be the case if there were fewer, larger producers.

Dependence develops rapidly with crack. The rapid, intense high lasts only a few minutes and is followed by depression. Another dose produces another rapid high, followed by greater depression. Even though a single dose may not be terribly expensive, users can spend increasing, and eventually huge, sums of money on crack. The rapid development of strong dependence was a surprise to everyone, and treatment centers were flooded with clients trying to break the vicious circle of emotional highs and lows. Most of the

well-known residential centers had long waiting lists by the summer of 1986, and initial indications from those who had been through treatment was that the relapse rate is high.[39]

What appears to be happening is a sociocultural shift: while fewer middle-class and upper-middle-class people are using cocaine and more of them are aware of its dangers, the use of the more dangerous crack by poor, urban teenagers has increased. Of those calling the nationwide cocaine hotline 1-800-COCAINE, the typical caller has changed from 1983 (college educated, earn as much as $25,000 annually) to 1987 (unemployed, crack user).[40]

The rapid growth in demand for crack, coupled with the ease of entry into production and marketing of this substance, promises to result in an ever-increasing flow of cocaine into the United States, in spite of enormous and expensive efforts by federal law-enforcement agencies to reduce cocaine trafficking. At the same time, we realize that as people experience the agonies and expense of dependence, and as the death toll of famous athletes and entertainers and of friends and acquaintances rises, more and more people will learn to fear the dangers of cocaine and will turn away from it. At what level these two opposing forces will level out remains to be seen. How many Americans will use cocaine, how many will enjoy it, how many will become severely dependent, and how many will die?

One of the foremost historians of heroin use and control pointed out in 1986[38] that we are in a sense reliving an earlier cycle of cocaine use that occurred around the turn of the century. As you know, when cocaine was first introduced the experts were mostly positive about its effects, and it was regarded as a fairly benign substance. Then, as more and more people used cocaine, its dangers and side effects became well known. In the third stage, in the early 1900s, society turned against this and other mind-altering drugs and passed laws to control them. After many years with little cocaine use, the drug had the reputation of being fairly benign and not truly addicting. We now appear to be in the second stage in which wide-

---

Issue: movies, the media, and miami vice

There is no question that our perception of which drugs are "in," as well as which ones are threats, have a lot to do with the way these substances are portrayed in the mass media. We read in the sports pages about professional athletes with big cocaine habits, we read news stories about young people smoking crack, and we see television news reports of huge bundles of money being confiscated from cocaine dealers. We get mixed messages from all this—cocaine is a problem for people with too much money and not enough sense, cocaine may be a danger to large numbers of kids, and cocaine is glamorous.

The violence of cocaine dealers has been a popular theme for movies such as *Mike's Murder, Scarface,* and *Against All Odds.* Obviously, most cocaine dealers don't get involved in much violence on a regular basis or we'd have fewer dealers than we have. But the show must go on! One popular television series, *Miami Vice,* is about two vice detectives who spend quite a bit of their time chasing cocaine dealers. What kinds of subtle messages come across about the cocaine business in this show? Is it only chance that for these two characters to be worthy opponents for the cocaine dealers they themselves must be "ultra-cool," drive expensive cars and boats, and wear the latest fashions?

---

spread use has begun to make us all aware of the dangers. How will our society react in the predicted turn away from cocaine?

Summary

The most potent CNS stimulants are represented by amphetamine and similar drugs and by cocaine. All of these substances have many effects in common: they are capable of reversing the effects of fatigue, of maintaining wakefulness, and of temporarily elevating the mood of the user.

Amphetamine is a synthetic drug that was developed as a bronchodilator and has been used illicitly almost since its introduction in 1932. Chemically similar to the catecholamine neuro-transmitters, it appears to act by stimulating catecholamine pathways in the brain.

Amphetamines are currently used to treat narcolepsy, attention deficit disorder in children, and in short-term weight reduction programs. They are much less widely prescribed now than they were in the early 1960s.

Amphetamines can produce improved performance on both mental and physical tasks, but they can also impair performances. The effect depends on the dose, the task, and the state of the individual before taking the drug.

Amphetamine can produce profound dependence, based on the dose and route of administration. Taken intravenously, amphetamine can be quite addicting. Although overdose deaths are not common even with quite large doses, there is concern that amphetamine may precipitate violent behavior. At high doses, psychotic reactions are common, although they usually clear up when the drug wears off.

Cocaine is derived from the coca plant and has been used in that form for centuries. Cocaine itself was introduced into medicine in the 1860s both as a local anesthetic and for its CNS stimulant effects. Because of rapid tolerance, rebound depression as the drug wears off, and psychotic reactions to high doses, cocaine is no longer used for its CNS effects. It has only limited use as a local anesthetic.

Cocaine is used illicitly by three main routes: it may be snorted into the nose, injected intravenously, or smoked as the freebase. Both IV injection and smoking produce rapid and powerful effects and result in rapid and potent dependence. The widespread presence of a new form of smokable cocaine, crack, is of concern because so many people have adopted this very addicting pattern of use.

REFERENCES

1. Benzedrine alert, Air Surgeon's Bulletin 1(2):19-21, 1944.
2. On a bender with Benzedrine, Everybody's Digest 5(2):50, 1946.

3. Monroe RR and Drell HJ: Oral use of amphetamines obtained from inhalers, Journal of the American Medical Association 135:909-915, 1947.

4. Hemmi T: How we have handled the problem of drug abuse in Japan. In Sjöqvist F and Tottie M, editors: Abuse of central stimulants, New York, 1969, Raven Press.

5. Kato M: A bird's eye view of the present state of drug abuse in Japan, Drug and Alcohol Dependence 11:55-56, 1983.

6. Brecher EM: Licit and illicit drugs, Boston, 1972, Little, Brown and Co.

7. Journal of the American Medical Association 183:363, 1963.

8. Baker JN, and others: The newest drug war, Newsweek, April 3, 1989, pp 20-22.

9. FDA orders curbs on amphetamine claims, American Druggist 162:16, August 24, 1970.

10. Crout JR: Statement before US Senate Subcommittee on Monopoly, Select Committee on Small Business, November 19, 1976.

11. Physician's Desk Reference, ed 43, Oradell, NJ, 1989, Medical Economics Company.

12. Diagnostic and Statistical Manual, ed 3, revised, American Psychiatric Association, 1987.

13. Kolata G: Consensus on diets and hyperactivity, Science 215:968, February 19, 1982.

14. Safer DJ, Allen RP and Barr E: Growth rebound after termination of stimulant drugs, Journal of Pediatrics 86:113-116, 1975.

15. Safer DJ and Krager JM: A survey of medication treatment for hyperactive/inattentive students, Journal of the American Medical Association 26:2256-2258, 1988.

16. Shaywitz SE: Increased medication use in attention-deficit hyperactivity disorder: regressive or appropriate? Journal of the American Medical Association 26:2270-2272, 1988.

17. Mandell AJ, Stewart KD, and Russo PV: The Sunday syndrome: from kinetics to altered consciousness, Federation Proceedings 40:2682-2688, 1981.

18. Laties VG and Weiss B: The amphetamine margin in sports, Federation Proceedings 40:2689-2692, 1981.

19. Smith GM and Beecher HK: Amphetamine sulfate and athletic performance, Journal of the American Medical Association 170:542-557, 1959.

20. Griffiths RR, Brady JV and Bradford LD: Predicting the abuse liability of drugs with animal self-administration procedures: psychomotor stimulants and hallucinogens. In Thompson T and Dews P, editors: Advances in behavioral pharmacology, vol 2, New York, 1979, Academic Press, Inc.

21. Kramer JC: In Amphetamines, Fourth report by the Select Committee on Crime, House Report No 91-1807, Washington, DC, 1971, US Government Printing Office.

22. Ellinwood EH: Assault and homicide associated with amphetamine abuse, American Journal of Psychiatry 127(9):90-95, 1971.

23. Greenberg SW: The relationship between crime and amphetamine abuse: an empirical review of the literature, Contemporary Drug Problems, Summer 1976, pp 101-130.

24. Bell DS: The experimental reproduction of amphetamine psychosis, Archives of General Psychiatry 29:35-40,1973.

25. Seiden LS and Vosmer G: 6-Hydroxydopamine is formed from dopamine in vivo after administration of methylamphetamine, Society for Neuroscience Abstracts 10:1200, 1984.

26. Taylor N: Plant drugs that changed the world, New York, 1965, Dodd, Mead & Co.

27. Taylor N: Flight from reality, New York, 1949, Duell, Sloan & Pearce.

28. Freud S: On the general effect of cocaine, lecture before the Psychiatric Union on March 5, 1885. (Reprinted in Drug Dependence 5:17, 1970.)

29. Holmstedt B: Historical survey. In Efron DH, editor: Ethnopharmacologic search for psychoactive drugs, Public Health Service Publication No 1645, Washington, DC, 1967, US Government Printing Office.

30. Doyle AC: The sign of the four. In The complete Sherlock Holmes, New York, 1938, Garden City Publishing Co.

31. Perry C: The star-spangled powder, Rolling Stone, p 26, August 17, 1972.

32. Ashley R: Cocaine its history, uses and effects, New York, 1976, Warner Books, Inc.

33. White PT: Coca—an ancient herb turns deadly, National Geographic 175:3-47, 1989.

34. Jones RT: The pharmacology of cocaine. In Grabowski J, editor: Cocaine: pharmacology, effects, and treatment of abuse, NIDA Research Monograph No 50, Washington DC, 1984, US Government Printing Office.

35. Jatlow, P: Cocaine: analysis, pharmacokinetics, and metabolic disposition, Yale Journal of Biology and Medicine 61:105-113, 1988.

36. Johanson, CE: Assessment of the dependence potential of cocaine in animals. In Grabowski J, editor: Cocaine: pharmacology, effects, and treatment of abuse, NIDA Research Monograph No 50, Washington DC 1984, US Government Printing Office.

37. Gawin FH and Kleber HD: Evolving conceptualizations of cocaine dependence, Yale Journal of Biology and Medicine 61:123-136, 1988.

38. Cocaine use in the US follows pattern of days gone by, professor says, The Denver Post, July 8, 1986.

39. Coming back from crack, Newsweek 107:52-53, June 30, 1986.

40. Isikoff M: Two-tier drug culture seen emerging, The Washington Post, January 3, 1989.

Chapter 8

Sedatives and Hypnotics

OBJECTIVES

After reading this chapter, you should be able to:

Distinguish among barbiturates, benzodiazepines, and other classes of depressant drugs and know something of the history of each major group.

Explain the mechanism of action of the barbiturates and the benzodiazepines in relation to the neurotransmitter GABA.

Describe the usefulness and some of the practical limitations of these drugs in treating anxiety, insomnia, and epilepsy.

Discuss the ability of these drugs to produce both psychological and physical dependence and be able to describe the withdrawal syndrome.

Discuss the ability of these drugs to produce both behavioral and physiological toxicity.

Describe two common patterns of sedative abuse.

Downers, depressants, sedatives, hypnotics, gin-in-a-pill. Known by many names, these drugs all have a widespread effect in the brain that can be summed up as decreased neural activity. The behavioral effects? As suggested by one of the proposed names, if you know what alcohol does, you know what these drugs do. They come from several different chemical classes but are grouped together because of their common psychological effects. At low doses these drugs may be prescribed for daytime use to reduce anxiety (as "**sedatives**"). At higher doses many of the same drugs are prescribed as sleeping pills (**"hypnotics"**). This group of drugs is often referred to as "sedative-hypnotics." The most widely used drug in this general category is alcohol, which is discussed in detail in a separate chapter. The **barbiturates,** which have been in medical use for over 80 years, will serve as an example of this class of drugs.

HISTORY AND PHARMACOLOGY
Nonbarbiturates

There are three CNS depressants with a longer history than the barbiturates that are rarely prescribed today. **Chloral hydrate** and **paraldehyde** have chemical and pharmacological characteristics much like alcohol, while the **bromides** are different.

Chloral hydrate was synthesized in 1832 but

was not used clinically until about 1870. It is rapidly metabolized to trichloroethanol, which is the active hypnotic agent. When taken orally, chloral hydrate has a short onset period (30 minutes), and 1 to 2 g will induce sleep in less than an hour. This agent does not cause as much depression of the respiratory and cardiovascular systems as a comparable dose of the barbiturates and has fewer aftereffects.

In 1869 Dr. Benjamine Richardson introduced chloral hydrate to Great Britain. Ten years later he called it "in one sense a beneficient, and in another sense a maleficient substance, I almost feel a regret that I took any part whatever in the introduction of the agent into the practice of healing. . . . "[1] He had learned that what man can misuse, some men will abuse. As early as 1871 he referred to its nontherapeutic use as "toxical luxury" and lamented that chloral hydrate addicts had to be added to "alcohol intemperants and opium-eaters." Chloral hydrate addiction is a tough way to go, since its major disadvantage is that it is a gastric irritant, and repeated use causes considerable stomach upset. A solution of chloral hydrate was used before 1900 as the famous "knockout drops" or "Mickey Finn"—a "few" drops in a sailor's drink, and before he woke up, he was shanghaied onto a boat at sea for a long trip to the Orient.

No such use ever occurred with paraldehyde, which was synthesized in 1829 and introduced clinically in 1882. Paraldehyde would probably be in great use today because of its effectiveness as a CNS depressant with little respiratory depression and a wide safety margin, except for one characteristic. It has a most noxious taste and odor that permeates the breath of the user.

The bromides are little used today, now that they have been removed from OTC sleep preparations. Bromides accumulate in the body, and the depression they cause builds up over several days of regular use. There are serious toxic effects with repeated hypnotic doses of these agents. Dermatitis and constipation are minor accompaniments; with increased intake, motor disturbances, delirium, and psychosis develop.

Barbiturates

Over 2500 barbiturates have been synthesized. Some of the best are among the oldest, although barbital (Veronal), the first to be used clinically in 1903, is little used today. It did start the practice of giving barbiturates names ending in -al. The second barbiturate in clinical use, phenobarbital (Luminal), was introduced in 1912. Amobarbital (Amytal) in 1923, as well as pentobarbital (Nembutal) and secobarbital (Seconal), both introduced in 1930, are well-established examples of the barbiturates.

As Table 8-1 indicates, barbiturates are typically grouped on the basis of the duration of their activity. In general, the drugs that are the most lipid soluble are the ones that have both the shortest time of onset (they are absorbed and enter the brain rapidly) and the shortest duration of action (they leave the brain quickly and tend to be more rapidly metabolized).[2]

Although a large fraction of phenobarbital is excreted unchanged in the urine, the majority of this drug and virtually all of the shorter-acting drugs are metabolized in the liver. The barbiturates are one of the classes of drugs that stimulate the activity of the microsomal enzymes of the liver. Some of the tolerance that develops to the barbiturates is the result of an increased rate of deactivation caused by this stimulation of microsomal enzymes.

The induction of these enzymes by the barbiturates might also cause the more rapid metabolism of other drugs, perhaps requiring an adjustment of the dose.

A typical dose of a barbiturate for daytime sedation would be 30 to 50 mg. This is intended to relax a person and reduce disruptive levels of anxiety without producing drowsiness or lethargy. For the hypnotic (sleep-inducing) effect, 100 to 200 mg is more usual. The short-acting barbiturates may be less useful for maintaining daytime sedation, since it is necessary to take them several times a day. Thus 30 mg of phenobarbital would have been a typical sedative prescription before the introduction of newer drugs for this purpose (e.g., diazepam [Valium]). On the other hand,

Table 8-1		
Groupings of available barbiturates		
Type	**Time to onset**	**Duration of action (hours)**
Short-acting	15 minutes	2 to 3
Pentobarbital (Nembutal) Secobarbital (Seconal)		
Intermediate-acting	30 minutes	5 to 6
Aprobarbital (Alurate) Amobarbital (Amytal) Butabarbital (Butisol)		
Long-acting	1 hour	6 to 10
Mephobarbital (Mebaral) Phenobarbital (Luminal)		

such a long-acting drug has disadvantages as a sleeping pill, since it may be difficult to wake up refreshed after 7 or 8 hours of sleep if the drug is still active. A more typical sleeping pill prescription would have been 100 or 200 mg amobarbital or secobarbital.

These drugs were widely used for both purposes, although they have gradually been replaced to a great extent by newer agents. Tolerance can develop to the barbiturates as well as both psychological and physical dependence. In addition, they do depress respiration and, in large doses or in combination with alcohol, can completely stop one's breathing. For many years these drugs were chosen above all others by those wishing to commit suicide. In addition, accidental overdoses occurred when sleeping pills were taken after an evening of heavy drinking.

Although the majority of individuals who took barbiturates were not harmed by them, there was a great deal of concern about both the addiction liability and the danger of overdose. These concerns led to the ready acceptance of new sedative or hypnotic agents that appeared to be safer.

Meprobamate

The modern antianxiety agents (*anxiolytics*) developed from a muscle relaxant called mephenesin, which was patented in 1946 and was a commercial success but had a short duration of action. One compound patented in 1952 was not only longer lasting but believed to be a unique type of CNS depressant. Clinical trials in 1953 supported this belief and the compound was approved by the FDA and released for prescription use in 1955. Meprobamate, the generic name, became Miltown to the public, and it represented the drug revolution of the 1950s to most people.

The boom in meprobamate use is difficult to see in perspective. In the year it was introduced, sales of Miltown went from $7500 in May to over $500,000 in December. The happy pills had arrived! A publicity agency and excessive prescribing by physicians combined to make Miltown a public nuisance as well as the unnamed object of comment concerning overuse by the American Psychiatric Association and the World Health Organization in 1957. Miltown became such a common word that physicians began prescribing meprobamate under its other brand name, Equanil.

It gradually became clear that meprobamate, like the barbiturates, can also produce both psychological and physical dependence. One review suggested that daily doses above 3200 mg for over 2 months can result in physical dependence.[3] Available tablets contain 400 to 600 mg, to be taken two or three times per day. Thus, physical dependence can result from taking a bit more than twice a normal daily dose. In 1970 meprobamate became a Schedule IV controlled substance, which limits the number of times a prescription for it can be refilled.

Although reports of overdose deaths from meprobamate alone are rare, in retrospect it seems ironic that the medical community so readily accepted meprobamate as being safer than barbiturates. Meprobamate was sold only in anxiolytic doses for daytime sedation. Barbiturates produce physical dependence at doses above 400 mg, or twice a maximum *hypnotic* dose. If barbiturates had been sold only as 30 mg phenobarbital for daytime sedation, many fewer cases of physical dependence or overdose would have been reported. Let this be an object lesson: by deciding that the "barbiturates" were addicting and deadly, the focus was on the chemical class, rather than on the dose and the manner in which the drug was used. Thus a new, safer chemical was accepted without considering that its safety was not being judged under the same conditions. This mistake has occurred frequently with psychoactive drugs. In fact, it occurred again as physicians began to turn away from meprobamate.

Benzodiazepines

The first of this class was chlordiazepoxide, which was marketed under the trade name Librium (because it "liberates" one from anxieties?). Chlordiazepoxide was synthesized in 1947, but it was 10 years before its value in reducing anxiety was suggested, and it was not sold commercially until 1960. The discovery of this class of drugs is a triumph for behavioral research; a drug company pharmacologist found that mice given the right dose of chlordiazepoxide would loosen their grip on an inclined wire screen and fall to the floor of the test cage. When this experiment had been done with barbiturates, the mice promptly fell asleep. With Librium, the relaxed mouse continued to walk around sniffing the cage in a normal manner.[4] This drug was marketed as a more selective "antianxiety" agent that produced less drowsiness than the barbiturates and had a much larger safety margin before overdose death occurred in animals. Clinical practice bore this out; physical dependence was almost unheard of and overdose seemed not to occur except in the presence of alcohol or other depressant drugs. Even strong psychological dependence seemed rare with this drug. The conclusion was reached that

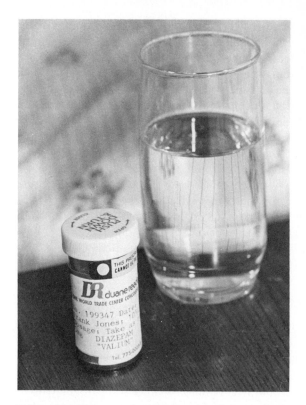

Valium is still among the most commonly prescribed drugs in the United States.

the "benzodiazepines" were as effective as the barbiturates and much safer. Librium became not only the leading psychoactive drug in sales, but the leading prescription drug of all. It was supplanted in the early 1970s by diazepam (Valium) a more potent (lower dose) agent made by the same company. From 1972 until 1978 Valium was the leading seller among all prescription drugs. As concerns about overprescription of Valium became widespread and as other benzodiazepines became available, sales of Valium have decreased.

Concerns about overprescribing Valium? Yes, it seems that many people were developing psychological dependence on Valium, and, rarely, withdrawal symptoms similar to those seen with alcohol or barbiturates were reported. Diazepam was one of the most frequently mentioned drugs in the DAWN system coroner's reports, although almost always in combination with alcohol or other depressants. What happened to the big difference between the barbiturates and the benzodiazepines? One possibility is that it may not be the chemical class of drugs that makes the big difference, but the dose and time course of the individual drugs.

Fig. 8-1 gives a schematic picture of the time course of the depressant actions of some of these drugs. Secobarbital, a short-acting barbiturate, has a relatively rapid onset that should make it more likely than other barbiturates to produce psychological dependence. Also, because its depressant action is terminated fairly quickly, withdrawal symptoms would be quite dramatic if the person had been taking large doses. Phenobarbital, a long-acting barbiturate, has a slower onset of action that should be less likely to produce psychological dependence. Because the depressant action is terminated more slowly, drug withdrawal occurs slowly and withdrawal symptoms are minimized. It has long been recognized that the short-acting barbiturates are the most likely to produce withdrawal symptoms. Since secobarbital, with its rapid onset and termination, was also prescribed in large, sleeping pill doses, both psychological and physical dependence were more common than with phenobarbital, which was usually prescribed in lower sedative doses.

The first benzodiazepine was chlordiazepoxide (Librium), which was sold in low doses for daytime use, has a slow onset of action and an even longer duration of action than phenobarbital. Librium produced few problems with either compulsive use or withdrawal symptoms. Diazepam has a more rapid onset than Librium, but because of slow metabolism and the presence of active metabolites, it also has a long duration of action. We might expect a drug with these characteristics to produce more psychological dependence than Librium, but only rarely to produce withdrawal symptoms. This is exactly what happened.

To summarize this pharmacology object lesson, there may be greater differences among the barbiturates and among the benzodiazepines than there are between these two classes.

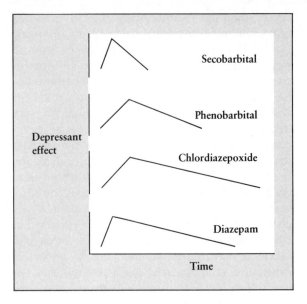

Figure 8-1. Schematic diagram of the relative time courses of two barbiturates and two benzodiazepines after oral administration.

Methaqualone

Even after benzodiazepines had taken over the daytime role of the barbiturates, secobarbital and amobarbital continued to be widely prescribed as sleeping pills. The market was wide open for a sleeping pill that would be less addicting and less dangerous. Maybe it was too wide open.

The methaqualone story is one where everyone was wrong—the pharmaceutical industry, the FDA, the DEA, the press, the physicians. No one can say he was without sin. Methaqualone was originally synthesized in India, tested and found to be ineffective as an antimalaria drug. But it was a good sedative, so in 1959 it was introduced as a prescription drug in Great Britain. It never sold well, but after the thalidomide disaster there was increased interest in a "safe" nonbarbiturate sleeping pill. Mandrax, 250 mg methaqualone and 25 mg of an antihistamine, promised to be that when it was introduced in 1965 in a massive advertising campaign to physicians. The campaign worked, and there were 2 million prescriptions issued for

Mandrax in 1971 in Great Britain. Even before that the drug had found its way into the street where it was widely abused: by heroin users, by high school students, by anyone who wanted a cheap but potent "down." Misuse was so great by 1968 that Great Britain tightened controls on it in 1970 and then again in 1973. After that the methaqualone problems subsided as other drugs came to prominence.

Germany introduced methaqualone in 1960 as a nonprescription drug, had its first methaqualone suicide in 1962, and discovered that 10% to 22% of the drug overdoses treated in this period were a result of this drug. In 1963 Germany reduced the problem by making methaqualone a prescription drug. In this 1960-1964 period Japan experienced a major epidemic of methaqualone abuse, causing over 40% of all overdoses admitted to mental hospitals. Japan tightened controls almost to the maximum possible on methaqualone and stemmed the tide.

In 1965, after 3 years of testing, Quaalude and Sopors, brand names for methaqualone, were introduced in the United States as prescription drugs with the package insert, "Addiction potential not established." Methaqualone was *not* a schedule drug; there were no monitoring rules or restrictions on the number of times the prescription could be refilled. In June 1966, the FDA Committee on the Abuse Potential of Drugs decided that there was no need to monitor methaqualone, since there was no evidence of abuse potential! Thus, from 1967 to 1973, the package insert read, "Physical dependence has not clearly been demonstrated," although by 1969 the evidence was very clear that methaqualone was an addicting drug.

In the early 1970s in this country, "ludes" and "sopors" (from *Quaaludes* and *Sopors*) were familiar terms in the drug culture and in drug treatment centers. Physicians were overprescribing what they believed to be a drug that was safer than the barbiturates, as well as nonaddicting. Most of the methaqualone sold on the street was legally manufactured and then either stolen or obtained through prescriptions. At any rate, sales

---

Your turn: a laughing matter?

Milton Berle, that famous comedian of the early years of television, was introduced at least once during the 1950s as "Miltown" Berle, a reference to the then popular Miltown (meprobamate). As we have seen, Miltown was displaced by Librium, then by Valium, but one of these sedatives has always been essentially a household word.

Try to think of some of the humorous comments you've heard or read about sedatives, such as Valium, methaqualone (Quaalude), or similar depressants. Write down as many jokes, asides, etc. as you can think of, whether from public media or from conversations. Is there a common theme to these jokes?

Jokes often serve some social purpose, such as reminding us of potential dangers by depicting someone in a humorously distressing situation. Do you think that joking about these drugs can serve such a purpose, or does "making light" of drug-induced impairments possibly encourage irresponsible drug use?

---

zoomed, and front-page reporting of its effects when misused helped build it as a drug of abuse.

Finally, 8 years after it was introduced into this country, 4 years after American scientists were saying it was addicting, 11 years after the first suicide, methaqualone was put on Schedule II October 4, 1973. By 1985 methaqualone was no longer available as a prescription drug, and it is now listed on Schedule I.

Was methaqualone really very different from the barbiturates? For a while, physicians thought so. Street users referred to it as the "love drug" (one of many drugs to have been called this) or "heroin for lovers," implying an **aphrodisiac** effect. In reality the effect is probably not different from the disinhibition produced by alcohol or other depressants. Because methaqualone causes the same kind of motor incoordination as alcohol and the barbiturates, one of its street names was "wallbanger" (after a popular mixed drink of the 1970s). Both psychological and physical dependence can develop to methaqualone as easily and rapidly as with the barbiturates, and for a few years methaqualone was also near the "top of the charts" for drug-related deaths (DAWN coroner's reports). If it's different, it isn't much different.

MECHANISM OF ACTION

An important key to understanding the effects of these sedative-hypnotic agents was found in 1977 when it was reported that radioactive diazepam (Valium) molecules had a high affinity for specific receptor sites in brain tissue.[5] Other benzodiazepine-type sedatives also bound to these receptors, and the relative affinities of these various molecules was highly correlated with their behavioral potencies in humans and other animals. These benzodiazepine receptors did not bind any of the known neurotransmitters, nor did they bind any of the barbiturates. However, it was soon noticed that the benzodiazepine receptors were always in close proximity to receptors for the amino acid neurotransmitter, gamma-aminobutyric acid (GABA). It now appears that when benzodiazepines bind to their receptor site, they enhance the normally inhibitory effects of GABA on its receptors. The barbiturates appear to act at a separate binding site nearby and also increase the actions of GABA on its receptors. The picture emerges of a GABA receptor complex, which includes the barbiturate binding site and the benzodiazepine receptor.[6] Drug companies are now developing new drugs based on their ability to bind to these sites, and we can expect to see a number of new sedative-hypnotics reaching the market over the next several years.

Although there have been intensive efforts to isolate an endogenous Valium-like substance from brain tissue, so far none has succeeded. A diazepam-binding inhibitor (DBI) peptide has been isolated from brain tissue,[7] but when this substance is administered it has effects opposite to those of diazepam, apparently producing excitement and increased anxiety in some animal tests. This promises to be an exciting area of research that can lead to increased understanding of brain function and drug actions.

BENEFICIAL USES
As Sedatives

> Raze out the written troubles of the brain,
> and with some sweet oblivious antidote
> Cleanse the stuff'd bosom of that perilous stuff
> Which weighs upon the heart . . .

As the lines from Shakespeare's *Macbeth* reveal, humans have often sought a "sweet oblivious antidote" to the cares and woes of living. Alcohol has most frequently been used for that purpose, but the sedative drugs also play a major role in modern society. In the United States in recent decades, the barbiturates, then meprobamate, and then the benzodiazepines have been among the most widely prescribed medications. Although no single brand of benzodiazepine dominates the market as Valium did, several benzodiazepines are now found among the top 50 drugs in sales. In 1987, Xanax was the most popular of these, ranking fourth. Also, both diazepam and lorazepam are among the most popular generic drug prescriptions (Table 8-2). The combined sales of the benzodiazepines make them easily the most widely prescribed drug class. Why? Most psychiatrists refer to the benzodiazepines as antianxiety agents, or anxiolytics. And most psychiatrists seem to accept the widely held view that various type of *neurotic* behavior (e.g., phobias, panic attacks, obsessive-compulsive disorders, or psychosomatic problems) may result from various forms of psychological stress that can be lumped under the general classification of "anxieties." So, if anxieties produce neurotic behavior and these drugs can reduce anxieties, then they will be useful in the treatment of neurotic psychiatric patients. In fact, the neuroses are now officially referred to as "anxiety disorders" (see Chapter 13). While this approach seems logical, in reality not all of these conditions respond well to antianxiety drugs, and for such things as simple phobia (e.g., of spiders) behavior therapy is a better treatment. Also, these drugs should probably be used to reduce acute anxiety and should not be taken on a chronic basis.[8] Most of the prescriptions for these antianx-

Table 8-2

Some popular benzodiazepines

Type	Half-life (hours)
Anxiolytics	
Alpraxolam (Xanax)	6-20
Chlorazepate (Tranxene)	30-200
Chlordiazepoxide (Librium)	5-30
Diazepam (Valium)	20-100
Lorazepam (Ativan)	10-20
Oxazepam (Serax)	5-15
Hypnotics	
Flurazepam (Dalmane)	40-250
Temazepam (Restoril)	5-25
Triazolam (Halcion)	1.7-3

in any individual case it may be impossible to know whether the patient feels better because of a specific antianxiety effect or because the drug might make anybody feel better. We cannot solve this therapeutic dilemma, but we can make a prediction: based on past history, there will continue to be a very large and profitable market for prescription sedatives.

As Sleeping Pills

While one or two beers might relax a person and reduce inhibitions a bit, the effect of larger amounts is more dramatic. If you consume several beers in an active, noisy party situation you may become wild and reckless. But if you consume the same number of beers, go to bed and turn off the lights, you will probably fall asleep fairly quickly. This is essentially the principle on which hypnotic drug therapy is based: the drug is not given in an anesthetic dose, but in a large enough amount to help you get to sleep more quickly.

Insomnia is a fairly common symptom, and one nationwide household survey found that about one out of three adults reported some trouble falling asleep, staying asleep, or both.[9] About half these people felt that their insomnia was serious, but fewer than 10% had used a prescription hypnotic drug within the past year. You should be aware that people who complain of insomnia often overestimate how long it takes them to get to sleep and underestimate how much time they actually sleep.[10] Partly because physicians know this and partly because of concern about tolerance, rebound insomnia, dependence, and "hangover" effects, fewer hypnotics are prescribed than 20 years ago, and they are usually taken for only 1 or 2 nights at a time rather than continually.

Since 1976, when flurazepam (Dalmane) became the leading hypnotic agent, the benzodiazepines have increasingly displaced the barbiturates in the sleeping pill market. In the late 1980s, the shorter-acting drug triazolam (Halcion) became the most commonly prescribed brand of hypnotic. There is an interesting story in this: When bar-

iety medications are not written by psychiatrists and are not written for patients with obviously neurotic conditions. In addition, many of these patients do take the drugs on a daily basis. What is being treated? Galen, the second century Greek physician, estimated that about 60% of the patients he saw had emotional and psychological, as opposed to physical, illness. Current estimates are that for a typical general practitioner about half the patients have no treatable physical ailment. Many of these patients who complain of nervousness or distress or of vague aches and pains will be given a prescription for a sedative such as Valium. One way to look at this is that the patients may be suffering from a low-level generalized anxiety disorder, and the sedative is therapeutic. A more cynical way of looking at it is that some patients are asking to be protected from the cares and woes of daily living. The physician prescribes something that is relatively safe and may make the patient feel better in a nonspecific way. The patient doesn't complain as much and comes back for more pills, so everyone is happy. While most physicians would agree that the benzodiazepines are probably overprescribed,

biturates are used they produce a fairly rapid tolerance, so that after a few nights of regular use they are no longer effective. To regain the hypnotic effect it became necessary to increase the dose, leading to concerns about addiction. One reason that Dalmane became the hypnotic drug of choice was that research indicated that it still produced hypnotic effects after 4 weeks of daily use. Dalmane, however, has an active metabolite with a long half-life (well over a day; see Table 8-2). With nightly use there is a buildup of this metabolite in the body. Perhaps the reason Dalmane still works after 4 weeks is that the total dose of metabolite plus Dalmane is quite large by that time. There is concern that this buildup of Dalmane plus its metabolite may impair the individual's performance during the daytime. Halcion has replaced Dalmane because it has a short half-life, no active metabolite, and should not build up in the body. Most patients are instructed to avoid daily use, but in some cases of severe insomnia chronic use is indicated. Can the short-acting benzodiazepines work under chronic treatment conditions without tolerance or withdrawal symptoms (rebound insomnia)? There are conflicting reports, but one large study indicated that short-acting benzodiazepines could still be effective after 3 months of chronic use, with no evidence of rebound insomnia on withdrawal.[11]

If you or someone you know has trouble sleeping, before resorting to the use of medication it would be wise to follow the suggestions given in Table 8-3. These tricks will probably help most people deal with their concerns about sleeplessness.

Anticonvulsant Effects

A thorough description of seizure disorders (the **epilepsies**) is beyond the scope of this book. However, you should know that both the barbi-

Table 8-3
"Sleep hygiene" techniques for patients with insomnia

Careful adherence to the following rules can lead to substantial improvement in sleep and can help prevent the development of chronic intractable insomnia.

- Establish and maintain a regular bedtime and a regular arising time. Try to wake up and get out of bed at the appointed time, even if you had trouble sleeping the night before. Avoid excessive sleep during holidays and weekends.
- When you get into bed, turn off the lights and relax. Avoid reviewing in your mind the day's stresses and tomorrow's challenges.
- Exercise regularly. Follow an exercise routine, but avoid heavy exercise late in the evening.
- Prepare a comfortable sleep environment. Too warm a room disturbs sleep; too cold a room does not solidify sleep. Occasional loud noises can disturb sleep without fully awakening you. "White noise" may be useful for masking a noisy environment.

- Watch what you eat and drink before bedtime. Hunger may disturb sleep, as may caffeine and alcohol. A light snack may promote sleep, but avoid heavy or spicy foods at bedtime.
- Avoid the use of tobacco.
- Do not lie awake in bed for long periods of time. If you cannot fall asleep within 30 minutes, get out of bed and do something relaxing before trying to fall asleep again. Repeat this as many times as necessary. The goal is to avoid developing a paired association between being in bed and restlessness.
- Do not nap during the day. A prolonged nap following a night of insomnia may disturb the next night's sleep.
- Avoid the chronic use of sleeping pills. While sedative-hypnotics can be effective when used as part of a coordinated treatment plan for certain types of insomnia, chronic use is ineffective at best and can be detrimental to sound sleep.

From Golden RN and James SP: Insomnia: clinical assessment and management of the patient who can't sleep, *Postgraduate Medicine* 83(4):251-258, 1988.

turates and the benzodiazepines are widely used for the control of epileptic seizures. They are effective in reasonably low doses and are often combined with other anticonvulsant drugs for even better effectiveness. There are some practical problems associated with this use, and by now you could guess what some of them are.

Anticonvulsant medications are given chronically, so there is a tendency for tolerance to develop. The dose should be kept high enough to control the seizures without producing undesirable drowsiness. Abrupt withdrawal of these drugs is likely to lead to seizures, so medication changes should be done carefully. In spite of these problems, the sedative drugs are currently a necessary and useful treatment for epilepsy.

CAUSES FOR CONCERN

Dependence Liability

Psychological dependence. Most people who have used either barbiturates or benzodiazepines have not developed habitual use patterns. However, it was clear with the barbiturates that some individuals did become daily users of intoxicating amounts. Again, the short-acting barbiturates seemed to be the culprits. When Librium, the first benzodiazepine, was in its heyday relatively little habitual use was reported. As Librium was displaced by the newer, more potent Valium, we saw increasing reports of habitual Valium use, perhaps because its onset, although slower than that of the short-acting barbiturates, is more rapid that that of Librium.

Animals given the opportunity to press a lever that delivers intravenous barbiturates will do so, and the short-acting types work best for this. Animals will also self-inject several of the benzodiazepines, but at lower rates than with the short-acting barbiturates.[12] When human drug abusers were allowed an opportunity to work for oral doses of barbiturates or benzodiazepines on a hospital ward, they developed regular patterns of working for the drugs. When given a choice between pentobarbital and diazepam, the subjects generally chose pentobarbital.[13] These experi-

ments indicate that these sedative drugs can serve as reinforcers of behavior, but that the short-acting barbiturates are probably more likely to lead to dependence than are any of the benzodiazepines currently on the market.

Physical dependence. A characteristic withdrawal syndrome can occur after chronic use of large enough doses of any of the sedative-hypnotic drugs. This syndrome is different from the narcotic withdrawal syndrome and similar to the alcohol withdrawal syndrome. An early description of the withdrawal from barbiturates will serve as an excellent example:

Upon abrupt withdrawal of barbiturates from individuals who have been ingesting 0.8 gm. or more daily of one of the shorter-acting barbiturates (secobarbital, pentobarbital, amobarbital), signs of barbiturate intoxication disappear in the first 8-12 hours of abstinence, and, clinically, the patient seems to improve. Thereafter, increasing anxiety, insomnia, tremulousness, weakness, difficulty in making cardiovascular adjustments on standing, anorexia, nausea and vomiting appear. One or more convulsions of **grand mal** type usually occur during the second or third day of abstinence. Following the seizures, a psychosis characterized by confusion, disorientation in time and place, agitation, tremulousness, insomnia, delusions and visual and auditory hallucinations may supervene. The psychosis

┌───┐

Your turn: drug advertising

If you have access to medical journals, either in a university library or possibly at a nearby hospital, leaf through some of them and find a few advertisements for Valium, Xanax, Tranxene, or Ativan. What kinds of messages do these advertisements send to the physicians who are their audience? Are the same ads found in specialist journals, such as the *American Journal of Psychiatry,* as are published for the broader audience in more general publications (*Journal of the American Medical Association* or *Modern Medicine*)?

Often these advertisements have descriptions, photographs, or drawings of patients. What are your attitudes toward a patient as depicted in one of these advertisements?

└───┘

clinically resembles alcoholic delirium tremens, usually begins and is worse at night, and terminates abruptly with a critical sleep.[14]

It should be pointed out that this syndrome is longer lasting and probably more unpleasant than the narcotic withdrawal syndrome. In addition, withdrawal from the sedative-hypnotics or alcohol is potentially life-threatening, with death occurring in as many as 5% of those who withdraw abruptly after taking large doses.

There has been considerable controversy over the frequency, nature, and severity of withdrawal symptoms after chronic use of the benzodiazepines. Animal experiments using large intravenous doses show clearly that a barbiturate-like withdrawal syndrome can be produced with benzodiazepines, with an onset that varies with the half-life of the drug. With Librium and Valium, especially when used in low doses, clinical reports of withdrawal were rare. Several reports have now generated sufficient data for us to be sure that benzodiazepine withdrawal symptoms can occur in patients, especially in those who have been taking the drug for a year or more. Although the use of short half-life benzodiazepines began much later than the use of the longer half-life forms, there are a few studies indicating more rapid and more severe withdrawal after the shorter half-life compounds, as would be expected.[15] The symptoms are rarely as severe as those seen with barbiturates, and often consist of increased anxiety, irritability, or insomnia, which may be confused with a return to predrug conditions of anxiety or insomnia for which the drug was initially prescribed.

Because there is a cross-dependence among the barbiturates, the benzodiazepines, and alcohol, it is theoretically possible to use any of the drugs to halt the withdrawal symptoms from any other depressant. Drug treatment is often used, and a general rule is to use a long-acting drug, given in divided doses until the withdrawal symptoms are controlled. One authority recommends using phenobarbital to treat any barbiturate dependence and diazepam in cases of alcohol or benzodiazepine dependence.[16]

Toxicity

The major areas of concern with these depressant drugs are the behavioral and physiological problems encountered when high doses of the drug are present in the body (acute toxicity). Behaviorally, all these drugs are capable of producing alcohol-like intoxication, with impaired judgment and coordination. Obviously, such an impaired state vastly multiplies the dangers involved in driving or other activities, and the effects of these drugs combined with alcohol are additive, so that the danger is further increased. There have also been reports of barbiturate-induced violence, which may be similar to the well-known effect of alcohol on aggression. On the physiological side the major concern is the tendency of these drugs to depress the rate of respiration. With large enough doses, as in accidental or intentional overdose, breathing ceases entirely. Again, the combination of these depressants and alcohol is quite dangerous. Although diazepam (Valium) is usually quite high on the list of drugs associated with deaths in the DAWN coroner's reports, in almost every case the culprit is diazepam in combination with alcohol, rather than diazepam alone.

Patterns of Abuse

Almost all of the abuse of these sedative-hypnotic agents has historically involved the oral use of legally manufactured products. Two characteristic types of abusers were associated with barbiturate use, and these two major types probably still characterize a large fraction of sedative abusers. The first type of abuser may be an older adult who obtains the drug on a prescription, either for daytime sedative use or as a sleeping pill. Through repeated use, tolerance develops and the dose is increased. Even though some of these individuals visit several different physicians to obtain prescriptions for enough pills to maintain this

---

Issue: valium and pregnancy

Valium is one of the most widely used prescription drugs in the country. Although it is generally good practice for pregnant women to avoid the use of any drug during the first 3 months of pregnancy and there is no absolute proof that Valium and other benzodiazepines can cause birth defects, because of the drug's popularity and the widely held belief that it is "safe," you should be aware that several studies have reported cases of cleft palate in children born to mothers who were taking benzodiazepines early in pregnancy.

Other case studies have reported something referred to as "floppy infant sydrome" in infants whose mothers took benzodiazepines late in pregnancy or while nursing. In these cases the infants seemed to have reduced muscle tone. Infants whose mothers were taking larger doses of benzodiazepines late in pregnancy may also experience withdrawal symptoms.

Because the need for the use of these drugs is rarely urgent, it seems that anyone taking a benzodiazepine who becomes pregnant should either stop the drug immediately or, in the case of epilepsy, withdraw as rapidly as possible.

---

level of use, many would vehemently deny that they were "drug abusers." This type of chronic use may lead to physical dependence. The other major group tends to be younger and consists of people who obtain the drugs simply for the purpose of "getting high." Sleeping pills may be taken from the home medicine cabinet, or the drugs may be purchased on the street. These younger abusers tend to take relatively large doses or to mix several drugs or to drink alcohol with the drug, all for the purpose of becoming intoxicated. With this type of use, the possibility for acute toxicity is particularly high.

Summary

The barbiturates, benzodiazepines, and other depressant drugs all have many effects in common with each other and with alcohol. These drugs may be prescribed in low doses for their sedative, or antianxiety, effect. In higher doses, the same or similar drugs are sometimes prescribed as sleeping pills (hypnotics). Over the past 20 years the barbiturates have been mostly displaced by the benzodiazepines, which are associated with fewer reports of dependence and perhaps with fewer overdose deaths. The benzodiazepines are the most widely prescribed type of psychoactive drug,

and most of these prescriptions are as sedatives. There may be overprescribing of the sedatives, but the drugs do appear to be effective for many people.

Although most research on insomnia suggests that drugs should only rarely be used to induce sleep, and then not on a repeated basis, in practice many prescriptions are still being written for sleeping pills. Benzodiazepines have largely replaced barbiturates for this use, also. The barbiturates and benzodiazepines both act to increase the inhibitory neural effects of the neurotransmitter GABA.

These drugs can produce both psychological and physical dependence. The short-acting barbiturates are more likely to produce both kinds of dependence than are the benzodiazepines, but that difference may be a result of the slower onset and longer duration of action of current benzodiazepines. Overdoses of these depressant drugs can cause death by inhibiting respiration, particularly if the drug is taken in combination with alcohol.

REFERENCES

1. Richardson BW: Chloral and other narcotics. I. Popular Science Monthly 15:492, 1879.
2. Goth A: Medical pharmacology, St. Louis, 1981, The CV Mosby Company.
3. Berger PA and Tinklenberg JR: Treatment of abusers of alcohol and other addictive drugs. In Psychopharmacology from theory to practice, 1977, Oxford University Press.

4. Rosenblatt S and Dobson R: Beyond Valium, New York, 1981, G.P. Putnam's Sons.

5. Squires RF and Braestrup C: Benzodiazepine receptors in rat brain, Nature 226:732-734, 1977.

6. Feldman RS and Guenzer LF: Fundamentals of neuro-psychopharmacology, Sunderland, Mass, 1984, Sinauer.

7. Alho H and others: Diazepam-binding inhibitor: a neuropeptide located in selected neuronal populations of rat brain, Science 229:179-182, 1985.

8. Gelenberg AJ: Anxiety. In Bassuk EL, Schoonover SC, and Gelenberg AJ, editors: The practitioner's guide to psychoactive drugs, ed 2, New York, 1983, Plenum Press.

9. Mellinger GD, Balter MB, and Uhlenhuth EH: Insomnia and its treatment: prevalence and correlates, Archives of General Psychiatry, 42:225-232, 1985.

10. Miller RR: A guide to the use of hypnotic drugs, Medical Times 107(6):28, 1979.

11. Allen RP, Mendels J, Nevins DB and others: Efficacy without tolerance or rebound insomnia for midazolam and temazopam after use for one to three months, Journal of Clinical Pharmacology 27:768-775, 1988.

12. Griffiths RR and others: Self-injection of barbiturates and benzodiazepines in baboons, Psychopharmacology 75:101-109, 1981.

13. Griffiths RR, Bigelow G, and Liebson I: Human drug self-administration: double-blind comparison of pentobarbital, diazepam, chlorpromazine and placebo, Journal of Pharmacology and Experimental Therapeutics 210:301-310, 1979.

14. Fraser HF, Shaver MR, Maxwell ES and others: Death due to withdrawal of barbiturates, Annals of Internal Medicine 38:1319-1325, 1953.

15. Roy-Byrne PP and Hommer D: Benzodiazepine withdrawal: overview and implications for the treatment of anxiety, The American Journal of Medicine 84:1041-1052, 1988.

16. Sellers EM: Alcohol, barbiturate and benzodiazepine withdrawal syndromes: clinical management, Canadian Medical Association Journal 139:113-120, 1988.

Chapter 9

Alcohol

OBJECTIVES

After reading this chapter, you should be able to:

Describe how alcohol is fermented and distilled and how these processes are used to produce various alcoholic beverages.

Discuss the history of regulation of alcoholic beverages and the current trends in sales of beer, wine, and liquor.

Explain how alcohol is absorbed and broken down in the body, and how blood alcohol level relates to changes in behavior.

Describe some of the important medical and social problems caused by alcohol use.

Discuss the factors that go into describing an individual as an alcoholic.

Alcohol—social lubricant, adjunct to a fine meal, or demon rum? People today are no different from people throughout the centuries in that many of them use alcohol, whereas many others condemn its use. This love-hate relationship with alcohol has been going on for a long time. There does seem to be a swing of the pendulum right now: health-conscious Americans are opting for low-alcohol drinks, bartenders are having contests to see who can make the best nonalcoholic cocktail, and we receive frequent reminders to use alcohol responsibly, not to drink and drive, and not to let our friends drive if they've been drinking. Let's take a closer look at the world's number one psychoactive substance.

ALCOHOLIC BEVERAGES
Fermentation and Fermentation Products

Many thousands of years ago, Neolithic man discovered "booze." Beer and berry wine were known and used about 6400 BC, while grape wine dates from 300 to 400 BC. Mead, which is made from honey, may be the oldest alcoholic beverage; some authorities suggest it appeared in the Paleolithic Age, about 8000 BC. Early use of alcohol seems to have been worldwide: beer was drunk by the American Indians whom Columbus met.

Fermentation forms the basis for all alcoholic beverages. Certain yeasts act on sugar in the presence of water, and this chemical action is fermentation. Yeast recombines the carbon, hydrogen, and oxygen of sugar and water into ethyl alcohol and carbon dioxide. Chemically, $C_6H_{12}O_6$ (glucose) + H_2O (water) is transformed to C_2H_6O (ethyl alcohol) + CO_2 (carbon dioxide).

Most fruits, including grapes, contain sugar, and addition of the appropriate yeast (which is pervasive in the air wherever plants grow) to a mixture of crushed grapes and water will begin the fermentation process. The yeast has only a limited tolerance for alcohol, so that when the concentration reaches 15%, the yeast dies, and fermentation ceases.

Cereal grains can also be used to produce alcoholic beverages. However, cereal grains contain starch rather than sugar, and, before fermentation can begin, the starch must be converted to sugar. This is accomplished by means of enzymes formed during a process called *malting*. In American beer, the primary grain is barley, which is malted by steeping it in water and allowing it to sprout. The sprouted grain is then slowly dried to kill the sprout but preserve the enzymes formed during the growth. This dried, sprouted barley is called malt, and, when crushed and mixed with water, the enzymes convert the starch to sugar. Only yeast is needed then to start fermentation.

Distilled Products

To obtain alcohol concentrations above those that can be reached by fermentation, distillation must be used. **Distillation** is a process in which the solution containing alcohol is heated and the vapors are collected and condensed into liquid form again. Since alcohol has a lower boiling point than water, there is a higher percentage of alcohol in the distillate (the condensed liquid) than there was in the original solution.

There is still debate over who discovered the distillation process and when the discovery was made, but many authorities place it in Arabia around 800 AD. The term **alcohol** is from an Arabic word meaning "finely divided spirit" and originally referred to that part of the wine collected through distillation—the essence of the wine! Only fermented beverages were used in Europe until the tenth century, when the Italians first distilled wine, thereby introducing "spirits" to the western world. These new products were formally and informally studied and used in the treatment of many illnesses, including senility. The prevalent feeling about their medicinal value is best seen in the name given these condensed vapors by a thirteenth century Professor of Medicine at the French University of Montpellier: *aqua vitae,* the water of life. Around the end of the seventeenth century the more prosaic Dutch called the liquid *brandy,* meaning burnt wine.

The name "whiskey" comes from the Irish-Gaelic equivalent of aqua vitae and was already commonplace around 1500. The distillation of whiskey in America started on a large scale toward the end of the eighteenth century. The chief product of the area just west of the Appalachian Mountains—western Pennsylvania, western Virginia, eastern Kentucky—was grain. It was not profitable for the farmers to ship the grain or flour across the mountains to the markets along the eastern seaboard. Since 10 bushels of corn could be converted to 6 barrels of flour, which could then be converted to 1 barrel of whiskey, which could be profitably shipped east, distillation started on a grand scale.

In the United States the alcoholic content of distilled beverages is indicated by the term *proof.* The percentage of alcohol by volume is one half the proof number, that is, 90-proof whiskey is 45% alcohol. The term **proof** developed from a British Army procedure to gauge the alcohol content of distilled spirits before there were modern techniques. The liquid was poured over gunpowder and ignited. If the alcohol content was high enough, the alcohol would burn and ignite the gunpowder, which would go "pooff" and explode! That was proof that the beverage had an acceptable alcohol content, about 57%.

REGULATION OF ALCOHOL USE

Alcohol is different from most of the recent psychoactive drugs in western civilization in that the problem has never been to prevent its introduction—it has always been everywhere! There have been repeated attempts to control its use and, on occasion, to eliminate its availability. Throughout Europe and America, from the fourteenth through the twentieth century, all attempts to suppress alcohol have failed.

Early attempts at regulation of alcohol consumption in England consisted of edicts handed down by religious authorities. Some of these were recorded as early as the sixth century AD. The first national English legislation to curb intemperance was passed in 1327; it tried to limit the number of establishments that could sell alcoholic beverages. It was rapidly repealed, and a different approach was tried over 150 years later in 1494. This was the first licensing law; it gave justices of the peace authority to determine where alcoholic drinks could be sold. Nothing succeeded. The consumption of alcohol in one form or another continued.

In 1688 distillation was opened wide in England; upon paying a small tax, anyone could become a distiller. The crowding of urban central-city poverty areas with the workers of the industrial revolution, coupled with low-cost, easily available alcohol, contributed to the increase in alcohol consumption and in public drunkenness.

The Temperance Movement

At no time did drinking in the United States reach the epidemic levels it had in England. An expanding frontier, fewer overcrowded slum areas, and a pioneer ideology resulted in almost everyone in the colonial period drinking, but moderately. As society changed in the early part of the nineteenth century, heavy drinking increased, and with each new public drunkard, there appeared two or three **temperance** workers. Temperance movements were everyhwere in this period, acquiring national status with the formation of the American Temperance Society in 1827, which, it is important to note, advocated temperance, not abstinence. The changing pattern of alcohol use in this period is indicated in Table 9-1. In 1834 Congress provided the plot for a thousand western movies by passing a law forbidding the sale of liquor to Indians. The evidence is mixed on whether Indians differ in the way they metabolize alcohol. Perhaps Indians are most sensitive to the CNS effects of alcohol. Perhaps, though, they learned to drink from the early fur trappers and explorers, whose drinking pattern was to get "bombed." This is still an open question.

In the second half of the nineteenth century things changed. Up to this time there had been little commercial nondistilled alcohol consumed in the United States. It was only with the advent of artificial refrigeration and the addition of hops, which helped preserve the beer, that there was an increase in the number of breweries. The waves of immigrants who entered the country in this period provided the necessary beer-drinking consumers.

At first, encouraged by temperance groups who preferred beer consumption to the use of liquor, breweries were constructed everywhere. Surprisingly, it was the great number of breweries that made abstainers out of temperants and brought about the second wave of state prohibition statutes that evolved into the national prohibition in 1920.

Table 9-1			
Estimated alcoholic beverage consumption (gallons per person 15 years of age and older)			
Year	Distilled spirits	Beer*	Wine
1800	7.2	32	0.6
1850	4.2	3	0.5
1900	2.0	24	0.7
1915	2.0	29	0.7

*In 1800 "beer" is mostly hard cider.

Prohibition

The first state **prohibition** period began in 1851 when Maine passed its prohibition law. Between 1851 and 1855 13 states passed statewide prohibition laws, but by 1868 nine had repealed them. The National Prohibition Party, organized in 1874, provided the impetus for the second wave of statewide prohibition that developed in the 1880s. From 1880 to 1889 seven states adopted prohibition laws, but by 1896 four had repealed them.

In 1899 a group of educators, lawyers, and clergymen described the saloon as the "workingman's club, in which many of his leisure hours are spent, and in which he finds more of the things that approximate luxury than in his home. . . ." They went on to say: "It is a centre of learning, books, papers, and lecture hall to them. It is the clearinghouse for common intelligence, the place where their philosophy of life is worked out, and their political and social beliefs take their beginnings."[1] pp.215-217

Truth lay somewhere between those statements and the sentiments expressed in a sermon:

The liquor traffic is the most fiendish, corrupt and hell-soaked institution that ever crawled out of the slime of the eternal pit. It is the open sore of this land. . . . It takes the kind, loving husband and father, smothers every spark of love in his bosom, and transforms him into a heartless wretch, and makes him steal the shoes from his starving babe's feet to find the price for a glass of liquor. It takes your sweet innocent daughter, robs her of her virtue and transforms her into a brazen, wanton harlot. . . .

The open saloon as an institution has its origin in hell, and it is manufacturing subjects to be sent back to hell. . . .[2] pp.66-67

Prohibition was not just a matter of "wets" versus "drys," or a matter of political conviction or health concerns. Intricately interwoven with these factors was a middle-class, rural, Protestant, evangelical concern that the good and true life was being undermined by ethnic groups with a different religion and a lower standard of living and morality. One way to strike back at these groups was through prohibition.

Between 1907 and 1919, 34 states enacted legislation enforcing statewide prohibition, while only two states repealed their prohibition laws. By 1917, 64% of the population lived in dry territory, and in the 1908 to 1917 period over 104,400 licensed bars were closed.

It should also be remembered that the fact that there was a state prohibition law did not mean that the residents did not drink. They did, both legally and illegally. They drank illegally in speakeasies and other private clubs. They drank legally from a variety of the many patent medicines that were freely available. A few of the more interesting ones were Whisko, "a nonintoxicating stimulant" at 55 proof; Golden's Liquid Beef Tonic, "recommended for treatment of alcohol habit" with 53 proof; and Kaufman's Sulfur Bitters, which "contains no alcohol" but was in fact 20% alcohol (40 proof) and contained no sulfur!

1917 was the beginning of the end. In January the U.S. Supreme Court upheld a law passed by Congress in 1913 forbidding interstate shipment of alcoholic beverages into areas where the manufacture and sale of liquor was illegal.[1] In March Congress passed an antiliquor advertising bill, which prohibited the use of the U.S. mail to advertise "spirituous, vinous, malted, fermented, or other intoxicating liquors of any kind" in an area that locally restricted their advertising. At this time, although only 64% of the population was dry, 90% of the land area was, so this law effectively stopped all but local advertising.

In August, 1917, the Senate adopted the resolution authored by Andrew Volstead, which submitted the national prohibition amendment to the states. The House of Representatives concurred in December, and 21 days later on January 8, 1918, Mississippi became the first state to ratify the Eighteenth Amendment. A year later, January 16, 1919, Nebraska was the thirty-sixth state to ratify the amendment, and the deed was done!

As stated in the amendment, a year after the thirty-sixth state ratified it, national prohibition came into effect: January 16, 1920. The amendment was simple, with only two operational parts:

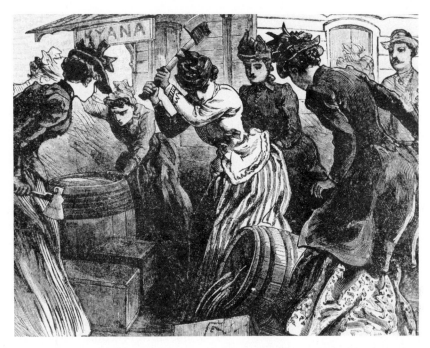

Carrie Nation became a symbol of the temperance movement with her "hachetations," which also led to her being arrested over 30 times.

Section 1. After one year from the ratification of this article the manufacture, sale or transportation of intoxicating liquors within, the importation thereof into, or the exportation thereof from the United States and all territory subject to the jurisdiction thereof for beverage purposes is hereby prohibited.

Section 2. The Congress and the several States shall have concurrent power to enforce this article by appropriate legislation.

The Eighteenth Amendment was not passed by just a few bible-thumpers—after all, it is not easy to amend the U.S. Constitution, as supporters of the Equal Rights Amendment know. It seems that most of the people in the United States supported some type of federal control over alcohol.[3] The law did not result in an alcohol-free society, and this came as quite a surprise to most people. Apparently the assumption was that the prohibition would be so widely accepted that little enforcement would be necessary. Along with saloons, breweries, and distilleries, hospitals that had specialized in the treatment of alcoholics closed their doors, presumably because there would no longer be a need for them.[4]

It soon became clear that people were buying and selling alcohol illegally and that enforcement of this law was going to be a big problem. It may be that the majority of the population supported the idea of prohibition, but such a large minority insisted on continuing to drink that speakeasies, hip flasks, and "bathtub gin" became household words. Organized crime became both more organized and vastly more profitable as a result of prohibition. The popular conception is that prohibition was a total failure, leading to its repeal. That is not the whole picture.

Prohibition did have the apparent effect of reducing overall alcohol intake. Hospital admissions for alcoholism, as well as deaths from alcoholism, declined sharply at the beginning of prohibition. However, during the decade of the 1920s it appears that the prohibition laws were increasingly violated, particularly in large eastern cities like New York, and the rates of alcoholism and alcohol-related deaths began to increase.[5] Even toward the end of the "noble experiment" as prohibition was called by its detractors, alcoholism and alcohol-related deaths were still lower than before prohibition.

Concern about the widespread and highly publicized disrespect for the law and the growth of organized crime led many people to call for repeal. The Depression, which began in 1929, also made people consider the value of tax revenues—better that liquor sales provide a profit for the government than for Al Capone and other gangsters.

The Eighteenth Amendment was repealed by the Twenty-first Amendment proposed in Congress on February 20, 1933 and ratified by 36 states by the fifth of December of that year. So ended an era. The Twenty-first Amendment was also short and sweet:

Section 1. The eighteenth article of amendment of the Constitution of the United States is hereby repealed.
Section 2. The transportation or importation into any State, Territory, or possession of the United States for delivery or use therein of intoxicating liquors, in violation of the laws thereof, is hereby prohibited.

When national prohibition ended, America did not return overnight to the pre-1920s levels of alcohol consumption. Sales increased rapidly until after World War II, at which point per capita consumption was approximately what it had been before prohibition. Thus, prohibition of alcohol, much like the current prohibitions of marijuana and heroin, did work in that it reduced alcohol availability, use, and related problems. On the other hand, it did not work to eliminate alcohol from America and it encouraged organized crime and created expensive enforcement efforts.

Since 1933

After national prohibition, control over alcohol was returned to the states. Each state has since had its own means of regulating alcohol. Although a few states remained totally "dry" following national prohibition, most allowed at least beer sales. Thus the temperance sentiment that beer was a safer beverage continued to influence policy. In many cases, beer containing no more than 3.2% alcohol by weight was allowed as a nonintoxicating beverage. Even states that remained dry, like Kansas and Oklahoma, allowed 3.2 beer. As we shall see, alcohol is alcohol, and 3.2 beer *is* intoxicating.

Over the years, the general trend was for a relaxation of laws: states that did not allow sales of liquor became fewer until in 1966 the last dry state, Mississippi, became wet. Until 1970, when the national voting age was lowered to 18, all states except New York and Louisiana had minimum ages of 21 for the purchase of alcoholic beverages. During the 1970s, 30 states lowered the drinking age to 18 or 19. Per capita consumption rates, which were relatively stable during the 1950s, increased steadily from 1965 through 1980. However, times have changed; pushed by concerns over young people dying in alcohol-related traffic accidents, Congress authorized the Transportation Department to withold a portion of the federal highway funds for any state that did not raise its minimum drinking age to 21. In 1988, the final state (Wyoming) raised its drinking age, making 21 the uniform drinking age all across the United States.

Taxation

Federal taxes on alcoholic beverages are a significant means of gathering money for the federal government. Although most of the federal revenue comes from individual income taxes, taxes on alcohol do represent about 1% of the total collections by the Internal Revenue Service.[6] This amounted to over $5 billion each year from 1972 through 1986. In October 1985 the federal tax on distilled spirits was raised from $10.50 to $12.50 per gallon. This increased cost may contribute slightly to the already decreasing sale of distilled spirits, but its major purpose was to increase federal revenues.

The states also collect over $1 billion each year

in excise taxes and license fees for alcoholic beverages. When all these are added up, over half the consumer's cost for an average bottle of distilled spirits represents taxes.

ALCOHOL AS A CONSUMER ITEM

Alcoholic beverages are of considerable economic importance in the United States. In the late 1980s Americans were spending over $50 billion a year, buying about 24 gallons of beer, 1.6 gallons of distilled spirits, and over 2 gallons of wine for every man, woman, and child. (Some per capita alcohol figures are based on all ages, some on those 21 and over, and some on the "drinking age" population, assumed to be over the age of either 14 or 15.) Total sales of distilled spirits reached a peak in 1980-1981 and declined each year from 1982-1987. Total beer sales, which had been increasing through 1980, were essentially level from 1981-1987. Wine is the only segment of the alcoholic beverage industry that continued to grow through 1987.[6]

Beer

Beer is made by adding barley malt to other cereal grains, such as ground corn or rice. The enzymes in the malt change the starches in these grains into sugar, then the solids are filtered out before the yeast is added to the mash to start fermentation. Hops (dried blossoms from only the female hop plant) are added with the yeast to give beer its distinctive, pungent flavor. One-fourth pound of hops is enough to flavor a 31-gallon barrel of beer. Most of the beer sold today in America is *lager,* from the German word *lagern,* meaning to store. To brew lager, a type of yeast is used that settles to the bottom of the mash to ferment. After fermentation, and before packaging, the beer is stored for a period to age. In most commercial beers today, alcohol content is a little over 4%. Since the majority of American beer is sold in bottles or cans, the yeast must be removed to prevent it from spoiling after packaging. This is usually accomplished by heating it (pasteurization),

but some brewers use microfilters to remove the yeasts while keeping the beer cold. The carbonation is added at the time of packaging.

Ale requires a top-fermentation yeast, warmer temperatures during fermentation, and more malt and hops, which produce a more flavorful beverage. *Malt liquor* is brewed much like lager but is aged longer, has less carbonation, more calories, and 1% to 3% more alcohol.

If you were asked to produce a "light" beer, with fewer calories, a lighter taste, and less alcohol, what would you do—add water? That's only part of the answer, since light beers have about 10% less alcohol and 25% to 30% fewer calories. The mash is fermented at a cooler temperature for a longer time so that more of the sugars are converted to alcohol. *Then* the alcohol content is adjusted by adding water, resulting in a beverage with considerably less remaining sugar and only a bit less alcohol. In the late 1980s Japanese brewers introduced "dry" beers, which are made by a similar process, are less sweet, and, in Japan, contain more alcohol. They were a big success, and one major American brewer introduced a "dry" beer that also showed promising early sales (even though its alcohol content is about the same as in their regular beer).

The beer-drinking, free-lunch saloon with nickel beer and bucket-of-suds-to-go disappeared forever with prohibition. And so did a couple of thousand breweries. Two years after prohibition ended there were only 750 brewers, and by 1941 that had dwindled to 507. From 1960 to the mid-70s about 10 beer makers vanished each year, until in 1976 there were less than 50. This declined to about 40 in the early 1980s, and then began to increase again as small, local "boutique" breweries began to sprout up, especially on the west coast.

Table 9-2 points to a couple of trends: first, you might notice that the lion's share of beer sales goes to a small number of brewers. As a result of mergers and consolidations during the 1980s, there are now five major brewing companies in the United States. The industry leader, Anheuser-Busch, continues to gain and now controls over 40% of the

Table 9-2		
Largest selling beer brands (1988)		
Brand	**Brewer**	**Sales***
Budweiser	Anheuser-Busch	50.4
Lite	Miller	19.3
Bud Light	Anheuser-Busch	9.7
Coors Light	Adolph Coors	8.9
Busch	Anheuser-Busch	8.6
Miller High Life	Miller	8.4
Old Milwaukee	Stroh	7.0
Coors	Adolph Coors	6.3
Milwaukee's Best	Miller	5.7
Michelob	Anheuser-Busch	4.4

*Millions of barrels.

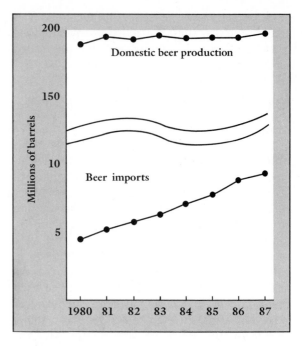

Figure 9-1. Recent trends in U.S. beer production and imports for foreign beer to the United States.

total market. In fact, their top-selling beer, Budweiser, accounts for over 25% of all beer sales. The only top-five brewer not accounted for in Table 9-2 is Heileman, which also sells Carling and several other brands. The other trend to notice is that three of the top five beers are now "light" beers—in 1978 there were no light beers among the top five.

Figure 9-1 shows the recent trends in domestic production and importation of beer. From 1980 to 1987, domestic production increased by only 4%, while imports more than doubled. [6] Asian and Australian imports increased fourfold during that period, while imports of Mexican beer increased by more than seven times. In spite of this increased appetite for foreign beers, they still represent only 5% of total U.S. sales. One way to look at what happened to the beer market in the 1980s is that the specialty beers produced by new, small breweries combined with increased numbers and variety of imports to add much in the way of choice for the beer fancier, but Budweiser alone outsold all the imports and boutique beers combined.

Americans drink almost 25 gallons of beer for every man, woman, and child each year, and that didn't change much during the 1980s. We're somewhat behind the Irish and Australians at over

30 gallons, and the Germans and Czechs who drink about 40 gallons per capita. On a per-capita basis, Mexicans and Japanese drink less than half the amount of beer consumed by Americans.

Wine

Wine is one of mankind's oldest beverages, a drink that has been praised as a gift from heaven and condemned as a work of the devil for generations. Although a large volume of wine is now produced in mechanized, sterilized wine "factories," there is still a greater variety among the various types of wine than exists among beers or whiskeys. There are many small wineries that operate alongside the industry giants, and the tradition continues that careful selection and cultivation of grapevines, good weather, precise timing of the harvest, and careful monitoring of fermentation and aging can result in wines of noticeably higher quality. An interesting ecological story resulted from the fact that most American wine grapes were originally transplanted from France and Spain. After a late nineteenth century disease destroyed almost all the European vineyards, it became necessary to transplant American vines, which had been protected by isolation, back into Europe. Today most of the French, Italian, and Spanish wine grapes are grown from descendants of those American vines.

There are two basic types of American wines. *Generics* usually have names taken from European land areas where the original wines were produced: Chablis, Champagne, Burgundy, Bordeaux, and Rhine are examples. These are all blended wines, made from whatever grapes are available, and during processing they are made to taste something like the traditional European wines from those regions. However, there is little guarantee of quality in these generic names among American wines. *Varietals* are named after one variety of grape that by law must make up at least 51% of the grapes used in producing the wine. Chardonnay, pinot noir, and zinfandel are some examples. There are many varietal wines, and traditionally they have been sold in individual bottles and are more expensive than the generics. To clarify the varietal-generic distinction with an example, in France the name Chablis is carefully protected by law. A French Chablis must come from the Chablis region and be made only from the chardonnay grape. In America, most inexpensive dry white wines are called Chablis, and they are likely to include a considerable amount of juice from table grapes such as the Thompson seedless. One varietal that seems to be uniquely Californian is zinfandel. This variety of red grape has been so widely planted that the wine is often packaged in large jugs or boxes and marketed more like a generic.

Most white wines are made from white grapes, although it is possible to use red grapes if the skins are removed before fermentation. Red wines are made from red grapes by leaving the skins in the crushed grapes while they ferment. Rose (pronounced rose-ay) wines were traditionally made by leaving the skins in for only a day or two, but

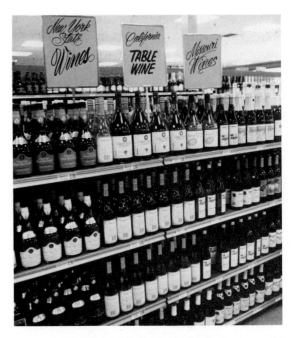

Wines from the United States.

most inexpensive American rose wine is made by mixing generic red and white wines. During the 1980s "blush" wines, such as white zinfandel, became quite popular. With the zinfandel grape, which is red, there may be enough staining of the juice because some of the grapes are crushed during transport, or the skins may be left in the crushed grapes for a short while, resulting in a wine that is just slightly pink.

Besides red vs. white and generic vs. varietal, another general distinction is "dry" vs. sweet. Most table wines are relatively dry, but some are sweeter than others. Also, the sweeter wines are likely to have a "heavier" taste overall, with the sweetness balancing out flavors that might be considered harsh in a dry wine. As a general rule lighter foods, such as broiled fish, call for a light, dry, white wine. With Thanksgiving turkey a Rhine or a blush wine would be appropriate, and a steak would go well with a red wine.

Because carbon dioxide is produced during fermentation, it is possible to produce naturally carbonated sparkling wines by adding a small amount of sugar as the wine is bottled and then keeping the bottle tightly corked. French champagnes are made in this way, as are the more expensive American champagnes, which may be labelled "naturally fermented in the bottle," or "methode Champagnoise." A less expensive way is to do the secondary fermentation in a large sealed tank and then maintain pressure while the wine is put in a bottle. A still cheaper method is used on inexpensive American champagnes and sparkling burgundies: Carbon dioxide is injected into a generic wine during bottling. Champagnes vary in their sweetness, also, with brut being the driest (dry and extra dry are not as dry).

It was discovered many years ago in Spain that if enough brandy is added to a newly fermented wine, the fermentation will stop and the wine will not spoil. Sealing the wine in charred oak casks for aging further refined its taste, and soon "sherry" was in great demand throughout Europe. Other fortified wines, all of which have an alcohol content near 20%, include port, Madeira, and Muscatel. Dry sherry is typically consumed before dinner, whereas the sweeter fortified wines may be drunk as a dessert wine.

In the 1960s Americans consumed less wine than they do now, and most of it consisted of dessert wines. Sales of the sweet wines have decreased, and sales of the drier table wines have increased to several times their 1960 level, bringing total wine sales up with them. The trend to increased wine drinking continued during the 1980s, as Figure 9-2 demonstrates. Part of this increase in per capita wine consumption is due to the introduction of the *wine cooler*.

These were derived from a popular low-alcohol mixed drink, a mixture of white wine and 7-up. Various 12-ounce bottles containing mixtures of wines with carbonated fruit-flavored drinks appeared with names like California Cooler, Sun Country Cooler, and Bartles and James (actually made by the wine industry giant, Ernest and Julio Gallo). These sweet, bubbly drinks look and taste a lot like soda pop, a fact that has not been lost

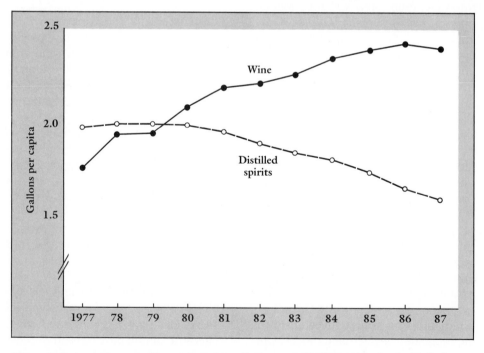

Figure 9-2. Annual per capita consumption of wine and distilled spirits in the United States. (Data from the Brewers' Almanac.[6])

on the marketers. Matilda Bay Original Fruit Cooler, and then others, began to be sold in 2-liter plastic bottles resembling soft drink bottles. They are popular with young drinkers who may not be aware that they contain both more alcohol and more calories than a bottle of beer. First introduced in 1981, sales really took off in 1984 and 1985, then continued to climb until by 1987 wine cooler sales represented 25% of the dollar sales for the American wine industry.[7] It appears likely that these coolers will replace beer as the most common "gateway" alcoholic beverage for beginning drinkers.

Distilled Spirits

Although brandy, distilled from wine, was probably the first type of "spirits" known to Europeans, the Celts of Ireland and the Scottish highlands were distilling a crude beverage known as *uisgebaugh*—water of life—before 1500. Today's

Scotch whisky (without the "e"; it's whiskey in the United States and in Ireland, whisky in Scotland and Canada) is the distillate of fermented malted barley. The distinctive smoky flavor comes from two sources: The malted barley is dried in kilns in which burning peat provides the heat, and some of the distinctive characteristics of peat are probably picked up by the malt. With so many casks of sherry wine being sent to the British Isles after the seventeenth century, the ever-frugal Scots began to use the empty casks to age their whisky, and current practice calls for this storage in old sherry casks for at least 3 years. Pure malt whisky of this type is more popular in the Highlands than elsewhere because of its strong flavors. Most commerical Scotch whisky is blended with lighter-tasting grain spirits to provide a more pleasing drink.

In America, the economics of trade resulted in an expanding production of spirits distilled from grain just as our new federal government was

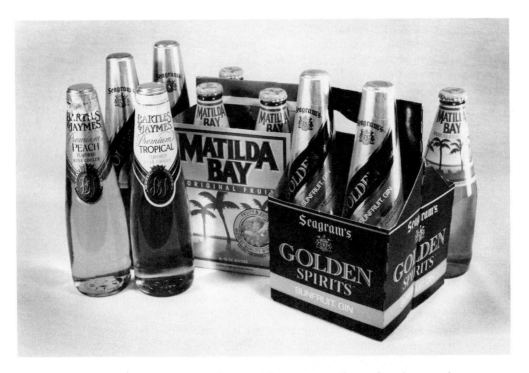

Wine coolers are accounting for a rapidly increasing share of total wine sales.

Your turn: wine coolers

Are wine coolers replacing beer as the first type of beverage most young people drink on their own? Their sweetness and relative lack of an alcohol taste would seem to make them an ideal transition beverage from soft drinks. One thing to think about is whether making the initiation to drinking easier might eventually lead to more young people drinking than before.

Try to get two or three young people to help you with a project: do a small survey among a group of college students, making sure to sample various ages. Ask if they can remember the first time they drank alcohol outside their own home and without adult supervision. What beverage was involved? If you are able to ask 20 or more at each age group, you may be able to see a trend with age. One prediction is that older students will have been more likely to have begun their drinking with beer and that younger students will be more likely to have begun with wine coolers. Also be sure to look for a sex difference.

---

forming. In 1789 one of the early distillers who established a good reputation was Elijah Craig, a Baptist minister living in what was then Bourbon County, Kentucky. He began storing his whiskey in charred new oak barrels, originating a manufacturing step still used with most American whiskeys.

By the seventeenth century improved distillation techniques made possible the production of relatively pure alcohol. Today's standard product from many large commercial distilleries is 95% pure alcohol (190 proof). Into the process goes whatever grain is available at a cheap price, tank loads of corn syrup, or other sources of sugars or starches. Out the other end comes *grain neutral spirits*, a clear and essentially tasteless liquid (other than the strong alcohol taste), which may be sold in small quantities as Everclear, or for use in medicine or research. More often, it is processed in bulk in various ways. For example, large quantities of grain neutral spirits are now being added to gasoline in some areas, to produce a less polluting fuel that also helps out the American

farmer. Besides other industrial uses for ethyl alcohol, in cleaners and solvents, bulk grain neutral spirits is also used in making various beverages. We have already mentioned its use in blended Scotch whiskys. One of the first beverages to be made from straight grain neutral spirits was gin. By filtering the distillate through juniper berries and then diluting it with water, a medicinal-tasting drink was produced. First called "jenever" by the Dutch and "genievre" by the French, the British shortened the name first to "geneva" and then to gin. This became a popular beverage in England, and now forms the basis for many an American martini.

Another major use for bulk grain neutral spirits is in the production of *vodka*. All American vodkas, and most vodkas from other countries, are simply a mixture of grain neutral spirits and water, adjusted to the desired proof. You may wonder why vodkas of the same proof are priced differently if they are all identical—and they are. The best answer to that question was given by an official of Heublein's, a company that produces both the high-priced *Smirnoff* vodka and a medium-priced vodka. "That's a very embarrassing question. Shall we say it's a difference in pricing policy?" Yes, we shall say that—maybe one label costs more?

The proof at which distillation is carried out influences the taste and other characteristics of the liquor. When alcohol is formed, other related substances, known as congeners, are also formed. These may include alcohols other than ethanol, oils, and other organic matter. Luckily they are present only in small amounts, because some of them are quite toxic. Grain neutral spirits contain relatively few congeners and none of the flavor of the grains used in the mash. Whiskey is usually distilled at a lower proof, not more than 160, and thus the distillate contains more congeners as well as some of the flavor of the grain used. If 51% or more of the grain used was rye, then the product is labeled *straight rye* whiskey. When corn constitutes over 51% of the grain in the mash, the liquor is called *bourbon*. (To be called *corn whiskey* requires that the mash be 80% or more corn.)

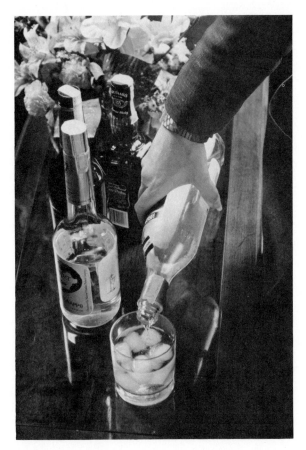

Sophisticated consumers have turned away from bourbon toward the lighter, more mixable vodka and blended whiskeys.

Both rye and bourbon are then diluted to 120 to 125 proof and aged in new, charred oak barrels for at least 2, and usually more, years. Whiskey accumulates congeners during aging, at least for the first 5 years, and it is the congeners and the grain used that provide the variation in taste among whiskeys.

Until prohibition almost all whiskey consumed in the United States was straight rye or bourbon manufactured in the United States. Prohibition introduced smuggled Canadian and Scotch whisky to American drinkers, and they liked them. World War II sent American men around the world, further exposing them to this different type of liquor.

Scotch and Canadian whiskys are lighter than American whiskey, which means lighter in color and less heavy in taste. They are lighter because Canadian and Scotch whiskys are typically *blended* whiskys, made from about two-thirds straight whisky and one-third grain neutral spirits. After World War II, U.S. manufacturers began selling more blended whiskey. Seagram's 7-Crown has been one of the most popular blended American whiskeys. If you were so inclined, you could make your own blended whiskey by mixing two bottles of straight bourbon with one bottle of vodka, which would soften the whiskey flavor and lighten the color.

Liqueurs, or cordials, are similar in some ways to the fortified wines. Originally the cordials were made from brandy, but rather than mixing the brandy with wine, it was mixed with other flavorings derived from herbs, berries, or nuts. After dilution with sugar and water, the beverages were highly flavored, sweet and usually about 20% to 25% alcohol. Some of the old recipes are still closely guarded secrets of a particular group of European monks. The 1980s saw an increase in popularity for these drinks, which are usually consumed in small amounts and have only about half the alcohol content of vodka or whiskey. Many new types were introduced, from Bailey's Irish Cream to an amazing variety of schnapps. Modern American peppermint, peach, and other types of schnapps are made from grain neutral spirits, which is diluted, sweetened, and flavored with artificial or natural flavorings.

Americans have changed their tastes in distilled spirits. For many years domestic whiskey dominated sales, but the trend toward lighter taste and increased "mixability," which began with imported and domestic blended whiskeys, also led to increased sales of gin, vodka, and rum. In 1983 domestic vodka production finally passed domestic whiskey to become the leading single type of distilled spirits consumed by Americans. Sales of imported whisky have declined more slowly, and 1983 also marked the first time in recent years that domestic whiskey sales fell behind imports. Sales of vodka, gin, and rum reached a peak in

1983 and have declined somewhat since then. Only those "yuppie" beverages among the distilled spirits continued to show increases through 1987; tequila and cordials (liqueurs), each of which accounts for a small share of the total market.[8] The resulting trend in overall *per capita* consumption of distilled spirits was downward during the 1980s, as shown in Figure 9-2.

WHO DRINKS? AND WHY?

There are clear differences even between primitive tribes that use alcohol only sparingly and those referred to as drinking tribes. The more sober tribes live in settled communities with structured social systems that spell out social level and social rights and obligations. The drinking tribes typically have a much looser social structure, with property being held communally and few ties to land. These tribes frequently are nomadic or survive by hunting rather than by growing crops. In brief, in primitive societies if one has to account for his behavior, provide for himself, and receive according to his output, drinking is usually well controlled. If there is no need for self-control, then heavy drinking is not atypical.

Comparing current alcohol use in various cultures around the world gives us a chance to look at ethnic and social factors that lead to differences in patterns of alcohol use. For example, both the Irish and the Russian cultures are associated with heavy drinking, especially of distilled spirits. This has been attributed to several factors, including early invasions by the hard-drinking Vikings at a time when each of these regions was beginning to develop a national identity. Also, both regions experienced frequent famine, and they were not exposed to the notion of individual potential that characterized the Renaissance, or to the notions of individual responsibility and sobriety that came with the Protestant reformation.[9] Americans of Irish descent have been studied and found to have higher rates of alcohol-related problems than other ethnic groups. A comparison of Irish-Americans with Italian-Americans is of interest: the Irish forbid children and adolescents from learning

to drink, but they seem to expect adult men to drink large quantities. They value hard liquor more than beer, and promote drinking in pubs, away from family influences. By contrast, Italian families give their children wine from an early age, in a family setting, but disapprove of intoxication at any age.[10]

Since the French drink primarily wine, and consume it in the family setting and with meals, it might be expected that they would not have many heavy drinkers or drinking-related problems. Unfortunately, the French consume more alcohol per capita than any other nation, and also have the highest rates of alcoholism, suicide, and of deaths from cirrhosis of the liver.[11] The French associate wine drinking with virility, and French working men have traditionally consumed large amounts of wine during the work day (it is not unusual for a French laborer to consume a liter of wine with lunch). The French government has had campaigns to promote responsible drinking of wine and the drinking of alternative beverages. That, combined with a greater tendency to stay home and watch television instead of going to a bistro in the evenings, has led to a decrease in wine consumption, but it is still high relative to other countries.

In the United States, it has been true for many years that about one-third of the adult population label themselves as abstainers. The two-thirds who use alcohol consume an amount that averages out to about three drinks for every day of the year. Most of us don't drink anything near that amount—in fact, another consistent finding is that half the alcohol is consumed by about 10% of the drinkers.

Whites are more likely to drink than blacks, Northerners than Southerners, younger than older, Catholics and Jews than Protestants, nonreligious than religious, urban than rural, large city than small city, and college educated than those with only a high school or grade school education.

Fig. 9-3 shows estimated overall alcohol consumption combining beer, wine, and distilled spirits (about half the total U.S. alcohol consumption

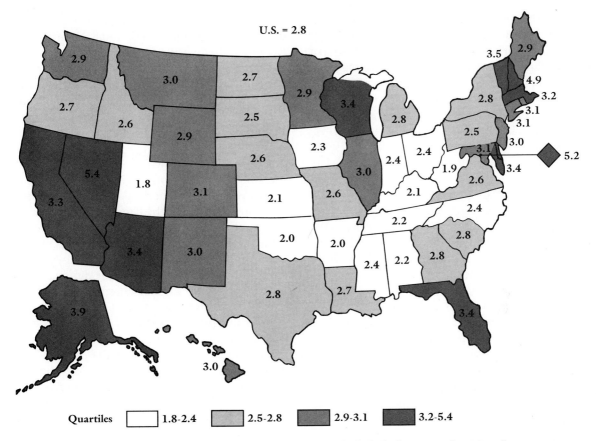

U.S. = 2.8

Quartiles □ 1.8-2.4 ▨ 2.5-2.8 ▨ 2.9-3.1 ■ 3.2-5.4

Figure 9-3. Apparent consumption of ethanol from all alcoholic beverages in U.S. gallons per capita of the population age 14 and older.

comes from beer) for each state, based on sales.[8] Nevada and the District of Columbia have by far the highest per-capita sales, followed by New Hampshire. The District of Columbia is the leader in consumption of both wine and spirits, while New Hampshire consumes the most beer. Nevada comes in second in all three. Note the generally low consumption in the southern states and the generally higher consumption in the western states, with the notable exception of Utah, which has a large Mormon population. These differences in per capita sales reflect differences in the proportion of drinkers in various parts of the country. If the sales figures are divided by the estimated number of drinkers rather than by the total adult

population, it appears that southern drinkers may consume at higher levels than northern drinkers.[12]

One theory of heavy drinking proposes that those populations of people who experience a great deal of social stress and tension (as in cities) and approve of the use of alcohol to release tension and relieve stress will drink more and have more drinking problems. One study compared the various states with regard to such stress indicators as business failures, unemployment, divorces, abortions, disasters, percentage of new residents, and high school dropout rates. On the overall state stress index, Nevada and Alaska scored the highest, Iowa and Nebraska the lowest. Alcohol norms were rated based on the percentage of fundamentalist or Mormon church members, the percentage of dry areas in the state, the number of liquor outlets per capita, and the number of hours per week allowed for drinking in bars. On this scale, Mississippi and Utah were the most restricted, Nevada and Wisconsin the least. Overall, both the stress index and the drinking norms were significantly correlated with indicators of heavy drinking and alcohol-related arrests.[13]

Looking at individual people, efforts to relate personality factors to drinking have not been terribly enlightening. Recently people have been studying the learned expectancies each of us has about what alcohol is for and what it does. We learn much of what we expect alcohol to do even before we take our first drink, from books, movies, and other people. One study reported that males who have strong expectations that alcohol will lead to increased social and physical pleasure and to sexual enhancement are most likely to drink heavily, whereas among females the heaviest drinkers were those who believed that alcohol would reduce tension.[14] You can see how these different expectancies might lead to different types of drinking in different situations, thus complicating attempts to predict simply who drinks and how much.

ALCOHOL PHARMACOLOGY
Absorption

Alcohol is unique in that it requires no digestion and can be absorbed unchanged from the stomach and, more rapidly, from the small intestine. In an empty stomach the overall rate of absorption depends on the concentration of alcohol. Even though concentration is the primary factor, the absorption rate can be altered. For example, alcohol taken with or after a meal is absorbed more slowly. This is because the food remains in the stomach for digestive action, and the protein in the food retains the alcohol with it in the stomach.

Plain water, by decreasing the concentration, slows the absorption of alcohol, but carbonated liquids speed it up. The carbon dioxide acts to move everything quite rapidly through the stom-

ach to the small intestine. It is this emptying of the stomach and the more rapid absorption of alcohol in the intestine that give Champagne and sparkling Burgundy a faster onset of action than wine. Once absorbed into the bloodstream, alcohol passes almost immediately through the liver.

Central Nervous System Effects

Alcohol is like any other general anesthetic: it depresses the central nervous system. It was used as an anesthetic until the late nineteenth century, when nitrous oxide, ether, and chloroform became more widely used. However, it was not just new compounds that decreased alcohol's use as an anesthetic; it has some major disadvantages. In contrast to the gaseous anesthetics, alcohol is almost completely metabolized in the body, and the rate of oxidation is slow. This gives alcohol a long duration of action that cannot be controlled. A second disadvantage is that the dose effective in surgical anesthesia is not much lower than the dose that causes respiratory arrest and death. Finally, alcohol slows the blood clotting time.

The exact mechanism for the CNS effect of alcohol is not clear. Until the mid-1980s the most widely accepted theory was that alcohol acted on all neural membranes, perhaps altering their electrical excitability. However, with increased understanding of the role of the GABA receptor complex in the actions of other depressant drugs (Chapter 8), there are many scientists who believe that the same receptor complex might play a special role in the action of alcohol. The study of GABA receptors led to the discovery of an experimental drug, RO 15-4513, that appeared to be a specific antidote or antagonist for many of the behavioral effects of alcohol. In a dramatic demonstration, intoxicated rats that had been unable to roll over and stand up appeared, within 2 minutes after an injection of RO 15-4513, to be "sober," and walking normally.[15] There has been great controversy over the issue of whether this drug is a selective blocker of alcohol's effects or simply a very powerful CNS stimulant that is able

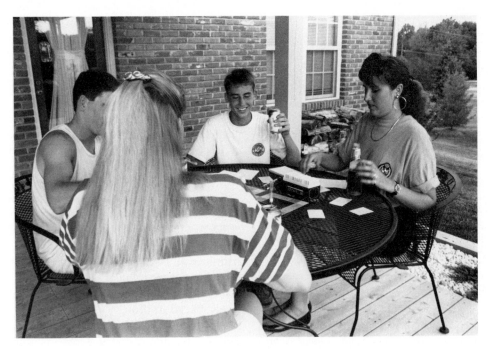

Drinking, especially of beer, sometimes begins at a young age.

to overcome some of the depressant actions of alcohol, but at this point it does not look as if a "sober-up" pill will be on the market at any time soon (see Issue box).

At the lowest effective blood levels, complex, abstract, and poorly learned behaviors are disrupted. As the dose increases, better learned and simpler behaviors are also affected. Inhibitions may be reduced with the result that performance might actually improve under certain conditions. Even though there may be an increase in activity, most scientists would not call alcohol a stimulant. Rather, the increased behavioral output is usually attributed to decreased inhibition of behavior.

If the alcohol intake is "just right," most people experience a "high," a happy feeling. Below a certain **blood alcohol level** (BAL) there are no mood changes, but at some point we become uninhibited enough to enjoy our own charming selves and uncritical enough to accept the clods around us. The point seems to occur when the alcohol has disrupted social inhibitions and im-

paired good judgment but has not depressed most behavior. We become witty, clever, true continentals! Fortunately, most of those around us at this time also have impairment of judgment, so they can't say any differently!

Another factor contributing to the feeling of well-being is the reduction in anxieties as a result of the disruption of normal critical thinking. The reduction in concern and judgment may range from not worrying about who'll pay the bar bill to being sure that you can beat the train to the crossing. A final effect of alcohol that may make the older person feel better is the anesthetizing of minor aches and pains.

No blood levels were suggested for the points at which an individual begins to feel good or happy or becomes amorous, or when sensory and motor functions are seriously impaired. BALs are reported as the number of grams of alcohol in each 100 ml of blood and are expressed as a percentage. Since 100 g in 100 ml would be 100%, 100 mg of alcohol in 100 ml of blood is reported as 0.1%.

Issue: a sober-up pill?

In 1986, it was reported that a drug had been found that was capable of counteracting the intoxicating effects of alcohol in rats.[15] This experimental compound, RO 15-4513, had been developed by chemists at Hoffman-LaRoche who were studying the benzodiazepine receptor by which such drugs as Valium act to enhance the inhibitory actions of the neurotransmitter GABA. They were at first very excited that this drug might save many lives. Their first disappointment was that the drug could not block the lethal effects of high doses of alcohol. If a rat were made intoxicated just to the point of immobility, it would walk again soon after RO 15-4513 administration, but higher doses would still kill the animal. Also, the drug would not prevent such long-term consequences of heavy drinking as brain and liver damage. Might it still be useful to help someone who had consumed too much at a bar? In theory, such a person could take the drug a few minutes before driving home and "sober up" for the drive. On the other hand, there was the fear that a person might drink to the point of intoxication, take a pill, and then continue drinking, leading to the threat of tissue damage or even death from overdose.

The company decided not to pursue the drug as a marketable product. Consider the legal questions that would arise if someone had a blood alcohol level of 0.20, took the pill, felt sober, drove, and caused an accident. If you owned the patent on this drug, would you consider selling it? If so, under what conditions?

Before suggesting blood alcohol level/behavioral change relationships, two factors must be mentioned. One is that the rate at which the blood alcohol rises is a factor in determining behavioral effects. The more rapid the increase, the greater the behavioral effects. Second, it is well to note that a classic study using a variety of simple visual, motor, and visual-motor tests showed disruption of performance at an average blood level of 0.05% in abstainers, 0.07% in moderate drinkers, and 0.1% in heavy drinkers.[16]

These results show clearly that behavioral and CNS tolerance to alcohol does develop. They also indicate that the better performance of the heavy drinker compared to the moderate drinker after equal amounts of alcohol is not caused by the greater rate of alcohol metabolism in heavy drinkers. A higher BAL is necessary to impair the performance of a chronic heavy drinker than to impair a moderate drinker's performance!

A partial explanation might be that the heavy drinker is better motivated to conceal the alcohol-induced impairment and probably has had more practice. Performance differences may only reflect the extent to which the two groups have learned to overcome the disruption of nervous system functioning. Another explanation may be that the CNS in the heavy drinker develops a tolerance to alcohol that does not exist in the moderate drinker. It is established that neural tissue becomes tolerant to alcohol, and tolerance can apparently develop even when the alcohol intake is well spaced in time.

Any dose-response curve contains considerable variability, and Table 9-3 reports some general behavior. These relationships are approximately correct for moderate drinkers. There are some reports that changes in nervous system function have been obtained at blood levels as low as 0.03% to 0.04%.

There is reason to believe that performance impairment in the 0.1% BAL range is the result of a decrement in decision-making capability. The integration of information and behavior seems to be the critical factor. It should be noted, however, that some changes in stimulus processing may occur even at low dose levels. One study presented a mild shock stimulus to the skin. The response elicited in the brain showed an increase in variability and a decrease in magnitude after alcohol ingestion.[17]

The vomiting reflex may be activated by alcohol at a blood level of about 0.12% or even lower, but only if that level is approached rapidly. With slow steady drinking the blood level increases gradually; and at high concentrations the vomiting center is depressed. The individual can then continue drinking up to lethal levels if he remains conscious!

The surgical anesthesia level and the minimum

Table 9-3	
Blood alcohol level and behavioral effects	
Percent blood alcohol level	**Behavioral effects**
0.05	Lowered alertness, usually good feeling, release of inhibitions, impaired judgement
0.10	Slowed reaction times and impaired motor function, less caution
0.15	Large, consistent increases in reaction time
0.20	Marked depression in sensory and motor capability, decidedly intoxicated
0.25	Severe motor disturbance, staggering, sensory perceptions greatly impaired, smashed!
0.30	Stuporous but conscious—no comprehension of the world around them
0.35	Surgical anesthesia; about LD 1, minimal level causing death
0.40	About LD 50

lethal level are perhaps the two least precise points in the table. In any case they are quite close, and the safety margin is less than 0.1% blood alcohol. Death resulting from acute alcohol intoxication usually is the result of respiratory failure when the medulla is depressed.

The blood alcohol level and behavior relationship is similarly but more enjoyably described in the following, which is modified from Bogen.[18]

At less than 0.03%, the individual is dull and dignified.
At 0.05%, he is dashing and debonair.
At 0.1%, he may become dangerous and devilish.
At 0.2%, he is likely to be dizzy and disturbing.
At 0.25%, he may be disgusting and disheveled.
At 0.3%, he is delirious and disoriented and surely drunk.
At 0.35%, he is dead drunk.
At 0.6%, the chances are that he is dead.

The relationship between BAL and alcohol intake, the oral consumption of an alcoholic beverage, is not simple but is reasonably well understood. Remember, alcohol is not appreciably excreted from, or stored anywhere in, the body before metabolism. When taken into the body, alcohol is distributed throughout the body fluids, including the blood.

However, alcohol does not distribute much into fatty tissues, so a 180-pound lean person will have a lower blood alcohol level than a 180-pound fat person who drinks the same amount of alcohol.

Table 9-4 demonstrates the relationships among alcohol intake, blood alcohol level, and body weight for hypothetical *average* males and females. The chart distinguishes between the sexes, because the average male has a lower proportion of body fat and therefore, for a given weight, has more volume in which to distribute the alcohol. It's worth spending a bit of time to try to understand this table, because you can learn a lot about how much you can probably drink to avoid going above a specified BAL.

First, Table 9-4 makes the simplifying assumption that all the alcohol is absorbed quickly and "in one hour," so that there is little opportunity for metabolism. If the 150-pound female had a tank of about 100 pounds (12.5 gallons or 45 liters) of water and just dumped 1 ounce (28.3 g) into it and stirred it up, the concentration would be about 0.6 g/liter, or 0.06 mg/100 ml (0.06%). Fig. 9-4 shows a schematic of such a tank. The 150-pound average male has a "tank" with more water in it, so his alcohol concentration is about 0.05%. The major factor determining individual differences in BAL is the volume of distribution, so find your own weight on this chart and estimate how many drinks could be poured into your "tank" to obtain a BAL of 0.05%.

Second, notice that several beverages are equated to ½ ounce of absolute alcohol. A 12-ounce can or bottle of beer at about 4.2% alcohol contains 12 × 0.042 = ½ ounce of alcohol. This same amount is found in a glass of wine containing about 4 ounces of 12% alcohol, 1 ounce of 100-proof spirits, or 1.25 ounces of 80-proof spir-

Table 9-4							
Relationships among sex, weight, oral alcohol consumption, and blood alcohol level							
Absolute alcohol (ounces)	**Beverage intake***	**Blood alcohol levels (g/100 ml)**					
		Female (100 lb)	**Male (100 lb)**	**Female (150 lb)**	**Male (150 lb)**	**Female (200 lb)**	**Male (200 lb)**
½	1 oz spirits† 1 glass wine 1 can beer	0.045	0.037	0.03	0.025	0.022	0.019
1	2 oz spirits 2 glasses wine 2 cans beer	0.090	0.075	0.06	0.050	0.045	0.037
2	4 oz spirits 4 glasses wine 4 cans beer	0.180	0.150	0.12	0.100	0.090	0.070
3	6 oz spirits 6 glasses wine 6 cans beer	0.270	0.220	0.18	0.150	0.130	0.110
4	8 oz spirits 8 glasses wine 8 cans beer	0.360	0.300	0.24	0.200	0.180	0.150
5	10 oz spirits 10 glasses wine 10 cans beer	0.450	0.370	0.30	0.250	0.220	0.180

*In 1 hour.
†100-proof spirits.

its. Each of these can be equated as a standard "drink."

Now, we have not taken either absorption or metabolism into account, and these are both important factors. However, we also have a simple way of looking at them. As we will see in the next section, alcohol is removed by the liver at essentially a constant rate of 0.25 to 0.3 ounce of ethanol per hour. There are some individual differences in this rate, but most people fall within this range, no matter what their body size or drinking experience, unless they have consumed so much alcohol that their liver is damaged. To be on the safe side, estimate that you can metabolize about 0.25 ounce per hour, and note that this is one half of one of our standard drinks (one beer, one shot, or one glass of wine). Over the course of an evening, if your rate of intake equals your rate of

metabolism, you will maintain a stable BAL. If you drink faster than one drink every 2 hours, your BAL will climb. The extra drinks, those over the one every 2 hours, will be added to your tank. Let's take an example from the chart: a 150-pound male goes to the bar at 8 P.M. and consumes six beers before midnight. During that 4 hours, his liver metabolized the alcohol from two of the beers, so he still has four drinks, or 2 ounces of ethanol, in his system. His BAL at midnight should be about 0.10%, making him legally intoxicated and unfit to drive home. If he had had two fewer beers (four over the 4-hour period), his BAL would be about 0.05%. In other words, once the two drinks for 4 hours of metabolism are accounted for, you simply add up the extra drinks and look up the estimated BAL on the chart. Note that a 100-pound female who had kept up with

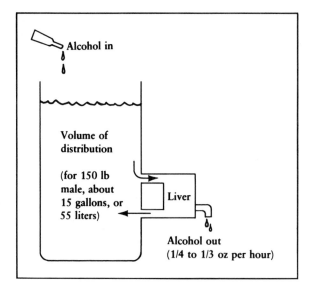

Alcohol in

Volume of
distribution

(for 150 lb
male, about
15 gallons, or
55 liters)

Liver

Alcohol out
(1/4 to 1/3 oz per hour)

Figure 9-4. The relationship between blood alcohol level and alcohol intake.

ever, so the best rule is to learn about your own sensitivity and not to feel compelled to keep up with anyone else's drinking. And alcohol-induced impairment is dose related and depends on what you're trying to do. Carrying on bar conversation places fewer demands on your nervous system than driving on a Los Angeles freeway during rush hour, where any alcohol at all might interfere.

BAL gives a good estimate of the alcohol concentration in the brain, and the concentration of alcohol in the breath gives a good estimate of the alcohol concentration in the blood. The concentration in the blood is almost exactly 2100 times the concentration in air expired from the lungs, making it possible to use breath samples as an accurate indicator of BAL. Such breath samples are easily collected by police and can form the basis for conviction as a drunk driver in most states.

our six-pack consuming friend would be in really bad shape at almost 0.20%. If he were driving home in a "dangerous and devilish" state, she might be too "dizzy and disturbed" to notice.

Let's take a brief look at some other-than-standard drinks. What if our male friend had been drinking 3.2 beer? Each 12-ounce beer at 3.2% has almost 0.4 ounce of alcohol instead of 0.5, so six of them contain 2.3 ounces. After metabolizing 1 ounce, his tank has 1.3 ounce or enough to put him at about 0.65%. He's better off than when he drank the six regular beers, but it's wrong to say that 3.2 beer is not intoxicating. Alcohol is alcohol, no matter what beverage it comes from. As an exercise, figure out how many 3.2 beers it would take to put this guy over the 0.10% line. Wine coolers contain 12 ounces of about 5% alcohol, more than one of our standard drinks.

What's a safe BAL? After we remember that nothing in this world is totally safe, let's say that if you are going to drink and want to remain in reasonable control of your faculties you should probably stay below 0.05%. Individuals do differ considerably in their sensitivities to alcohol, how-

Driving under the Influence

Attention was focused in the early 1980s on the large number of traffic fatalities involving alcohol. The total number of traffic fatalities in 1980 was over 50,000, but by 1983 that had dropped to nearer 40,000. There have been slight increases in the number of fatalities since then, but we hope it will be many years before we again reach the number of traffic deaths we were experiencing in the late 1970s. It is difficult to estimate exactly how many of those fatalities are *caused* by alcohol, but we can obtain some relevant information. Many states mandate that all fatally injured drivers have blood alcohol measurments done by the coroner. Based on those measurements, estimates have been made for data collected by the federal Fatal Accident Reporting System of the proportion of fatally injured drivers who were intoxicated (BAL >0.10). The results for several years are given in Table 9-5. It appears that about half of fatally injured drivers had been intoxicated in 1980, but the fraction is now about 40%.[19]

Several studies have demonstrated that the danger of combining alcohol with automobiles is dose related.[20] The relative risk of being involved

Table 9-5								
Alcohol involvement in fatal traffic accidents								
Driver BAL	1980 (%)	1981 (%)	1982 (%)	1983 (%)	1984 (%)	1985 (%)	1986 (%)	1987 (%)
BAL > .10	50	49	49	46	43	41	40	39

in a fatal crash is about three times as great as a sober driver at a BAL of 0.08 and about 15 times as great at 0.12. (Note how close these figures are to the commonly used value for intoxication of 0.10.) Similarly, the risk of involvement in a personal injury crash increases with BAL, as does the risk of involvement in a fatal pedestrian accident. As with other dose-response curves, these data provide strong evidence that the relationship between drinking and accidents is causal and not merely related to the lifestyles of individuals who drink.

There are some other interesting facts that have emerged from studies of alcohol and accidents. Alcohol-related traffic fatalities are not a random sample of all fatalities. Single-vehicle fatalities are more likely to involve alcohol than are multiple-vehicle fatalities in which the fatally injured person was driving the striking vehicle. The probability of alcohol involvement is lower if the fatally injured individual was driving a vehicle that was struck by another driver. Alcohol-related fatalities are a greater proportion of the fatalities occurring during dark hours than during daylight and are a greater proportion of fatalities occurring on the weekend than during the week. In fact, if someone is killed in a struck vehicle during daylight hours on Monday through Thursday, the odds are less than 1 in 10 that the victim was impaired by alcohol. The odds are more like 9 in 10 for a single vehicle accident occurring in the early morning hours on a weekend.[20,p.16]

When you hear that about 90% of all the fatally injured drivers who had been drinking were male, that sounds like a big difference, and it is. But it is important to remember that over 80% of all fatally injured drivers are male, whether or not drinking is involved. That males are more likely to be involved in alcohol-related traffic fatalities reflects two important facts: any given car is more likely to have a male than a female driver, and male drivers are more likely to have been drinking than female drivers.

Who's responsible for all these alcohol-related traffic accidents? One question is whether there are certain individuals, such as problem drinkers, responsible for much of the drunk driving. Of the drivers involved in fatal crashes in 1981 who had BALs of 0.10 or more, 11% had previous convictions for driving under the influence (DUI).[20,p.34] Problem drinkers, although a relatively small fraction of the drinking population, are more likely on a given day to be driving around with a high BAL. On the other hand, almost 90% of those involved in fatal crashes and who were by definition driving while intoxicated when it happened had at least never been convicted of DUI in the past. Therefore, whereas individual problem drinkers cause more than their share of traffic accidents, the majority of alcohol-related traffic accidents are caused by individuals who have not been identified as problem drinkers. Anyone who drinks and drives is a potential threat.

Younger drivers have more than their share of alcohol-related accidents. In 1981, those aged 16 to 24 made up 16.5% of the U.S. population, yet were involved in 44.6% of the alcohol-related traffic accidents.[20,p.30]

What can be done about this problem? Current efforts may be seen mainly on three fronts: identifying repeat offenders and keeping them off the roads, publicizing in all the mass media the dan-

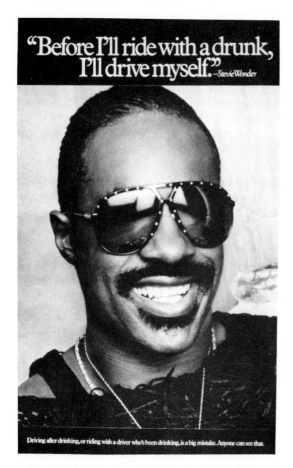

"Before I'll ride with a drunk, I'll drive myself." —Stevie Wonder

Driving after drinking, or riding with a driver who's been drinking, is a big mistake. Anyone can see that.

Stevie Wonder and other celebrities have helped carry the message to avoid drinking and driving.

gers of drinking and driving, and increasing the minimum drinking age. Although it is impossible to determine the effectiveness of any one of these measures, Table 9-9 indicates that the total effort is working to reduce alcohol-related fatalities.

Suicide and Homicide

The relationship between alcohol use and homicides is well known to police and the judicial system. One review of the world literature[21] did not deal with background factors but noted several studies that found that in at least 50% of the homicides the slayer, the victim, or both had measur-

> ### Your turn: alcohol and violence
>
> One of the interesting things about alcohol's involvement in accidents or violence is that it is so common it is not newsworthy. For example, a recent newspaper reported an incident that occurred in the wee hours of a Saturday morning in which one man stabbed another over a piece of leftover meatloaf. The article didn't mention alcohol involvement, but it seemed so likely that someone was drunk that the example was used in class. One of the class members happened to be a sheriff's deputy and was able to get a copy of the arrest report. Sure enough, both men had high BALs (one was over 0.20).
>
> Such incidents are more common than you might think: another example was a man in Los Angeles who was being taunted by bystanders because he was having trouble parking his car in front of a nightclub. He proceeded to shoot one of the taunters. The news account didn't mention that he was drunk, but what do you think?
>
> Check the Saturday and Sunday morning newspapers for 2 or 3 weeks and see how many reports you can find in which it seems likely that alcohol was involved. Does the news article state or imply that drinking was involved or avoid the issue entirely?

able blood alcohol levels. Drinking *is* involved in homicide, but alcoholism is not. Most homicides occur between friends or acquaintances—family quarrels, neighborhood disputes—so the relationship to drinking is easy to understand.

Suicide and suicide attempts seem to have a different background, but most agree that alcohol is involved in about one-third of all suicides. Alcoholism is second only to depression as the diagnosis in suicide attempters, and there are some who believe that all alcoholics are seriously depressed. A report on "Alcoholism, Alcohol Intoxication, and Suicide Attempts"[22] studied a group of suicide attempters, 75% of whom were drinking at the time of the attempt, and identified two types of alcohol-suicide situations. One type, the most common and most likely to succeed, involves the solitary, chronic heavy use of alcohol accompanied by increasing depression and withdrawal.

The second type consists of individuals who become intoxicated quite rapidly in a situation involving interpersonal aggression and activity. It is probable that the superficial explanation has considerable validity in these two types: the use of alcohol increases the chronic drinker's feelings of being no-damn-good, and the disinhibiting effect of alcohol allows the aggressive drinker to turn his anger on himself.

Blackouts

Alcohol-induced blackouts are periods of time during alcohol use in which the individual appears to function normally but later, when the individual is sober, the events cannot be recalled. The drinker may drive home or dance all night interacting in the usual way with others. When the individual cannot remember the activities, the people, or anything—that's a blackout. Most authorities include it as one of the danger signs suggesting excessive use of alcohol. Amazingly, it has not been studied extensively. An 1884 article titled "Alcoholic Trance" refers to the syndrome:

> This trance state is a common condition in inebriety, where . . . a profound suspension of memory and consciousness and literal paralysis of certain brain-functions follow.
>
> This trance state may last from a few moments to several days, during which the person may appear and act rationally, and yet be actually a mere automaton, without consciousness or memory of his actual condition.[23]

Sexual Behavior

> Lechery, sir, it provokes, and
> unprovokes; it provokes the desire,
> but it takes away the performance.[24]

Alcohol, since it is a depressant drug, decreases inhibitions and at least makes the thought of sexual activity more likely. It may be that the amount of sexual behavior increases following moderate alcohol intake but there is considerable anecdotal evidence that the quality decreases.

A 1970 survey of *Psychology Today* readers found that men were equally divided as to whether alcohol use increased or decreased sexual pleasure. Women reported that alcohol use increased sexual pleasure by a 3 to 1 margin. A 1974 survey of male business executives found a positive relationship between reported frequency of alcohol use and whether the respondent said that alcohol acted as a sexual stimulant. It was also true that those who drank less also engaged in less sexual activity.[25] In the absence of other data these findings are explained more parsimoniously as a result of different lifestyles rather than supporting the idea that alcohol is a sexual stimulant.

A sophisticated and well-designed study[26] using college females as subjects explored the relationships among the dose of alcohol ingested (0.05, 0.25, 0.50, 0.75 g/kg), self-reports of sexual arousal, and vaginal vasocongestion. There were two experimental conditions—watching an erotic-pornographic film and watching a nonerotic film of a tour of a computer facility—and two sets of instructions—one suggesting that alcohol would increase sexual arousal and the other suggesting that alcohol would decrease sexual arousal. The subjects were tested about 40 minutes after alcohol intake. Each subject was tested under each alcohol dose and in each session both the erotic and nonerotic films were viewed.

Several results are worthy of note. The instructional set did not generally alter the *expected* effect of alcohol: most of the college females expected alcohol to increase sexual arousal. On the self-report measure: (1) sexual arousal increased with alcohol intake and (2) the percent of subjects reporting arousal to the erotic film increased as the amount of alcohol ingested increased.

The erotic film elicited much greater vaginal vasocongestion than the computer film, providing some validity to vaginal vasocongestion as a measure of sexual arousal. Importantly, the amount of increase in vaginal vasocongestion decreased as the dose of alcohol increased. For women, increased alcohol intake results in self-reports of increased sexual arousal along with a decrease in a physiological measure of arousal.

A similar study[27] was carried out on college

males by the same research team. The physiological measure of arousal was also vasocongestion—speed, amount, and duration of penile erection. The doses of alcohol ingested were 0.08, 0.4, 0.8, and 1.2 g/kg. All three measures of penile vasocongestion decreased as the dose of alcohol was increased. Self-reports of degree of arousal were highly correlated with the extent of vasocongestion.

In the infrequent, social user of alcohol the body returns to normal as the alcohol is metabolized and leaves the body. The alcoholic is not as fortunate. It has long been known that heavy alcohol users and alcoholics suffer from a variety of sexual problems and show atrophy of the testicles and impaired sperm production. One report found that 8% of male alcoholics were impotent, and in half of those the condition persisted during years of sobriety.[28] There may be, of course, a large psychological factor in impotence, so it is of some interest that there seems now to be a physiological basis for it in alcoholism. One biochemical study in humans required volunteers to drink about 3 g of alcohol per kilogram of body weight a day for 4 weeks.[29] A twofold to fivefold increase was found in the activity of the liver enzyme that metabolizes testosterone. There was not an increased production of testosterone, and reduced levels of this male sex hormone could, over time, result in the physical and behavioral changes mentioned earlier. Don't panic, guys—to achieve the level of alcohol intake used in the experiment would require you to drink about a quart of distilled spirits a day. Note, however, that a dose-response curve was not done, and no information is available about the effects on testosterone of prolonged low-level alcohol intake.

A January 1982 report in *Medical World News* told of the reversal of alcoholic impotence with daily doses of oral androgen—even though the predrug testosterone levels of these nondrinking alcoholic men were normal. Further work is needed but this finding may be a major breakthrough. It may also be a useful adjunct to alcoholic rehabilitation programs. As motivation to keep the alcoholic from drinking, the discoverer

of this approach said, "If you tell someone you're going to fix his liver, he'll just shrug his shoulders. But it you tell him you're going to fix his gonads, he'll pay attention."

Physiological Effects

Peripheral blood effects.   One effect of alcohol on the CNS is the dilation of the peripheral blood vessels. This increases the heat loss from the body but makes the drinker feel warm. The heat loss and cooling of the interior of the body are enough to cause a slowdown in some biochemical processes. It is this dilation of the peripheral vessels that argues against the use of alcohol in individuals in shock or extreme cold. Under these conditions blood is needed in the central parts of the body, and heat loss must be diminished if the person is to survive.

Hangovers

The Germans call it "wailing of cats" (Katzenjammer), the Italians "out of tune" (stonato), the French "woody mouth" (gueule de boise), the Norwegians "workmen in my head" (jeg har tommeermenn) and the Swedes "pain in the roots of the hair" (hont i haret).[30]

Hangovers aren't much fun. And they aren't very well understood, either. The symptoms are well known to a high percentage of even moderate drinkers who occasionally overindulge: upset stomach, fatigue, headache, thirst, depression, anxiety, general malaise.

Some authorities believe that the symptoms of a hangover are the symptoms of withdrawal from a short- or long-term addiction to alcohol. The pattern certainly fits. Some alcoholics report continuing to drink just to escape the pain of the hangover. This behavior is not unknown to moderate drinkers, either: many believe that the only "cure" for a hangover is some of "the hair of the dog that bit you"—alcohol. And it may work to minimize symptoms, since it spreads them out over a longer period of time. There is no evidence that any of the "surefire-this'll-fix-you-up" remedies are effective. An analgesic for the headache, rest, and time are the only known "cures." Some of the ways to reduce the probability and the severity of a hangover will be evident from the following.

A study titled "Experimental Induction of Hangover,"[31] provided support for two factors contributing to the hangover syndrome: (1) the higher your BAL, the more likely you are to have a hangover, and (2) with the *same* BAL, bourbon drinkers were more likely (two out of three) than vodka drinkers (one out of three) to have a hangover. This fits with the belief that some hangover symptoms are reactions to congeners. Congeners are natural products of the fermentation and preparation process, some of which are quite toxic. Congeners make the various alcoholic beverages different in smell, taste, color, and, possibly, hangover potential. Beer, with a 4% alcohol content, has only a 0.01% congener level, whereas wine has about 0.04% and distilled spirits between 0.1% and 0.2%. Gin, being a mixture of almost pure alcohol and water, has a congener content about the same as wine, while a truly pure mixture of alcohol and water (vodka) has the same congener level as beer. Aging distilled spirits does not decrease the level of congeners but, in fact, increases their level about threefold.

Still other factors contribute to the trials and tribulations of the "morning after the night before." One of the actions of alcohol on the brain is to decrease the output of the antidiuretic hormone responsible for retaining fluid in the body. This action probably means that the body excretes more fluid than is taken in with the alcoholic beverages. However, this does not seem to be the only basis for the thirst experienced the next day. Another cause may be that alcohol causes fluid inside cells to move outside the cells. This cellular dehydration, without a decrease in total body fluid, is known to be related to, and perhaps to be the basis of an increase in thirst.

The nausea and upset stomach typically experienced can most likely be attributed to the fact that alcohol is a gastric irritant. The consumption of even moderate amounts causes local irritation of the mucosa covering the stomach. It has been suggested that the accumulation of acetaldehyde, which is quite toxic even in small quantities, contributes to the nausea and headache. The headache may also be a reaction to fatigue. Fatigue sometimes results from a higher than normal level of activity while drinking. Increased activity frequently accompanies a decrease in inhibitions, a readily available source of energy, and a high blood sugar level. One of the effects of alcohol intake is to increase the blood sugar level for about an hour after ingestion. This may be followed several hours later by a low blood sugar level and an increased feeling of fatigue. Although hangover cures may be just around the corner, for now the only sure cure is time.

When alcohol intake occurs regularly and in large quantities over a period of years, physical dependence on the drug follows. Abrupt withdrawal from alcohol results in dangerous changes in body physiology. Before the addiction to alcohol reaches this point, physical symptoms sometimes develop, with facial appearance the first to be affected. The capillaries around the conjunctiva of the eyes become enlarged, and the skin of the face, forehead, and under the eyes becomes puffy and filled with fluid.

In an individual with a fair complexion, the skin may appear continually flushed and, after prolonged use, a "whiskey nose" may develop. The frequent hoarseness of the alcoholic results from the accumulation of fluid in the mucous membranes of the nose, pharynx, larynx, and vocal cords. Continual ingestion of alcohol leads to an inflamed stomach associated with nausea and loss of appetite.

The relationship of alcohol use to many diseases has been studied extensively and still continues. One long-term study of white middle-aged males (40 years and over) with good jobs showed that there was an increased mortality from all causes only ". . . at the level of six or more drinks per day."[32,p.78] Keeping all of this in mind, let's review some of the major health concerns discussed in the NIAAA's 1987 report to Congress.[12] As a general rule, we can say that heavy alcohol use, either directly or indirectly, affects every organ system in the body. The alcohol or its primary metabolite, acetaldehyde, may irritate and damage tissue directly. Because alcohol provides "empty" calories, many heavy drinkers do not eat well and chronic malnutrition leads to tissue damage.

Perhaps the biggest concern is the damage to brain tissue that is seen in chronic alcoholics. It has been reported for years that the brains of deceased alcoholics demonstrate an obvious overall loss of brain tissue: the ventricles (internal spaces) in the brain are enlarged, and the fissures (sulci) in the cortex are widened. Modern imaging techniques, first CT scans and then PET and MRI, have demonstrated this tissue loss in living alcoholics as well. Two particular regions demonstrate cell loss that is associated with the classical *Wernicke's disease*: the mammillary bodies of the hypothalamus and the medial and frontal nuclei of the thalamus. When these areas are damaged, the patient probably has been exhibiting *Korsakoff's psychosis*, which is characterized by impaired memory and a loss of contact with reality. This Wernicke-Korsakoff syndrome has traditionally been reported in individuals with a long history of very heavy drinking. Some important questions arise: Is the brain damage due to alcohol or to malnutrition? How much alcohol intake is required to produce less obvious brain damage? Can the damage be reversed if one stops drinking? Experiments have replicated the neuronal damage in animals fed adequate diets, thus implying that the damage is caused directly by the alcohol. One experiment used CT scans and reported evidence of brain damage in 31 of 39 drinkers who consumed less than 5 ounces of alcohol per day. Most of these people also showed some deficits on tests of psychomotor functioning, thus implying that damage may result from levels of drinking lower than those previously demonstrated to be dangerous. Some studies have now reported both behavioral improvement and apparent regrowth of brain size in alcoholics after 4 months of abstinence. However, not all such studies find improvement, and some have found improvement in some types of mental tasks but not in others. There is some room for hope, especially in younger alcoholics.

Another area of concern is the effect of alcohol on the heart and circulation. There is no doubt that heavy alcohol use is associated with increased mortality due to heart disease. Much of this is due to damage to the heart muscle (cardiomyopathy), but there is also an increased risk of the more typical heart attack due to coronary artery disease. Heavy drinkers are also more likely to suffer from high blood pressure and strokes. An interesting twist to this story is that several studies have found a *lower* incidence of heart attacks in moderate drinkers than in abstainers, and for several years there has been discussion about this "protective" effect of moderate alcohol consumption and the possible mechanism for it. However, some recent studies have pointed out that the middle-aged and elderly men who do not drink include a substantial fraction of people who once drank, some of whom may be abstinent alcoholics, and others of whom may have quit drinking on their doctor's advice because of poor health. That may explain at least part of why abstinent people have more heart attacks than moderate drinkers. Whether or not moderate drinking actually has a protective effect against heart attacks, none of the studies indicate that moderate drinkers are more healthy overall, since the decreased number of heart attacks may be offset by increased mortality from cancer and stroke.

Alcohol use is associated with cancers of the mouth, tongue, pharynx, larynx, esophagus, stomach, liver, lung, pancreas, colon, and rectum. There are many possible mechanisms for this, from direct tissue irritation to nutritional deficiencies to the induction of enzymes that activate other carcinogens. There is a particularly nasty interaction with cigarette smoking to increase the incidence of cancers of the oral cavity, pharynx, and larynx. Also, suppression of the immune system by alcohol, which occurs to some extent every time intoxicating doses are used, probably increases the risk of cancer from some viruses.

The immune deficits seen in chronic alcoholics are associated with at least some increase in the frequency of various infectious diseases, including tuberculosis, pneumonia, yellow fever, cholera, and hepatitis B. It is not yet clear whether alcoholics are also more likely to show rapid progression of AIDS-related disorders if they become infected with HIV.

After all is said and done, there is no evidence that occasional drinking of one or two drinks has overall negative effects on the physical health of most individuals. An important exception to this statement may be during pregnancy.

Fetal Alcohol Syndrome

The unfortunate condition of infants born to alcoholic mothers was noted in an 1834 report to the British Parliament: they have a "starved, shriveled, and imperfect look." Until recently most scientists and physicians believed that any effects on the offspring of heavy alcohol users were the result of poor nutrition or poor prenatal care. In 1973 an article reported that:

Eight unrelated children of three different ethnic groups, all born to mothers who were chronic alcoholics, have a pattern of craniofacial, limb, and cardiovascular defects associated with prenatal-onset growth deficiency and developmental delay. This seems to be the first reported association between maternal alcoholism and aberrant morphogenesis in the offspring.[33]

That publication signaled the recognition of **fetal alcohol syndrome** (FAS), a collection of physical and behavioral abnormalities that seems to be caused by the presence of alcohol during development of the fetus. There are three primary criteria for diagnosing FAS, at least one of which *must* be present:
1. Growth retardation occurring before and/or after birth
2. A pattern of abnormal features of the face and head, including small head circumference, small eyes, or evidence of retarded formation of the midfacial area, including a flattened bridge and short length of the nose and flattening of the vertical groove between the nose and mouth (the philtrum)
3. Evidence of central nervous system abnormality, including abnormal neonatal behavior, mental retardation, or other evidence of abnormal neurobehavioral development.[34,p.70]

Each of these features can be seen in the absence of alcohol exposure, and other features may also be present in FAS, such as eye and ear defects, heart murmurs, undescended testicles, birthmarks, and abnormal fingerprints or palmar creases. Thus the diagnosis of FAS is a matter of judgment, based on several symptoms and often on the physician's knowledge of the mother's drinking history.

A large number of animal studies have now been done in a variety of species, and they point rather clearly to the fact that FAS is related to the peak BAL and to the duration of alcohol exposure, even when malnutrition is not an issue. With increasing amounts of alcohol there is an increase in mortality, a decrease in infant weight, and increased frequency of soft tissue malformation in mice and other animal models.

By no means do *all* infants born to drinking mothers show abnormal development. If they did, it would not have taken so long to recognize FAS as a problem. Estimates of the prevalence of FAS in the overall population have ranged from 0.4 per 1000 births to 2.9 per 1000. Estimating the prevalence among problem drinkers or alcohol abusers is more of a problem. Not only is there the difficulty of diagnosing FAS, but also of diagnosing alcohol abuse. If the physician knows that the mother is a heavy drinker, this may increase the probability of noticing or diagnosing FAS, thus inflating the prevalence statistics among drinking mothers. FAS itself seems to occur in 23 to 29 per 1000 births among women who are problem drinkers. If all alcohol-related birth defects are counted, the rate among these women is higher, from 80 to a few hundred per 1000. It may be that maternal alcohol abuse is the most frequent known environmental cause of mental retardation in the Western World.[34]

In addition to the risk of FAS, the fetus of a mother who drinks heavily risks not being born at all. Spontaneous abortion early in pregnancy is perhaps twice as likely among the 5% of women

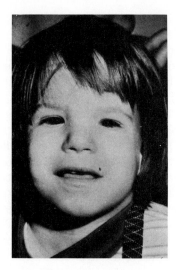

This photograph shows some of the symptoms of fetal alcohol syndrome. Note the small eyes, flattened bridge of the nose, and flattening of the vertical groove between the nose and mouth.

who are the heaviest drinkers. The data on later pregnancy loss (stillbirths) are not as clearly related to alcohol, for either animals or humans.

An important question, and one that can never be answered in absolute terms, is whether there is an acceptable level of alcohol consumption for pregnant women. The data we do have on drinking during pregnancy rely on self-reports by the mothers, who are assumed to be at least as likely as everyone else to underreport their drinking. In addition, almost every study that has been done has used different definitions of heavy drinking, alcohol abuse, or problem drinking. It is clear that the heaviest drinkers in each study are the most at risk for alcohol-related problems with their children, but we don't really know if the large number of light or moderate drinkers are causing significant risks. Based on the dose-related nature of birth problems in animal studies, one might argue that any alcohol use at all produces some risk, but at low levels the increased risk is too small to be revealed except in a large-scale study. In 1981 the Surgeon General recommended that "pregnant women should drink absolutely no alcohol be-

cause they may be endangering the health of their unborn children." Maybe that's going a bit too far. The bottom line is this: scientific data do not demonstrate that occasional consumption of one or two drinks definitely causes FAS or other alcohol-related birth defects. On the other hand, the data neither prove that low-level alcohol use is safe nor do they indicate a safe level of use. Remember from Chapter 6 that it is not within the realm of science to declare something totally safe, so it will be impossible ever to set a safe limit on alcohol use. It is good to know that most women decrease their alcohol use once they have become pregnant, and many decrease it further as pregnancy progresses.[34,p.76]

Metabolism

As a "food" item, alcohol has a couple of unusual characteristics. First, it requires no digestion and is absorbed unchanged into the bloodstream. Second, although alcohol does contain usable calories (it produces energy when it is metabolized), alcohol itself cannot be stored nor can it be converted into lipids or protein so that this energy can be stored for later use. You might think that this means that alcohol itself cannot contribute to weight gain, but that is not so. With alcohol in the system, other calories that might be burned are not.

Once absorbed, alcohol remains in the bloodstream and other body fluids until it is metabolized, and over 90% of this metabolism occurs in the liver. A small amount of alcohol, less than 2%, is normally excreted unchanged, some in the breath, some through the skin, and some in the urine. This small loss has almost no effect on BAL.

The primary metabolic system is a simple one: the enzyme *alcohol dehydrogenase* converts alcohol to *acetaldehyde*. Acetaldehyde is then coverted fairly rapidly to acetic acid. With most drugs a constant *proportion* of the drug is removed in a given amount of time, so that with a high blood level the amount metabolized is high. With alcohol, the amount that can be metabolized is constant at about 0.25 to 0.3 ounces per hour, regardless of the BAL. The major factor determining the rate of alcohol metabolism is the activity of the enzyme alcohol dehydrogenase. Since exercise, drinking coffee, and so on have no effect on this enzyme, the sobering-up process is essentially a matter of waiting for this enzyme to do its job at its own speed.

Acetaldehyde may be more than just an intermediate step in the oxidation of alcohol. Acetaldehyde is quite toxic and, even though blood levels are only one one-thousandth of those of alcohol, may in fact be the cause of some of the physiological effects now attributed to alcohol. Although more work needs to be done in this area, it is an intriguing finding that acetaldehyde blood levels are higher in alcoholic patients than in non-alcoholic.[35] The danger in heavy alcohol use may be in the higher blood levels of acetaldehyde.

The second enzyme system is much more complicated and, at this time, has many more known ramifications. The liver responds to chronic intake of alcohol by increasing production of a certain type of membrane: endoplasmic reticulum. This increase in endoplasmic reticulum is associated with increased levels of the *microsomal drug metabolizing enzymes* (Chapter 6). This gives rise to some interesting situations. In the long-term, heavy-alcohol-intake person there is an increase in the activity of the microsomal enzymes. As long as there is alcohol in the system, alcohol gets preferential treatment and the metabolism of other drugs is slower than normal. When heavy alcohol use stops and the alcohol has disappeared from the body, the high activity level of the enzymes continues for 4 to 8 weeks. During this time drugs are metabolized *more* rapidly. To obtain therapeutic levels of the drugs metabolized by this enzyme system (for example, the benzodiazepines) it is necessary to administer *less* drug to the drinking alcoholic and more drug to the just-nondrinking alcoholic.

One of the enzymes that increases is the *microsomal ethanol oxidizing system* (MEOS). Thus alcohol increases the activity of one of the two enzyme systems responsible for its own oxidation. The increased activity of this MEOS pathway may

be a partial basis for the tolerance to alcohol that is shown by heavy users of alcohol.

Another reason why it is important to know about the MEOS is that it is part of the indirect cause of the *fatty liver* that develops in alcohol consumers. For most of us this is not a serious problem. Fatty acids are the usual fuel for the liver. When alcohol is present, it has higher priority and is used as fuel. As a result, fatty acids (lipids) accumulate in the liver and are stored as small droplets in liver cells. Sometimes the droplets increase in size to the point where they rupture the cell membrane (and pour lipids into the bloodstream, which may have serious effects on the cardiovascular system), causing death of the liver cells. Up to the point where the liver cells die, a fatty liver is completely reversible and usually of minor medical concern. If alcohol input ceases, the liver uses the stored fatty acids for energy.

Sometimes, with prolonged and/or high-level alcohol intake, another phase of liver damage is observed. This is alcoholic hepatitis, which is a serious disease and includes both inflammation and impairment of liver function. Usually this occurs in areas where there are dead and dying liver cells, but it is not known if an increasingly fatty liver leads to alcoholic hepatitis. It is known that you can have alcoholic hepatitis in the absence of a fatty liver.

Cirrhosis is the liver disease everyone knows is related to high and prolonged levels of alcohol consumption. It's not easy to get cirrhosis from drinking alcohol—you have to work at it. Usually it takes about 10 years of steady drinking of the equivalent of a pint or more of whiskey a day. Not all cirrhosis is alcohol related, but a high percentage is, and cirrhosis is the seventh leading cause of death in the United States. In large urban areas it is the fourth or fifth leading cause of death in men ages 25 to 65. In cirrhosis, liver cells are replaced by fibrous tissue, which changes the structure of the liver. These changes decrease blood flow and, along with the loss of cells, result in a decreased ability of the liver to function. When the liver does not function properly, fluid accumulates in the body, jaundice develops, and cancer may develop in the liver. The yellow color of the jaundiced individual is the result of bile pigment distributed through the body, but, most importantly, it is a sign that the liver is not functioning properly, and toxins are beginning to accumulate in the blood. Cirrhosis is not reversible, but stopping the intake of alcohol will retard its development and decrease the serious medical effects. The liver has a large reserve capacity and is able to function adequately with mild cirrhosis. One of the important, unanswered questions is why not all alcoholics develop cirrhosis.

This is a good place to clear up some possible confusion over the role of diet, vitamin deficiency, alcohol intake, and impairment of liver function. For many years it was believed that the negative effects of alcohol consumption on the liver were secondary to vitamin deficiency. Since some people take in over half their daily calories through alcohol, they usually eat poor diets—and have vitamin deficiencies. It was thought that protein and perhaps vitamin deficiency caused the liver damage. There was support for this from animal research: animals fed diets severely deficient in vitamins and proteins developed liver disease in the absence of alcohol. The other side of the coin also matched: animals fed alcohol *and* adequate diets did not develop liver disease.

That position was altered considerably, if not reversed, with the use of new behavioral techniques and the finding that baboons[36] would develop liver disease—fatty liver, alcoholic hepatitis, and cirrhosis—if the alcohol intake was high enough, even though they had adequate diets. Both dietary deficiencies and alcohol consumption probably interact in most cases to cause human liver disease. It seems now that protein and vitamin deficiencies by themselves are not enough to damage the liver.

Alcohol Withdrawal—Delirium Tremens

The physical dependence associated with prolonged heavy use of alcohol is best seen when alcohol intake is stopped. *The abstinence syndrome that develops is medically more severe and more likely to cause death than withdrawal from narcotic drugs.* In untreated advanced cases, mortality may be as high as one in seven. Withdrawal symptoms do not appear until the BALs drop below the intoxication level, and these withdrawal symptoms alone may be enough to keep the drinker drinking.

One physician[37] has described the progression of withdrawal, the abstinence syndrome, in the following way:

Stage 1: Tremors, excessively rapid heartbeat, hypertension, heavy sweating, loss of appetite, and insomnia.
Stage 2: Hallucinations—auditory, visual, tactile, or a combination of these; and, rarely, olfactory signs.
Stage 3: Delusions, disorientation, delirium, sometimes intermittent in nature and usually followed by amnesia.
Stage 4: Seizure activity.

The belief was expressed that the term **delirium tremens** should be used only when the syndrome progresses through all four stages. In fact, medical treatment is usually sought in either stage 1 or 2, and rapid intervention will prevent stage 3 or 4 from occurring.

Tremors are one of the most common physical changes associated with alcohol withdrawal and may persist for a long period after alcohol intake has stopped. The classic drunk, bending over to sip from his cup, attests to the frequency of tremors. Anxiety, insomnia, feelings of unreality, nausea, vomiting, and many other symptoms are also common.

The withdrawal symptoms do not develop all at the same time or immediately after abstinence begins. The initial signs may develop within a few hours (tremors, anxiety), but the individual is relatively rational. Over the next day or two, hallucinations appear and gradually become more terrifying and real to the individual. Huckleberry Finn described these quite vividly in his pap.[38]

Pap took the jug, and said he had enough whisky there for two drunks and one delirium tremens. . . He drank and drank. . . .

I don't know how long I was asleep, but . . . there was an awful scream and I was up. There was pap looking wild, and skipping around every which way and yelling about snakes. He said they was crawling up on his legs; and then he would give a jump and scream, and say one had bit him on the cheek—but I couldn't see no snakes. He started and run round . . . hollering "Take him off! he's biting me on the neck!" I never see a man look so wild in the eyes. Pretty soon he was all fagged out, and fell down panting; then he rolled over . . . kicking things every which way, and striking and grabbing at the air with his hands, and scream-ing . . . there was devils a-hold of him. He wore out by and by . . . He says. . .

"Tramp-tramp-tramp; that's the dead; tramp-tramp-tramp; they're coming after me; but I won't go. Oh, they're here; don't touch me—don't! hands off—they're cold; let go. . ."

Then he went down on all fours and crawled off, begging them to let him alone. . .

By and by he . . . jumped up on his feet looking wild . . . and went for me. He chased me round and round the place with a claspknife, calling me the Angel of Death, and saying he would kill me, and then I wouldn't come for him no more . . . Pretty soon he was all tired out . . . and said he would rest for a minute and then kill me. . . .

In one double-blind, multiple hospital study, 7% of the patients given placebos suffered con-vulsions during withdrawal, while 6% showed de-lirium tremens.[39] In another study convulsions were reported in 12% of the patients, delirium tremens in 5%, and hallucinations in 18%.[40]

The symptoms that do develop seem to result from the fact that the cells of the body, and par-ticularly the CNS, have been functioning reason-ably normally in spite of the depressant action of alcohol. When the alcohol is reduced, the cells become hyperactive. Released from the depression induced by the drug, the cells overreact and be-come hyperexcitable.

Optimal treatment of the patients seems to be the administration of antianxiety agents such as chlordiazepoxide or diazepam (Chapter 8). In comparing the effectiveness of several compounds in blocking withdrawal symptoms, chlordiaz-epoxide reduced the incidence of convulsions and

delirium tremens to less than 1%.[39] This is a result of a high degree of cross-dependence between al-cohol and chlordiazepoxide, so one drug can be substituted for the other and withdrawal contin-ued at a safer rate. The use of drugs to decrease alcohol withdrawal signs is clearly only symptom-atic treatment. To keep the alcoholic from resum-ing drinking is a difficult task that will be discussed in Chapter 18.

WHO IS AN ALCOHOLIC?

Defining alcoholism is not an easy thing to do. The term has different meanings to different au-thorities, so picking any one of them gets you into a discussion right away. In Chapter 18 we will see that how one defines alcoholism has important implications for the approaches that are taken in treatment, the treatment goals, and how one mea-sures success. Our immediate concern is how many and what types of people will be included in the group defined as alcoholics.

When we see a man who drinks to the point of drunkenness every day, who has lost his job and family, who has a damaged liver, and who will suffer from delirium tremens if he doesn't drink for a day, then everyone can agree that we have an alcoholic. Some definitions have focused on the *physiological* aspects of this model alcoholic, and define alcoholism on the basis of obvious liver or brain damage, tolerance, or withdrawal symp-toms. Other definitions have focused on the *psy-chosocial* aspects, using criteria such as daily use or interference with personal, social, or occupa-tional behavior. The problem arises when we leave the stereotype, model alcoholic and start looking at ourselves and our friends and neigh-bors. There are lots of people who do not have obvious symptoms of liver or brain damage and who don't get the "shakes" if they don't drink on a given day, but who drink regularly, depend on drinking at least as an important aspect of their individual and social lives, and who suffer some level of interference with their personal, social, or occupational life. In fact, it is probably true that almost anyone who drinks at all will occasionally drink too much and have a hangover at work, be embarrassed socially, or fail to accomplish some personal goal on that day. How do we decide when such a person becomes an alcoholic? As far as this text is concerned, we don't. The term has too many meanings to too many people for us to be at all specific in our definition and still do justice to this important topic. What we will do is describe several of the ways in which this issue has been addressed.

Probably the most significant influence on American attitudes about alcoholism is a 50-year-old book called *Alcoholics Anonymous*. This book described the experiences of a small group of people who formed a society whose "only requirement for membership is a desire to stop drinking." That society has now grown to include more than 1.5 million members in over 100 countries. A central part of their belief system is that alcoholism is a progressive disease characterized by a loss of control over drinking, and can never be cured. People who do not have the disease may drink and even become intoxicated, but they do not "lose control over alcohol." There is a suspicion that the alcoholic may be different even before the first drink is taken. The only treatment is to arrest the disease by abstaining from drinking. This *disease model* of alcoholism has received support from many medical practitioners and has been endorsed by the American Medical Association and other professional groups. In one sense, this description of alcoholism as a disease is a reaction against long-held notions that excessive drinking is only a symptom of some other underlying pathology, such as depression or some type of personality defect. Traditional psychoanalysts practicing many years ago might have treated the alcoholic by trying to discover the unconscious conflicts or personality deficiencies that caused the person to drink. One important consequence of defining alcoholism as a *primary* disease is to recognize that the drinking itself may be the problem, and that treatment and prevention should be aimed directly at alcoholism.

However, there are many scientific critics of the disease concept. If alcoholism is a disease, what is its cause? How are "alcoholics" different from "nonalcoholics," except that they tend to drink a lot and have many alcohol-related problems? Let's accept for the purpose of discussion that those who go into hospitals or treatment programs with a primary diagnosis of alcoholism are alcoholics. What are their characteristics? Although sequential stages have been described for this "progressive disease," most individual alcoholics don't seem to fit any single set of descriptors. Some don't drink alone, some don't drink in the morning, some don't go on binges, some don't drink every day, and some don't report strong cravings for alcohol. Experiments have shown that alcoholics do retain considerable control over their drinking, even while drinking—it's not that they completely lose control when they start drinking, but they may have either less ability or less desire to control their drinking, because they do drink excessively. Although an "alcoholic personality" has been defined that characterizes many alcoholics who enter treatment, the current belief is that these personality factors (impulsive, anxious, depressed, passive, dependent) reflect the years of intoxication and the critical events that led to the decision to enter treatment, rather than being pre-exising abnormalities that caused the alcoholism.

The American Psychiatric Association's Diagnostic and Statistical Manual of Mental Disorders, third edition, revised (DSM-III-R, 1987)[41] is probably the closest thing we have to a single official, widely accepted set of labels for behavior disorders, including substance abuse and dependence (see Chapter 2). The DSM-III-R does not separately define these for alcohol, but includes it as one of the psychoactive substances. This manual implies, but does not directly state, that the term alcoholism may refer either to alcohol abuse, which is defined in psychosocial terms (a maladaptive pattern of use indicated by either continued use despite knowledge of having persistent problems caused by alcohol), or alcohol dependence, which describes more serious psychosocial characteristics and includes the physiological factors of tolerance and withdrawal among the possible symptoms.

In 1989, it may have appeared that the U.S. Supreme Court had finally decided the issue of whether alcoholism is or is not a disease. Two veterans of the armed services had filed for educational benefits after the 10 year eligibility period following their service had elapsed. The Veterans Administration denied their benefits, even though extensions of the eligibility period can be granted if the individual was delayed in education by physical or mental disorders "not the result of their own willful misconduct." These individuals argued that they were alcoholics and, since alcoholism is a disease over which they had no control, they should be allowed the extension. Newspapers, magazines, and television commentators widely touted the case as deciding once and for all whether alcoholism is "truly" a disease or whether it should be considered more akin to misbehavior (willful misconduct). On one side were legions of treatment professionals and alcoholics (or ex-alcoholics, if there can be such a thing) who believe very strongly in the disease model upon which most programs of treatment and recovery are based. On the other side were a smaller number of professionals and academics who argued that we have gone too far in the "medicalization" of alcohol, with every wife-beater and criminal claiming the illness and being sent off for treatment. They argued that people must be held accountable for their behavior and misbehavior regarding alcohol.[42] The Supreme Court ruled in favor of the Veterans Administration, but we cannot conclude from that that alcoholism is not "truly" a disease. We should recognize by now that alcoholism is one of those complex concepts that means different things to different people in different contexts, not something that can be defined perfectly and absolutely. "Disease" is the same kind of concept. We could pick an official definition of alcoholism, which we should recognize as being somewhat arbitrary, and an official definition of disease, similarly somewhat arbitrary, and then match them up to see if alcoholism is "truly" a disease. A more sensible conclusion would be that there are probably contexts in which it makes sense to think of alcoholism as a disease, other contexts in which it

How can you tell if you have a drinking problem?

There have been many self-tests published for people to use to determine if they are alcoholics or if they have a drinking problem. None of them should be taken as an absolute test or as providing a definite answer to that question, because in most cases it is a complex, subjective judgment as to whether someone should seek help. One of the best popularly printed self-tests appeared in a "Dear Abby" column, and it is offered here as a possible guide. If these questions seem to indicate that you or a friend need to seek help, we recommend a visit to a counselor, psychologist, or physician who is experienced in the assessment of chemical dependency. An assessment would probably include the use of a more professional questionnaire such as the Michigan Alcoholism Screening Test (MAST) or the Alcohol Dependency Scale (ADS).

Check those that apply to you:

( ) 1. Have you ever decided to stop drinking for a week or so, but only lasted for a couple of days?
( ) 2. Do you wish people would stop nagging you about your drinking?
( ) 3. Have you ever switched from one kind of drink to another in the hope that this would keep you from getting drunk?
( ) 4. Have you had a drink in the morning in the past year?
( ) 5. Do you envy people who can drink without getting into trouble?
( ) 6. Have you had problems connected with drinking during the past year?
( ) 7. Has your drinking caused problems at home?
( ) 8. Do you ever try to get "extra" drinks at a party because you did not get enough to drink?
( ) 9. Do you tell yourself you can stop drinking anytime you want to, even though you keep getting drunk when you don't mean to?
( )10. Have you missed days at work (or school) because of drinking?
( )11. Do you have "blackouts"?
( )12. Have you ever felt that your life would be better if you did not drink?

If you checked four or more of these, it would be a good idea to seek the guidance of a specialist in chemical dependency or to seek help directly through Alcoholics Anonymous or a similar organization. It's perfectly acceptable to go to an open AA meeting, listen to what is being said, and decide for yourself if their program would be useful to you.

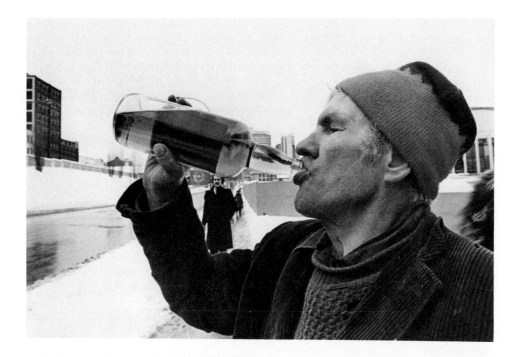

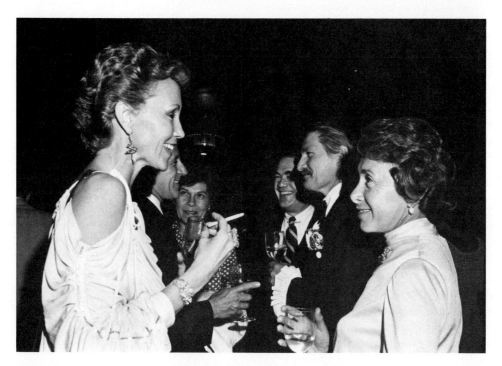

The street wino fits our idea of an alcoholic, but most alcoholics are not so easy to spot.

probably does not make sense to think that way, and perhaps many contexts in which it is not at all clear.

The most important definition may be the one that the individual drinker places on his or her own drinking behavior. A good example is provided by an interview with TV and movie actor Dick Van Dyke. As with every member of Alcoholics Anonymous, he is an alcoholic because he decided he was an alcoholic:

Van Dyke: I didn't miss work ever because of drinking. And I never drank at work. Never drank during the day—only at home and only in the evenings. . . .

I never craved a drink during the day. I was never a morning drinker—I didn't want one then. The idea made me as sick as it would make anyone else. But evening drinking is a form of alcoholism, just like periodic drinking is a form of alcoholism.

Question: Did your drinking problem have a big effect on your home life?

Van Dyke: It was a funny thing. My 19-year-old daughter was on the Tom Snyder "Tomorrow Show." . . . Tom asked my daughter about my drinking—my alcoholism—"How did that affect you?" She said, "I never knew it. My father was so quiet about it, never made any noise. As a matter of fact, some of the best talks we ever had were when my father was drinking." Which is a very strange reaction. When I asked her afterwards, she said, "I never knew a thing about it."

Question: For 5 years you had a drinking problem without really admitting it to yourself. What finally happened to make you realize that you were an alcoholic?

Van Dyke: I don't know. . . . I said to myself, "What am I doing?" My wife had long gone to bed. I was sitting alone, drinking, lost in what I took to be deep thought. I realized suddenly, "Why, I am thinking gibberish here—my mind is completely out of it." When I woke up the next morning, I got up and went to a hospital. Went straight into a treatment center.[43]

At the other end of the spectrum is the person who could be officially labeled as suffering from alcohol dependence, but who repeatedly refuses treatment because he won't admit to being an alcoholic:

This 45-year-old white male had 8 years of education and 2 years in the army. He started drinking at 18 and, although he was court martialed three times and spent 6 months in the stockade for alcohol-related offenses, he says his drinking has been a problem only for the last 10 years.

His drinking sprees now last 3 to 4 weeks and occur about six times a year. During these sprees he reports consuming at least a quart of whiskey, a gallon of wine, and 1 to 3 six-packs of beer every day. He has had blackouts, extreme shakes, and hallucinations on a "few" occasions. He has had more arrests for public drunkenness than he can remember.

On his first admission to the hospital 5 years ago he said he only drank a few beers a day, but his wife brought him to the hospital because he was talking to the TV, hearing strange music, and seeing bugs and snakes. On his next admission 2 years later, he said he was ready for treatment but managed to miss all of his scheduled appointments. When confronted, he dressed and left the hospital.

Factors Predisposing to Alcoholism

Whether or not alcoholism represents a single disease state, for many years we have wondered why some people seem to be able to drink in moderation all their lives while others repeatedly become intoxicated, suffer from alcohol-related problems, and continue to drink excessively. So far, no single factor and no combination of multiple factors has been presented that allows us to predict which individuals will become alcoholics. Multiple theories exist, including biochemical, psychoanalytic, and cultural approaches. At this period of scientific history, probably the most attention is being focused on understanding two types of factor: cognitive and genetic.

The importance of cognitive factors with regard to alcohol's effects is perhaps best demonstrated by a series of experiments conducted by Marlatt and his colleagues on "loss of control" in alcoholics and social drinkers.[44] The experimental subjects are given drinks that either do or do not contain alcohol, and half of each group are told that the drinks do contain alcohol whereas the other half of each group are told that the drinks do not have alcohol in them. Both alcoholics and social drinkers are "fooled" by the instructions, and report more intoxication and consume more drinks when they are told the drinks have alcohol, regardless of the actual alcohol content. It is important that alcoholics given alcohol to drink did not report becoming intoxicated and did not increase their drinking if they were led to expect that the drink contained no alcohol. If alcoholics do lose control when they begin drinking, it may be because they have come to believe that they will lose control if they drink (this is sometimes referred to as the Abstinence Violation Effect). These experiments have been replicated several times by others. In such experiments, which contrast the pharmacological effects of alcohol with the cognitive effects of expecting to drink alcohol, typically alcohol itself can be shown to impair information processing ability and motor performance regardless of expectation. Expectancy of alcohol increases alcohol consumption, sexual arousal, and aggressiveness.[45] The most obvious interpretation of such results is that alcohol use provides a social excuse for behaving in certain ways that would otherwise be considered inappropriate, and it is enough for one to believe that he or she has drunk alcohol for such behaviors to be released. These experiments have led to a broader study of expectancies about alcohol: how do we learn what to expect about alcohol's effects, and how do different sets of expectations relate to differences in drinking practices? So far, evidence indicates that our expectancies are culturally and experientially influenced, and may be largely formed even before we first drink. Those who believe more strongly that alcohol is likely to have desirable consequences (make them more sexual, more outspoken or even aggressive, more talkative, feel good) are more likely to be heavy drinkers.[46] One interesting question is why some of these expectancies about what alcohol does for people are so strongly developed that even years of negative consequences from drinking do not change the expectancies of some alcoholics.

There is considerable evidence in support of the idea that some degree of vulnerability to alcoholism may be inherited.[47] Alcoholism does tend to "run in families," but some of that could be due to similar expectancies developed through similar cultural influences and children learning from their parents. Studies on twins provide one way around this problem. Monozygotic (one-egg, or identical) twins share the same genetic material, whereas dizygotic (two-egg or fraternal) twins are no more genetically related than any two siblings. Both types of twins are likely to share very similar cultural and family learning experiences. If one adult twin is diagnosed as alcoholic, what is the likelihood that the other twin will also receive that diagnosis (are the twins concordant for the trait of alcoholism)? Almost all such studies report that the concordance rate for monozygotic twins is higher than that for dizygotic twins, and in some studies is as high as 50%. These results imply that inheritance plays a strong role, but is far from a complete determinant of alcoholism. Another important type of study looks at adopted sons whose biological fathers were alcoholics. These reports consistently find that such adoptees have a much greater than average chance of becoming alcoholics, even though they are raised by nonalcoholic parents. Although these studies again provide clear evidence for a genetic influence, it is important to remember that most children of alcoholics do not become alcoholics— they simply have a statistically greater risk of doing so. For example, in one study 18% of adopted-away sons of alcoholics became alcoholic, compared to 5% of adopted-away sons whose parents had not received the diagnosis of alcoholism.

Further evidence for an inherited risk factor in alcoholism comes from experiments on young men (because alcoholism is more common in men) who are drinking but have not yet demonstrated alcoholism. If these young men had an alcoholic parent, they were less affected by a dose of alcohol than were control subjects with no family history of alcoholism. The argument is that these vulnerable individuals may drink more alcohol because they are less able to detect the initial effects of alcohol. Another type of study examined electrical brain-wave responses recorded from the scalp in response to repeated auditory stimuli. Al-

---

Issue: advertising alcohol

After prohibition, purveyors of distilled spirits did not advertise on radio, and later, on televison. This has been a voluntary ban by the radio and television and liquor industries. Now a group called SMART (Stop Marketing Alcohol on Radio and Television) is seeking a mandatory ban on the broadcasting of beer and wine advertisements. When such a ban was placed on cigarette advertising, the industry switched to advertising mainly in newspapers and magazines.

Involved are the constitutional issues of freedom of speech (limited in the area of "commerical" speech, and further limited by FCC licensing of broadcasters), as well as the practical issues: Would the ban reduce alcohol use or not? What would the economic effects be on broadcasters, print media, and beer and wine producers?

---

coholic men as a group have a smaller response at a particular time point after the stimulus (the P300 wave). In addition, young men who have never themselves drunk alcohol but whose fathers are alcoholics, as a group show a similarly reduced P300 wave.[48]

Once again, it is important to realize that these significant effects are derived from groups of people, and do not characterize each individual in the group. There is currently a growing industry based on dealing with the needs of "adult children of alcoholics" (ACOAs), which seems sometimes to be based on the notion that all such children must be permanently abnormal, either genetically or psychologically. While there may be some benefit in awareness and watchfulness on the part of such individuals, one should be wary of any approach that tends to characterize all ACOAs as being the same.

Summary

Alcohol, the ancient excretion product of yeasts, has been used by humans since before recorded history. Its social, economic, and psychological importance is reflected in the history of govern-mental attempts at regulation and in the myriad federal, state, and municipal taxes and laws affecting what may be sold, when, where and to whom, and how it may be advertised.

In present-day America about two-thirds of the adults drink alcohol in the form of beer, wine, and distilled spirits. Changing attitudes toward health have reduced the consumption of distilled spirits and increased the sales of low-alcohol and no-alcohol adult beverages.

The major factor determining how much liquor one can "hold" is the volume of distribution, based mainly on body weight. The rate of metabolism of alcohol is fairly constant for an individual, so there are no magic formulas for "sobering up."

Alcohol has been implicated as a cause of many deaths in traffic accidents, and also contributes to murder and suicide. Its effects on sexual behavior are complex, but it may generally be said to increase one's interest in sex but to interfere with physiological functions important to arousal.

Alcoholism is our most significant drug addiction, yet we have been unable to develop a consensus defining alcoholism. Both psychological and biological factors have been indentified that seem to predispose some individuals to alcoholism, and the evidence for heritability is increasing.

REFERENCES

1. Koren J: Economic aspects of the liquor problem, New York, 1899, Houghton, Miffllin & Co.
2. Clark NH: The dry years: prohibition and social change in Washington, Seattle, 1965, University of Washington Press.
3. Kyvig DE: Sober thoughts: myths and realities of national prohibition after fifty years. In Kyvig DE, editor: Law, alcohol and order, Westport, Conn, 1985, Greenwood Press.
4. Keller M: Alcohol problems and policies in historical perspective. In Kyvig DE, editor: Law, alcohol and order, Westport, Conn, 1985, Greenwood Press.
5. Emerson H: Alcohol and man, New York, 1932, The MacMillan Co,. Reprinted by Arno Press, 1981, New York.
6. The brewers almanac, Washington DC, 1988, United States Brewers Association.
7. Montgomery A: The cooler illusion, Nutrition Action Healthletter, August, 1988, pp 8-9.
8. Sales data provided by the Distilled Spirits Council of the United States, Inc, Washington, DC.

9. Segal BM: The Soviet heavy-drinking culture and the American heavy-drinking subculture. In Babor TF, editor: Alcohol and culture: comparative perspectives from Europe and America, New York Academy of Sciences, 1986.

10. Vaillant G: Cultural factors in the etiology of alcoholism: a prospective study. In Babor TF, editor: Alcohol and culture: comparative perspectives from Europe and America, New York Academy of Sciences, 1986.

11. Geddes D: France sets records in suicide, alcoholism and anxiety, The Times (London), June 14, 1986, p 9.

12. Sixth special report on alcohol and health, DHHS Publication No (ADM) 87-1519. Washington, DC, US Government Printing Office, 1987.

13. Linsky AS and others: Social stress, normative constraints and alcohol problems in American states, Social Science in Medicine, 24:875-883, 1987.

14. Mooney DK and others: Correlates of alcohol consumption: sex, age, and expectancies relate differentially to quantity and frequency, Addictive Behaviors, 12:235-240, 1987.

15. Kolata G: New drug counters alcohol intoxication, Science, 234:1198-1199, 1986.

16. Goldberg L: Quantitative studies on alcohol tolerance in man, Acta Physiologica Scandinavica 5(suppl 16):1-128, 1943.

17. Salamy A: The effects of alcohol on the variability of the human evoked potential, Neuropharmacology 12:1103-1107, 1973.

18. Bogen E: The human toxicology of alcohol. In Emerson H, editor: Alcohol and man, New York, 1932, The MacMillan Co.

19. IHHS facts 1988, Insurance Institute for Highway Safety, Washington, DC.

20. Alcohol and highway safety 1984: a review of the state of the knowledge, Washington, DC, 1985, Department of Transportation Publication No DOT-HS-806-569, US Government Printing Office.

21. Goodwin DW: Alcohol in suicide and homicide, Quarterly Journal of Studies on Alcohol 34:144-156, 1973.

22. Mayfield DG and Montgomery D: Alcoholism, alcohol intoxication, and suicide attempts, Archives of General Psychiatry 27(3):349-353, 1972.

23. Crothers TD: Alcoholic trance, Popular Science Monthly 26:189, 191, 1884.

24. Shakespeare W: Macbeth, Act II, Scene 1.

25. Wilson GT: Alcohol and human sexual behavior, Behavior Research and Therapy 15:239-252, 1977.

26. Wilson GT and Lawson DM: Effects of alcohol on sexual arousal in women, Journal of Abnormal Psychology 85(5):489-497, 1976.

27. Briddell DW and Wilson GT: Effects of alcohol and expectancy set on male sexual arousal, Journal of Abnormal Psychology 85(2):225-234, 1976.

28. Lemere F and Smith JW: Alcohol-induced sexual impotence, American Journal of Psychiatry 130(2):212-213, 1973.

29. Rubin E and others: Prolonged ethanol consumption increases testosterone metabolism in the liver, Science 191:563-564, 1976.

30. Brody J: Personal health, New York Times, December 27, 1976, p. C13.

31. Chapman LF: Experimental induction of hangover, Quarterly Journal of Studies on Alcohol, Suppl 5, pp. 67-86, March 10, 1970.

32. Dyer AR and others: Alcohol consumption and 17-year mortality in the Chicago Western Electric Company Study, Preventive Medicine 9:78-90, 1980.

33. Jones KL and others: Pattern of malformation in offspring of chronic alcoholic mothers, Lancet, 1(7815):1267-1271, June 9, 1973.

34. Fifth special report on alcohol and health, DHHS Publication No. (ADM) 84-1291, Washington, DC, US Government Printing Office, 1984.

35. Screening tests for alcoholism? Lancet, p 1117-1118, November 22, 1980.

36. Rubin E and Lieber CS: Fatty liver, alcoholic hepatitis and cirrhosis produced by alcohol in primates, New England Journal of Medicine 290:128-135, 1974.

37. High degree of morbidity, mortality found in acute alcohol withdrawal, Alcohol and Health Notes, p 2, October 1973.

38. Twain M: The adventures of Huckleberry Finn, 1885.

39. Kaim SC, Klett CJ, and Rothfeld B: Treatment of the acute alcohol withdrawal state: a comparison of four drugs, American Journal of Psychiatry 125:1640-1646, 1969.

40. Victor M and Adams RD, Cited by Fraser HF: Tolerance to and physical dependence on opiates, barbiturates and alcohol, Annual Review of Medicine 8:427-440, 1957.

41. Diagnostic and Statistical Manual of Mental Disorders, third edition, revised Washington, DC, 1987, American Psychiatric Association.

42. Alcoholism a disease or foible? Denver Post, December, 1988.

43. Even my kids didn't know I was an alcoholic: an interview with Dick Van Dyke, The Drinking American, Publication No (ADM) 76-348, Department of Health, Education, and Welfare, Washington, DC, 1976, US Government Printing Office.

44. Wilson GT: Cognitive studies in alcoholism, Journal of Consulting and Clinical Psychology 55:325-331, 1987.

45. Hull JG and Bond CF: Social and behavioral consequences of alcohol consumption and expectancy: a meta-analysis, Psychological Bulletin 99:347-360, 1986.

46. Critchlow B: A utility analysis of drinking, Addictive Behaviors 12:269-273, 1987.

47. Biological and genetic factors in alcoholism, Research Monograph No 9. Rockville, Md, 1983, National Institute on Alcohol Abuse and Alcoholism.

48. Schuckit MA: Biological vulnerability to alcoholism, Journal of Consulting and Clinical Psychology 55:301-309, 1987.

Chapter 10

Nicotine

OBJECTIVES

After reading this chapter, you should be able to:

State some facts about the history of tobacco and the spread of its use around the world.

Describe how cigarettes are made and how they have changed over the years.

Discuss the increased use of smokeless tobacco and the fad involving clove cigarettes.

List some facts about the consequences of smoking for cancer, heart disease, obstructive lung disease, and pregnancy.

Discuss the pharmacology of nicotine and evidence indicating that it is the dependence-producing agent in tobacco.

Describe drug and nondrug approaches to smoking cessation.

TOBACCO

Tobacco was a plant just waiting for civilization to discover it—so it could conquer civilization. Long before Columbus stumbled onto the Western Hemisphere, the Indians here were using tobacco. It was one of the many contributions of the New World to Europe: corn, sweet potatoes, white potatoes, chocolate, and—so you could lie back and enjoy it all—the hammock. Christopher Columbus recorded that the natives of San Salvador presented him with tobacco leaves on October 12, 1492. A fitting birthday present.

In 1497 a monk who had accompanied Columbus on his second trip wrote a book on native customs that contained the first printed report of tobacco smoking. It wasn't called tobacco, and it wasn't called smoking. Inhaling smoke was called drinking. In that period you either "took" (used snuff) or "drank" (smoked) tobacco.

The word tobacco came from one of two sources. "Tobaco" referred to a two-pronged tube used by natives to take snuff. Some early reports confused the issue by applying the name to the plant they incorrectly thought was being used. Another idea is that the word developed its current usage from the province of Tobacos in Mexico where everyone used the herb. Be that as it may, in 1598 an Italian-English dictionary published in London translated the Italian "Nicosiana" as the herb "Tobacco," and that spelling and usage gradually became dominant.

One member of Columbus's party was the poor fellow who introduced tobacco drinking to Europe. He was also the first European to touch Cuba and possibly the first to smoke tobacco. When he continued his habit in Portugal, his friends were convinced the devil had possessed him as they saw the smoke coming out his mouth and nose. The priest agreed, and Rodrigo spent the next several years in jail, only to find on his release that people were doing the same thing for which he had been jailed!

Early Medical Uses

Tobacco was formally introduced to Europe as an herb useful for treating almost anything. A 1529 report[1] indicated that tobacco was used for "persistant headaches," "cold or catarrh," "abscesses and sores on the head." Between 1537 and 1559, 14 books mentioned the medicinal value of tobacco.

Jean Nicot was sent to Lisbon, Portugal in 1559 to arrange a royal marriage that never took place, but he became enamored with the medical uses of tobacco. He tried it on enough people to convince himself of its value and sent glowing reports of the herb's effectiveness to the French court. He was successful in "curing" the migraine headaches of Catherine de Medicis, Queen of Henry II of France, which made tobacco use very much "in." It was called the *herbe sainte,* holy plant, and the *herbe a tous les maux,* the plant against all evils. The French loved it, and, although tobacco had been introduced earlier to Paris, Nicot received the credit. By 1565 the plant had been called nicotiane, and Linnaeus sanctified it in 1753 by naming the genus *Nicotiana.* When a pair of French chemists isolated the active ingredient in 1828, they acted like true nationalists and called it nicotine.

In the late sixteenth century

it was more likely than not that . . . the doctor would prescribe tobacco . . . Did the patient suffer from flatulence? The remedy was a tobacco emetic . . . A heavy cough? Smoke of tobacco, deeply inhaled. Pains accompanying gestation or labor? Place a leaf of tobacco, very hot, on the navel. If a form of delirium ensued, blow smoke up the nostrils[2,pp.38-39]

In this period Sir Anthony Chute[1,p.238] summarized much of the earlier material and said, "Anything that harms a man inwardly from his girdle upward might be removed by a moderate use of the herb." Others, however, felt differently: "If taken after meals the herb would infect the brain and liver," and, "Tobacco should be avoided by (among others) women with child and husbands who desired to have children."[1,p.238]

A few years later in 1617 Dr. William Vaughn phrased the last thought a little more poetically:

Tobacco that outlandish weede
It spends the braine and spoiles the seede
It dulls the spirite, it dims the sight
It robs a woman of her right.[3]

Special note must be made of a series of experiments reported in 1805 by Dr. D. Legare, since his work pushed back the boundaries of ignorance and clearly disproved an old folk remedy. Beyond the shadow of a doubt, Dr. Legare personally proved that, contrary to general opinion, blowing tobacco smoke into the intestinal canal did *not* resuscitate drowned animals or people!

The slow advance of medical science through the eighteenth and nineteenth centuries gradually removed tobacco from the doctor's black bag, and nicotine was dropped from *The United States Pharmacopeia* in the 1890s.

Tobacco Use Spreads

In the sixteenth century the English had real heroes to love and to emulate, men like Sir Walter Raleigh (who wasn't always a pipe tobacco) and Sir Francis Drake (who never was). They sailed the seven seas and, unlike most sailors of the day, took up pipe smoking. During the Elizabethan era, smoking became a national pleasure for the English, even though few people on the continent smoked.

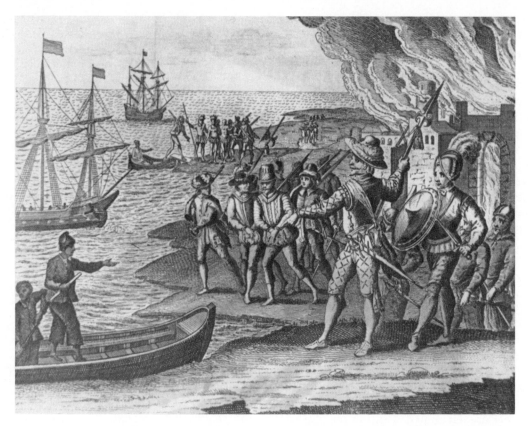

During the swashbuckling days of Sir Walter Raleigh, most sailors took up pipe smoking.

To fully appreciate the history of tobacco you must know that there are over 60 species of *Nicotiana*, but only two major ones. **Nicotiana tobacum,** the major species grown today in over 100 countries, is large leafed. Most importantly, *tobacum* was indigenous only to South America, so the Spanish had a monopoly on its production for over a hundred years. **Nicotiana rustica** is a small-leaf species and was the plant existing in the West Indies and eastern North America when Columbus arrived.

The Spanish monopoly on tobacco sales to Europe was a thorn in the side of the British. When the settlers returned to England in 1586 after failing to colonize Virginia, they brought with them seeds of the *rustica* species and planted them in England, but this species never grew well. The English crown again attempted to establish a tobacco colony in 1610 when they sent John Rolfe as leader of a group to Virginia. From 1610 to 1612 Rolfe tried to cultivate *rustica* but the small-leafed plant was weak, poor in flavor, and had a sharp taste.

In 1612 Rolfe's wife died, but, more important, he somehow got hold of some seeds of the Spanish *tobacum* species. This species grew beautifully and sold well in 1613. The colony was saved, and every available plot of land was planted with *tobacum*. By 1619, as much Virginia tobacco was sold in London as Spanish tobacco. That was also the year that King James prohibited the cultivation of any tobacco in England and declared the tobacco trade a royal monopoly.

Tobacco became one of the major exports of

the American colonies to England. The Thirty Years' War spread smoking throughout central Europe, and nothing stopped its use. Measures such as one in Bavaria in 1652 probably slowed tobacco use, but only momentarily. This law said that "tobacco-drinking was strictly forbidden to the peasants and other common people . . . " and made tobacco available to others only on a doctor's prescription from a druggist.[4,pp.112-114]

During the eighteenth century smoking gradually diminished, but the use of tobacco did not. Snuff replaced the pipe in England. At the beginning of that century the upper class was already committed to snuff. The middle and lower classes only gradually changed over, but by 1770 very few people smoked. The reign of King George III (1760 to 1820) was the time of the big snuff. His wife Charlotte was so addicted to the powder that she was called "Snuffy Charlotte," although for obvious reasons not to her face. On the continent Napoleon had tried smoking once, gagged horribly, and returned to his 7 pounds of snuff a month.

Tobacco in Early America

Trouble developed in the colonies, which, being democratic, made the richest man in Virginia (perhaps the richest in the colonies) commander in chief of the Revolutionary Army. In 1776 George Washington said in one of his appeals, "if you can't send money, send tobacco."[5,p.73] Tobacco played an important role in the Revolutionary War, since it was one of the major products for which France would lend the colonies money. Knowing the importance of tobacco to the colonies, one of Cornwallis' major campaign goals in 1780 and 1781 was the destruction of the Virginia tobacco plantations.

After the war, the American man in the street rejoiced and rejected snuff as well as tea and all other things British. The aristocrats who organized the republic were not as emotional, though, and installed a communal snuff box for members of Congress. Only in the mid-1930s did this remembrance of things past disappear. However, to emphasize the fact that snuff was a nonessential, the new Congress put a luxury tax on it in 1794.

> If you don't smoke and you don't snuff
> How can you possibly get enough?

By chewing, which gradually increased in the United States. Chewing was a suitable activity for a country on the go; it freed the hands, and the wide open spaces made an adequate spittoon. There were also other considerations: Boston, for example, had passed an ordinance in 1798 forbidding anyone from being in possession of a lighted pipe or "segar" in public streets. The original impetus was a concern for the fire hazard involved in smoking, not the individual's health, and the ordinance was finally repealed in 1880. Today it is difficult to appreciate how much of a chewing country we were in the nineteenth century. In 1860 only seven of 348 tobacco factories in Virginia and North Carolina manufactured smoking tobacco. The amount of tobacco for smoking did not equal the amount or chewing until 1911 and did not surpass it until the 1920s. Even as cigarettes began developing in Europe, American chewing tobacco was expanding.

The Civil War shut southern **bright** (that is, light colored when cured) tobacco out of northern markets, but Ohio and Kentucky had a different variety of tobacco, *burley,* that was darker and better suited for chewing. Burley had a low sugar content and thus could absorb up to 25% of its weight in licorice, rum, and molasses, whereas the bright tobacco from Virginia and North Carolina could absorb only 4% of its weight. The tobaccos from west of the Appalachian Mountains reached their peak in the period 1890 to 1910. The 1890s particularly were times of price wars and intense competition. By selling at less than cost, consumption of chewing tobacco increased so that by 1897 one half of all tobacco in the United States was prepared for chewing. The names of some of the brands suggest the savageness of the competition: "Battle Ax," "Scalping Knife," "Crossbow."

The high level of chewing tobacco production during the Industrial Age led to occasional accidents, as suggested by a quote from a 1918 decision of the Mississippi Supreme Court:

> We can imagine no reason why, with ordinary care, human toes could not be left out of chewing tobacco, and if toes are found in chewing tobacco, it seems to us that somebody has been very careless.[2,p.303]

The turn of the century was the approximate high point for chewing tobacco, the sales of which slowly declined through the early part of the century as other tobacco products became more popular. In 1945 cuspidors were removed from all federal buildings. Perhaps they should have been saved for the 1990s!

Cigars and Cigarettes

The transition from chewing to cigarettes had a middle point, a combination of both smoking and chewing: cigars. Cigarette smoking was coming, and the cigar manufacturers did their best to keep cigarettes under control. They suggested that cigarettes were drugged with opium so you could not stop using them and that the paper was bleached with arsenic and thus was harmful to you. They had some help from Thomas Edison in 1914:

> The injurious agent in Cigarettes comes principally from the burning paper wrapper . . . . It has a violent action in the nerve centers, producing degeneration of the cells of the brain, which is quite rapid among boys. Unlike most narcotics, this degeneration is permanent and uncontrollable. I employ no person who smokes cigarettes.[2,p.274]

Most cigars had been hand rolled or at least made by hand shaping in a mold, but as sales increased, machines had to be used. Today, a good worker hand rolls about 200 cigars in an 8- to 9-hour day. There was an aversion to machine-made cigars, so some advertising was educational in nature. As an example of the high level of advertising before television and Madison Avenue:

> Spit is a horrid word, but it's worse on the end of your cigar. Why run the risk of cigars made by dirty yellowed fingers and tipped in spit?.[2,p.273]

The efforts of the cigar manufacturers worked for a while, and cigar sales reached their highest level in 1920, when eight billion were sold. As sales increased, though, so did the cost of the product. The whole world knows that "what this country *needs* is a really good five-cent cigar," but how many know that this statement was made by a vice president of the United States as an aside in the Senate when one of the members was going on at great length about the needs of the country?

Thin reeds filled with tobacco had been seen by the Spanish in Yucatan in 1518. In 1844 the French were using them, and the Crimean War circulated the cigarette habit throughout Europe. The first British cigarette factory was started in 1856 by a returning veteran of the Crimean War, and in the late 1850s an English tobacco merchant, Phillip Morris, began producing handmade cigarettes. In the continent the use of this new dose form must have developed fairly rapidly. One company in Austria began making double cigarettes in 1865—both ends had a mouthpiece, and the consumer cut them in two—and sold 16 million in 1866.

In the United States cigarettes were being produced during the same period (14 million in 1870), but it was in the 1880s that their popularity increased rapidly. The date of the first patent on a cigarette-making machine was 1881, and by 1885 over a billion cigarettes a year were being sold.

Not even that great he-man, boxer John L. Sullivan could stem the tide, though in 1905 his opinion of cigarette smokers was pretty clear:

> Smoke cigarettes? Not on your tut-tut . . . . You can't suck coffin-nails and be a ring-champion . . . . You never heard of . . . a bank burglar using a cigarette, did you? They couldn't do it and attend to biz. Why, even drunkards don't use the things . . . . Who smokes 'em? Dudes and college stiffs—fellows who'd be wiped out by a single jab or a quick undercut. It isn't natural to smoke cigarettes. An American ought to smoke cigars . . . . It's the Dutchmen, Italians, Russians, Turks and Egyptians who smoke cigarettes and they're no good anyhow.[2,p.259]

By the turn of the century there was a preference for cigarettes with an aromatic component, that is, Turkish tobacco. A new cigarette in 1913 capitalized on the lure of the Near East while rejecting it in actuality. Camels were a blend of burley and bright with just a hint of Turkish tobacco—you had the camel and pyramid on the package, what more could you want? Besides, eliminating most of the imported tobacco made the price lower. Low price was combined with a big advertising campaign: "The Camels are coming. Tomorrow there'll be more CAMELS in town than in all of Asia and Africa combined." By 1918 Camels had 40% of the market and stayed in front until after World War II.

The year 1919 was marked by the first ad showing a woman smoking. To make the ad easier to accept, the woman was oriental looking and the ad was for Turkish-type cigarettes. King-size cigarettes appeared in 1939 in the form of Pall Mall, which became the number one seller. Filter cigarettes as filter cigarettes, not cigarettes that happen to have filters along with a mouthpiece, appeared in 1954 with Winston, which rapidly took over the market and continued to be number one until the mid-1970s. Filter cigarettes captured an increasing share of the market, and now represent over 90% of all U.S. cigarette sales.

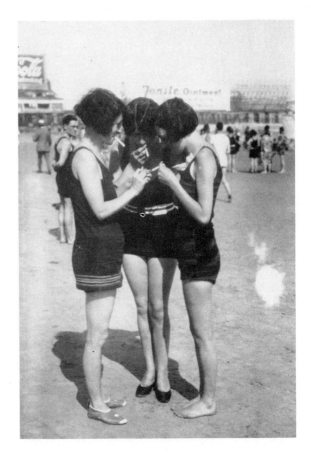

As women boldly began to show more skin, their smoking habits also went public.

CURRENT TOBACCO PRODUCTS
From Farm to Fag

Tobacco is grown on about 180,000 American farms, most with only a few acres devoted to tobacco. There's a lot of hand labor involved, requiring about 250 man-hours for each harvested acre (compared with about 3 man-hours per acre for wheat).[6] Tobacco seeds are started in seed beds and transplanted, 5000 to 10,000 plants an acre, when they are 6 to 8 inches high. In 2 to 3 months, when the tobacco is ready to harvest, the leaves will be 1 to 2½ feet long, and a typical **burley** tobacco plant will have 10 leaves. The nicotine content of a raw tobacco leaf ranges from 0.3% to 7% and varies with the variety, climatic conditions, fertilizer used, and many other factors.

Nicotine levels can be manipulated during processing to any desired level.

Burley is one of the major tobaccos used in cigarettes. It is harvested by cutting the stalk close to the ground, then hanging the entire stalk in a curing barn for 4 to 6 weeks. The plant uses its stored food, dies, and loses about 80% of its weight through moisture loss. This is "air-curing," the method used for most cigarette tobacco grown west of the Appalachians. East of the mountains "flue-curing" is used to produce **bright** tobacco. Tobacco that is to be flue-cured has the leaves separated from the stalks during harvesting, and heat is added to the curing barn so that the process is complete in less than a week.

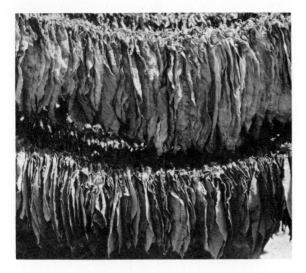

Before tobacco is sold for smoking it is "cured."

After curing, the burley leaves are removed from the stalk and sorted on the basis of color, size, and stalk position. Almost all tobacco is still sold at one of the 163 auction houses in this country. The farmer's hard work is well rewarded, with an average gross income of over $3,000 per acre (compared with less than $100 per acre for wheat). Overall tobacco is America's sixth largest legal cash crop.

When the tobacco reaches the buyer's processing plant, modern technology takes over. Here the tobacco leaves are shredded, dried, picked, blown clean of foreign matter and stems, remoisturized to a particular level, and packed in huge wooden barrels called *hogsheads*. The hogsheads are placed in storehouses, where the tobacco ages for 2 to 3 years.

Proper aging is one of the secrets to good tobacco. Aging allows fermentation to occur so that the tobacco gets darker and loses moisture, as well as nicotine (probably about one third of its original level) and other volatile substances. When the aging is complete, moisture is again added, and various types of tobacco are blended. During the blending process (top secret!), other substances are also added. Glycerine is used to stabilize the moisture content, and a variety of flavorants are

included. A 1972 publication by the Reynolds Tobacco Company listed 1290 flavorants that could be added to tobacco, including such common tastes as chocolate, licorice, and sugar. The blended material is compressed and then cut into hangnail-size strips to prepare it for the cigarette machine.

A century ago James Buchanan Duke thought his cigarette girls were doing very well if they could consistently roll four cigarettes a minute. In 1881 he started the cigarette revolution by using a machine that had just been patented. It produced 200 cigarettes a minute! He would love today's machine. It starts with a roll of cigarette paper 3½ miles long, makes a continuous clothesline-like tube filled with tobacco, cuts it to length, weighs the cigarette, rejecting those over or under the correct weight, and checks it for uniformity. It does everything but salute, and still turns out 3600 cigarettes a minute. Filter cigarettes are made by adding a machine that attaches a double-size filter between two cigarettes and then cuts them apart at the same rapid rate.

Toward a Less Hazardous Cigarette

The cigarette of the 1950s was quite different from the cigarette of the 1980s. For one thing, in the 1950s, it required 2¾ pounds of leaf tobacco to produce 1000 cigarettes. Now only about 1¾ pounds are required to produce the same number. Besides the addition of filters, two other technological changes have decreased the amount of leaf tobacco per cigarette. One is the use of reconstituted sheets of tobacco. Parts of the tobacco leaf and stems that had been discarded in earlier years are now ground up, combined with many added ingredients to control such factors as moisture, flavor, and color, and then rolled out as a flat, homogenized sheet of tobacco. After shredding, this material is combined with normally processed leaf tobacco. Today about 20% of all cigarette tobacco is reconstituted sheet.

The second development that reduced the need for tobacco in cigarettes is "fluffing." Tobacco is freeze dried, and an inert gas, such as Freon, is

Your turn: who buys tobacco?

Many young people begin smoking at the age of 12 or so; some boys begin using chewing tobacco at the age of 10 or 11, and it is clear that a significant fraction of teenagers smoke or chew regularly. Most states have laws preventing minors from purchasing tobacco, yet it appears that these laws are often not enforced. Is this the case in your community?

The first step in evaluating the situation would be to find out what the law actually is. It may be posted on cigarette machines or near sales locations in some states. Another source of information would be the library at a law school, if you are near one. Also, one could ask the police or the prosecuting attorney's office.

Then it would be interesting to get an estimate of the distribution of ages of tobacco purchasers. Post yourself near a machine in a public area or, if possible, near enough to a sales counter in a convenience store to see if tobacco is being purchased. Estimate as best you can the age and sex of every person you see who purchases tobacco. If you want to do this in a cooperative venture with some friends, you might observe several different types of sales outlets. By the way, be prepared to tell the store's proprietor what you're doing if asked, and then be prepared to leave the premises if asked.

used to expand the tobacco cells so that they take up more space and absorb more additives. One low-tar cigarette introduced in the early 1970s was able to reduce by 35% the tobacco in each cigarette because of its process to "fluff" the tobacco. Fluffing, of course, reduces the **tar, nicotine,** and **carbon monoxide** content of a cigarette, but it also reduces smoking time, perhaps by 15%.

For many years the Federal Trade Commission (FTC) measured the tar and nicotine content of cigarettes and published a listing of the results by brand name and type. These were measured by standardized smoking machines. The machine contained a filter, and the word tar refers to a complex mixture that remains on the filter after moisture and nicotine have been removed. As you might suspect, cigarettes with less tobacco have less tar and less nicotine, and measurements across brands found very high correlations between the two. Thus it is possible to speak of the tar and nicotine (T/N) content of a cigarette. The FTC has stopped this monitoring project because of its cost, and the industry's Tobacco Institute is now carrying out the analyses with FTC oversight.

Because of the previously mentioned changes in cigarette manufacturing, T/N levels declined regularly from the 1950s to the 1980s (Fig. 10-1). Low T/N cigarettes are associated with a lower health risk, and low T/N became a significant factor in advertising and in brand selection. However, there are a few things you should know about low T/N cigarettes. First is that the measurements are made by machine that smokes each cigarette in a standard manner (e.g., to within 3 mm of the filter "overwrap"). Manufacturers were able to reduce T/N content by manipulations such as using a longer overwrap or putting airholes around the filter. Smokers could and did smoke differently from the machine (for instance, covering some or all of the air holes while puffing), thus obtaining more tar and nicotine. It seems that smokers aim for a certain nicotine input, and when switched to a low T/N brand they take more puffs and inhale more deeply so as to largely compensate for the change in cigarettes.[7] Obviously, if a smoker compensates in this manner there might be little value in switching. Also, there is a limit to how low a T/N level the consumer will accept, as there is a decrease in satisfaction. At some point (about 8 mg tar and 0.3 mg nicotine) smokers begin to lose interest.

Trends in Smoking Behavior

The health warnings and the educational programs have certainly had an effect (Fig. 10-2). After World War II cigarette sales increased, both on a per capita basis and in total sales. The peak year for per capita sales was 1963. After that, the postwar baby boom generation began to influence the 18-and-over statistics because a large number of young people were less likely to have begun smoking. Also, in 1964 the Surgeon General's re-

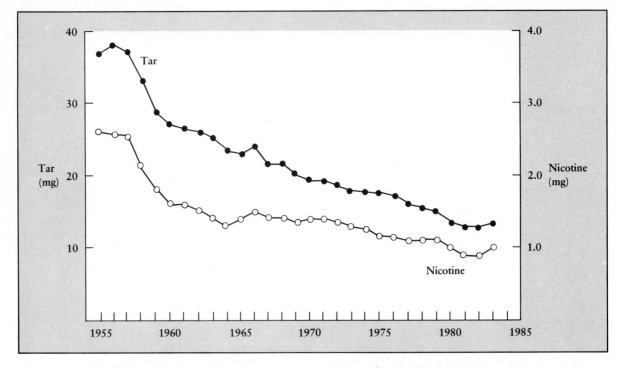

Figure 10-1. U.S. sales-weighted average tar and nicotine yields (all domestic brands on U.S. market). Data from Federal Trade Commission (last collected in 1983).

port on Smoking and Health declared that smoking is a health hazard. For the next several years per capita sales decreased, with a more rapid decrease after 1973. Because of the expanding adult population, total cigarette sales continued to climb slowly even while per capita sales dropped. This trend continued until 1981, when the peak was reached with sales of over 640 billion cigarettes. For the past several years both total and per capita sales have declined. In 1987, per capita sales were 3201 cigarettes, the lowest since World War II.

For many years a much greater percentage of adult men smoked than adult women. The 1970s saw an alarming increase in smoking among young females: for the first time, in 1976, more female than male high school seniors reported smoking (Fig. 10-3). Since then, fewer high school seniors of both sexes have been smoking, but the decrease has been greater among males than females, which has widened the females' lead.

Among adult smokers, males still slightly outnumber females, however, the trend is toward equality. Please note at this point that women are also moving toward equality with men in lung cancer, heart disease, and overall life expectancy.

Smokeless Tobacco

In the early 1970s many cigarette smokers apparently began to look for alternatives that would reduce the risk of lung cancer. Pipe and cigar smoking enjoyed a brief, small increase followed by a long period of decline. Sales of **smokeless** tobacco products, specifically, different kinds of chewing tobacco, began to increase. Once limited to western movies and the baseball field as far as public awareness was concerned, smokeless tobacco use has grown to the extent that it is now a matter of public concern.

The most common types of oral smokeless to-

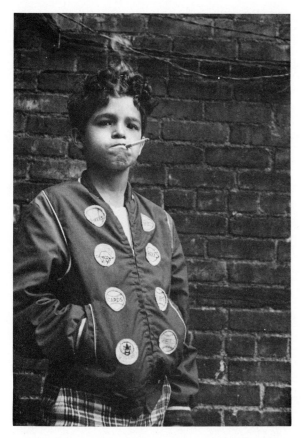

Would tougher laws or enforcement of laws against selling tobacco to minors prevent kids like this from getting cigarettes?

comes in a little teabag type of packet, so that loose tobacco fragments don't stray out onto the teeth. Moist snuff, which has its traditional popularity base in the rural west, continued to show large sales gains into the late 1980s. With all forms of oral smokeless tobacco, nicotine is absorbed through the mucous membranes of the mouth into the bloodstream, and users achieve blood nicotine levels comparable to those of smokers.

At the moment smokeless tobacco enjoys many competitive advantages over smoking. First, it is unlikely to cause lung cancer. Smokeless tobacco is much less expensive than cigarettes, with an average user spending only a couple of dollars a week. In spite of the Marlboro advertisements, a cowboy or anyone else who is working outdoors finds it more convenient to keep some tobacco in his mouth than to try to light cigarettes in the wind and then have ashes blowing in his face. And, believe it or not, chewing may be more socially acceptable than smoking under most circumstances. After all, the user doesn't blow smoke all around, and most people don't even notice when someone is chewing, unless the chewer has one of those huge wads in his mouth or spits frequently. Many users can control the amount of tobacco they put in their mouths so that they don't have to spit very often. What they do with the leftover **quid** of tobacco is a different story and often not a pretty sight.

Since the use of chewing tobacco had never completely died out in rural areas, its resurgence has been strongest there. It is primarily a male phenomenon, and surveys of high school students in Oregon, Colorado, and Louisiana have found 20% to 25% of the boys reporting smokeless tobacco use. In one survey of Wyoming junior high school students, about 25% of the boys reported being current users of smokeless tobacco, compared to only 1.2% of the girls. For the boys, the median reported age of first use was 11 years.[8] Although these studies indicate high rates of regional use, increased sales of smokeless tobacco are not limited to the rural west and south. Promoted by sports celebrities, increased advertising budgets, and sponsorship of auto racing, college

bacco in the United States are loose leaf (Red Man, Levi Garrett, Beech Nut), which is sold in a pouch, and **moist snuff** (Copenhagen, Skoal), which is sold in a can. When you see a baseball player on TV with a big wad in his cheek, it is probably composed of loose-leaf tobacco. Sales of loose leaf tobacco, growing from a traditional base in the southeast and midwest, increased by about 50% during the decade of the 1970s, and then remained stable or declined slightly through the 1980s. Moist snuff is not "snuffed" into the nose in the European manner; a small pinch is dipped out of the can and placed beside the gum, often behind the lower lip. One form of moist snuff also

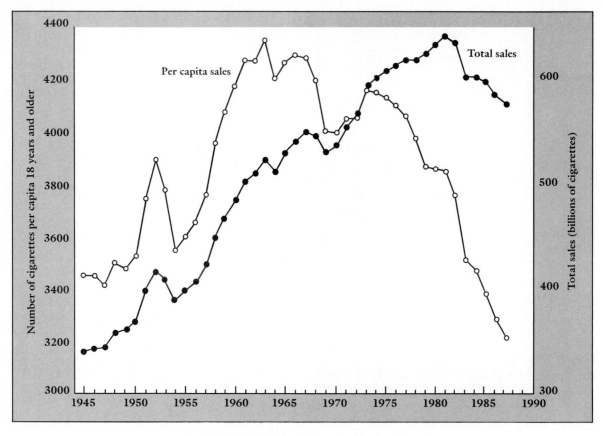

Figure 10-2. Trends in cigarette sales since 1945.

rodeo, and skiing, smokeless tobacco use appears to be increasing among young men in many parts of the country.

Some authors have actively promoted smokeless tobacco as a substitute for the more dangerous habit of cigarette smoking.[9] However, smokeless tobacco is not without its hazards. The one of most concern is the increased risk of cancer of the oral cavity, pharynx, and esophagus. In spite of the fact that snuff and chewing tobacco are not burned during use, they do contain potent carcinogens, including high levels of tobacco-specific **nitrosamines.** Many users experience tissue changes in the mouth, with **leukoplakia** (a whitening, thickening, and hardening of the tissue) a relatively frequent finding. Leukoplakia is considered

to be a precancerous lesion, that is, a tissue change that may develop into cancer. The irritation of the gums can cause them to become inflamed or to recede, exposing the teeth to disease. The enamel of the teeth may also be worn down by the abrasive action of the tobacco. In short, dentists are also becoming more aware of the destructive effects of oral tobacco.

Concerns about these oral diseases led to the Surgeon General's office sponsoring a conference and producing a report on that conference, "The Health Consequences of Using Smokeless Tobacco."[10] This report went into some depth in reviewing epidemiological, experimental, and clinical data, and concluded that ". . . the oral use of smokeless tobacco represents a significant health

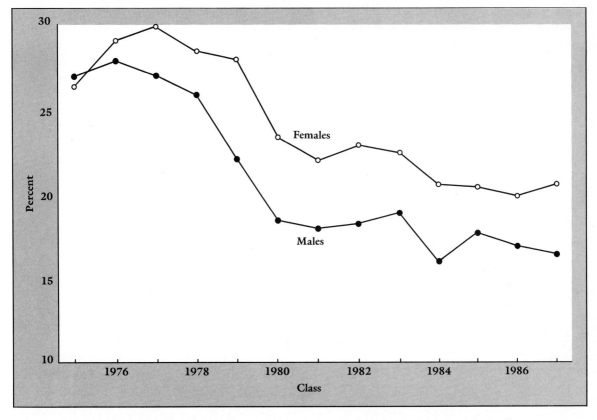

Figure 10-3. Percentage of high school seniors reporting daily use of cigarettes in the last 30 days: 1975-1987. Data from NIDA and University of Michigan's Institute for Social Research.

risk. It is not a safe substitute for smoking cigarettes. It can cause cancer and a number of noncancerous oral conditions and can lead to nicotine addiction and dependence." Packages of smokeless tobacco now carry a series of rotating warning labels describing these dangers.

Clove Cigarettes

In the 1980s young Americans discovered **kretek:** Indonesian clove cigarettes. In 1980, 12 million clove cigarettes were sold, mostly on the West Coast. By 1984 the market had grown to 150 million and spread across the country.[11] The cigarettes are expensive and aromatic. Many of the young users believe these cigarettes to be tobacco free and therefore safer than regular cigarettes. The fact is, these kretek contain 60% to 70% tobacco and generate more tar, nicotine, and carbon monoxide than standard American cigarettes.

Some users have had unusual lung reactions to the clove cigarettes, which researchers believe may be due to eugenol, the organic chemical that gives cloves their aroma. Eugenol tends to anesthetize the back of the throat, reducing the apparent harshness of the smoke and allowing deeper inhalation. However, the Centers for Disease Control recorded 10 severe illnesses and two deaths in a little over a year that were associated with the smoking of clove cigarettes. Fluid in the

That's Jake

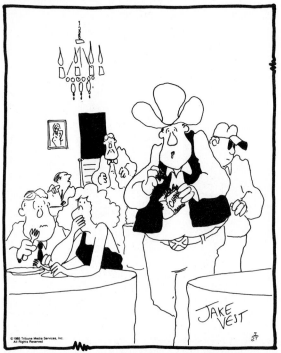

'The sign said this was the No Smoking section
but I can't find a sign of a spittoon.'

lungs, wheezing, and bloody phlegm have been
reported by users, along with the less serious
symptoms of shortness of breath, nausea, vomiting, and respiratory tract infections. New Mexico
was the first state to ban sales of clove cigarettes.

A SOCIAL AND ECONOMIC DILEMMA

It is now clear that cigarette smoking is deadly,
but acceptance of the facts may have been slowed
to some extent because tobacco, like alcohol and
other substances, has long been the subject of
emotional diatribes. In 1604 King James of England (the same one who had the Bible translated)
wrote and published a strong antitobacco pamphlet stating that tobacco was "harmefull to the
braine, dangerous to the lungs." Never one to let
morality or health concerns interfere with business, he also supported the growing of tobacco in

Virginia in 1610, and when the crop prospered,
he declared the tobacco trade a royal monopoly.

New York City made it illegal in 1908 for a
woman to use tobacco in public, and in the Roar-
ing Twenties women were expelled from schools
and dismissed from jobs for smoking. You must
appreciate that these concerns were partly for society and partly to protect women from themselves!

Smoking by women and even young girls must be
considered from a far different standpoint than smoking
by men, for not only is the female organism by virtue
of its much more frail structure and its more delicate
tissues much less able to resist the poisonous action of
tobacco than that of men, and thus, like many a delicate
flower, apt to fade and wither more quickly in consequence, but the fecundity of woman is greatly impaired
by it. . . . authorities cannot be expected to look on un-
moved while a generation of sterile women, rendered
incapable of fulfilling their sublime function of moth-
erhood, is being produced on account of the immod-
erate smoking of foolish young girls.[12,pp.39-40]

The effect of cigarette smoking on fertility could
not have been too great since in the 1930s the
antitobacco people said:

Fifty percent of our insanity is inherited from parents
who were users of tobacco. . . . Thirty-three percent of
insanity cases are caused direct from cigarette smoking
and the use of tobacco . . . .[13,p.97]

Those who have lived through the marijuana
era of the late 1960s and the 1970s have heard
similar statements. In 1931:

Judge Gimmill, of the court of Domestic Relations
of Chicago, declared that, without exception, every boy
appearing before him that had lost the faculty of blush-
ing was a cigarette fiend. The poison in cigarettes has
the same effect upon girls: it perverts the morals and
deadens the sense of shame and refinement . . . .

The bathing beaches have become resorts for women
smokers, where they go to show off with a cigarette in
their mouths. The bathing apparel in the last ten years
has been reduced from knee skirts to a thin tight-fitting
veil that scarcely covers two-thirds of their hips. Many
of the girl bathers never put their feet in the water, but
sit on the shore, show their legs and smoke cigarettes.[13,p.187]

Besides people's tendency to be suspicious of anticigarette claims, there are other potent forces that work to keep billions of cigarettes going up in smoke. Everyone knows that the tobacco industry has a lot of clout. It was tobacco that founded the English colonies and that funded the American revolution, but more significant is the continued economic importance of these products. Recent downturns in total sales have largely been offset by increased prices and reduced manufacturing costs, so that making and selling tobacco products is still a highly profitable business, with net income representing about 18% of sales.[14] It is perhaps not surprising that these companies were involved in some of the largest corporate mergers and leveraged buyouts of the 1980s.

A lot of people make their living, either directly or indirectly, from tobacco. Besides the farmers and manufacturers, there are about 2500 wholesalers. Tobacco products are sold in almost a million retail outlets, more than half of which are vending machines. Grocery stores sell more cigarettes than any other outlet, and recently sales in gasoline stations have been increasing while vending machine sales have dropped. Cigarette companies were the largest advertisers on television and radio until such ads were banned in 1971. Now they spend their advertising money on magazine and newspaper ads. It has been pointed out that most magazines need those revenues to survive, and they are therefore not likely to print many articles about the dangers of smoking.[15] After the American Medical Association's House of Delegates voted to oppose all advertising of tobacco products, the tobacco industry spent most of 1987 successfully lobbying against legislation that would have banned advertising of cigarettes in magazines and newspapers.

Governments, too, derive significant income from tobacco taxes. In 1987, the U.S. government received $4.8 billion, an amount that was equalled by the total state tobacco tax revenues. Also, at a time in which the trade deficit is of such concern, it is important to remember that the value of exports exceeded imports by over $2 billion. In all,

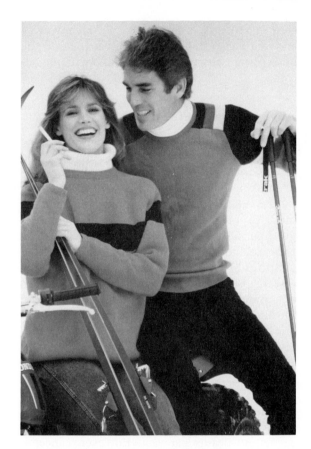

Some cigarette ads make an obvious effort to counter the unhealthy image of cigarette smoking.

the tobacco industry estimates that it directly generates over $40 billion of the gross national product and employs over 700,000 people.[16]

CAUSES FOR CONCERN

As early as 1939 a major authority on cancer stated that "the increase in the incidence of pulmonary carcinoma is due largely to the increase in cigarette smoking."[16]

Although the first clear scientific evidence linking smoking and lung cancer appeared in the 1950s, acceptance was slow. Each decade brought clearer evidence and more forceful warnings from the Surgeon General. By now it is abundantly clear that tobacco is America's true "killer weed," and is a bigger public health threat than all the other drug substances combined, including alcohol.

Adverse Health Effects

Each year the Public Health Service of the United States reviews the world scientific literature and reports to Congress on the health consequences of smoking.

The 1982 report focused on cancer in great detail.[17] In that report, considerable attention was given to nitrosamines, a type of chemical known to be carcinogenic. Four **tobacco-specific nitrosamines (TSNAs)** have been characterized, and research is going forward with those chemicals to determine how carcinogenic they are. The subject of the 1983 report was cardiovascular disease,[18] and the 1984 report covered **chronic obstructive lung diseases** (chronic bronchitis and **emphysema**).[19] If we add it all up it comes out like this: although lung cancer is not common, almost all lung cancers occur in smokers. Among deaths resulting from all types of cancer, smoking is estimated to be related to 30%, or about 129,000 premature deaths per year. However, cancer is only the second leading cause of death in the United States. It now appears that smoking may also be related to about 30% of deaths from the leading killer, coronary heart disease, or about 170,000 premature deaths per year. In addition, cigarette smoking is the cause of 80% to 90% of deaths resulting from chronic obstructive lung disease—another 62,000 cigarette-related premature deaths per year. The total from these three causes is over 360,000 per year in the United States. No wonder these reports keep saying that "cigarette smoking is the chief, single, avoidable cause of death in our society and the most important public health issue of our time."

It is important not to engage in overkill (a bad phrase in this context). Too much doomsaying may result in people just avoiding the facts. One final comment: think of anything related to good physical health; what the research says is that cig-arette smoking will impair it! The earlier the age at which you start smoking, the more smoking you do, the longer you do it—the greater the impairment (see Fig. 10-4). Smoking doesn't do any part of the body any good, at any time, under any conditions (Fig 10-5).

There is no bright side, but there is a less dark side. The 1981 report of the Surgeon General[20] focused on the low tar/nicotine cigarettes. The conclusions:

1. There is no such thing as safe smoking or a safe cigarette.
2. Smoking low T/N cigarettes reduces the risk of lung cancer and improves life expectancy—if you don't smoke more of the lower T/N cigarettes than you did of the higher T/N cigarettes.
3. No evidence yet exists about the effects of low T/N cigarettes on other diseases.
4. Additives may be a big health problem, particularly in the low T/N cigarettes.

Your best bet? Don't smoke. Save your money, save your health, and give yourself the gift of 7 years of life!

Passive Smoking

There has been a great deal said and written about **passive smoking,** that is, nonsmokers who inhale cigarette smoke from their environment. The importance of this issue can best be demonstrated by a couple of court cases. In 1976 the Superior Court of New Jersey ruled in favor of a Mrs. Shimp, a telephone company employee who was allergic to cigarette smoke and who worked in a small office along with some smokers. The judge's opinion established several principles:

The evidence is clear and overwhelming. Cigarette smoke contaminates and pollutes the air creating a health hazard not merely to the smoker but to all those around her who must rely upon the same air supply. The right of an individual to risk his or her own health does not include the right to jeopardize the health of those who must remain around him or her in order to properly perform the duties of their jobs. The portion of the population which is especially sensitive to ciga-

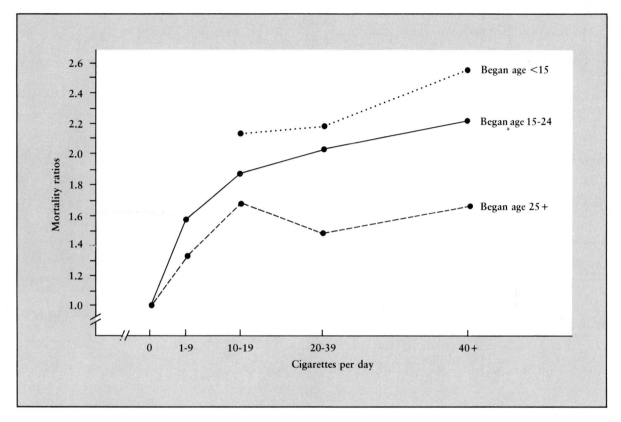

Figure 10-4. Mortality ratios (total deaths, mean ages, 55 to 64) as a function of the age at which smoking started and the number of cigarettes smoked per day.

rette smoke is so significant that it is reasonable to expect an employer to foresee health consequences and to impose upon him a duty to abate the hazard which causes the discomfort.

In determining the extent to which smoking must be restricted the rights and interests of smoking and nonsmoking employees alike must be considered. The employees' rights to a safe working environment makes it clear that smoking must be forbidden in the work area. The employee who desires to smoke on his own time, during coffee breaks and lunch hours should have a reasonably accessible area in which to smoke.[20]

On the other hand, a 1985 ruling prohibited the Wisconsin Revenue Department from implementing rules that completely forbid smoking in the workplace, even in smoking areas.[21] Cases are being heard all around the country, and it may be years before a workable set of rules is forged in the courts.

It is obvious that cigarette smoke can be irritating to others, but is it damaging? Besides the cases of individuals who have lung disorders or are allergic to smoke, is there evidence that cigarette smoke is harmful to exposed nonsmokers? Research is going forward, but it is complicated; the smoke rising from the ash of the cigarette **(sidestream smoke)** is higher in many carcinogens than is the mainstream smoke delivered to the smoker's lungs. Of course, it is also more diluted. How many smokers in the room? How much do they smoke? How good is the ventilation? These variables make definitive research dif-

SURGEON GENERAL'S WARNING: Smoking Causes Lung Cancer, Heart Disease, Emphysema, And May Complicate Pregnancy.

SURGEON GENERAL'S WARNING: Quitting Smoking Now Greatly Reduces Serious Risks to Your Health.

SURGEON GENERAL'S WARNING: Smoking By Pregnant Women May Result in Fetal Injury, Premature Birth, And Low Birth Weight.

SURGEON GENERAL'S WARNING: Cigarette Smoke Contains Carbon Monoxide.

Figure 10-5. Cigarette packages and advertisements are required to "rotate" among different warning labels.

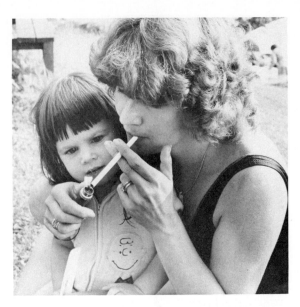

How damaging is this mother's cigarette smoking to her child's health?

ficult. The 1986 report, "The Health Consequences of Involuntary Smoking,"[22] tackled this complex issue, reviewing the available evidence in over 300 pages, and came to three main conclusions:

1. Involuntary smoking is a cause of disease, including lung cancer, in healthy nonsmokers.
2. The children of parents who smoke compared with the children of nonsmoking parents have an increased frequency of respiratory infections, increased respiratory symptoms, and slightly smaller rates of increase in lung function as the lung matures.
3. The simple separation of smokers and nonsmokers within the same air space may reduce, but does not eliminate, the exposure of nonsmokers to environmental tobacco smoke.

These concerns have led to many more restrictions on smoking in the workplace and in public. Several states and municipalities now have laws prohibiting smoking in public conveyances and requiring the establishing of smoking and non-smoking areas in public buildings and restaurants. A few employers have gone so far as to either encourage or attempt to force their employees to quit smoking both on the job and elsewhere, citing health statistics indicating more sick days and greater health insurance costs. This conflict between smoker and nonsmoker seems destined to get worse before it gets better. Although to some this battle may seem silly, it represents a very basic conflict between individual freedom and public health.

Smoking and Health in Other Countries

Cigarette smoking is a social and medical problem worldwide. The mid-1970s showed the start of many government programs to reduce smoking. This leads to interesting situations since in many countries cigarettes are a state monopoly (for example, France and Japan) and a source of great amounts of revenue. As sales level and decline in

Your turn: profit vs conscience

Try to place yourself in the position of a tobacco company executive. By now the evidence is overwhelming that cigarette smoking can be dangerous, and it is also clear that there will be increasing restrictions placed on advertising and on smoking in public areas. Tobacco taxes are high and could go higher, and it is likely that as per capita sales continue to decline, so will profits from tobacco sales. You have a social conscience and are concerned about the health issue, the farmers, the workers, and the tobacco dealers whose livelihood depends on tobacco, and you are of course concerned about the financial health of your company.

Looking ahead, how would you propose that the company proceed, given that it wants to be a good "corporate citizen" while continuing to make a profit? Assume that various changes may have to be phased in over a period of years.

Table 10-1

Governmental actions on smoking

1964	Surgeon General's report on smoking and health determines that cigarette smoking is a health hazard.
1966	Federal Cigarette Labeling and Advertising Act requires, as of January 1, cigarette packs to carry statement: CAUTION: CIGARETTE SMOKING MAY BE HAZARDOUS TO YOUR HEALTH.
1967	Federal Communications Commission rules that the "Fairness Doctrine" applies to cigarette advertising, and TV and radio must carry antismoking messages.
1970	Cigarette pack statement changed to WARNING: THE SURGEON GENERAL HAS DETERMINED THAT CIGARETTE SMOKING IS DANGEROUS TO YOUR HEALTH.
1971	Radio and TV ads banned as of January 2. Interstate Commerce Commission restricts smoking to rear five rows of interstate buses.
1972	All cigarette advertising must carry the same health warning as on packs, as well as the tar and nicotine content of a cigarette. The Consumer Product Safety Act specifically excludes cigarettes from being considered under the act.
1973	Arizona becomes first state to prohibit smoking in all elevators, indoor theaters, libraries, art galleries, museums, concert halls, and buses; all airlines required to designate smoking and no smoking areas in planes.
1978	Civil Aeronautics Board bans cigar and pipe smoking on all American commercial airlines.
1984	The Comprehensive Smoking Education Act requires that cigarette packages and adversising begin to carry new rotational label statements as of October 12, 1985.
1988	Smoking banned on U.S. commercial flights under 2 hours in duration.

developed countries, advertising and promotions in Third World countries ("the great taste of America") resulted in large increases in exports of American exports throughout the 1970s and 1980s. Asians in particular seem to want American cigarettes, and one of the major efforts has been to open Japanese, Taiwanese, and Korean cigarette markets to U.S. imports.[23] There are *no* warnings printed on the packs we sell to them! (Shades of patent medicines in the late nineteenth century.) Realize that these are mostly underdeveloped countries with lots of preventable disease and high infant mortality, and then listen to the World Health Organization: ". . . the control of cigarette smoking could do more to improve health and prolong life in these countries than any single action in the whole field of preventive medicine."[24]

Smoking and Pregnancy

The nicotine, hydrogen cyanide, and carbon monoxide in a smoking mother's blood also reach the developing fetus and have significant negative consequences there. On the average, babies born to smokers are about half a pound lighter than babies born to nonsmokers. This basic fact has been known for almost 30 years and has been

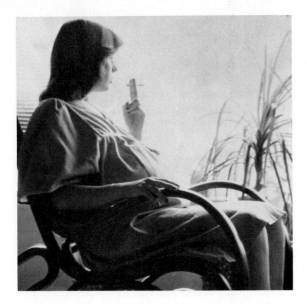

Smoking, especially during the last months of pregnancy, is likely to result in growth retardation in the fetus.

confirmed in almost 50 studies.[25] There is a dose-response relationship: the more the woman smokes during pregnancy, the greater the reduction in birth weight. Is the reduced birth weight the result of an increased frequency of premature births or of retarded growth of the fetus? Smoking shortens the gestation period by only an average of 2 days, and when gestation length is accounted for, the smokers still have smaller babies. Ultrasonic measurements taken at various intervals during pregnancy show smaller fetuses in smoking women for at least the last 2 months of pregnancy. The babies of smokers are normally proportioned, are shorter and smaller than the babies of nonsmokers, and have smaller head circumference. The reduced birth weight in smokers is not related to how much weight the mother gains during pregnancy, and the consensus is that reduced availability of oxygen is responsible for the diminished growth rate. Women who give up smoking early in pregnancy (by the fourth month) have babies of similar weight to those of nonsmokers.

Besides the developmental effects evident at birth, several studies indicate small but consistent differences in body size, neurological problems, reading and mathematical skills, and hyperactivity at various ages. It therefore appears that smoking during pregnancy may have long-lasting effects on both the intellectual and physical development of the child. Several studies have also found an increased risk of Sudden Infant Death Syndrome if the mother smokes, but it is not clear if this is related more to smoking during pregnancy or to passive smoking (the infant breathing smoke) after birth.

So far we have been talking about normal deliveries of babies. Spontaneous abortion (miscarriage) has also been studied many times in relation to smoking and with consistent results: smokers have more spontaneous abortions than nonsmokers (perhaps between 1.5 and 2 times as many). As far as congenital malformations are concerned, the evidence for a relationship to maternal smoking is not as clear. If there is a small effect here, it may be either related to or obscured by the fact that many smokers also drink alcohol and coffee. One study indicated an increased risk of facial malformations associated with smoking by the father. Neonatal death rates are higher among children of smoking mothers, and this effect is much greater among older women of low socioeconomic status who have had more than three pregnancies.

In addition to these demonstrated effects are the concerns about increased risk of childhood cancer, which has not yet been fully explored. The overall message is very, very clear. There are definite, serious risks associated with smoking during pregnancy. If a woman smoker discovers herself to be pregnant, that should be a clear signal to quit smoking.

PHARMACOLOGY OF NICOTINE

Nicotine is a naturally occurring liquid alkaloid that is colorless and volatile. On oxidation it turns brown and smells much like burning tobacco. Tolerance to its effects develops, along with the dependency that led Mark Twain to remark how easy it was to stop smoking—he'd done it several times!

Nicotine was isolated in 1828 and has been studied irregularly since then. It has no therapeutic actions, so no drug company has exhaustively looked at its effects. Since it has proved to be a valuable pharmacological tool for studying synaptic functions, as well as being the active ingredient in tobacco, there is some relevant information. The structure of nicotine is shown in Fig. 10-6; it should be noted that there are both *d* and *l* forms, but they are equipotent. It is of some importance that nicotine in smoke has two forms, one with a positive charge and one that is electrically neutral. The neutral form is more easily absorbed through the mucous membranes of the mouth, nose, and lungs.

Absorption and Metabolism

Inhalation is a very effective drug-delivery system, with 90% of inhaled nicotine being absorbed. The physiological effects of smoking one cigarette have been mimicked by injecting about 1 mg of nicotine intravenously.

Acting with almost as much speed as cyanide, nicotine is well established as one of the most toxic drugs known. In humans, 60 mg is a lethal dose, and death follows intake within a few minutes. A cigar contains enough nicotine for two lethal doses (who needs to take a second one?), but not all of the nicotine is delivered to the smoker or absorbed in a short enough period of time to kill a person.

Nicotine is primarily deactivated in the liver, with between 80% and 90% being modified before excretion through the kidneys. Part of the tolerance that develops to nicotine may result from the fact that either nicotine or the tars increase the activity of the liver microsomal enzymes which are responsible for the deactivation of drugs. These enzymes increase the rate of deactivation and thus decrease the clinical effects of the benzodiazepines and some antidepressants and analgesics. The final step in eliminating deac-

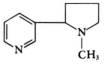

Figure 10-6. Nicotine (1-methyl-2-[3-pyridyl] pyrrolidine).

tivated nicotine from the body may be somewhat slowed by nicotine itself, since it acts on the hypothalamus to cause a release of the hormone that acts to reduce the loss of body fluids.

Physiological Effects

Nicotine.   The effect of nicotine on areas outside the CNS has been studied extensively. Nicotine mimics acetylcholine by acting at the nicotinic type of cholinergic receptor site and stimulating the dendrite. Nicotine is not rapidly deactivated, and continued occupation of the receptor prevents incoming impulses from having an effect, thereby blocking transmission of information at the synapse. Thus nicotine first stimulates and then blocks the synapse. This blockage of cholinergic synapses is responsible for some of its effects, but others seem to be the result of a second action.

Nicotine also causes a release of adrenaline from the adrenal glands as well as from other sympathetic sites and thus has in part a sympathomimetic action. An additional action that should be identified is that it stimulates and then blocks some sensory receptors, including the chemical receptors found in some large arteries and the thermal pain receptors found in the skin and tongue.

The symptoms of low-level nicotine poisoning are well known to beginning smokers and small children behind barns and in alleys: nausea, dizziness, and a general weakness. In acute poisoning, nicotine causes tremors that develop into convulsions, terminated frequently by death. The cause of death is suffocation resulting from paralysis of the muscles used in respiration. This paralysis stems from the blocking effect of nicotine on the cholinergic system that normally activates the muscles. With lower doses there is actually an increase in respiration rate because the nicotine stimulates oxygen-need receptors in the carotid artery. At these lower doses of 6 to 8 mg there is also a considerable effect on the cardiovascular system as a result of the release of adrenaline. Such release leads to an increase in coronary blood flow, along with vasoconstriction in the skin and increased heart rate and blood pressure. The increased heart rate and blood pressure increase the oxygen need of the heart but not the oxygen supply. Another action of nicotine with negative health effects is that it increases platelet adhesiveness, which increases the tendency to clotting.

Within the CNS, nicotine seems to act at the level of the cortex to increase somewhat the frequency of the electrical activity, that is, to shift the EEG toward an arousal pattern.

Smoking.   Many effects of nicotine are easily discernible in the smoking individual. The heat releases the nicotine from the tobacco into the smoke. Inhaling while smoking one cigarette has been shown to inhibit hunger contractions of the stomach for up to 1 hour. That finding, along with a very slight increase in blood sugar level and a deadening of the taste buds, may be the basis for a decrease in hunger after smoking.

In line with the last possibility, it has long been an old wive's tale that when a person stops smoking, he or she begins to nibble food and thus gains weight. In addition, there is evidence that smoking may increase metabolism rate, so that a weight gain upon quitting might be partially due to less energy utilization by the body. The very complex interactions between smoking, eating, and body weight have been reviewed by one of the major contributors to our understanding of smoking behavior.[26]

In a regular smoker, smoking results in a constriction of the blood vessels in the skin along with a decrease in skin temperature and an increase in blood pressure. The blood supply to the skeletal muscles does not change with smoking, but a routine finding in a regular smoker is a higher than normal amount of carboxyhemoglobin (up to 10% of all hemoglobin) in the blood. All smoke contains carbon monoxide, with cigarette smoke being about 1% carbon monoxide, pipe smoke, 2%, and cigar smoke, 6%. The carbon monoxide combines with the hemoglobin in the blood so that it can no longer carry oxygen. It is this effect of smoking, a decrease in oxygen-carrying ability of the blood, that probably explains the shortness of breath smokers experience when they exert themselves.

It is probable that the decrease in oxygen-carrying ability of the blood and the decrease in placental blood flow is related to the many results showing that pregnant women who smoke greatly endanger their unborn children.

Behavior Effects

In spite of all the protests and the cautionary statements you may read or hear, the evidence is overwhelming that nicotine is the primary, if not the only, reinforcing substance in tobacco. Monkeys will work very hard when their only reward consists of regular intravenous injections of nicotine. The more nicotine in a cigarette, the lower the level of smoking. Intravenous injections and oral administration of nicotine will decrease smoking under some conditions—but not all.

An ongoing debate—in smokers as well as researchers—is whether nicotine acts to arouse and activate the smoker or whether it calms and tranquilizes the drug user. One review of the literature pointed very nicely to the paradoxical effects of nicotine, ". . . a substantial number of studies have shown that nicotine increases heart rate, blood pressure, and numerous other indices of autonomic arousal; yet rather than producing expected increases of emotional behavior and feelings, it usually decreases emotions.[27,p.657]

Most people smoke in a fairly consistent way, averaging one to two puffs per minute, with each puff lasting about 2 seconds with a volume of 25 cc. This rate delivers to the individual about 1 to 2 μg/kg of nicotine with each puff. There must be something optimal or unique about this dose, since smokers could increase the dose by increasing the volume of smoke with each puff or puffing more often.

A study in cats suggested that this dose rate is optimal in causing a release of acetylcholine from the cortex and an increase in EEG activation. When cats were given 2 µg/kg of nicotine intravenously every 30 seconds, 70% of the animals showed EEG activation, more than with other tested doses or delivery times. The similarity of this nicotine dose and administration interval to the human self-selected dose and interval was intentional. Thus it may be that one of the rewards a smoker receives that keeps him smoking is cortical arousal and an alerting of functions.

Several recent British studies have shown that smokers are able to sustain their attention to a task requiring rapid processing of information from a computer screen much better if they are allowed to smoke before beginning the task. This could either be because the nicotine produces a beneficial effect on this performance or because when the smokers were not allowed to smoke they were suffering from some sort of withdrawal symptom. Subsequent experiments on both smokers and nonsmokers using an oral nicotine tablet established that nicotine improved performance in both groups, at least for a few minutes.[28]

Addiction to Nicotine

Evidence that nicotine is a reinforcing substance in nonhumans, and that most people who smoke want to stop and can't, and that when people do stop smoking they gain weight and exhibit other withdrawal signs, and that people who chew tobacco also have trouble stopping, all led by 1988 to a need for a thorough look at the addicting properties of nicotine. The 1988 Surgeon General's report provided it, in the form of a 600-page tome.[29] This had been a traditionally difficult subject: not that many years ago psychiatrists were arguing that smoking fulfilled unmet needs for oral gratification and therefore represented a personality defect. The tobacco industry still argues that smoking is simply a matter of personal choice

and that many people have been able to quit. As we should know by now, one can choose to try something but, while theoretically able to choose to stop, have a very difficult time doing so because of the potent reinforcing properties of the substance. That is the case with nicotine. The 1988 report reviewed nicotine pharmacology and tolerance in great detail, examined evidence for withdrawal and reinforcement, and came to some pretty strong conclusions:

1. Cigarettes and other forms of tobacco are addicting.
2. Nicotine is the drug in tobacco that causes addiction.
3. The pharmacologic and behavioral processes that determine tobacco addiction are similar to those that determine addiction to drugs such as heroin and cocaine.

Obviously this statement, while based on an exhaustive review of scientific data, is at one level a political message. It says to Congress and the American people that heroin and cocaine are not in some fundamental way more evil than tobacco. That message has met with some predictably negative reactions from the tobacco industry and from some tobacco-state politicians.

SMOKING—HOW NOT TO

When you're young and healthy it's difficult, if not impossible, to think about death, being chronically ill, or having emphysema so bad you can't get enough oxygen to walk across the room without having to stop to catch your breath. By the time you start to think and worry about those things it's difficult to change your health habits.

Think about these things. If you smoke about a pack a day you probably increase the probability of dying of lung cancer 1100%, of any other cancer 200%, of respiratory disease 400%, and of other causes 200%. Looked at another way: smoking two packs of cigarettes a day you decrease the remaining years of your life by 20% if you're 35, by 24% if you're 45, 29% at 55, and 35% at 65.[30]

Issue: smoker's face

In an article in the *British Medical Journal (December 1985, p. 1760)* Dr. Douglas Model reported that he was able to predict which patients did or did not smoke by looking at their faces. His criteria for "smoker's face" were the following: lines or wrinkles on the face, typically radiating at right angles from the upper and lower lips or corners of the eyes, deep lines on the cheeks, or numerous shallow lines on the cheeks and lower jaw; a subtle gauntness of the facial features with prominence of the underlying bone contours; a slightly pigmented grey appearance of the skin; and a florid, slightly orange, purple, and red complexion. Dr. Model detected what he considered to be smoker's face in 19 of 41 current smokers, three of 37 past smokers, and in none of the 38 nonsmokers in his sample—not perfect, but rather impressive statistically, given that he did not know the smoking history of these people and judged their faces from several feet away.

This report raises some interesting questions. Obviously judging smoker's face is not reliable enough to be used as a validation of self-reports of smoking. And it is clear that other factors such as age, race, exposure to sunlight, and general health will interact with smoking to alter a person's appearance. But why should some people who smoke have more wrinkles and either grey or florid skin? Is the gauntness related to the fact that smokers may be thinner than nonsmokers? Does the lower rate of smoker's face among past smokers indicate that the changes are reversible and if so, how long does it take? It might be interesting to see if you can learn to spot smoker's face, first by looking at the faces of people who are smokers and then by predicting that someone is a smoker and either asking or waiting to see if they light up.

A lot of people want to stop smoking. A lot of people have already stopped. Are there ways to efficiently and effectively help those individuals who want to stop smoking to stop? With any form of pleasurable drug use it is easier to keep people from starting to use the drug than it is to have them stop once they have started. All the educational programs have had an effect on our society and on our behavior. There are now over 40 million former smokers in the United States, and about 90% of them report that they quit smoking without formal treatment programs. There is some indication that those who quit on their own may do better than those who have been in a treatment program, but then those who quit on their own also tend not to have been smoking as much or for as long.

One reason it is so hard for people to stop is that a pack-a-day smoker puffs at least 50,000 times a year. That's a lot of individual nicotine "hits" reinforcing the smoking behavior. There are a variety of behavioral treatment approaches to assisting smokers who want to quit, and hundreds of research articles have been published on them. Although most of these programs are able to get almost everyone to quit for a few days, by 6

months 70% to 80% of them are smoking again. Some of the programs that combine multiple approaches seem to have better success, with up to 40% remaining abstinent for 1 year.[29,p.488]

If nicotine is the critical thing, why not provide nicotine without the tars and carbon monoxide? Chewing gum is now available by prescription containing 2 mg nicotine, and it has been shown to be a useful adjunct to smoking cessation programs. In 1984 and 1985, the first 2 years this gum was available, over 5 million prescriptions were written for it.[31] There is money to be made helping people quit smoking, especially if it could be done painlessly, with a substitute. One problem is that with gum the nicotine is absorbed slowly, whereas smoking delivers a rapid rise in blood nicotine levels. Other approaches under consideration include lozenges, nose drops, sprays, and a patch that can be applied directly to the skin. Also, there have been efforts to introduce smokeless cigarettes, as much for the convenience of a smoker who can't light up as an aid to cutting down or quitting. They have not been readily accepted by consumers, however.

Is there a nondrug program that can be recommended to others, or used on one's self? Yes and no. A review of programs and techniques, "Behavioral Treatment of Smoking Behavior,"[32] made two points that are relevant here: There is a lot of variability in the effect of a given program—some people do very well, some very poorly and if one program won't work for an individual, maybe another one will. Fact is, we don't know enough yet to place a smoker in a program that is best for him. If you want—that is, are *really* motivated—to stop smoking, keep trying programs; odds are you'll find one that works . . . eventually.

It *is* possible to stop and it's well worth the effort. After everything has been said, stopping smoking—or any other habit—depends on the motivation to stop, the conviction that it's possible to stop, and the availability of a substitute or an adequate reward for stopping. All the rehabilitation, therapy, behavior modification, and other procedures are just devices to make the process easier. But remember, if one technique doesn't work, try another, and another, and . . . .

Summary

Tobacco has been used in many forms throughout history, but in modern America cigarette smoking has been the most important form of tobacco use. A decreasing percentage of the American population is now smoking, and the cigarettes they do smoke have decreased in tar and nicotine content. Two areas of concern have been increased smoking among young women and the more recent use of smokeless tobacco by young men.

Smoking shortens an individual's life expectancy considerably, and cigarettes are associated with over 350,000 premature deaths each year in the United States. In addition, there are risks to the developing fetus if the mother smokes during pregnancy.

The reason people find it so difficult to stop smoking is a dependence on nicotine, which appears to have both relaxing and alerting properties. Nicotine gum is one approach that has been used to assist people who want to stop smoking.

REFERENCES

1. Stewart GG: A history of the medicinal use of tobacco, 1492-1860, Medical History 11:228-268, 1967.
2. Brooks JE: The mighty leaf, Boston, 1952, Little, Brown & Co.
3. Vaughn W: Quoted in Dunphy EB: Alcohol and tobacco amblyopia: a historical survey, American Journal of Ophthalmology 68:573, 1969.
4. Corti: A history of smoking, London, 1931, George G Harrap & Co. Ltd.
5. Heimann RK: Tobacco and Americans, New York, 1960, McGraw-Hill Book Co.
6. Tobacco industry profile, 1988, The Tobacco Institute, Washington, DC.
7. Russell MAH: Nicotine intake and its regulation by smokers. In Martin WR and others, editors: Tobacco smoking and nicotine: a neurobiological approach, New York, 1988, Plenum Press.
8. Gritz ER, Ksir C, and McCarthy, WJ: Smokeless tobacco use in the United States: present and future trends, Annals of Behavioral Medicine 7:2, 24-27, 1985.
9. Russell MAH and others: A new age for snuff? Lancet 1:474-475, March 1, 1980.
10. The health consequences of using smokeless tobacco: a report of the advisory committee to the Surgeon General, NIH publication no. 86-2874. Washington, DC, 1986, US Government Printing Office.
11. Beware those spicy cigarettes, Consumer Reports 50:641, 1985.
12. Lorand A: Life shortening habits and rejuvenation, Philadelphia, 1927, FA Davis Co.
13. Eaglin J: The CC cough-fin brand cigarettes, Cincinnati, 1931, Raisbeck & Co., Printers.
14. US Public Health Service Office on Smoking and Health: Smoking, tobacco and health: a fact book. Washington, DC, 1987, US Government Printing Office.
15. Okie S: The press and cigarette ads: smoke gets in their eyes, New York, 1987, HealthLink, National Center for Health Education.
16. Ochsner A: Comment at the International Cancer Congress of 1939, cited in news release of the American Cancer Society, December 1970.
17. The health consequences of smoking for cancer: a report of the Surgeon General, DHHS Publication No. (PHS) 82-50179. Washington, DC, 1982, US Government Printing Office.
18. The health consequences of smoking: cardiovascular disease: a report of the Surgeon General. DHHS Publication No. (PHS) 84-50204, Washington, DC, 1983, US Government Printing Office.
19. The health consequences of smoking: chronic obstructive lung disease: a report of the Surgeon General. DHHS Publication No. (PHS) 84-50205, Washington, DC, 1984, US Government Printing Office.

20. *Shimp v. New Jersey Bell Telephone Company,* Superior Court of New Jersey, Chancery Division, Salem County, Docket No. C-2904-75, filed December 22, 1976.

21. Smoker wins in Wisconsin, The Tobacco Observer 10(1):1, 1985.

22. The health consequences of involuntary smoking, a report of the Surgeon General, DHHS Publication (CDC) 87-8398. Washington, DC, 1987, US Government Printing Office.

23. Jain M: Foreign tobacco firms puffing way into Asian market. Associated Press newspaper report, January 17, 1988.

24. Broady JE: Personal health, New York Times, July 8, 1981, p. C18.

25. The health consequences of smoking for women: a report of the Surgeon General, Washington DC, 1981, US Government Printing Office.

26. Jarvik ME: Does smoking decrease eating and eating increase smoking? In Martin WR and others, editors: Tobacco smoking and nicotine: a neurobiological approach, New York, 1988, Plenum Press.

27. Gilbert OG: Paradoxical tranquilizing and emotion-reducing effects of nicotine, Psychological Bulletin 86(4): 643-662.

28. Wesnes K: Nicotine increases mental efficiency: but how? In Martin WR and others, editors: Tobacco smoking and nicotine: a neurobiological approach, New York, 1988, Plenum Press.

29. The health conseqeunces of smoking: nicotine addiction, a report of the Surgeon General, DHHS Publication No. (CDC)88-8406. Washington, DC, 1988, US Government Printing Office.

30. Rogot E: Smoking and life expectancy among U.S. veterans, Public Health Briefs, American Journal of Public Health 68(10):1023-1025, 1978.

31. Findlay WS: Nicotine gum triples chances to stop smoking, USA Today, November 5, 1985.

32. Glasgow RE and Bernstein DA: Behavioral treatment of smoking behavior. In Prokop CK and Bradley LA, editors: Medical Psychology, New York, 1981, Academic Press, Inc.

Chapter 11

Caffeine

OBJECTIVES

After reading this chapter, you should be able to:

Describe three plant sources and several other dietary and medical sources for caffeine and approximately how much caffeine is obtained from each.

Discuss the time course of caffeine's action in the body and the mechanism by which it acts.

Describe several physiological and behavioral effects of caffeine.

Explain the concerns that have been expressed about caffeinism and the potential toxicity of caffeine.

How many drugs can lay claim to divine intervention in their introduction to mankind? The **xanthines,** of which caffeine is the best known, have three such legends, and that fact alone tells you that this has been an important class of drugs throughout the ages. Caffeine is the psychoactive agent in coffee.

CAFFEINE CONTAINING PLANTS
Coffee

The legends surrounding the origin of coffee are at least geographically correct. The best concerns an Arabian goatherd named Kaldi who couldn't understand why his goats were bouncing around the hillside. One day he followed them up the mountain and ate some of the red berries the goats were munching. "The results were amazing. Kaldi became a happy goatherd. Whenever his goats danced he danced and whirled and leaped and rolled about on the ground." Kaldi took the first coffee trip! A holy man took in the scene, and "that night he danced with Kaldi and the goats." The legend continues with Mohammed telling the holy man to boil the berries in water and have the brothers in the monastery drink the liquid so they could keep awake and continue their prayers.[1]

Around 900 AD an Arabian medical book suggested that coffee was good for just about everything, including measles and reducing lust. Once something gets into the literature, it's very difficult to change people's minds; women in England argued against the use of coffee over 700 years later. They published a 1674 pamphlet titled "The Women's Petition Against Coffee, representing to public consideration the grand inconveniences accruing to their sex from the excessive use of the drying and enfeebling liquor." The women claimed men used too much coffee, and as a result the men were as "unfruitful as those *Desarts* whence that unhappy *Berry* is said to be brought." The women were *really* unhappy, and the pamphlet continued:

Our Countrymens pallates are become as *Fanatical* as their Brains; how else is't possible they should *Apostatize* from the good old primitive way of Ale-drinking, to run a *Whoreing* after such variety of distructive Foreign Liquors, to trifle away their time, scald their *Chops,* and spend their *Money,* all for a little *base, black, thick, nasty bitter stinking, nauseous* Puddle water. . . .[2]

Some men probably sat long hours in one of the many coffeehouses composing "The Men's Answer to the Women's Petition Against Coffee," which said in part:

Why must innocent COFFEE be the object of your Spleen? That harmless and healing Liquor, which Indulgent Providence first sent amongst us. . . . Tis not this incomparable fettle Brain that shortens Natures standard, or makes us less Active in the Sports of Venus, and we wonder you should take these Exceptions. . . .[2]

We can all rest easier today and discuss over a cup of coffee the fact that gradually became clear: there is no truth to the idea that coffee diminishes sexual excitability or reduces lust. It is doubtful that the Arabians believed it either, since the use of coffee spread throughout the Muslim world. In Mecca people spent so much time in coffeehouses that the use of coffee was outlawed, and all supplies of the coffee bean were burned. Prohibition rarely works, and coffee speakeasies began to open. Wiser heads prevailed, and the prohibition was lifted.

The middle of the seventeenth century saw the same play enacted but with a new cast of characters and a different locale. Coffeehouses began appearing in England (1650) and France (1671), and a new era began. Coffeehouses were all things to all people: a place to relax, to learn the news of the day, to seal bargains, to plot! This last possibility made Charles II of England so nervous that he outlawed coffeehouses, labeling them "hotbeds of seditious talk and slanderous attacks upon persons in high stations." King Charles was no more successful than the women. In only 11 days the ruling was withdrawn, and the coffeehouses developed into the "penny universities" of the early eighteenth century. For a penny a cup you could listen to and learn from most of the great literary and political figures of the period. Lloyds of London, the insurance house, started in Edward Lloyd's coffeehouse around 1700.

Across the channel, cheap wine made the need for another social drink less essential in France than in England. French coffeehouses made at least one contribution to Western culture, the cancan! French cabaret owners were not ready to turn the other cheek, and they fought back: one owner was able to persuade his cancan girls to perform without any bloomers! In spite of this, coffeehouses survived, and coffee consumption increased. In 1974 France was consuming almost 12 pounds of coffee per person per year.

Across the Atlantic, coffee drinking increased in the English colonies, although tea was still their thing. Cheaper and more available than coffee, tea had everything, including, beginning in 1765, a 3-pence-a-pound tax on its importation!

The British Act that taxed tea helped fan the fire that lit the musket that fired the shot heard around the world. That story is better told in connection with tea, but the final outcome was that to be a tea drinker was to be a Tory. Coffee became the new country's national drink.

Coffee use expanded as the West was won, and the amount consumed by each person showed steady increases. Some experts became worried about the tendency to "have another cup of coffee," although they believed they could explain it. One wrote:

The absolute coercion which is imposed on the Americans of the United States by the Prohibition Act with respect to alcohol has necessarily had the result of greatly increasing the use of other excitants and also narcotics. . . . The consumption of coffee has also developed in an undreamt-of manner. In 1919 929.2 million pounds were consumed and in 1920 as many as 1,360 million pounds. The consumption therefore increased from 9 to 12.9 pounds per head per year, and is approaching the threshold of abuse.[3,p.253]

Funny thing: prohibition went away, the coffee consumption continued to rise. We must have been well over the "threshold of abuse" in 1946 when coffee consumption reached an all-time high of 20 pounds per person. The trend has been downhill since then (although the population growth has blunted the impact of decreased use): the United States consumed 10 pounds of coffee per person in 1986.[4]

Some of the decrease can be attributed to changing life-styles—sun and fun and convenient canned drinks seem to fit together better and soft drinks seem to go with fast food. Table 11-1 shows the percentage of Americans over the age of 10 who drank different beverages on typical days from 1950 to 1985. The biggest changes are the drop in coffee use and the increase in soft drinks, so that more people are now choosing soft drinks than coffee.

If the national drink is not as national as it once was, neither is it as simple. Kaldi and his friends could just munch on the coffee beans or put them in hot water and be content. Somewhere in the dark past, probably when the warehouses were burned down, the Middle East discovered that roasting the green coffee bean did not ruin it but, in fact, improved the flavor, aroma, and color of the drink made from the bean. For years housewives, storekeepers, and coffeehouse owners bought the green bean, then roasted and ground it just before use. Commercial roasting started in 1790 in New York City, and the process gradually spread through the country. One problem is that, while the green bean can be

Table 11-1					
Consumption of beverages					
	1950 %	1962 %	1976 %	1981 %	1985 %
Coffee	75	75	59	56	55
Milk, milk drinks	51	53	50	50	47
Juices	33	41	44	48	46
Soft drinks	29	33	49	52	59
Tea	24	25	26	33	31

stored indefinitely, the roasted bean deteriorates seriously within a month. Ground coffee can be maintained at its peak level in the home only for a week or two, and then only if it is in a closed container and refrigerated. Vacuum packing of ground coffee was introduced in 1900, a process that maintains the quality until the seal is broken.

Coffee growing spread worldwide when the Dutch began cultivation in the East Indies in 1696. Latin America had an ideal climate for coffee growing, and with the world's greatest coffee-drinking nation just up the road several thousand miles, it became the world's largest producer. Different varieties of the coffee tree and different growing and processing conditions provide many opportunities for varying the characteristics of coffee.

No one really went commercial with a combination of different coffee beans until J.O. Cheek developed a blend in 1892 and introduced it through a famous Nashville hotel: Maxwell House. The coffee was so well received that the hotel owners let the coffee be named after the hotel.

In the early 1950s about 94% of American coffee was from Latin America, but that percentage has steadily declined; today less than half is grown in this hemisphere. Brazil is the principal exporter to the United States, with Colombia second. Both countries grow **arabica,** which has a caffeine content of about 1%. **Robusta,** with a caffeine level

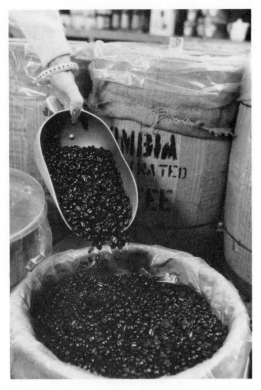

Americans buy their coffee in many forms. Some connoissuers prefer to buy the roasted beans in bulk and grind them just before brewing.

inexpensive African coffee beans to use in manufacturing instant coffee, since they believe that their coffee is too good to be used in that way.

Americans are drinking more decaffeinated coffee and less regular coffee, in keeping with the health-conscious style of the 1980s.[5] There are several ways of removing caffeine from the coffee bean. In the process used by most American companies, an organic solvent of some type is used, and there have been concerns about residues of the solvent that remain in the coffee. The most widely used solvent has been methylene chloride, but studies have shown that high doses of that solvent can cause cancer in laboratory mice. In 1985 the FDA banned the use of methylene chloride in hair sprays, which can be inhaled during use, but proposed to allow the solvent to be used in decaffeination as long as residues did not exceed 10 parts per million. Decaffeinated coffees contain considerably lower amounts than that, so the assumption is that the risk is minimal. The Swiss water process, which is not used on a large commercial scale in the United States, removes more of the coffee's flavor. By the way, the caffeine that is taken out of the coffee is used mostly in soft drinks. One of the largest decaffeinating companies is owned by Coca-Cola.

at 2%, is the variety grown in Africa and is usually of a lower grade and price.

The economics of coffee (it is number two in international trade, far behind oil) have as much to do with coffee consumption as does our changing life-style. A price increase in the early fifties—to a dollar a pound!—shifted us from a 40-cups-per-pound to a 60-cups-per-pound nation. This dilution reduced the cost but also the quality of the beverage. Two things happen when prices go up: the quality of the coffee decreases and people drink less coffee. Instant coffee has been around since before the turn of the century, but sales began their marked increase in the hustle and bustle following World War II: another decrease in the quality of the beverage, but an increase in the convenience. Interestingly, Brazil imports many

Tea

Tea and coffee are not like day and night, but their differences are reflected in the legends surrounding their origins. The bouncing goatherd of Arabia suggests that coffee is a boisterous, blue-collar drink. Tea is a different story: much softer, quieter, more delicate. According to one legend, Daruma, the founder of Zen Buddhism, fell asleep one day while meditating. Resolving that it would never happen again, he cut off both eyelids. From the spot where his eyelids touched the earth grew a new plant. From its leaves a brew could be made that would keep a person awake. Appropriately the tea tree, *Thea sinensis* (now classed as **Camellia sinensis**) is an evergreen, and *sinensis* is the Latin word for Chinese.

The first report of tea that seems reliable is in

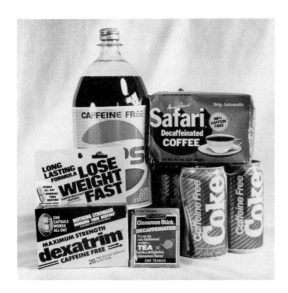

Caffeine-free has become a big selling point for health-conscious consumers in the 1980s, not only in decaffeinated coffee, but also in caffeine-free colas and herbal teas.

a Chinese manuscript around 350 AD when it was primarily seen as a medicinal plant. The nonmedical use of tea is suggested by a 780 AD book on the cultivation of tea, but the real proof that it was in wide use in China is that a tax was levied on it in the same year. Before this time Buddhist monks had carried the cultivation and use of tea to Japan.

Europe had to wait eight centuries to savor the herb that was "good for tumors or abscesses that come from the head, or for ailments of the bladder . . . it quenches thirst. It lessens the desire for sleep. It gladdens and cheers the heart." The first European record of tea, in 1559, says "One or two cups of this decoction taken on an empty stomach removes fever, headache, stomach-ache, pain in the side or in the joints. . . ." It was 50 years later in 1610 that the Dutch delivered the first tea to the continent of Europe.

An event occurred 10 years before that which had tremendous impact on the history of the world and on present patterns of drug use. In 1600 the English East India Company was formed, and

Queen Elizabeth gave the company a monopoly on everything from the east coast of Africa across the Pacific to the west coast of South America! In this period the primary imports from the Far East were spices, and the company prospered. A major conflict developed between the Dutch and English trade interests over who belonged where in the East. In 1623 a resolution "gave" the Dutch East India Company the islands (the Dutch East Indies), while the English East Indian Company had to be content with India and other countries on the continent!

The English East India Company concentrated on importing spices, so the first tea was brought to England by the Dutch. As the market for tea increased, the English East India Company expanded its imports of tea from China. Coffee had arrived first, so most tea was sold in coffeehouses. Even as tea's use as a popular social drink expanded in Europe, there were some prophets of doom. A 1635 publication by a physician claimed that, at the very least, using tea would speed the death of those over 40 years old. The use of tea was not slowed, though, and by 1657 tea was being sold to the public in England. This was no more than 10 years after the English had developed the present word for it: tea. Although spelled *tea*, it was pronounced *tāy* until the nineteenth century. Prior to this period the Chinese name *ch'a* had been used, anglicized to either *chia* or *chaw*.

With the patrons of taverns off at coffeehouses living it up with tea, coffee, and chocolate, tax revenues from alcoholic beverages declined. To offset this loss, coffeehouses were licensed, and a tax of 8 cents was levied on each gallon of tea and chocolate sold. To keep the profits from the expanding tea trade at home, Britain banned Dutch imports of tea in 1669, which gave the English East India Company a monopoly. Profit from the China tea trade colonized India, brought about the Opium Wars between China and Britain, and induced the English to switch from coffee to tea. In the last half of the eighteenth century, the East India Company carried out a "Drink Tea" campaign unlike anything ever seen before that time. Advertising, patriotism, low cost on tea, and high taxes on alcohol made Britain a nation of tea drinkers.

It was the same profit motive that led to the American Revolution. Because the English East India Company had a monopoly on importing tea to England and thence to the American colonies, the British government imposed high duties on tea when it was taken from warehouses and offered for sale. But, as frequently happens, when taxes went up, consumption did not go down, but smuggling increased. It reached the point in Britain where more smuggled tea than legal tea was being consumed. The American colonies, though, ever loyal to the king, were becoming big tea drinkers, which helped the king and the East India Company stay solvent. The Stamp Act in 1765, which included a tax on tea, changed everything. Even though the Stamp Act was repealed in 1766, it was replaced by the Trade and Revenue Act of 1767, which did the same thing.

These measures made the colonists unhappy over paying taxes they had not helped formulate (taxation without representation), and in 1767 this resulted in a general boycott on the consumption of English tea. Coffee use increased, but the primary increase was in the smuggling of tea. The drop in legal tea sales filled the tea warehouses and put the East India Company in financial trouble. To save the company, in 1773 Parliament gave the East India Company the right to sell tea in the American colonies without paying the tea taxes. The company was also allowed to sell the tea through its own agents, and this would eliminate the profits of the merchants in the colonies.

Several boatloads of this tea, which would be sold cheaper than any before, sailed toward different ports in the colonies. The American merchants would not have made any profit on this tea, and they were the primary ones who rebelled at the cheap tea. Some ships were just turned away from port, but the beginning of the end came with the 342 chests of tea that turned the Boston harbor into a teapot on the night of December 16, 1773.

The revolution in America and the colonists' rejection of tea helped tea sales in Great Britain, since to be a tea drinker was to be loyal to the Crown. Many factors contributed to change the English from coffee to tea drinkers, and the preference for tea persists today. Although their use of coffee increases yearly and that of tea declines, the English are still tea drinkers. In 1981 the per capita consumption in the United Kingdom was 8 pounds of tea, second in the world only to Ireland. Oddly enough, over 80% of the coffee sold in the United Kingdom is instant coffee. In 1984 Americans averaged about 7/10 of a pound of tea (enough for 140 cups); this has remained fairly constant for several years.

From plant to pot. Most of the tea (about 70%) that comes to America starts life on a 4- to 5-foot bush high in the mountains of Sri Lanka (Ceylon), India, or Indonesia. Unpruned, the bush would grow into a 15- to 30-foot tree, which would be difficult to pluck, as picking tea leaves is called. The pluckers select only the bud-leaf and the first two leaves at each new growth; these are the "tiny little tea leaves." The bud-leaf is called flowering orange pekoe, the second leaf is larger and called orange pekoe, and the third and largest is pekoe (pekoe is pronounced "peck-ho," *not* "peak-o"). Orange pekoe is not a variety of tea but rather a size and quality of tea leaf, since generally the bud-leaf is of the highest quality and the third leaf of lowest quality.

In one day a plucker will pluck enough leaves to make 10 pounds of tea in the grocery store. Plucking is done every 6 to 10 days in warm weather as new growth develops on the many branches. The leaves are dried, rolled to crush the cells in the leaf, and placed in a cool, damp place for fermentation (oxidation) to occur. This oxidation turns the green leaves to a bright copper color. Nonoxidized leaves are packaged and sold as green tea, the type used in Chinese restaurants in this country. Oxidized tea is called black tea and accounts for about 98% of the tea Americans consume. Oolong tea is greenish-brown, since it consists of partially oxidized, fermented leaves.

The Tea Importation Act of 1897 was designed to set minimum standards of quality in the tea

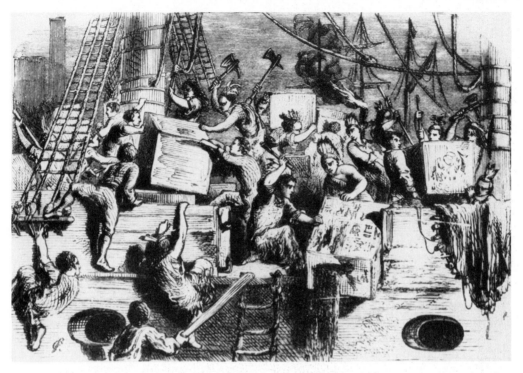

The famous "Boston Tea Party" was a reaction by American merchants to the English Parliament's special concessions to the East India Company.

that could be sold in the United States. This may have been the earliest of the consumer protection laws. The 1897 Act required that samples be taken of each tea shipment, and only those that exceeded a certain minimum quality could be released for sale.

How do you determine the quality of a tea? Right, you taste it. The FDA has three official tasters, one each in New York, San Francisco, and Boston, and they brew many cups of tea a day from samples taken from arriving shipments. The mixture is composed of 5 ounces of boiling water and ¼ ounce of tea, which they slurp from (you guessed it) a teaspoon. After swirling it in the mouth, they spit it out and go on to the next cup. The taste test tells the taster if the tea meets minimum taste standards that are established each year in February. Separate standards for each of the seven types of tea are now recognized by the

FDA. Tastes in tea change, as does the way in which people like to take their tea.[6]

Until 1904 the only choices available were sugar, cream, and lemon with your hot tea. At the Louisiana Purchase Exposition in St. Louis in 1904, iced tea was sold for the first time. It now accounts for 75% of all tea consumed in America. Tea lovers found 1904 a very good year. Fifteen hundred miles east of the fair, a New York City tea merchant decided to send out his samples in hand-sewn silk bags rather than tin containers. Back came the orders—send us tea, and send it in the same little bags you used to send the samples. From that inauspicious beginning evolved the modern tea bag machinery that cuts the filter paper, weighs the tea, and attaches the tag: all this at a rate of 150 to 180 tea bags per minute.

Pound for pound, loose black tea actually contains a greater concentration of caffeine than coffee beans. However, because about 200 cups of tea can be made from each pound of dry tea leaves, compared to 50 or 60 cups of coffee per pound, a typical cup of tea has less caffeine than a typical cup of coffee. The caffeine content of teas varies widely, depending upon brand and the strength of the brew. Most instant teas have 50 to 60 mg of caffeine per cup; Table 11-2 describes the caffeine content of several types of tea bag teas.[7]

Most tea is sold in tea bags these days, and the market has been flooded with a variety of tea products. Instant teas, some containing flavorings and sweeteners, are popular for convenience. Flavored teas, which contain mint or spices or other substances along with tea, offer other options. The biggest boom in recent years has been in so-called herbal teas, which mostly contain no "tea" at all. These teas are made up of mixtures of other plant leaves and flowers for both flavor and color, and have become quite popular among people who avoid caffeine.

It can only gladden and cheer the hearts of real tea drinkers to know that the largest seller of tea in America is a company named after a man, born in Scotland of Irish parents, who emigrated to America, became rich and famous in England, and believed in ships with sails right up to the end: Sir Thomas Lipton (1850-1931).

Although tea contains another chemical that derived its name from the tea plant, theophylline ("divine leaf") is present only in very small, nonpharmacological amounts in the beverage. Theophylline is very effective at relaxing the bronchial passages, and is widely prescribed for use by asthmatics.

Chocolate

Long before Columbus landed on San Salvador, Quetzalcoatl, Aztec god of the air, gave man a gift from paradise: the chocolate tree. Linnaeus was to remember this legend when he named the cocoa tree **Theobroma,** food of the gods. The Aztecs treated it as such, and the cacao bean was an important part of their economy, with the cacao bush being cultivated widely. Montezuma, em-

Table 11-2

Caffeine content (mg) in tea (strength established by color comparison)

Brand	Weak	Medium	Strong
Red Rose	45	62	90
Salada	25	60	78
Lipton	25	53	70
Tetley	18	48	70
Twining's English Breakfast	26	78	107

peror of Mexico in the early sixteenth century, is said to have consumed nothing other than 50 goblets of chocolatl every day. The chocolatl (from the Mayan words *choco* [warm] and *latl* [beverage]) was flavored with vanilla but was far from the chocolate of today. It was a thick liquid like honey that was sometimes frothy and had to be eaten with a spoon. The major difference was that it was bitter; the Aztecs didn't know about sugar cane.

Cortez introduced sugarcane plantations to Mexico in the early 1520s and supported the continued cultivation of the *Theobroma cacao* bush. When he returned to Spain in 1528, Cortez carried with him cakes of processed cocoa. The cakes were eaten, as well as being ground up and mixed with water for a drink. Although chocolate was introduced to Europe almost a century before coffee and tea, its use spread very slowly. Primarily this was because the Spanish kept the method of preparing chocolate from the cacao bean a secret until the early seventeenth century. When knowledge of the technique spread, so did the use of chocolate.

During the seventeenth century chocolate drinking reached all parts of Europe, primarily among the wealthy. Maria Theresa, wife of France's Louis XIV, had a "thing" about chocolate, and this furthered its use among the wealthy and fashionable. Gradually it became more of a social drink, and by the 1650s chocolate houses were open in England, although usually the sale of chocolate was added to that of coffee and tea in the established coffeehouses.

In the early eighteenth century there were health warnings against the use of chocolate in England, but use expanded. Its use and importance is well reflected in a 1783 proposal in Congress that the United States raise revenue by taxing chocolate as well as coffee, tea, liquor, sugar, molasses, and pepper.

Although the cultivation of chocolate never became a matter to fight over, it too has spread around the world. The New World plantations were almost destroyed by disease at the beginning of the eighteenth century, but cultivation had already begun in Asia, and today a large part of the crop comes from Africa.

Until 1828 all chocolate sold was a relatively undigestible substance obtained by grinding the cacao kernels after processing. The preparation had become more refined over the years, but it still followed the Aztec procedure of letting the pods dry in the sun, then roasting them before removing the husks to get to the kernel of the plant. The result of grinding the kernels is a thick liquid called chocolate liquor. This is baking chocolate. In 1828 a Dutch patent was issued for the manufacture of "chocolate powder" by removing about two thirds of the fat from the chocolate liquor. The chocolate powder was the forerunner of today's breakfast cocoa.

The fat that was removed, cocoa butter, became important when someone found that if it was mixed with sugar and some of the chocolate powder, it could easily be formed into slabs or bars. In 1847 the first chocolate bars appeared, but it was not until 1876 that the Swiss made their contribution to the chocolate industry by inventing milk chocolate, which was first sold under the Nestlé label. By FDA standards, milk chocolate today must contain at least 12% milk solids, although better grades contain almost twice that amount.

If we are to have cigarettes without tobacco and coffee without caffeine, does it surprise you that you may be eating chocolate without chocolate?

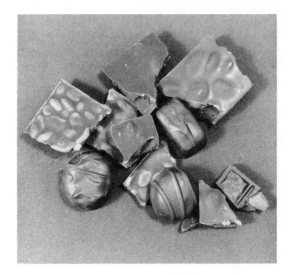

Chocolate candy contains only a small amount of caffeine.

The "true taste of chocolate made entirely without chocolate" is only the beginning. Check your next Valentine's Day box of chocolates, and you may find you have also bought a variety of artificial flavors, antioxidants (to increase shelf life), and stabilizers.

When chocolate turns white, it may still be all right to eat, but it is probably old, since the white color comes from the separation of the cocoa butter. Someday when you have the time, you can check on whether your piece of chocolate is all chocolate and properly manufactured. Put it on your tongue: it should melt at body temperature. But be careful! One chocolate lover has said, "Each of us has known such moments of orgastic anticipation, our senses focused at their finest, when control is irrevocably abandoned. Then the tongue possesses, is possessed by, what it most desires; the warm, liquid melting of thick, dark chocolate."[8]

The active ingredient in chocolate is **theobromine.** It has physiological actions that closely parallel those of caffeine but is much less potent in its effects on the central nervous system. The average cup of cocoa contains about 4 mg of caffeine

Table 11-3

Caffeine in beverages and foods

Item	Caffeine (mg) Average	Range
Coffee (5 oz cup)		
Brewed, drip method	115	60-180
Brewed, percolater	80	40-170
Instant	65	30-120
Decaffeinated, brewed	3	2-5
Decaffeinated, instant	2	1-5
Tea (5 oz cup)		
Brewed, major U.S. brands	40	20-90
Brewed, imported brands	60	25-110
Instant	30	25-50
Iced (12 oz glass)	70	67-76
Cocoa beverage (5 oz cup)	4	2-20
Chocolate milk beverage (8 oz glass)	5	2-7
Milk chocolate (1 oz)	6	1-15
Dark chocolate, semi-sweet (1 oz)	20	5-35
Baker's chocolate (1 oz)	26	26
Chocolate flavored syrup (1 oz)	4	4

Your turn: caffeine in soft drinks

What sorts of regulations, if any, should govern the inclusion of caffeine in soft drinks? Remember that some very young children currently obtain considerable doses of caffeine from these drinks. The maximum amount found in a 12-ounce can has crept up from around 45 mg in the mid-1970s to almost 60 mg. There is no requirement that the caffeine content be printed on the label, and products can and do change their caffeine content from time to time.

Taking into account the concerns of parents, consumers, and producers, as well as the objective evidence for potential problems associated with caffeine, propose a regulatory change that would be fair and effective.

---

but over 200 mg of theobromine. Table 11-3 compares the caffeine contents of various forms of coffee, tea, and chocolate.

OTHER SOURCES OF CAFFEINE
Soft Drinks

Since the beginning and early history of cola drinks is not shrouded in the mists that veil the origins of the other xanthine drinks, there is no problem in selecting the correct legend. And that's what the story of Coca-Cola is: a true legend in our time. From a green nerve tonic in 1886 in Atlanta, Georgia, that did not sell well at all, Coca-Cola has grown into . . . but you *know* what it is—everyone does everywhere! Unbelievable, it must be "the real thing" and provide "the pause that refreshes," or else it couldn't sell over 1.5 billion cases a year worldwide. And that includes mainland China where it's called "Ke Koy Ke Le"—which translated means "tasty happiness."[9] Yes, Coke is it!

Dr. J.C. Pemberton's tonic contained caramel, fruit flavoring, phosphoric acid, caffeine, and a secret mixture called Merchandise No. 5. A friend, F.M. Robinson, suggested the name by which it is still known: Coca-Cola. The unique character of Coca-Cola and its later imitators is a blend of fruit flavors that makes it impossible to identify any of its parts.

An early ad for Coca-Cola suggests its varied uses:

The "INTELLECTUAL BEVERAGE" and TEMPERANCE DRINK contains the valuable TONIC and NERVE STIMULANT properties of the Coca plant and Cola (or Kola) nuts, and makes not only a delicious, exhilarating, refreshing and invigorating Beverage, (dispensed from the soda water fountain or in other carbonated

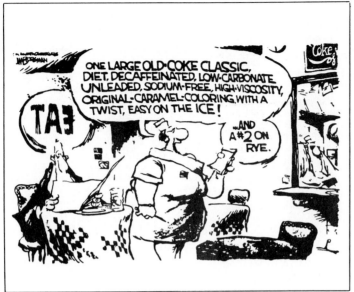

Reprinted with special permission of King Features Syndicate, Inc.

Soft-drink manufacturers each offer a wide variety of products these days to take advantage of every corner of the market.

beverages), but a valuable Brain Tonic, and a cure for all nervous affections—SICK HEADACHE, NEURALGIA, HYSTERIA, MELANCHOLY, &c.[10,p.138]

Coca-Cola was touted as "the new and popular fountain drink, containing the tonic properties of the wonderful coca plant and the famous cola nut." You must remember that this was the period of Sherlock Holmes, Sigmund Freud, and patent medicine—all saying very good things about the product of the coca plant: cocaine. The company admitted to small amounts of cocaine in its beverage in 1903, but a government analysis of Coca-Cola in 1906 did not find any.

The name Coca-Cola was originally conceived to indicate the nature of its two ingredients with tonic properties. The suggeston of the presence of extracts of coca leaves and cola (kola) nuts in the beverage was supposed to be furthered by the use on each bottle of a pictorial representation of the leaves and nuts. Unfortunately the artist-glass blower didn't know that the coca and cacao plants were different, so the bottle had kola leaves and cacao pods! In 1909 the FDA seized a supply of Coca-Cola syrup and made two charges against the company. One was that it was misbranded because it contained "no coca and little if any cola" and second, that it contained an added poisonous ingredient, caffeine.

Before the 1911 trial in Chattanooga, Tennessee, the company paid for some research into the physiological effect of caffeine, and when all the information was in, the company won, and the government appealed the decision. In 1916 the Supreme Court of the United States upheld the lower court by rejecting the charge of misbranding, stating that the company has repeatedly said that "certain extracts from the leaves of the coca shrub and the nut kernels of the cola tree were used for the purpose of obtaining a flavor" and that "the ingredients containing these extracts" with the cocaine eliminated is called Merchandise No. 5. The way this is done today is that coca leaves are imported by a pharmaceutical company in New Jersey. The cocaine is extracted for medical use and the decocainized leaves are shipped to the Coca-Cola plant in Atlanta, Georgia, where Merchanidse No. 5 is produced. A 1931 report indicated that Merchandise No. 5 contained an extract of three parts coca leaves and one part cola nuts, but to this day it remains a secret formula.

Then there was the problem of the caffeine:

. . . it is clear that the only queston arising under section 7 is whether the caffeine in the Coca Cola is an "added poisonous or other added deleterious ingredient which may render such article injurious to health.". . .[11]

The question of whether caffeine was an "added poisonous ingredient" was not so readily resolved. Caffeine was added, but it was an essential part of the Coca-Cola formula. In that respect it was not added above and beyond the essential ingredients; it was one of them. The Supreme Court said that the lower courts should decide if the caffeine made the drink injurious to health.[11] At that time the company substantially reduced the amount of caffeine in its syrup, and the government never felt it had a case worth pursuing beyond that point.

In 1981 the FDA changed its rules so that a "cola" no longer has to contain caffeine. If it does contain caffeine it may not be more than 0.02%, which is 0.2 mg/ml, or a little less than 6 mg per ounce. There are some consumer and scientist groups that believe that all cola manufacturers should indicate on the label the amount of caffeine the beverage contains. This is in keeping with the trend toward providing more information to the consumer and seems highly probable. The same labeling would probably also be required of coffee, tea, and chocolate, although in these beverages the caffeine is not an added ingredient.

Table 11-4 lists some popular soft drinks along with their caffeine content in a 12-ounce serving. Diet soft drinks, now mostly sweetened with aspartame, and caffeine-free colas are commanding a larger share of the market, but regular colas are still the single most popular type of soft drink. As

---

> **Your turn: how much caffeine do you use?**
>
> How many different products do you use that contain caffeine (see Tables 11-3 to 11-5)? Keep a complete record of your own intake of coffee, tea, soft drinks, and so on for a typical 3-day period (72 hours). From that record, estimate as closely as you can your total caffeine intake in milligrams. Then compare that figure with the averages reported in the 1985 *New England Journal of Medicine* (see Table 11-6).

---

with beers and some other products, the modern marketing strategy seems to be for each company to try to offer products of every type, so as to cover the market. We saw earlier that soft drinks have become increasingly popular. In 1985, per capita soft drink consumption was 45 gallons, up from 14 in 1960 and 24 in 1970.

Over-the-Counter Drugs

Few people realize that, in addition to the caffeine contained in beverages, many nonprescription drugs also include caffeine, some in quite large amounts. Table 11-5 lists the caffeine content of some of these drugs. Presumably many people who buy "alertness tablets" such as No Doz are aware that they are buying caffeine. But many buyers of such things as Excedrin may not realize how much caffeine they are getting. Imagine the condition of someone who took a nonprescription water-loss pill, a headache tablet, and a cold tablet all containing caffeine, and who then drank a couple of cups of coffee!

A 1985 report[12] described a study in which 400 men and women were asked to report on their consumption over a 3-day period of all foods, beverages, and medications that might contain caffeine. Only 11 of the 400 did not take in any caffeine at all, and the total intake averaged around 400 mg per day. The sources of this intake in both men and women are reported in Table 11-6.

Table 11-4	
Caffeine in popular soft drinks	
Brand	**Caffeine* (mg)**
Sugar-Free Mr. Pibb	58.8
Moutain Dew	54.0
Mello Yello	52.8
Tab	46.8
Coca-Cola	45.6
Diet Coke	45.6
Shasta Cola	44.4
Mr. Pibb	40.8
Dr. Pepper	39.6
Big Red	38.4
Pepsi-Cola	38.4
Diet Pepsi	36.0
Pepsi Light	36.0
RC Cola	36.0
Diet Rite	36.0
Canada Dry Jamica Cola	30.0
Canada Dry Diet Cola	1.2

*Per 12-ounce serving.

Table 11-5	
Caffeine content of OTC drugs	
Drug	**Caffeine (mg)**
Stimulants	
No Doz	100
Vivarin	200
Analgesics	
Anacin	32
Excedrin	65
Goody's Headache Powders	32.5
Midol	32.4
Vanquish	33
Cold remedies	
Coryban-D	30
Triaminicin	30
Diuretics	
Aqua-Ban	100
Maximum-strength Aqua-Ban plus	200

CAFFEINE PHARMACOLOGY

Xanthines are the oldest stimulants known. Xanthine is a Greek word meaning yellow, the color of the residue if the xanthines are heated with nitric acid until dry. The three xanthines of primary importance are caffeine, theophylline, and theobromine.

These three chemicals are methylated xanthines and are closely related alkaloids, as can be seen in Fig. 11-1. Most alkaloids are insoluble in water, but these are unique, since they are slightly water soluble.

These xanthines have similar effects on the body, with caffeine having the greatest and theobromine almost no stimulant effect on the central nervous system and the skeletal muscles. Theophylline is the most potent, and caffeine the least potent, agent on the cardiovascular system. Caffeine, so named because it was isolated from coffee in 1820, has been the most extensively studied and, unless otherwise indicated, is the drug under discussion here.

Time Course

In humans absorption of caffeine is rapid after oral intake; peak blood levels are reached 30 minutes after ingestion. Although maximal CNS effects are not reached for about 2 hours, the onset of effects may begin within half an hour after intake. The half-life of caffeine in humans is about 3 hours, and no more than 10% is excreted unchanged.

Cross-tolerance exists among the methylated xanthines; loss of tolerance may take more than 2 months of abstinence. The tolerance, however, is low grade, and, by increasing the dose two to four times, an effect can be obtained even in the tolerant individual. There is less tolerance to the CNS stimulation effect of caffeine than to most of its other effects. The direct action on the kidneys, to increase urine output, and the increase of salivary flow do show tolerance.

Dependence on caffeine is real. While people who are not coffee drinkers or who have been drinking only decaffeinated coffee often report un-

Table 11-6						
Caffeine consumption during a 72-hour period among 173 men and 228 women						
	Men			**Women**		
	Caffeine consumption			Caffeine consumption		
Source	**(mg)**	**(% of total caffeine intake)**	**Reported use during study period (%)**	**(mg)**	**(% of total caffeine intake)**	**Reported use during study period (%)**
Coffee	914.86	79.2	79.29	970.07	76.2	83.8
Tea	111.75	9.7	34.7	125.58	9.9	40.8
Soft drinks	65.79	5.7	28.9	75.82	6.0	28.1
Chocolate beverages	2.43	0.2	10.4	4.32	0.3	18.0
Bar chocolate	7.19	0.6	23.7	5.73	0.5	22.4
Over-the-counter drugs	48.32	4.2	21.4	92.17	7.2	26.8
TOTAL	1150.34			1273.6		

pleasant effects (nervousness, anxiety) after being given caffeinated coffee, those who regularly consume caffeine report mostly pleasant mood states after drinking coffee. Various experiments have reported on the reinforcing properties of caffeine in regular coffee drinkers; one of the most clear-cut allowed patients on a research ward to choose between two coded instant coffees, identical except that one contained caffeine. Subjects had to choose at the beginning of each day which coffee they would drink for the rest of that day. Subjects who had been drinking caffeine-containing coffee prior to this experiment almost always chose the caffeine-containing coffee.[13] Thus, the reinforcing effect of caffeine probably contributes to psychological dependence.

There has long been clear evidence of physical dependence on caffeine as well. The most reliable withdrawal sign is a headache, which occurs on an average of 18 to 19 hours after the most recent caffeine intake. Other symptoms include increased fatigue and decreased sense of vigor. These withdrawal symptoms are strongest during the first 2 days of withdrawal, then decline over the next 5 or 6 days.[13]

Mechanism of Action

For years no one really knew the mechanism whereby the methylxanthines had their effects on the central nervous system. In the early 1980s evidence was presented that caffeine and the other xanthines block the brain's receptors for a substance known as **adenosine,** which may itself be some type of neurotransmitter or neuromodulator. Adenosine acts normally in several areas of the brain to produce behavioral sedation by inhibiting the release of neurotransmitters. Caffeine's stimulant action blocks the receptors for this inhibitory effect. Now that this mechanism is understood, it will allow for the rapid development of new chemicals having similar but perhaps more potent effects.[14]

Physiological Effects

A comparison of the actions of the xanthines is given in Table 11-7. The pharmacological effects on the CNS and the skeletal muscles are probably the basis for the wide use of caffeine-containing beverages.

With two cups of coffee taken close together

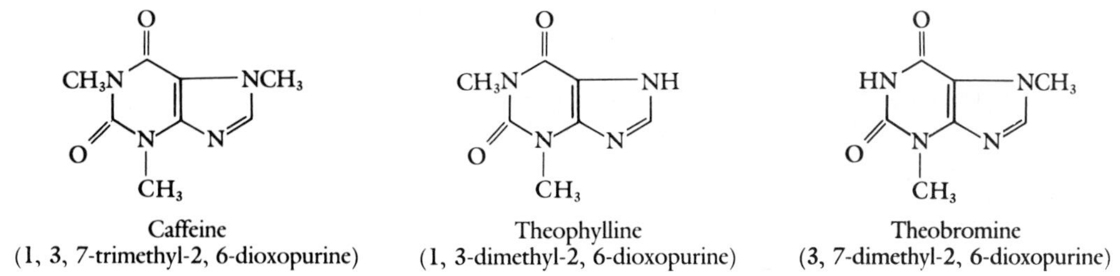

Caffeine
(1, 3, 7-trimethyl-2, 6-dioxopurine)

Theophylline
(1, 3-dimethyl-2, 6-dioxopurine)

Theobromine
(3, 7-dimethyl-2, 6-dioxopurine)

Figure 11-1. Methylated xanthines.

(about 200 mg of caffeine), the cortex is activated, the EEG shows an arousal pattern, and drowsiness and fatigue decrease. Some research suggests that this effect is the result of a direct action of caffeine on the cortex. Other results attribute the activation to the release of noradrenaline from the adrenal medulla and the brain. This CNS stimulation is also the basis for "coffee nerves," which can occur at low doses in sensitive individuals and in others when they have consumed large amounts of caffeine.

In the absence of tolerance, even 200 mg will increase the time it takes to fall asleep and will cause disturbances in the sleep. There is a good relationship between the mood-elevating effect of caffeine and the extent to which it will keep the individual awake.

Higher dose levels (about 500 mg) are needed to affect the autonomic centers of the brain, and heart rate and respiration may be increased at this dose. The direct effect on the cardiovascular system is in opposition to the effects mediated by the autonomic centers. Caffeine acts directly on the vascular muscles to cause dilation, while stimulation of the autonomic centers results in constriction of blood vessels. Usually dilation occurs, but in the brain the blood vessels are constricted, and this constriction may be the basis for caffeine's ability to reduce hypertensive headaches.

The opposing effects of caffeine, directly on the heart and indirectly through effects on the medulla, make it very difficult to predict the results of normal (that is, less than 500 mg) caffeine intake. At higher levels there is an increase in heart rate, and continued use of large amounts of caffeine may produce an irregular heartbeat in some individuals.

The basal metabolic rate may be increased slightly (10%) in chronic caffeine users, since 500 mg has frequently been shown to have this effect. This action probably combines with the stimulant effects on skeletal muscles to increase physical work output and decrease fatigue after use of caffeine.

Behavioral Effects

A hundred years ago the French essayist Balzac spoke with feeling and described the effects of coffee:

[It] causes an admirable fever. It enters the brain like a bacchante. Upon its attack, imagination runs wild, bares itself, twists like a pythoness and in this paroxysm a poet enjoys the supreme possession of his faculties; but this is a drunkenness of thought as wine brings about a drunkenness of the body.[15,p.65]

In the original French the description is even more stimulating and erotic. Unfortunately it does not refer to the effect most people receive from their morning cup of coffee.

Even today essayists sometimes take wing and soar away from the hard research data. One authoritative source[16,p.368] records that caffeine produces "a more rapid and clearer flow of thought . . . a greater sustained intellectual effort and a more perfect association of ideas." As I write this while drinking a cup of coffee, I'd like to

---

Table 11-7

Comparison of pharmacological activity of the xanthines

	CNS and respiratory stimulation	Cardiac stimulation and coronary dilation	Smooth muscle relaxation	Skeletal muscle stimulation	Diuresis
Caffeine	1*	3	3	1	3
Theophylline	2	1	1	2	1
Theobromine	3	2	2	3	2

*1 means most active.

---

believe that this is true. A number of studies have examined the effects of caffeine on information-processing tasks, memory, and mood. While varying results have been obtained, possibly owing to differences in the subjects' prior caffeine use, procedural differences in testing and so on, it does appear that caffeine can enhance auditory vigilance task performance (a measure of sustained attention) and performance on a fairly simple choice reaction time task over a wide range of doses (32 to 256 mg).[17] This is the sort of thing one would expect from a mild stimulant. More complex cognitive tasks are not reliably improved by caffeine.

There is considerable evidence that 200 to 300 mg of caffeine will partially offset fatigue-induced decrement in the performance of motor tasks. Like the amphetamines, but to a much smaller degree, caffeine prolongs the amount of time an individual can perform physically exhausting work.

Many studies have looked at the effect of caffeine on the behavior of hyperkinetic children (see Chapter 7) and most have not shown any therapeutic effect. One report[18] of the effects of 3 and 10 mg per kg of caffeine on normal 8- to 13-year-old boys showed decreased reaction times and increased vigilance along with increased motor activity. That's pretty much what might be expected from a mild stimulant.

Even the television ads tell you—make that "one last drink for the road" *coffee.* There is not a lot of evidence to support the value of this. Caffeine will not lower blood alcohol level—but it may arouse the drinker. As they say—put coffee in a sleepy drunk, you get a wide-awake drunk.

The best simple summary is that 150 to 300 mg of caffeine offsets fatigue-induced performance decrements in both physical and mental tasks, slows the development of boredom, and *may,* in a rested, interested individual, increase motor and mental efficiency above control levels.

CAUSES FOR CONCERN

Caffeine is one of those drugs that seem to always be in trouble. It's always suspected of doing bad things. Since it is probably the most widely used psychoactive drug in the world (it's acceptable to those in the Judaic-Christian as well as Islamic traditions), it is understandable that it would elicit both good and bad reports. Although it is important to point out that there is not yet clear evidence that moderate caffeine consumption is dangerous, the scientific literature has investigated the possible effects of caffeine in cancer, benign breast disease, reproduction, and heart disease. Part of the problem in knowing for certain about some of these things is that epidemiological research on caffeine consumption is difficult to do well. Coffee drinkers also tend to smoke more, for example, so the statistics have to correct for smoking behavior. Also, some studies have asked only how many cups of coffee people drink per day, without correcting for decaffeinated coffee, tea, colas, or other sources of caffeine, or without correcting for differences between weekend and weekday coffee drinking.[19]

Cancer

In the early 1980s there was a report that coffee drinkers have an increased risk of pancreatic cancers. However, the studies since then have criticized procedural flaws in that report and have found no evidence of such a link. The 1984 American Cancer Society nutritional guidelines indicated that there was no reason to consider caffeine a risk factor in human cancer.

Benign Breast Disease

A relationship has been suggested between use of the methylxanthines and *fibrocystic breast disease*. This is not a form of breast cancer, but a condition in which benign lumps form in womens' breasts. The condition can also be quite painful. The early studies have been criticized for not having proper controls, and in 1984 the AMA's Council on Scientific Affairs concluded that "there is currently no scientific basis for associating methylxanthine consumption with fibrocystic disease of the breast."

A large study[20] of all types of benign breast diseases found no significant relationship to caffeine use. This study, which appeared in 1985, was widely cited as indicating that there may be no such risk associated with caffeine. The author who originally reported the positive relationship continued to maintain that patients with fibrocystic disease who stop the use of coffee and other methylxanthines will improve.[21] However, a recent controlled clinical trial found no such improvement when patients were put on a caffeine-free diet.[22] The bottom line? As of yet, there seems to be no clear evidence that anyone not suffering from painful breasts with benign lumps should not drink coffee or colas in moderation. However, anyone who has received a diagnosis of sensitive benign breast disease would be wise to stop all coffee, tea, colas, and other sources of methylxan-

thines to see if this will help the condition to improve.

Reproductive Effects

Although studies in pregnant mice have indicated that large doses of caffeine may produce skeletal abnormalities in the pups, studies on humans have not found a relationship between caffeine and birth defects.[23] Recent studies do provide strong suggestions that caffeine consumption by a woman may reduce her chances of becoming pregnant,[24] increase the chances of spontaneous abortion (miscarriage),[25] and slow the growth of the fetus so that the baby may weigh less than normal at birth.[26] Although more research is needed to estimate the actual risks to reproduction, for now caution is definitely called for. If a woman wants to become pregnant, stay pregnant, and produce a strong, healthy baby, the list of drugs to avoid should include caffeine, in addition to alcohol, tobacco, and any other drug that is not absolutely necessary for her health.

Heart Disease

There are many reasons for believing that caffeine might increase the risk of heart attacks, including the fact that it increases heart rate and blood pressure. Until recently, there were about as many studies that found no relationship between caffeine use and heart attacks as there were studies that found such a relationship. One very interesting report used a somewhat different approach. Rather than asking people who had just had heart attacks about their prior caffeine consumption and comparing them to people who were hospitalized for some other ailment (the typical retrospective study), this study began in 1948 to track male medical students enrolled in the Johns Hopkins Medical School.[27] More than 1000 of these subjects were followed for 20 years or more after graduation, and periodically asked about various habits including drinking, smoking, and coffee consumption. Thus this was a prospective study, to see which of these habits might predict future

---

Issue: caffeine and panic attacks

The National Institute of Mental Health (NIMH) reported in 1985 that caffeine can precipitate full-blown *panic attacks* in some people.[31] Panic attacks are not common, but can be very debilitating for those who suffer them. They consist of sudden, irrational feelings of doom, sometimes accompanied by choking, sweating, and heart palpitations.

In an experiment conducted at NIMH laboratories in Maryland, a group of people who had previously suffered panic attacks were given 480 mg caffeine, equivalent to about 5 cups of brewed coffee. Panic attacks were precipitated in almost half of those people. In a group of 14 people who had never before experienced a panic attack, two suffered an attack after receiving 720 mg caffeine.

The results are interesting from a scientific point of view because they not only reveal individual differences in susceptibility to panic, but also because of the possible implications for an understanding of the biochemistry of panic disorders. The experiment may also have more immediate and practical implications in that if a person does experience a panic attack, caffeine consumption should be looked at as a possible cause.

---

health problems. Those who drank five or more cups per day were about 2.5 times as likely to suffer from coronary heart disease. This result and recent indications that coffee drinking may increase blood cholesterol levels has stimulated more research, including a large-scale retrospective study in which the incidence of nonfatal heart attacks in men under 55 years old was directly related to the amount of coffee consumed, among both smokers and nonsmokers. Those drinking five or more cups per day were about twice as likely to suffer a heart attack as those who drank no coffee.[28]

The latest information, then, gives a strong suggestion that caffeine may increase the risk of heart attacks. This would be of special concern to those with other risk factors (e.g., smoking, family history of heart disease, overweight, high blood pressure, high cholesterol levels).

Caffeinism

Caffeine is not terribly toxic, in that overdose deaths are extremely rare. It is estimated that over 10 g (equivalent to 100 cups of coffee) would be required to cause death from oral caffeine, and one person has died after an intravenous injection of 3.2 g.[29] Death is produced by convulsions, which lead to respiratory arrest.

However, high intake of caffeine can cause a variety of unpleasant symptoms, and because of caffeine's domesticated social status it may be overlooked as the cause. For example, nervousness, irritability, tremulousness, muscle twitching, insomnia, flushed appearance, and elevated temperature may all result from excessive caffeine use. There may also be palpitations, heart arrhythmias, and gastrointestinal disturbances. In several cases in which serious disease has been suspected, the symptoms have miraculously improved when coffee was restricted. There has been a report that high levels of caffeine consumption among college students are associated with lower academic performance![30]

Summary

The ancient plants, coffee, tea, and cacao, all contain caffeine and two related xanthines. In addition, Americans can derive a surprising amount of caffeine from soft drinks and nonprescription medicines.

Caffeine has a longer-lasting effect than many people realize and may help to keep you awake even several hours after it is taken in. It exerts a stimulating action in several brain regions by blocking inhibitory receptors. In regular caffeine users a headache may develop if caffeine use is stopped.

Caffeine is capable of reversing the effects of fatigue on both mental and physical tasks, but may not be able to improve the performance of a well-rested individual, particularly on complex tasks.

Excessive caffeine consumption, referred to as "caffeinism," can produce an anxiety-like reaction. The results of research on various possible adverse physiological effects of caffeine use are confusing and controversial at present, but caffeine use during pregnancy is not advised.

REFERENCES

1. Uribe Compuzano A: Brown gold, New York, 1954, Random House, Inc.
2. Meyer H: Old English coffee houses, Emmaus, Pa, 1954, The Rodale Press.
3. Lewin L: Phantastica narcotic and stimulating drugs, New York, 1931, EP Dutton & Co, Inc.
4. Statistical abstract of the United States, US Department of Commerce, Washington, DC, 1988, US Government Printing Office.
5. America's new abstinence, Fortune, March 18, 1985, pp. 20-23.
6. Dick RH and Hopkins H: Putting tea to the taste, FDA Consumer, pp. 18-27, September 1974.
7. Groisser DS: A study of caffeine in tea, The American Journal of Clinical Nutrition 31(10):1727-1731, October 1978.
8. Prial FJ: Secrets of a chocoholic, New York Times, May 16, 1979, p. C1.
9. Sterba JP: Coke brings "tasty happiness" to China, New York Times, April 16, 1981, p. A3.
10. Huisking CL: Herbs to hormones, Essex, Conn, 1968, Pequot Press, Inc.
11. Sixth Circuit Court of Appeals, 1914: 215 Federal Reporter 539, June 13, 1914.
12. Weidner G and Istvan J: Dietary sources of caffeine, New England Journal of Medicine 313:1421, 1985.
13. Griffiths RR and others: Human coffee drinking: reinforcing and physical dependence producing effects of caffeine, Journal of Pharmacology and Experimental Therapeutics 239:416-425, 1986.
14. Snyder SH and Sklar P: Behavioral and molecular actions of caffeine: focus on adenosine, Journal of Psychiatric Research 18:91-106, 1984.
15. Mickel EJ: The artificial paradises in French literature, Chapel Hill, NC, 1969, University of North Carolina Press. (Free translation from French.)
16. Goodman LS and Gilman A: The pharmacological basis of therapeutics, ed. 5, New York, 1975, Macmillan Publishing Co, Inc.
17. Lieberman HR and others: The effects of low doses of caffeine on human performance and mood, Psychopharmacology 92:308-312, 1987.
18. Elkins RN and others: Acute effects of caffeine in normal prepubertal boys, American Journal of Psychiatry 138(2):178-183, 1981.
19. Schreiber GB and others: Measurement of coffee and caffeine intake: implications for epidemiological research, Preventive Medicine 17:280-294, 1988.
20. Lubin F and others: A case-control study of caffeine and methylxanthines in benign breast disease, Journal of the American Medical Association 253:2388-2392, 1985.
21. Minton JP: Caffeine and benign breast disease, Journal of the American Medical Association 254:2408, 1985.
22. Allen SS and Froberg DG: The effect of decreased caffeine consumption on benign proliferative breast disease: a randomized clinical trial, Surgery, 101:720-730, 1987.
23. Dews P and others: Report of Fourth International Caffeine Workshop, Food Chemistry and Toxicology 22:163-169, 1984.
24. Wilcox A and others: Caffeinated beverages and decreased fertility, Lancet 1:1453-1455, 1988.
25. Srisuphan W and Bracken MB: Caffeine consumption during pregnancy and association with late spontaneous abortion, American Journal of Obstetrics and Gynecology 154:14-20, 1986.
26. Martin TR and Bracken MB: Association between low birth weight and caffeine consumption during pregnancy, American Journal of Epidemiology 126:813-821, 1987.
27. LaCroix AZ and others: Coffee consumption and the incidence of coronary heart disease, New England Journal of Medicine 315:977-982, 1986.
28. Rosenberg L and others: Coffee drinking and nonfatal myocardial infarction in men under 55 years of age, American Journal of Epidemiology 128:570-578, 1988.
29. Syed IB: The effects of caffeine, Journal of the American Pharmaceutical Association NS16:568-572, 1976.
30. Gilliland K and Andress D: Ad lib caffeine consumption, symptoms of caffeinism, and academic performance, American Journal of Psychiatry 138(4):512-514, 1981.
31. Stewart SA: Caffeine can push the panic button, USA Today, October 23, 1985.

Chapter 12

Over-the-Counter Drugs

OBJECTIVES

After reading this chapter, you should be able to:

Describe the process by which the FDA has reviewed OTC products for safety and effectiveness.

Discuss the effects of three types of OTC psychoactive drugs: stimulants, weight-control products, and sedatives.

Explain how aspirin and related products work to relieve pain.

Describe the causes of colds and which symptoms are treated with which type of ingredient.

List eight chemicals that are the main active ingredients in all the OTC products covered in this chapter.

Over-the-counter (OTC) drugs are those that are self-prescribed and self-administered for the relief of symptoms of self-diagnosed illnesses. There are certainly a lot of them. One estimate is that three out of every four individuals have the symptoms of some illness each month, but only one of those seeks professional help. The other two frequently turn to OTC drugs.

Americans are now spending over $7 billion a year on OTC products. That's not as much as we spend on prescription drugs or booze or cigarettes or illicit cocaine, but it's enough to keep several OTC drug manufacturers locked in fierce competition for those sales. The two biggest markets are for aspirin-like analgesics ($2 billion) and for the collection of cough, cold, and allergy products ($2.2 billion).[1] Do we really need all these nonprescription tablets, capsules, liquids, and creams? How much of what we buy is based on advertising "hype," and how much on sound decisions about our health? How are we as consumers to know the difference? The FDA is in the process of trying to help us with these decisions.

FDA REGULATION OF OTC PRODUCTS

The 1962 Kefauver-Harris amendment required that all drugs be evaluated for both safety and efficacy. The FDA was not only to set up criteria for new drugs entering the market, but also to establish a procedure for reviewing all the OTC drugs already on the market. At first glance this seemed an impossible task, since there were somewhere between 250,000 and 300,000 different products on the market (no one knew for sure). In addition, each product was likely to change its ingredients without warning, just like the "new" and "improved" soaps and toothpastes do. The FDA made the decision not to study individual products but to review their ingredients. The FDA set up advisory panels to review each of 26 classes of OTC products. Each panel was to look at the active ingredients contained in products in its class, to decide whether there was evidence indicating that each ingredient was safe and effective for its purpose, and also to decide what sorts of claims could be made for that ingredient on the label.

These classes of OTC Drugs were to be reviewed by the FDA:

1. Antacids
2. Antimicrobials
3. Sedatives and sleep aids
4. Analgesics
5. Cold remedies and antitussives
6. Antihistamines and allergy products
7. Mouthwashes
8. Topical analgesics
9. Antirheumatics
10. Hematinics
11. Vitamins and minerals
12. Antiperspirants
13. Laxatives
14. Dentifrices and dental products
15. Sunburn treatments and preventives
16. Contraceptive and vaginal products
17. Stimulants
18. Hemorrhoidals
19. Antidiarrheals
20. Dandruff and athlete's foot preparations
21. Bronchodilators and antiasthmatics
22. Antiemetics
23. Ophthalmics
24. Emetics
25. Miscellaneous internal products
26. Miscellaneous external products

Before the panel could begin work, some rules had to be laid down about what was meant by such terms as "safe" and "effective," keeping in mind that no drug is entirely safe and many may have only limited effectiveness. The FDA uses the acronym GRAS (Generally Recognized as Safe) to mean that, given the currently available information, people who are informed and qualified would agree that the ingredient should be considered safe. Safe means ". . . a low incidence of adverse reactions or significant side effects under adequate directions for use and warnings against unsafe use as well as low potential for harm which may result from abuse. . . ."[2]

Similar acronyms are used for two other important concepts: GRAE (Generally Recognized as Effective) and GRAHL (Generally Recognized as Honestly Labeled).

Effectiveness means a reasonable expectation that, in a significant proportion of the target population, the pharmacological effect of the drug, when used under adequate directions for use and warnings against unsafe use, will provide clinically significant relief of the type claimed.

Labeling shall be clear and truthful in all respects and may not be false or misleading in any particular. It shall state the intended uses and results of the product; adequate directions for proper use; and warnings against unsafe use, side effects, and adverse reactions. . . .[2]

Even this approach turned out to be a lot of work. The first panels were appointed in 1972, the last advisory panel report was completed in 1983, and the FDA began to publish "Tentative Final Monographs" on each category in 1985. The idea was to solicit comments from the public and the drug companies before publishing Final Monographs, but so far the amount of comment has been so great that revised Tentative Final Monographs are still appearing. It's not clear whether these are getting more Final or more Tentative as the process continues. They are certainly becoming longer, as they include more comments and responses to comments. This does not mean that there has been no regulation at all during this time; far from it. As advisory panels made tentative decisions, those were communicated to the manufacturers, who were encouraged to change their formulations. Because the process was taking so long, in 1980 the FDA Commissioner acted to speed up both the reviews and the effects of those reviews. Thus the FDA began publishing some brief advisory opinions banning certain products or combinations and sent letters to manufacturers and distributors of the products ordering them removed from the market immediately.

The advisory panel was to rule on each active ingredient and to place it in one of three categories:

Category I Ingredient is GRAS and GRAE.

Category II Ingredient is not GRAS and/or GRAE; the manufacturer has 6 months from the date of the panel report to prove the ingredient should be in Category I, or it may not be shipped in interstate commerce.

Category III Data insufficient to determine safety and/or effectivess. Manufacturers given 1 year from the date of the panel report to prove GRAS, or ingredient goes to Category II.

The overall result of this procedure can be seen by taking a trip to your neighborhood drugstore and looking at the lists of ingredients on a given type of medication. You should be struck that all the competing brands contain much the same few ingredients. In some categories there may be only one active ingredient in Category I, and then all competing brands will be essentially identical!

OVER-THE COUNTER VERSUS PRESCRIPTION DRUGS

You may remember that it was the 1938 Food, Drug, and Cosmetic Act that established a classification of drugs that would be available only by prescription. The rule is:

A drug shall be permitted for OTC sale and use by the laity unless, because of its toxicity or other potential for harmful effect or because of the method . . . nec-

---

> **Your turn: the medicine chest**
>
> The family medicine chest is often a treasure trove of old tablets, capsules, liquids, and lozenges. Start digging around and see how many different OTC drugs you can find in yours. How old do you think some of them might be? If any of them have expiration dates, have the dates passed?
>
> Because formulations change from year to year there's a good chance the medicines you now have are not the same as the ones being sold in the drugstore. Write down the formulations for a few of your medicine chest drugs. Then go to the drugstore and compare them with the current formulation for that same brand of product. Do you wonder if some of the old ingredients were removed from the market because the FDA no longer considers them to be safe?

---

essary to its use, it may safely be sold and used only under a practitioner's prescription.[2]

Sometimes the only difference between an OTC product and a prescription product is the greater amount of active ingredient in each prescription dose. More often, however, prescription drugs are chemicals that are unavailable OTC. Under the current regulations, once a manufacturer succeeds in activating a New Drug Application for a prescription drug, there is no automatic review to see if the drug could later be considered for OTC status. In general, there doesn't appear to have been much incentive for a drug manufacturer to try to get OTC status for a drug. Therefore most of the new drugs that have found their way onto the market in the past several years have stayed prescription drugs.

The FDA advisory panels that reviewed products in a given OTC category sometimes did more than was required of them. In some cases they recommended that higher doses be allowed in OTC preparations—and as a result we can now buy higher strength OTC antihistamines. And in several cases the suggestion was that prescription-only ingredients be sold OTC.

SOME PSYCHOACTIVE OTC PRODUCTS

Stimulants

This was one of the original FDA categories and turns out to be one of the simplest. The FDA allows these drugs to be sold to "help restore mental alertness or wakefulness when experiencing fatigue or drowsiness." If it sounds like caffeine could do this, you're right! No Doz, a well-known product that has been around for years, has the tried-and-true formula: 100 mg caffeine (about the equivalent of an average cup of brewed coffee). The recommended dose is 2 tablets initially, then one every 3 hours. Another well-known product, Vivarin, contains 200 mg caffeine, and the initial dose is 1 tablet. Thus, although the packages look different and different people make them, a smart consumer would choose between these two based on the price per milligram caffeine. Or choose a less expensive "store" brand, or buy coffee (usually more expensive), or just get enough rest and save your money. If you do buy these caffeine tablets, the labels warn you about using them with coffee, tea, or cola drinks. As far as the FDA is concerned, the only active ingredient allowed in OTC stimulants is caffeine.[3]

Look-Alikes

There is a reasonably brisk business in the semilegal field of selling caffeine tablets manufactured in either table or capsule form to resemble prescription stimulants, such as amphetamine. In fact, many "street" purchases of "speed" these days turn out to contain caffeine as their major ingredient. Some states have tried to ban the sale of these look-alikes, and the FDA has tried to regulate them, but it is tough, since caffeine itself is allowed. Mail-order advertisements for these products may be found in the back of various magazines (Chapter 7). While they no longer use such suggestive names as "speed" for the products, one does claim the brand name "Amphetrazine."

Some companies have manufactured combinations of caffeine with either **ephedrine** or **phenylpropanolamine (PPA).** You may remember from Chapter 7 that ephedrine is a **sympathomimetic** derived from a Chinese herbal tea and sold as a bronchodilator. The amphetamine molecule was derived from it. PPA has a similar structure to amphetamine and to ephedrine and is sold in weight-control preparations. Each of these has mild stimulant properties of its own. The FDA has ruled that OTC products labeled as stimulants that contain anything other than caffeine as an active ingredient could not be sold. They also outlawed OTC products labeled for any purpose that contained combinations of caffeine, ephedrine, or PPA. In 1985 the FDA took legal action against several mail-order distributors of such combination products.[4]

Weight-Control Products

The original FDA list of OTC drug categories did not include "appetite suppressants" or a similar term. Apparently the FDA didn't think they would be dealing with such a product, since at the time the use of the prescription amphetamines for this purpose was under widespread attack. However, data were presented that indicated the likelihood that phenylpropanolamine (PPA) was safe and effective, and by the late 1970s several products were being sold that contained PPA as their only active ingredient. Some studies indicated that caffeine could potentiate the appetite-suppressing effect of PPA, and for a brief period during the early 1980s several of the products included both PPA and caffeine. After the 1983 FDA ruling prohibiting such combinations on the grounds they might not be safe, all products returned to PPA.

The recommended dose for appetite suppression is 75 mg per day. The final decision on PPA has not yet been reached. There is some concern about the safety even of 75-mg doses, with the threat being increased blood pressure resulting from sympathetic stimulation. There is also some controversy about the effectiveness of PPA, since its effect, as with all appetite suppressant drugs,

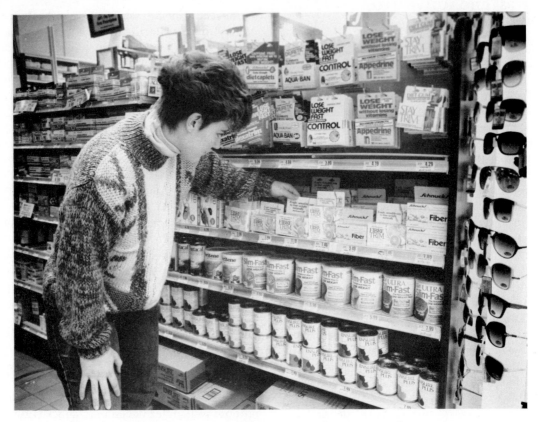

These weight-loss products rely on a single active ingredient.

is small and rather short-lived. For the moment, those large numbers of competing weight-control products in the drugstore are essentially the same: 75 mg PPA. (Many proudly proclaiming that they are caffeine free!) Some have only 25 or 37.5 mg and recommend taking them two or three times per day, some are in sustained-release capsules, and some include vitamin supplements (not considered an active ingredient by the FDA). An interesting aspect of this apparent competition can be seen in the fact that Appedrine, Control, Dexatrim, and Prolamine, all competing products containing PPA, are all made by the same company. These include tablets and capsules, with and without vitamin supplements, and varying amounts of PPA per tablet. The point of these different packages and products is obviously to cover the mar-

ket, but as far as the FDA is concerned the bottom line is the same for all of them: 75 mg PPA.

Just as the final word is not in on PPA, the FDA is still reviewing evidence on benzocaine-containing candies and gums. These products are supposed to numb the tongue, reducing the sense of taste. It has not yet been finally determined if this is an effective way to reduce food intake. The FDA has reviewed and ruled against several other products that have been advertised for weight control. Starch blockers, which were supposed to interfere with the absorption of carbohydrates from starchy foods, have never been proved to do so. The FDA asked for all sales to stop until safety and effectiveness could be established, and the government has seized the products after promoters failed to comply. Cholecystokinin (CCK) is a hormone that does decrease food intake when injected directly into the brains of experimental animals, but the chemical is quickly destroyed in the digestive tract if taken by mouth. Nevertheless, products claiming to include CCK have been advertised and sold, and the FDA has ordered this practice discontinued. Other unapproved products for weight reduction that have come under FDA scrutiny in the 1980s include DHEA, arginine and ornithine, spirulina, and glucomannan. None of these products has been demonstrated to be effective in weight loss, despite claims of "burning fat," "natural" weight loss, "Oriental weight-loss secret," and so on.[5]

Sedatives and Sleep Aids

A few years ago, the shelves contained a number of OTC sedative, or "calmative," preparations, including Quiet World and Compoz, which contained very small amounts of the anticholinergic scopolamine combined with the **antihistamine** methapyrilene. At the same time, sleep aids, such as Sleep-Eze and Sominex, contained just a bit more of the same two ingredients. The rationale for the scopolamine, particularly at these low doses, was under FDA investigation, but scopolamine had traditionally been included in many such medications in the past. With the antihistamines, it is quite clear that some of them do produce a kind of sedated state and may produce drowsiness. The FDA advisory panel accepted methapyrilene, but eventually rejected scopolamine. For a while all of these medications contained only methapyrilene. Then, in 1979 it was reported that methapyrilene caused cancer in laboratory animals, so it was no longer GRAS. Next came pyrilamine maleate, then doxylamine succinate, and then **diphenhydramine,** all antihistamines. The interesting thing about this whole process was that if you bought the same brand from one year to the next to the next, you would get a different formulation each time. But if you bought several different brands at the same time, you stood a good chance of getting the same formulation in all of them!

The category of "sedative" no longer exists for OTC products. One product, Miles Nervine, which went from a sedative containing bromide salts to a calmative containing whatever they all contained each year, is now Miles Nervine Nighttime Sleep-Aid, containing 25 mg diphenhydramine. Nytol is also a nighttime sleep aid containing the same ingredient. Sominex and Sleep-Eze are still around, and both also contain diphenhydramine.

As we said in Chapter 8, insomnia is perceived to be a bigger problem than it actually is for most people, and it is rare that medication is really required. These antihistamines can induce drowsiness, but not very quickly. If you do feel the need to use these to get you to sleep more rapidly, take them at least 20 minutes before retiring. Their sedative effects are potentiated by alcohol, so it is not a good idea to take them after drinking.

ANALGESICS
People and Pain

Pain is such a little word for such a big experience. Most people have experienced pain of varying intensities, from mild to moderate to severe to excruciating! Two major classes of drugs are used to reduce pain or the awareness of pain. Anesthetics (meaning "without sensibility") have this effect by reducing all types of sensation or by blocking consciousness completely. The barbiturates and the volatile anesthetics, such as ether, are good examples of this type of agent. Analgesics (meaning "without pain") are compounds that reduce pain without causing a loss of the senses. Narcotics are one group of drugs in this class, but this chapter will primarily discuss the OTC internal analgesics such as aspirin and acetaminophen.

One classification divides pain into two types, depending on its place of origin. Visceral pain, such as intestinal cramps, arises from nonskeletal portions of the body; narcotics are effective in reducing pain of this type. Somatic pain, arising from muscle or bone and typified by sprains, headaches, and arthritis, is reduced by salicylates (aspirin).

Pain is unlike other sensations in many ways,

mostly the result of the influence of nonspecific factors. The experience of pain varies with personality, sex, and time of day[6] and is increased with fatigue, anxiety, fear, boredom, and anticipation of more pain. Because pain is very susceptible to nonspecific factors, a brief comment is required on the effectiveness of a placebo in reducing pain. Classic studies have been done by Beecher, who has also summarized reports of many investigators on the effectiveness of placebos in the reduction of pain.[7] These were real situations with a variety of clinical causes ranging from postoperative pain to the aches associated with the common cold. About 35% of the patients in these studies had their pain "satisfactorily relieved" by placebos. That is, when individuals in pain were given an inactive substance along with the suggestion that it would reduce the pain, 35% of the patients obtained relief.

This 35% proportion is quite high when it is appreciated that morphine provides satisfactory relief of pain in only about 75% of patients. It was also found that placebos are most effective in reducing pain in stressful situations, whereas morphine has its smallest effect in these stressful situations. As might be expected from the last statement, placebos are more effective in real-life pain than in experimental pain. The internal analgesics mentioned in the next section have been repeatedly shown to be more effective at therapeutic doses than placebos for certain kinds of pain.

Aspirin

Salicylates are the most widely used class of internal analgesics. The word itself suggests their long heritage, coming from the Latin *salix,* meaning willow. Over 2400 years ago, the Greeks used extracts of willow and poplar bark in the treatment of pain, gout, and other illnesses. Aristotle commented on some of the clinical effects of similar preparations, and Galen also made good use of these formulations.

These remedies fell into disrepute, however, when St. Augustine declared that all diseases of Christians were the work of demons and thus a punishment from God. The American Indian, unhampered by this enlightened attitude, used a tea brewed from willow bark to reduce fever. The salicylates were not rediscovered in Europe until about 200 years ago when an Englishman, the Reverend Edward Stone, combined two bits of the best information then available and put the result to clinical test. The two pieces of data he combined were (1) listen to old wives' tales, and (2) plants acquire the characteristics of the place where they grow. The old wives kept saying willow bark is good for pain and whatever else ails you! Stone phrased the second attitude nicely:

> As this tree delights in a moist or wet soil where aches chiefly abound, the general maxim that many natural maladies carry their cures along with them, or that their remedies lie not far from their causes, was so very apposite to this particular case that I could not help applying it. That this might be the intention of Providence had some little weight with me.[8]

Stone prepared an extract of the bark and gave the same dose to 50 patients with varying illnesses and found the results to be "uniformly excellent."

In the nineteenth century the active ingredient in these preparations was isolated and identified as salicylic acid. In 1838 salicylic acid was synthesized, and in 1859 procedures were developed that made bulk production feasible. Salicylic acid and sodium salicylate were then used for many ills, especially arthritis.

In the giant Bayer Laboratories in Germany in the 1890s there worked a chemist named Hoffmann. His father had a severe case of rheumatoid arthritis, and only salicylic acid seemed to help. The major difficulty then, as today, was that the drug caused great gastric discomfort. So great was the stomach upset and nausea that Hoffmann's father frequently preferred the pain of the arthritis. Hoffmann studied the salicylates to see if he could find one with the same therapeutic effect as salicylic acid, but without the side effects.

In 1898 he synthesized **acetylsalicylic** acid and tried it on his father, who reported relief from pain without stomach upset. The compound was tested, patented, and released for sale in 1899 as

Aspirin. Aspirin was a trademark name derived from acetyl and spiralic acid (the old name for salicylic acid).

Aspirin was marketed for physicians and sold as a white powder in individual dosage packets, available only on prescription. It was immediately popular worldwide, and the U.S. market became large enough that it was very soon manufactured in this country. In 1915 the 5 gr (325 mg) white tablet stamped Bayer first appeared, and, also for the first time, Aspirin became a nonprescription item. The Bayer Company was on its way. It had an effective drug that could be sold to the public and was known by one name—Aspirin. And they had the name trademarked!

Before Feburary, 1917, when the patent on Aspirin was to expire, Bayer started an advertising campaign to make it clear that there was only one Aspirin, and its first name was Bayer. Several companies started manufacturing and selling Aspirin as aspirin, and Bayer sued. What happened after this is a long story, but you know who lost; aspirin is aspirin—or is it?

Therapeutic use.   Say what you will, aspirin is truly a magnificent drug. It is also a drug with some serious side effects. Aspirin has three effects that are the primary basis for its clinical use. It is an analgesic that effectively blocks somatic pain in the mild to moderate range. Aspirin is also **antipyretic:** it reduces body temperature when elevated by fever. Last, but not least aspirin is an **anti-inflammatory** agent. It reduces the inflammation and soreness in an injured area. This action is the basis for its extensive use in arthritis. It is difficult to find another drug that has this span of effects coupled with a relatively low toxicity. It does, however, have side effects that pose problems for some people.

Since the action of a drug depends on its concentration at the cellular site of action, much work has been done to see how aspirin gets there, how fast it gets there, and how long it stays. Aspirin is readily absorbed from the stomach but even faster from the intestine. Thus anything that delays movement of the aspirin from the stomach should affect absorption time. The evidence is mixed on whether taking aspirin with a meal, which delays emptying of the stomach, increases the time before onset of action. It is clear, however, that a water solution of aspirin is more rapidly absorbed than the tablet form and thus gives higher and earlier effective blood levels of the drug. Although the effervescent aspirins are absorbed more rapidly and result in earlier and higher blood levels of aspirin, there is no evidence that analgesia occurs sooner than with regular aspirin. Remember, too, that excessive use of these drugs disrupts the body's normal acid-base balance and creates other problems.

It is interesting that two famous compounds which the Bayer Laboratories in Germany were instrumental in introducing to the world are rapidly transformed to their original form after absorption. Both heroin and aspirin were first synthesized in the Bayer Laboratories. Aspirin, either in the gastrointestinal tract or in the bloodstream, is converted to salicylic acid. Taken orally, aspirin is a more potent analgesic than salicylic acid, since aspirin irritates the stomach less and is thus absorbed more rapidly.

The term *therapeutic dose* will be used repeatedly, with 600 to 1000 mg suggested as the dose range for aspirin. Most reports suggest that 300 mg is usually more effective than a placebo, while 600 mg is clearly even more effective. Many studies indicate that increasing the dose above that level does not increase aspirin's analgesic action, but some research indicates that 1200 mg of aspirin may provide greater relief than 600 mg.[9] In one study,[10] after ingestion of a 650-mg tablet of aspirin, headache and postpartum pain were not reduced significantly from placeo until 45 minutes had elapsed; maximum relief was obtained after 60 minutes. At 4 hours after intake, pain levels were equivalent in the drug and placebo groups, that is, the analgesia was gone. These reports agree with the salicylate blood levels measured in the same patients. At 45 minutes and at 4 hours the levels were the same.

At therapeutic doses aspirin does have analgesic actions that are fairly specific. First, and in marked contrast to narcotic analgesics, aspirin does not affect the impact of the anticipation of pain. It seems probable also that aspirin has its primary effect on the ability to withstand continuing pain. This no doubt is the basis for much of the self-medication with aspirin, since moderate, protracted pain is fairly common.

Other work suggests that aspirin is most effective as an analgesic against the middle range of pain. At low pain levels, it is difficult to show the effectiveness of any compound because of the extreme variability of patients' responses. At the level of "unbearable" pain, in experimental situations, aspirin does not increase the amount of time an individual can tolerate the high pain levels.[11] The salicylates do not block all types of pain. They are especially effective against headache and musculoskeletal aches and pains, less effective for toothache and sore throat, and almost valueless in visceral pain, as well as in traumatic (acute) pain.

The antipyretic (fever-reducing) action of aspirin does not lower temperature in an individual with normal body temperature. It has this effect only if the person has a fever. The mechanism by which the salicylates decrease body temperature is fairly well understood. They act on the temperature-regulating area of the hypothalamus to increase heat loss through peripheral mechanisms. Heat loss is primarily increased by vasodilation of peripheral blood vessels and by increased perspiration. Heat production is not changed, but heat loss is facilitated so that body temperature may go down.

More aspirin has probably been employed for its third major therapeutic use than for either of the other two. The anti-inflammatory action of the salicylates is the major basis for its use in rheumatoid arthritis.

Most tablets, including aspirin, develop a harder external shell the longer they sit. This hardening effect does not change the amount of the active ingredient, but it does make the active ingredient less effective because disintegration time is increased by the hard exterior coating. Along the same line, moisture and heat speed the de-

composition of acetylsalicylic acid into two other compounds: salicylic acid, which causes gastric distress, and acetic acid—vinegar. When the smell of vinegar is strong in your aspirin bottle, discard it!

For many years, some aspirin preparations have been *buffered* with additional ingredients meant to neutralize the acidity of aspirin. This is intended to have two effects: first, to reduce stomach irritation; second, by moving the aspirin more rapidly into the intestine, to produce faster relief. There is ample evidence that buffered aspirin does reach the blood somewhat more rapidly, but no one has ever been able to show that this results in faster or stronger pain relief. The problem with allowing companies to claim reduced stomach irritation is that while some reduced irritation may be experienced by some people, the FDA worries that people with ulcers or other stomach disorders will think it is all right to take buffered aspirin, which it is not. Both of these claims remain Category III (insufficient data).[12]

Various effects: adverse and otherwise

1. Aspirin increases bleeding time by inhibiting blood platelet aggregation. This is not an insignificant effect. Two or three aspirins can double bleeding time, the time it takes for blood to clot, and the effect may last for 4 to 7 days. In one study[13] bleeding time increased 40% 2 hours after 30 mg of aspirin was administered.

Two possibly big advantages of the anticoagulant effect are of particular interest to men. A *transient ischemic attack* (TIA) results when a tiny clot forms in the brain or the retina, temporarily cutting off the blood supply to a small region. This may precede a stroke, in which the loss of blood to a brain region results in permanent damage. You probably won't find this mentioned on aspirin bottles in the store, since the FDA doesn't want people self-diagnosing and self-treating TIAs or strokes, but the professional labeling (for physicians and pharmacists to read), says,

For reducing the risk of recurrent transient ischemic attacks (TIA's) or stroke in men who have transient ischemia of the brain due to fibrin platelet emboli. There is inadequate evidence that aspirin or buffered aspirin is effective in reducing TIA's in women at the recommended dosage. There is no evidence that aspirin or buffered aspirin is of benefit in the treatment of completed strokes in men or women.[12]

Perhaps even more importantly, evidence has been building for some time that men who have had one heart attack (myocardial infarction) and who take an aspirin tablet every other day, have a reduced risk of a second heart attack. The Canadian government approved aspirin to prevent second heart attacks in 1982, and the FDA tentatively approved this use in 1985. Two large-scale 1988 experiments, one British and one American, make it very clear that this is a real effect. The FDA will include in the *professional labeling only*, and not to the general public, an indication for aspirin "to reduce the risk of death and/or nonfatal myocardial infarction in patients with a previous myocardial infarction or unstable angina pectoris (chest pain)."[12] Again, the FDA doesn't want people self-diagnosing and self-treating heart attacks. What we don't know, because the study hasn't been done, is whether it would make sense for people who have not experienced angina or a heart attack but who have other risk factors (overweight, high incidence of heart disease in the family) to use aspirin to prevent heart attacks. The aspirin makers would probably like it if every male over the age of 40 started taking an aspirin every other day, and the television ads are becoming rather suggestive that you should "ask your doctor" about this. The FDA has gotten manufacturers to agree not to make advertising claims that aspirin can prevent a first heart attack, but publicity about the research results produced a 16% increase in the sales of Bayer aspirin in 1987.[1]

There's good and bad in the anticoagulant effect of aspirin. Its use before surgery may help prevent blood clots from appearing in patients at high risk for clot formation. For many surgical patients, however, facilitation of blood clotting is desirable,

and the rule is no aspirin or other salicylates for 7 to 10 days before surgery. The same principle— no aspirin—should hold for women in their last trimester of pregnancy. This may be particularly important, since aspirin does cross the placental barrier, and neither the short- nor long-term effects on the fetus are known.

2. "Ingestion of aspirin, in doses of 1 to 3 gm/ day, will induce occult gastrointestinal bleeding in about 70% of normal subjects."[14] In most cases this is only about 5 ml per day, but that is five times the normal loss. In some people the blood loss may be great enough to cause anemia. The basis for this effect is not clear but is believed to be a direct eroding by the aspirin tablets of the gastric mucosa. The rule is clear: drink lots of water when you take aspirin, or, better yet, crush the tablets and drink them in orange juice or other liquid.

3. Aspirin use increases the number of viruses produced in sufferers of the common cold.[15] If this result is broadly supported, it would mean that the aspirin user is more likely to "spread germs" or reinfect himself than the nonaspirin user. Fitting in with that is a report[16] showing that aspirin blocks the effect of interferon—a natural substance that makes cells resistant to viruses.

4. Aspirin is a leading cause of accidental poisoning deaths in children under 5 years of age, as it has always been since records have been kept. Household plants and household soaps have been the first and second causes of nonfatal accidental poisonings in young children for many years, but aspirin continues to lead in mortality.

5. Reye's syndrome. For several years there have been increasing concerns about the relationship of aspirin use to **Reye's syndrome**. This is a rare disease (190 cases in the United States in 1984). Almost all of the cases occur in people under the age of 20, usually after they have had a viral infection, such as influenza or chicken pox. The children begin vomiting continuously, then they may become disoriented, undergo personality changes, shout, or may become lethargic.

Some may enter comas, and some of those will either die or suffer permanent brain damage. The overall mortality rate is about 26%.[17]

No one knows what causes Reye's and it isn't believed to be *caused* by aspirin. However, there are data that suggest the disease is more likely to occur in children who have been given aspirin during the preceding illness. In late 1984 the results of a Centers for Disease Control pilot study were released, indicating that the use of aspirin may increase the risk of Reye's syndrome by as much as 25 times. In 1985 makers of all aspirin products were asked to put warning labels on their packages. These labels recommend that you consult a physician before giving aspirin to children or teenagers with chicken pox or flu.

In early 1986 it was reported that fewer parents in Michigan were giving aspirin to children for colds or influenza, and the incidence of Reye's syndrome had also decreased in Michigan.[18] Although there is still no indication as to how or why this effect occurs, the Michigan study lends further strength to the relationship between aspirin use and Reye's syndrome. Our advice is that no one under the age of 20 use aspirin in treating chicken pox, influenza, or even what might be suspected to be a common cold.

Some of the more incidental effects of aspirin need to be noted. At therapeutic doses these include an increase in fluid retention and blood volume, which sometimes results in a slight weight gain. Respiration is increased, as is oxygen consumption, and blood sugar levels increase in normal individuals but decrease in diabetic persons.

Mechanism of action.   Aspirin is now believed to have both a central and a peripheral analgesic effect. The central effect is not clear, but the peripheral effect is well on its way to being understood; it is now known that aspirin modifies the *cause* of pain.[19]

Prostaglandins are local hormones that are manufactured and released when cell membranes are distorted or damaged, that is, injured. The prostaglandins then act on the endings of the neurons that mediate pain in the injured areas. The prostaglandins sensitize the neurons to mechan-ical stimulation and to stimulation by two other local hormones, histamine and bradykinin, which are more slowly released from the damaged tissue. Aspirin blocks the synthesis of the prostaglandins. To summarize: (1) Prostaglandins are not stored but are rapidly synthesized and released from cells when injury occurs. (2) Prostaglandins sensitize the pain neurons to other damage-released local hormones. (3) Prostaglandin synthesis is blocked by aspirin. (4) Without the prostaglandin sensitization, impulses are not initiated in pain pathways by the other local hormones.

There is now abundant evidence to support this rough outline of the mechanism of the action of aspirin. For one, aspirin does not block the pain induced by injections of prostaglandins. Another is that aspirin has an analgesic effect only in tissues where prostaglandin formation is taking place. A similar explanation seems most reasonable and supportable as the basis for the anti-inflammatory action of aspirin.

The antipyretic action has also been spelled out: a specific prostaglandin acts on the anterior hypothalamus to decrease heat dissipation through the normal procedures of sweating and dilation of peripheral blood vessels. Aspirin blocks the synthesis of this prostaglandin in the anterior hypothalamus, and this is followed by increased heat loss.

Acetaminophen

There are two related analgesic compounds: **phenacetin** and **acetaminophen**. Phenacetin was the *P* in the APC tablets your parents know about (*A* is for aspirin and *C* is for caffeine). Soldiers knew well that at sick call the APC tablets were the Army's Perfect Cure—for everything. Phenacetin has now gone to the land of dead drugs: the review panel put it in Category II.

And it's about time. Phenacetin has been around since 1887 and has long been suspected of causing kidney lesions and dysfunction. In 1964, the FDA required a warning on all products containing phenacetin, which limited their use to 10 days, since the phenacetin might damage the kidneys. Anacin then dropped the *P* from its basic APC formulation, since it did not want to put the warning on the label.

The only real question is why everything took so long. Phenacetin was known to be rapidly converted to acetaminophen, which was the primary active agent. The mechanism of analgesic action of acetaminophen is not known, but it is equipotent with aspirin in its analgesic, as well as its antipyretic, effects. The antipyretic mechanism is similar to that of aspirin, but the analgesic effect may be additive to that produced by aspirin. Acetaminophen is not anti-inflammatory and thus is of minimal value in arthritis, gout, and the like.

Acetaminophen has been marketed as an OTC analgesic since 1955 but it was the big advertising pushes in the 1970s for two brand name products, Tylenol and Datril, that brought acetaminophen into the bigtime. It is usually advertised as having most of the good points of "that other pain reliever" and many fewer disadvantages. To a degree this is probably true: if only analgesia and fever reduction are desired, acetaminophen is probably the drug of choice. A 1977 review of its therapeutic and other effects commented that "there is also growing concern that increasing household availability and the public's lack of recognition of acetaminophen's acute toxicity will produce a new health hazard.[20]

That prediction came true in the 1980s, as more and more reports of acetaminophen-induced liver damage and deaths came in. Acetaminophen is now the seventh most likely drug to result in an emergency-room visit, and is tenth among drugs mentioned in drug-related deaths, according to the DAWN statistics (Chapter 2). The FDA doesn't want to advertise on the package that acetaminophen can be lethal, for fear of attracting suicide attempts. So they require a warning against overdose, and include the statement that "Prompt medical attention is critical for adults as well as for children even if you do not notice any signs or symptoms."[12] This statement reflects the fact that damage to the liver may not be noticed until 24 to 48 hours later, when the symptoms of impaired liver function finally emerge. You should remember that acetaminophen is not necessarily "safer" than aspirin, especially if the recommended dose is exceeded.

Ibuprofen

Since the discovery that aspirin and similar drugs work through inhibiting the synthesis of prostaglandins, the drug companies have been able to use that information to design new and sometimes more potent analgesics, most of which have been available only as prescription products. Ibuprofen, which was originally available by prescription, is now found in several OTC analgesics. In addition to its analgesic potency, ibuprofen is a potent anti-inflammatory, and has received wide use in the treatment of arthritis. Ibuprofen, unlike aspirin and acetaminophen, is not a very effective antipyretic. The most common side effects of ibuprofen are gastrointestinal: nausea, stomach pain, and cramping. There have been a few reports of fatal liver damage with overdoses of ibuprofen, so again it is wise not to exceed the recommended dose.

Table 12-1 contains a list of several OTC internal analgesics along with the amounts of each ingredient they contain. The FDA has been discussing whether or not to exclude products that contain both aspirin and acetaminophen, and they aren't yet sure about the value of including caffeine. Products containing ibuprofen warn against combining them with aspirin, since that mixture hasn't been thoroughly studied.

In 1987, aspirin products held 45% of this market, acetaminophen 38%, and ibuprofen 17%.[1] Over the short run, we can probably expect ibuprofen sales to increase slowly. Over the long run, we may expect to see new prostaglandin-synthesis inhibitors on the OTC market.

COLD AND ALLERGY PRODUCTS
The All-Too-Common Common Cold

There has to be something good about an illness that Charles Dickens could be lyrical about.

Table 12-1

Ingredients in OTC analgesics

Brand	Aspirin	Acetaminophen	Ibuprofen	Caffeine	Other
Anacin	400			32	
Advil			200		
Bufferin	325				Magnesium carbonate, calcium carbonate, magnesium oxide
Empirin	325				
Excedrin	250	250		65	
Mediprin			200		
Nuprin			200		
Vanquish	227	194		33	Magnesium hydroxide, aluminum hydroxide gel

I am at this moment
Deaf in the ears,
Hoarse in the throat,
Red in the nose,
Green in the gills,
Damp in the eyes,
Twitchy in the joints,
And fractious in temper
From a most intolerable
And oppressive cold.[21]

The common cold is caused by a virus—well, viruses, over a hundred have been identified—but in 40% to 60% of individuals with colds researchers cannot connect the infection to a specific virus. That makes it tough to find a cure. Two groups of viruses are known to be associated with colds—the **rhinoviruses** and the more recently identified (and less well-studied) **coronaviruses**. These viruses are clearly distinct from those that cause influenza, measles, and pneumonia. Success in developing vaccines against poliomyelitis and measles has made some experts optimistic about a vaccine for the common cold. Others are pessimistic because of the great variety of viruses and the fact that the rhinoviruses can apparently change their immunologic reactivity very readily.

One potential way to treat colds might be with *interferon*. Interferons are one of the body's lines of defense against infection and are naturally pro-duced by cells attacked by viruses. Interferons do not prevent viruses from entering cells but bind to receptors on cell surfaces and induce the synthesis of enzymes that inhibit viral replication. Interferon is being widely and rapidly studied—not just for the common cold but for cancer and other major infections. In one study volunteers were given "a nasal spray of interferon one day before and three days after they were exposed to common cold viruses."[22] *None* of those volunteers developed symptoms while 80% of the placebo control group did!

Viruses damage or kill the cells they attack. The rhinoviruses zero in on the upper respiratory tract, at first causing irritation that may lead to reflex coughing and sneezing. Increased irritation inflames the tissue and is followed by soreness and swelling of the mucous membranes. As a defense against infection, the mucous membranes release considerable fluid, which causes the "stuffed-up feeling."

Although the incubation period may be a week in some cases, the more common interval between infection and respiratory tract symptoms is 2 to 4 days. Prior to the onset of respiratory symptoms, the individual may just "feel bad" and develop joint aches and headaches. When fever does occur, it almost always develops early in the cold.

Most of us grew up believing that colds are

Your turn: learning about OTC drugs

There's no substitute for hands-on experience when it comes to understanding the makeup of OTC drugs. A good exercise is to take your book to the local drugstore, use it as a guide, and go through the products systematically. Read the ingredients on a label, then compare them with what you have learned about ingredients from this chapter. (Look for each ingredient in Table 12-3).

Look specifically for the five cold remedies in Table 12-2. Have the formulations changed since this table was prepared in 1989? If a different ingredient is present, is it found in only one or in several products?

If you also take a calculator, you can compare prices per milligram of active ingredient. You will no doubt find a wide range of costs, especially if the store carries its own or a generic brand.

One further exercise: see how many different formulations you can find with the same brand name. In other words, how many different kinds of Dristan or Contac or Anacin are there?

After this experience, the next time you go to a drug store to buy an OTC product, you should feel much more comfortable with your ability to make a good selection.

---

passed by airborne particles jet propelled usually through unobstructed sneezing. ("Cover your mouth! Cover your face!") The old wives—and the old scientists—were wrong. You need to know four things so you can avoid the cold viruses of others—and avoid reinfecting yourself:

1. Up to 100 times as many viruses are produced and shed from the nasal mucosa as from the throat.
2. There are few viruses in the saliva of a person with a cold, probably no viruses at all in about half of these individuals.
3. Dried viruses survive on dry skin and nonporous surfaces—plastic, wood, and so on—for over 3 hours.

Usually colds start by the fingers picking up viruses and then the individual rubs his eyes or picks his nose. In one study of adults with colds 40% had viruses on their hands but only 8% expelled viruses in coughs or sneezes.[23] The moral of the story is clear. To avoid colds: wash your hands frequently, and you may kiss, but not hold hands with your sweetheart! You don't have to worry about your pets—only man and some apes are susceptible to colds.[24]

The experimental animal of choice for studying colds has to be the human. In many studies with human volunteers, three types of findings seem to recur. First, not all who are directly exposed to a cold virus develop cold symptoms. In fact, only about 50% do. Second, in individuals with already existing antibodies to the virus, there may be only preliminary signs of a developing cold. These signs may last for a brief period (12 to 24 hours) and then disappear. The last finding crosses swords with the old wives, so it is best to quote:

Chilling experiments with volunteers did not show any particular influence on susceptibility to colds. Some volunteers were given an inoculation followed by a hot bath and made to stand in a draft in wet bathing suits. Some took walks in the rain and sat around in wet clothes. Other subjects were given the same chilling treatments with inoculations which contained no virus. No significant differences were found in these various well-controlled groups.[25]

Treating Cold Symptoms

Although there is no cure for a cold and no treatment that will reduce its duration, some of the symptoms can be relieved. Because these cold symptoms are fairly complex, most cold remedies have traditionally included several active ingredients, each aimed at a particular type of symptom. In some ways, the FDA's Cold, Cough, Allergy, Bronchodilator, and Antiasthmatic Advisory Review Panel probably had the most difficult job: multiple symptoms, many ingredients for each symptom, and rapid changes in scientific evidence during the time they have been studying these products. In the preliminary report, issued in 1976, the panel placed less than half the 119 ingredients it reviewed into Category I. Most went into Category III. The *Tentative Final Monograph* was published in 1985,[26] and several ingredients were recommended for approval or for shifting to OTC status that had not been available when the panel started its job.

There are three common types of ingredient in modern cold remedies: *antihistamines*, for the temporary relief of runny nose and sneezing; *nasal decongestants*, for temporary relief of swollen membranes in the nasal passages, and *analgesic-antipyretics*, for the temporary relief of aches and pains and to reduce fever. The 1985 FDA list included 10 antihistamines in Category I, but by far the most common antihistamine to be found on the shelves is **chlorpheniramine maleate**. The 1985 list had 13 Category I nasal decongestants. These are primarily sympathomimetics, including our old friend ephedrine and **pseudoephedrine**. The FDA deferred a decision on phenylpropanolamine (PPA), which is also found in OTC weight-control products, until a later date. In 1989 the most common nasal decongestants in cold remedies were pseudoephedrine and PPA. The anal-

gesic-antipyretic may be either aspirin or acetaminophen, but acetaminophen is the more common ingredient.

Table 12-2 gives recent formulations for five popular OTC cold remedies. Note that three of them also contain the cough suppressant **dextromethorphan**, which is the most common active ingredient in OTC cough medicines.

It is ironic that the one type of ingredient found in almost every cold remedy since before the FDA began its review continues to be under attack. The FDA advisory panel had serious questions about the data supporting the effectiveness of antihistamines in treating colds, and their first report relegated them to Category III. Although some studies have since reported that chlorpheniramine maleate is better than placebo at reducing runny noses, prompting the FDA to move several antihistamines to Category I, more recent controlled experiments have not found any benefit. A 1987 symposium of specialists concluded that ". . . anti-

---

Table 12-2

Ingredients in selected brand name OTC cold and allergy products

Brand	Sympathomimetic	Antihistamine	Analgesic	Cough suppressant	Other
Comtrex*	12.5 phenylpropanolamine HCl	2 chlorpheniramine maleate	325 acetaminophen	10 dextromethorphan hydrobromide	
Contac*	75 phenylpropanolamine HCl	8 chlorpheniramine maleate			
Tylenol Cold*	30 pseudoephedrine HCl	2 chlorpheniramine maleate	325 acetaminophen	15 dextromethorphan hydrobromide	
Dristan (capsules*)	5 phenylephrine HCl	2 chlorpheniramine maleate	325 acetaminophen		
NyQuil†	60 pseudoephedrine HCl	7.5 doxylamine succinate	1000 acetaminophen	30 dextromethorphan hydrobromide	25% alcohol

*mg/tablet.
†mg/adult dose (1 ounce).

histamines do not have a place in the management of upper respiratory infection, though they continue to be useful for allergy". In 1989, Consumer Reports magazine called on the FDA to remove antihistamines from cold remedies,[27] and that may happen.

Allergy and Sinus Medications

There are other related products on your pharmacists' shelves. In addition to the cough medicines, there are *allergy* relief pills that rely mainly on the same antihistamine, chlorpheniramine maleate, to slow down the runny nose. There are *sinus* medicines that use one of the sympathomimetic nasal decongestants (PPA or pseudoephedrine), often combined with an analgesic, to reduce swollen sinus passages and treat sinus headache.

CHOOSING AN OTC PRODUCT

By now you should be getting the idea that, thanks to the FDA's decision to review ingredients rather than individual formulations, you as a consumer can now review and choose among the great variety of products by knowing just a few ingredients

and what they are intended to accomplish. Table 12-3 lists only eight ingredients. Those eight are the major active ingredients to be found in different combinations in OTC stimulants, sleep aids, weight-control products, analgesics, cold, cough, allergy and sinus medications!

Want to treat your cold without buying a combination cold remedy? If you have aches and pains, take your favorite analgesic. For the vast majority of colds, the slight elevation in temperature should probably not be treated, as it is not dangerous and may even help to fight the infection.[28] Unless the body temperature remains at 103° F or above or reaches 105° F, fever is not considered dangerous. If you have a runny nose, you may or may not get relief from an antihistamine. Generic chlorpheniramine maleate or a store brand allergy tablet is an inexpensive source. These will probably give you a dry mouth and may produce some sedation or drowsiness (which, of course, is why some of the more sedating antihistamines are used in sleep aids). Stuffed-up nose? Pseudoephedrine nose drops will shrink swollen membranes for a time. Although oral sympathomimetics are also effective, nose drops are more effective. You can find these ingredients in sinus preparations (or weight-con-

---

Table 12-3

Common OTC ingredients

Ingredient	Action	Source
Acetylsalicylic acid (ASA; aspirin)	Analgesic-antipyretic	Headache remedies, arthritis formulas, cold and sinus remedies
Acetaminophen	Analgesic-antipyretic	Headache remedies, cold and sinus remedies
Caffeine	Stimulant	"Alertness" medications
Chlorpheniramine maleate	Antihistamine	Cold remedies, allergy products
Dextromethorphan	Antitussive	Cough suppressants, cold remedies
Diphenhydramine	Antihistamine	Sleep aids, some cold remedies
Phenylpropanolamine (PPA)	Sympathomimetic	Weight-control products, cold and sinus remedies
Pseudoephedrine	Sympathomimetic	Cold and sinus remedies

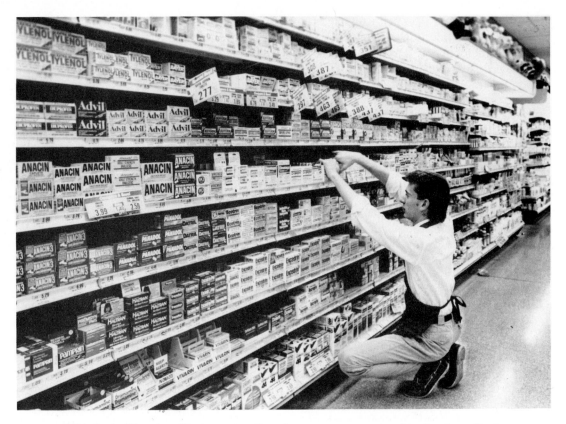

What looks like a bewildering array of products may represent only a few ingredients.

trol products!). However, these sympathomimetics should be used cautiously. There is a rapid tolerance to their effects, and, if they are used repeatedly, a rebound stuffiness may develop when they are stopped. Cough? Dextromethorphan can be obtained in cough medications.

Why not buy all this in one tablet or capsule? That's a common approach. But why treat symptoms you don't have? During the course of a cold, a runny nose might occur at one time, congestion at another, and coughing not at all. By using just the ingredients you need, when you need them, you might save money, and you have the satisfaction of being a connoisseur of colds. For many colds, no treatment at all might be the best treatment.

SUMMARY

OTC drugs are used by millions of Americans who take them for headaches, colds, and other mild ailments. A drug can be sold OTC only if it can be used safely when following the label directions. The FDA has been reviewing OTC ingredients for safety and efficacy, and the result has been that most of the various brands of medicines sold for a given use contain the same few ingredients.

Although psychoactive OTC drugs represent a relatively small share of the overall market, it is still an important share. The OTC stimulants and sleep aids are much less potent than the stimulant and depressant drugs covered in Chapters 7 and 8. The main ingredient in OTC weight-control

---

Issue: quackery and nutrition supplements

The May 1985 *Consumer Reports* contained an exposé entitled "Foods, Drugs or Frauds." In related articles the magnitude of the problem became clear: products are being sold as cancer treatments, for herpes prevention, and other health-related uses. However, because the products are marketed as "nutrition supplements" rather than as "drugs," the manufacturers have been selling them in health food stores and door-to-door without bothering to demonstrate effectiveness to the FDA. How do they get away with this? A product is considered to be a drug if it is "intended for use in the diagnosis, cure, mitigation, treatment, or prevention of disease in man or animal." The companies are careful not to print such claims directly on the label, because FDA regulations are quite explicit about claims made on a product label. Instead, the claims may be made in literature found in the store nearby, or they may be made verbally by the seller. This makes it more difficult for the FDA to prove that a nutrition supplement is being sold as a drug. Mail-order companies may use delivery services other than the U.S. Postal Service to avoid federal mail-fraud statutes.

Consumer Reports claimed that the FDA has "pretty much thrown in the towel" when it comes to prosecuting these companies. Of the agency's budget of over $350 million, about $1.8 million went to combat health quackery. This included public education programs and civil actions (seeking injunctions and seizing merchandise). In the 22 years before the 1985 article, the FDA had undertaken only two criminal prosecutions involving fraudulent nutrition supplements. Why? The FDA now has so much responsibility for reviewing and regulating the products of legitimate manufacturers that fighting quackery has become a lower priority.

---

products, PPA, is still under review by the FDA and may or may not receive final approval. Cold remedies may seem to represent a great variety of confusing products. However, when analyzed according to symptoms and ingredients, the picture is found to be much simpler. Currently an informed consumer can understand a large fraction of all the medicines in a drug store by knowing only eight ingredients.

REFERENCES

1. Up-front thrills and chills, Drug Topics April 18, 1988, pp. 34-50.
2. Edwards, CC: Closing the gap, FDA Papers Reprint, February 1973.
3. FDA: OTC stimulant drug products, final monograph, Federal Register February 29, 1988.
4. Summaries of court actions, FDA Consumer, May, 1985, p. 42.
5. Willis J: In FDA Consumer, July-August, 1985, pp. 27-29.
6. Glynn CJ: Factors that influence the perception of intractable pain, Medical Times 108(3):11s-26s, March 1980.
7. Beecher HK: Placebo effects of situations, attitudes and drugs: a quantitative study of suggestibility. In Rickels K, editor: Non-specific factors in drug therapy, Springfield, Ill., 1968, Charles C Thomas, Publisher.
8. Smith LH, Jr, Chairman, Medical Staff Conference: The clinical pharmacology of salicylates, California Medicine 110:411, 413, 1969.
9. Parkhouse J and others: The clinical dose response to aspirin, British Journal of Anaesthesiology 40:433-441, 1968.
10. Wiseman EH and Federici NJ: Development of a sustained-release aspirin tablet, Journal of Pharmaceutical Sciences 57:1535-1539, 1968.
11. Wolff BB and others: Response of experimental pain to analgesic drugs. III. Codeine, aspirin, secobarbital, and placebo, Clinical Pharmacology and Therapeutics 10:217-228, 1969.
12. FDA: Internal analgesic, antipyretic, and antirheumatic drug products for OTC human use; tentative final monograph. Federal Register November 16, 1988.
13. Amrein PC and others: Aspirin-induced prolongation of bleeding time and perioperative blood loss, Journal of the American Medical Association 245(18):1825-1828, 1981.
14. Weiss HJ: Aspirin—a dangerous drug? Journal of the American Medical Association 229:1221-1222, 1974.
15. Stanley ED and others: Increased virus shedding with aspirin treatment of rhinovirus infection, Journal of the American Medical Association 231:1248-1251, 1975.
16. Pottathil R and others: Establishment of the interferon-mediated antiviral state: role of fatty acid cyclooxygenase, Proceedings of the National Academy of Sciences of the USA 77(9):5437-5440, 1980.

17. Kolata G: Study of Reye's-aspirin link raises concerns, Science 227:392, 1985.

18. Remington PL and others: Decreasing trends in Reye's syndrome and aspirin use in Michigan—1979 to 1984, Pediatrics 77:93-98, 1986.

19. Vane JR: The mode of action of aspirin and similar compounds, Hospital Formulary, p. 628, November 1976.

20. Penna RP, project director: Handbook of nonprescription drugs, ed, 5, Project Drugs, Washington, D.C., 1977, American Pharmaceutical Association.

21. Dickens C: The collected letters of Charles Dickens, 1880, Chapman & Hall Ltd.

22. The big IF in cancer—will the natural drug interferon fulfill its early promise, Time, pp. 60-66, March 31, 1980.

23. Klumpp TG: The common cold—new concepts of transmission and prevention, Medical Times, 108(11):98, 1s-3s, November 1980.

24. Tyrell DAJ: Hunting common cold viruses by some new methods, Journal of Infectious Diseases 121:561-571, 1970.

25. Adams JM: Viruses and colds, the modern plague, New York, 1967, American Elsevier Publishing Co., Inc.

26. Federal Register 50:10, January 15, 1985.

27. Cold remedies: which ones work best? Consumer Reports, January, 1989, pp. 6-11.

28. FDA Consumer 19(9):16, November, 1985.

Chapter 13

Psychotherapeutic Drugs

OBJECTIVES

After reading this chapter, you should be able to:

Explain the medical model of mental disorders and how that model relates to drug therapy.

Describe the major symptoms associated with anxiety disorders, psychosis, and the mood disorders.

Discuss some of the approaches to drug treatment that were used before 1950.

List the names of some of the antipsychotic and antidepressant drugs and know how they work and how effective they are.

Explain why lithium was so slow in being introduced to the U.S. market and for what conditions it is now used.

For most of today's mentally ill, the primary mode of therapy has become drug therapy. Powerful psychoactive medications help to control psychotic behavior, depression, and mania in thousands of patients, reducing human suffering and health care costs. Yet these drugs are far from cures, and they often have undesirable side effects. Should mental disorders be approached with chemical treatments? Do these treatments actually work? How do they work? What can these drugs tell us about the causes of mental illness? Although we don't yet have complete answers to any of these questions, we do have partial answers for all of them.

MENTAL ILLNESS
The Medical Model

The use of a term such as **mental illness** seems for some to imply a particular model for behavioral disorders or dysfunctions. The medical model, which has been attacked by both psychiatrists (who are medical doctors) and psychologists (who generally hold a doctorate), is supposed to entail the following notions: a patient appears with a set of **symptoms,** and on the basis of these symptoms a **diagnosis** is made as to which **disease** the patient is suffering from. Once the disease is known, its **cause** can be determined and the patient provided with a **cure.** Such a model seems

---

Anxiety disorders

Panic disorder (with or without agoraphobia)

One or more panic attacks that were unexpected and not triggered by situations in which the person was the focus of others' attention. These panic attacks are characterized by such symptoms as shortness of breath, dizziness or faintness, palpitations or accelerated heart rate, trembling, sweating, choking, numbness, fear of dying, fear of going crazy or doing something uncontrolled.

The agoraphobia (fear of the marketplace) that often accompanies panic disorder is a fear of being in places or situations from which escape might be difficult or help might not be available in the event of a panic attack. The person may then avoid going outside the home alone, or be afraid of being in a crowded place or standing in a line.

Social phobia

These patients fear and avoid potentially embarassing situations (speaking in public, going into public restrooms).

Simple phobia

An irrational fear of a specific object or situation (e.g., claustrophobia, fear of heights, fear of some type of animal).

Obsessive-compulsive disorder

Recurrent, persistent ideas, images, or impulses that are perceived as involuntary intrusions into consciousness are referred to as obsessions. Compulsions are urgent repetitive behaviors, such as hand washing.

Post-traumatic stress disorder

The person has experienced an event that is outside the range of usual human experience and that would be markedly distressing to almost anyone. The traumatic event is persistently reexperienced through recurring recollections, dreams, a sudden feeling as if the event were occurring.

Generalized anxiety disorder

Unrealistic or excessive anxiety and worry about more than one life circumstance (e.g., finances, academics) for a period of 6 months or longer.

---

to fit well for a disease such as syphilis, in which sores and the presence of spirochetes lead to a specific diagnosis, and the use of antibiotics to kill the spirochetes rids the body of the disease. However, this simple illness model does not fit most behavioral disorders well. A person may be inactive, not say much, not sleep or eat well, and what little they do say might be quite negative. This behavior may lead us to call that person depressed. Does that mean that the person has *a disease* called depression, with a physical cause and a potential cure? Or is calling someone depressed more akin to calling them a name than it is to giving them a diagnosis? The behaviors that we refer to as indicating depression are varied and probably have many causes, most of them not known and we certainly have no cures for them as yet.

In spite of these attacks on the medical model, it still seems to guide much of the current thinking about behavioral disorders. The fact that psychoactive drugs can be effective in controlling symptoms, if not in curing diseases, has lent a great deal of strength to the disease concept. For if chemicals can help to normalize an individual's behavior, a natural assumption might be that the original problem resulted from some chemical imbalance in the brain. If that is so, then perhaps measurements of chemicals in urine, blood, or cerebrospinal fluid could provide more specific and accurate diagnosis and give direction to our efforts at drug therapy.[1] This kind of thinking gives scientists great hope, and many experiments have attempted to find the searched-for chemical imbalances, so far with very little success.

Classification of Mental Disorders

Because human behavior is so variable and because we do not know the causes of most mental disorders, classification of the mentally ill into diagnostic categories is difficult. Nevertheless, there are some basic divisions that are widely used and important for understanding the uses of psychotherapeutic drugs. In 1987 the American Psychiatric Association published the revised third edition of its *Diagnostic and Statistical Manual of Mental Disorders* (often referred to as the DSM-III-R).[2] This manual provides criteria for classifying mental disorders into hundreds of specific diagnostic categories. Partly because of the adoption of this classification system by major health insurance companies, its terms and definitions have become standard for all mental health professionals.

Anxiety is a normal and common human experience: anticipation of potential threats and dangers is often useful in helping to avoid them. When these worries become unrealistic, resulting in chronic uneasiness, fear of impending doom, or bouts of terror or panic, they may interfere with the individual's daily life. Physical symptoms may also be present, often associated with activation of the autonomic nervous system (flushed skin, dilated pupils, gastrointestinal problems, increased heart rate, or shortness of breath). Psychosomatic complaints, phobias, and obsessive-compulsive behaviors are among the symptoms that have often been referred to as **neurotic.** Perhaps because of the use of so-called antianxiety drugs (Chapter 8) in treating these problems, there is a tendency to think of anxiety not as a behavioral symptom but rather as an internal state that *causes* the disorders. The DSM-III-R refers to several types of primary anxiety disorders (see box on p. 254).

Psychosis refers to a major disturbance of normal intellectual and social functioning in which there is loss of contact with reality. Not knowing the current day, month, or year; hearing voices that aren't there; or believing that you are Napoleon or Christ are only some examples of the ways in which this withdrawal from reality may be seen. Many people refer to psychosis as reflecting a primary disorder of *thinking*, as opposed to emotion.

Again psychotic behavior may be viewed as a symptom that can have many possible causes. One important distinction that is made is between the *organic* and the *functional* psychoses. An organic illness is one that has a known physical cause, and psychosis may result from many such things, including brain tumors or infections, metabolic or

---

Schizophrenia

A. Presence of psychotic symptoms (1, 2, or 3) for at least 1 week:
1. Two of the following
   a. Delusions
   b. Prominent hallucinations
   c. Incoherence or marked loosening of associations (illogical)
   d. Catatonic behavior (decreased movement and reaction)
   e. Flat or grossly inappropriate affect (mood)
2. Bizarre delusions (i.e., totally unbelievable)
3. Prominent hallucinations of a voice or voices (long conversations or commentaries, not just a word or two)
B. Functioning in such areas as work, social relations, and self-care is markedly below the highest level achieved before the disturbance.
C. Any periods of depression or mania have been brief relative to the total duration of the disturbance.
D. Continuous signs of the disturbance for at least 6 months.

---

endocrine disorders, degenerative neurological diseases, chronic alcohol use, or high doses of stimulant drugs, such as amphetamine or cocaine. Functional disorders are simply those for which there is no known or obvious physical cause. A person suffering from a chronic psychotic condition for which there is no known cause will probably be diagnosed as **schizophrenic.** There is a popular misconception that schizophrenia means "split personality" and refers to individuals exhibiting multiple personalities. Instead, schizophrenia should probably be translated as *shattered mind.* The DSM-III-R criteria for schizophrenic disorder are given in the box above.

Mood disorders refers to the appearance of depressed and/or manic symptoms. Look back at Fig. 7-2 for one schematic representation of mood in which depression is shown as an abnormally low mood state and mania as an abnormally high mood state. The important distinction in DSM-III-R, and in drug treatment of mood disorders, is between *bipolar disorder*, in which periods of both

---

Mood disorders

I. Manic episode
  A. A distinct period of abnormally and persistently elevated, expansive, or irritable mood.
  B. During the mood disturbance, at least three of the following symptoms have persisted or have been present to a significant degree:
   1. Inflated self-esteem or grandiosity
   2. Decreased need for sleep
   3. More talkative than usual or pressure to keep talking
   4. Flight of ideas or feeling that thoughts are racing
   5. Distractibility
   6. Increase in activity
   7. Excessive involvement in pleasurable activities that have a high potential for painful consequences (shopping, sex, foolish investments)
  C. Mood disturbance sufficiently severe to cause marked impairment in functioning.
  D. No prolonged delusions or hallucinations in the absence of mood symptoms.
II. Major depressive episode
  A. At least five of the following symptoms have been present during a 2-week period and represent a change from previous functioning. At least one of the symptoms is either No. 1 or No. 2:
   1. Depressed mood most of the day, nearly every day
   2. Markedly diminished interest or pleasure in all, or almost all, activities most of the day, nearly every day
   3. Significant weight loss or weight gain or decrease or increase in appetite
   4. Insomnia or hypersomnia
   5. Psychomotor agitation (increased activity) or retardation (decreased activity)
   6. Fatigue or loss of energy
   7. Feelings of worthlessness or excessive guilt
   8. Diminished ability to think or concentrate
   9. Recurrent thoughts of death or suicide or a suicide attempt or plan for committing suicide
  B. Not due to a known organic factor or a normal reaction to the death of a loved one.
  C. No prolonged delusions or hallucinations in the absence of mood symptoms.

---

depression and mania have been observed at some time, and *major depression,* in which only depression is seen. The DSM-III-R criteria for mania and depression are described in the box "Mood Disorders."

You should keep in mind that individual human beings often don't easily fit the textbook definitions and that in many cases assigning a diagnosis and selecting a treatment are more matters of experience and art than they are of science. For example, a person may display both abnormal mood states and bizarre thinking. If it is assumed that the disturbance of thinking is the primary disorder, and that the abnormal mood is secondary, then the individual will likely be called a schizophrenic. Another professional might see the mood disorder as primary, with the crazy talk just supporting a negative view of the world and call the person depressed.

TREATMENT OF MENTAL DISORDERS
Before 1950

Over the centuries, mental patients have been subjected to various kinds of treatment, depending on the views held at the time regarding the causes of mental illness. Since we are concerned with drug therapy, a good place to begin our history is in 1917, when a physical treatment was first demonstrated to be effective in serious mental disease. In those days a great proportion of the psychotic patients were suffering from *general paresis,* a syphilitic infection of the nervous system. It was noticed that the fever associated with malaria often produced marked improvement, and so in 1917 "malaria therapy" was introduced in the treatment of general paresis. Of course, the later discovery of antibiotics that could cure syphilis have all but eliminated this particular type of organic psychosis.

In the 1920s some of the more wealthy patients could afford to go in for a course of "narcosis therapy," in which barbiturates and other depressants were used to induce sleep for as long as a week or more. Another use of sedative drugs was in conjunction with psychotherapy: an intravenous dose of sodium pentothal, a rapid-acting barbiturate, would relax a person and produce more talking during psychotherapy. The theory was that by reducing inhibitions the patient could bring out repressed thoughts; thus the term *truth serum* came to be used for sodium pentothal or for scopolamine, an anticholinergic drug used similarly. Anyone who has ever heard someone talking after drinking a good bit of alcohol will tell you that they may be less inhibited, but this doesn't necessarily always result in the truth being spoken. So-called truth sera apparently worked about as well.

In 1933, Manfred Sakel of Vienna induced coma in some schizophrenics by the administration of insulin. The resulting drop in blood glucose level caused the brain's neurons to first increase their activity and produce convulsions and then to decrease their activity and leave the patient in a coma. A course of 30 to 50 of these treatments over a 2- to 3-month period was said to be highly effective, and discharge rates of 90% were reported in the early years of insulin shock therapy. Later studies demonstrated that the relapse rate was quite high, and this treatment has been abandoned.

Ladislas von Meduna believed strongly that epilepsy and schizophrenia were mutually exclusive illnesses. He had observed, incorrectly, that no epileptic was schizophrenic, and no schizophrenic ever had epilepsy. Reasoning that the epileptic convulsions prevented the development of schizophrenia, he felt that inducing convulsions might have therapeutic value for these patients. His first convulsant drug was camphor, but it had disadvantages, the major one being a time lag of hours between injection and the convulsions. In 1934 he started injecting Metrazol (pentylenetetrazol), which induced convulsions in less than 30 seconds, and reported improvement rates in schizophrenics of 50% to 60%.

The use of a drug was not ideal for inducing convulsions, since the 30-second interval between injections and loss of consciousness (with the convulsion) produced much anguish in the patient. Ugo Cerletti, after experimenting on pigs in a slaughterhouse, developed the technique of using electric shock to induce convulsions. This method has the advantage of inducing loss of consciousness and convulsion at the moment the electric shock is applied.

Electroconvulsive therapy (ECT) is hardly ever used now with schizophrenics. Although early work in the 1930s and 1940s suggested high improvement rates, later studies found only about half showing a reduction of schizophrenic symptoms, and the relapse rates were high. ECT is still used with severely depressed patients.[3]

By the 1950s, probably the major drug in use for severely disturbed patients in the large mental hospitals was **paraldehyde,** a sedative introduced in Chapter 8. Although producing little respiratory depression and therefore safer than the barbiturates, the drug has a characteristic odor that is still well remembered by those who worked in or visited the hospitals of that era. Sedation of severely disturbed patients by drugs that make them drowsy and slow them down has been referred to as using a "chemical straitjacket."

Antipsychotics

A number of people were involved in the discovery that a group of drugs called the **phenothiazines** had special properties when used with mental patients. Credit is usually given to a French surgeon, Laborit, who tested these compounds first in conjunction with surgical anesthesia. He noted that the most effective of these phenothiazines, chlorpromazine, did not by itself induce drowsiness or a loss of consciousness, but it seemed to make the patients unconcerned about their upcoming surgery. He reasoned that this effect might reduce emotionality in psychiatric patients and encouraged its use with them. The first report of these French trials of chlorpromazine in mental patients mentioned that the patients were not only calmed, but the drug seemed to act on the psychotic process itself. This new type of drug action fairly quickly attracted a variety of names: in the United States the drugs were generally called tranquilizers, which some now think was an unfortunate term that focuses on the calming action and seems to imply sedation. Another term used was *neuroleptic,* meaning taking hold of the nervous system, a term implying an increased amount of control. Although both terms are still in wide use, most medical texts now refer to this group of drugs as **antipsychotics,** reflecting their special ability to reduce psychotic symptoms in schizophrenics and in other types of psychosis without necessarily producing drowsiness and sedation.

One of the early reports (1955) dealing with the side effects of chlorpromazine on a large number of hospitalized psychotic patients stated that:

> . . . [it] produces marked quieting of the motor manifestations. Patients cease to be loud and profane, the tendency to hyperbolic associations diminished, and the patients can sit still long enough to eat and to take care of normal physiological needs. . . .
>
> In the more chronic psychotic states, the effect of the drug is much less immediately dramatic, but, for those experienced with the relief of psychotic symptoms from other measures, the use of the drug produces results that are equally gratifying when compared with results in the more acute situations.[4]

This early evaluation was well founded, as suggested by the following statement made in 1976:

> Since chlorpromazine . . . and . . . subsequent antipsychotic drugs . . . have had profound effects on . . . psychiatry, reducing the lengths of hospitalization for schizophrenic patients and permitting many patients to be handled in the community in ways not heretofore even anticipated, it is remarkable that no Nobel Prize in medicine has been awarded to the discoverers of chlorpromazine.[5,p.13]

The tremendous impact of phenothiazine treatment on the management of hospitalized psy-

chotics is clear from a 1955 statement by the director of the Delaware State Hospital:

> We have now achieved . . . the reorganization of the management of disturbed patients. With rare exceptions, all restraints have been discontinued. The hydrotherapy department, formerly active on all admission services and routinely used on wards with disturbed patients, has ceased to be in operation. Maintenance EST [electroshock treatment] for disturbed patients has been discontinued . . . There has been a record increase in participation by these patients in social and occupational activities.
>
> These developments have vast sociological implications. I believe it is fair to state that pharmacology promises to accomplish what other measures have failed to bring about—the social emancipation of the mental hospital.[6,pp.83-84]

Treatment effects and considerations. Paralleling an increase in the use of phenothiazines in the treatment of the mentally ill was the increase in the sophistication of experimental programs that evaluate the effectiveness of various drugs. Results from these studies show clearly that phenothiazine-treated patients improve more than patients receiving placebo or no treatments. In an NIMH study, after 6 weeks 75% of acute schizophrenics receiving phenothiazines showed either moderate or marked improvement, whereas of those receiving placebos only 23% improved. One summary of the double-blind, controlled studies found that 106 studies reported that phenothiazine treatment of psychotics was more effective than placebo treatment, while only 24 found it to be no better than placebo treatment.[7] In each of the 24 studies where phenothiazines were not shown to be significantly better treatment than placebo, low doses of the drug were used. Even then there were nonsignificant trends favoring phenothiazine treatment.

"Ninety-five percent of acute schizophrenic patients treated with a drug given in an adequate dose will show some improvement within 6 to 8 weeks. More than 50% . . . will improve moderately to markedly . . . "[8,p.203] From the sixth to the twelfth week some improvement is still occurring, but beyond that there is little if any change. It is important to remember that the actions of the phenothiazines are much more specific than the term "tranquilizer" implies.

The inappropriateness of the term "tranquilizer" is evident when the pattern of response produced by antipsychotic drugs is examined. They certainly do more than simply calm patients or put them in a "chemical straitjacket." The core symptoms of schizophrenia are consistently improved: emotional withdrawal, hallucinations, delusions and other disturbed thinking, paranoid projection, belligerence, hostility and blunted affect. On the other hand, somatic complaints, anxiety and tension, symptoms which might ordinarily be favorably affected by a "tranquilizer," are not much changed . . . [9,p.4]

Another aspect of evaluating the effectiveness of drug treatment is determining the incidence of relapse or symptom recurrence when treatment is discontinued. It is most likely that discontinuation of drug therapy will lead to relapse in 75% to 95% of patients within a year and in more than 50% of patients in 6 months.[10] Almost all studies report that when medication is resumed, there is again a reduction in symptoms.[11] It has been shown that antipsychotic medication can be withdrawn 2 or 3 days a week without relapse occurring in "chronic schizophrenics on maintenance chemotherapy" in mental hospitals.[12]

Some patients respond to one phenothiazine and not to another, a few don't respond to any of them. No one is quite sure why. It may be that the phenothiazine does not get absorbed and thus does not reach the bloodstream and then the brain. Blood levels of the phenothiazines are difficult to do but a majority of the few studies that have been done show a relationship between blood levels and clinical effectiveness.[13] One review phrased the problem of "no effect with treatment" very briefly: "The most common cause of treatment failure in acute psychosis is an inadequate dose, and the most common cause of relapse is patient noncompliance."[8,p.202]

One study[14] is of particular interest, since within a single hospital, using five wards, it compared the effectiveness *and the cost* of each of five treatment methods in first-admission schizo-

---

Your turn: should a patient be forced to take a drug?

Should a person be forced to take medication against his or her will? It is often the case that psychotic patients are quite suspicious of the doctors and other personnel with whom they interact, and often the patient doesn't want to take medication. If the patient has been committed to the hospital, then the doctors are expected to give them appropriate medical care, even if this means physically restraining the individual while an injection of an antipsychotic drug is given.

These drugs are not without their side effects, and in an ideal world the individual patient could be given the pros and cons and allowed the choice. In this case, the more the patient needs the medication, the more obvious it is that he or she is incapable of making a rational choice. So patients are often cajoled into taking the medications or are given them against their will.

There are some who consider this forced drugging to be an unconscionable invasion of the person's body, akin to rape, and would never allow anyone to force another to take a drug. What's your opinion? Could you draw up a proposed set of rules and regulations establishing conditions under which a person could be forced to take a drug?

---

phrenics. The five methods were (1) individual psychotherapy, (2) phenothiazine medication, (3) methods 1 and 2, (4) electroshock, and (5) milieu, in which social interactions and support and understanding are the keystones. Effectiveness was measured by the release rate within a year of admission. The percent of patients discharged in each of the five groups was 64%, 95%, 96%, 79%, and 59%, respectively. Clearly medication was the most significant factor. The cost to treat each patient until discharge or for 1 year if not released is given here in rounded figures (the costs are for 1965): (1) $7,200, (2) $3,000, (3) $3,600, (4) $4,400, and (5) $6,200. All mental health workers know generally this state of affairs, but it seems important to emphasize it. The use of antipsychotic drugs in the treatment of schizophrenics is not only the most effective treatment, it is also the least expensive. One study[15] has shown that a *very* intensive (and thereby expensive) psychotherapy and psychosocial hospital treatment program can perhaps provide even more effective treatment than a program based on medication. The program unfortunately cannot be widely adopted because of its high requirement of professional time.

In the years since 1950, many new phenothiazines have been introduced, and several completely new types of antipsychotic drugs have been discovered. The ones on the U.S. market are listed in Table 13-1. These drugs vary considerably in how much sedation accompanies their antipsychotic effect, and physicians tend to select among the drugs depending partly on how much sedation they feel is called for. For example, in 1987 the two biggest selling antipsychotic brands were Mellaril, one of the most sedating, and Haldol, one of the least sedating.

Mechanism of antipsychotic action.   For several years it was difficult to know which of the many biochemical effects of these drugs was responsible for their antipsychotic action. The phenothiazines tend to block the receptors for norepinephrine, dopamine, acetylcholine, serotonin, and histamine. Since the antipsychotic drugs vary widely in how much it takes to produce a clinical response (clinical potency) and in biochemical affinity for these various receptors, it was possible to demonstrate a strong correlation between dopamine-receptor binding and clinical potency. It is therefore now accepted that the antipsychotic effect is a result of blockade of dopamine receptors.[16]

Side effects of antipsychotics.   Two positive aspects of the antipsychotics are that they are not addictive, and it is extremely difficult to use them to commit suicide. Some allergic reactions may be noted, such as jaundice or skin rashes. Some patients exhibit photosensitivity, a tendency for the skin to darken and burn easily in sunlight. These reactions have a low incidence and usually decrease or disappear with a reduction in dosage. *Agranulocytosis*, low white blood cell count of unknown origin, can develop in the early stages of

Table 13-1		
Antipyschotic drugs		
Generic name	Brand name	Usual dose range (mg/day)
Phenothiazines		
Chlorpromazine	Thorazine	100-2000
Triflupromazine	Vesprin	20-150
Thioridizine	Mellaril	100-600
Mesoridazine	Serentil	100-400
Trifluoperazine	Stelazine	5-60
Acetophenazine	Tindal	20-100
Fluphenazine	Permitil, Prolixin	5-60
Perphenazine	Trilafon	8-64
Proclorperazine	Compazine	10-150
Other chemical classes		
Clorprothixene	Taractan	100-600
Thiothixene	Navane	5-60
Haloperidol	Haldol	2-100
Loxapine	Loxitane	30-250
Molindone	Moban	10-225

treatment. It is extremely rare, but has a high mortality, perhaps 50%.

The most common side effects of antipsychotic medication involve the extrapyramidal motor system. The major extrapyramidal effects include a wide range of signs from facial tics to symptoms that resemble Parkinson's disease: tremors of the hands when they are at rest; muscular rigidity, including a mask-like face; and a shuffling walk. You may remember that Parkinson's disease results from damage to the dopamine neurons in the basal ganglia and that it is now treated with a dopamine precursor, L-dopa. The antipsychotic drug-induced pseudoparkinsonism is a result of the blockade of dopamine receptors in the basal ganglia. L-dopa is not used to treat these symptoms because it has a tendency to worsen psychotic symptoms. However, before the introduction of L-dopa, Parkinson's disease was treated with anticholinergic drugs that block receptors in the output pathways from the basal ganglia. These anticholinergic antiparkinson drugs are used to control the extrapyramidal side effects of the antipsychotic medications.

The antipsychotic medications vary considerably in their tendency to produce extrapyramidal symptoms, but we now realize this is because of the variance in the amount of anticholinergic activity that the drugs themselves possess. For example, thioridazine (Mellaril), which produces very few extrapyramidal side effects, is about seven times as potent an anticholinergic as chlorpromazine (Thorazine), which is about nine times as anticholinergic as trifluoperazine (Stelazine), which produces many extrapyramidal effects.[17] Haloperidol (Haldol) is almost purely a dopamine antagonist with little anticholinergic activity: it too produces a high incidence of extrapyramidal effects. While some clinicians prefer to use antipsychotic drugs that produce fewer extrapyramidal effects, others prefer to treat the psychotic symptoms with a more pure dopamine antagonist and to separately treat the extrapyramidal symptoms as necessary with an anticholinergic, such as benztropine (Cogentin).

Tardive dyskinesia is the most serious complication of antipsychotic drug treatment and its prevalence among inpatients treated with antipsychotic drugs is now about 25%. Although first observed in the late 1950s, it was not viewed as a major problem until the mid-70s, 20 years after these drugs were introduced.[18] The term *tardive dyskinesia* means "late-appearing abnormal movements" and refers primarily to "slow, rhythmical movements in the region of the mouth with protrusion of the tongue, smacking of the lips, blowing of the cheeks, and side-to-side movements of the chin, as well as other bizarre muscular activity."[19,pp.126-127] The fact that this syndrome usually occurs only after years of antipsychotic drug treatment and that the symptoms persist and sometimes increase when medication is stopped raised the possibility of irreversible changes. The current belief is that tardive dyskinesia is the result of supersensitivity of the dopaminergic receptors. Although reversal of the symptoms seems possible, the best treatment is prevention, which can be accomplished through early detection and an immediate lowering of the level of medication. There is still debate over the relative importance of age, dosage level, and years on medication in the onset of tardive dyskinesia.

Antidepressants

Monoamine oxidase inhibitors. The story of the antidepressant drugs starts with the fact that tuberculosis was a major chronic illness until about 1955. In 1952 preliminary reports suggested that a new drug, isoniazid, was effective in treating tuberculosis; isoniazid and similar drugs that followed were responsible for the emptying of hospital beds. One of the antituberculosis drugs was iproniazid, which was introduced simultaneously with isoniazid but was withdrawn as too toxic. Clinical reports on its use in tuberculosis hospitals emphasized that there was considerable elevation of mood in the patients receiving iproniazid. These reports were followed up, and the drug was reintroduced as an antidepressant agent in 1955 on the basis of early promising studies with depressed patients.

Iproniazid is a **monamine oxidase (MAO) inhibitor,** and its discovery opened up a new class of compounds for investigation. Although several MAO inhibitors were introduced over the years, toxicity and side effects have limited use and reduced their number. Iproniazid itself was removed from sale in 1961 after being implicated in at least 54 fatalities. Currently there are three MAO inhibitors on the U.S. market: isocarboxazid (Marplan), phenelzine (Nardil), and tranylcypromine (Parnate). A major limitation to the use of the MAO inhibitors is that they alter the normal metabolism of a dietary amino acid, tyramine, such that if an individual consumes foods with a high tyramine content while taking MAO inhibitors, a hypertensive (high blood pressure) crisis may result. Since aged cheeses are one source of tyramine, this is often referred to as the "cheese reaction." A severe headache, palpitations, flushing of the skin, nausea, and vomiting are some symptoms of this reaction, which has in some cases ended in death from a stroke (cerebrovascular accident). Besides other foods and beverages that contain tyramine (chianti wine, smoked or pickled fish, and many others), patients taking MAO inhibitors must also avoid sympathomimetic drugs, such as amphetamines, methylphenidate, and phenylpropanolamine (PPA).

MAO is an enzyme involved in the breakdown of serotonin, norepinephrine, and dopamine, and its inhibition results in increased availability of these neurotransmitters at the synapse. Just how such a change is translated into antidepressant action is not clear. Recently it has been determined that there are two types of MAO, called MAO-A and MAO-B. An experimental drug, chlorgyline, that selectively inhibits MAO-A seems to be a more effective antidepressant than drugs that act primarily on MAO-B.[20] Thus we may see the development of new and more effective antidepressant agents of this type.

Tricyclic antidepressants. Sometimes when you are looking for one thing, you find something entirely different. This happened with the phenothiazine antipsychotics, which were first tested as antihistamines. The MAO inhibitors were found among antituberculosis agents. The most important group of antidepressants was identified in a search for better antipsychotic agents.

The basic phenothiazine structure consists of three rings, with various side chains for the different drugs. Imipramine resulted from a slight change in the middle of the three rings and was tested in 1958 on a group of patients. The drug had little effect on psychotic symptoms, but improved the mood of depressed patients. This was the first **tricyclic** antidepressant, and many more have followed. In addition, other compounds have been introduced that do not have a tricyclic structure. Table 13-2 lists some current heterocyclic antidepressants. Although these drugs are not effective in all patients, most controlled clinical trials do find that depressive episodes are less severe and resolve more quickly if the patients are treated with one of these antidepressants than if they are given a placebo.

Table 13-2

Heterocyclic antidepressant drugs

Generic name	Brand name	Usual dose range (mg/day)
Tricyclics		
Imipramine	Tofranil, Janimine	150-300
Amitriptyline	Elavil, Endep	150-300
Nortriptyline	Aventyl, Pamelor	75-150
Desipramine	Norpramine, Pertofrane	75-200
Protriptyline	Vivactil	20-60
Doxepin	Sinequan, Adapin	150-300
Other chemical classes		
Amoxapine	Asendin	150-600
Maprotiline	Ludiomil	75-300
Trazodone	Desyrel	150-600

Mechanism of antidepressant action. The original tricyclics interfere with the reuptake into the terminal of the neurotransmitters norepinephrine and serotonin. This results in an increased availability of these neurotransmitters at the synapse. Since MAO inhibition also results in increased availability of the same neurotransmitters, there has been considerable speculation that the antidepressant actions of both classes of drugs result from increased synaptic availability of either norepinephrine or serotonin or both. However, the antidepressant effect of either the tricyclics or the MAO inhibitors exhibits a "lag period": the patients must be treated for about 2 weeks before improvement is seen. The biochemical effects on enzymes or reuptake occur in a matter of minutes. Also, some of the tricyclics are fairly selective inhibitors of the reuptake of norephinephrine, some selectively block reuptake of serotonin, and some have about equal effects on both neurotransmitters. Although it has been suggested that some patients might benefit more from one type than another, experiments have so far failed to reveal any rational basis for choosing among the drugs in any individual case, and overall the effectiveness of the drug does not seem to depend on which of the two neutrotransmitters is more affected.

Current theories of the antidepressant action of these agents focus less on the direct biochemical effects of the drugs than on the reaction of the neurons to those direct effects. For example, after prolonged exposure to all the antidepressants, there is a decreased number of receptors for both norepinephrine and serotonin, as well as other changes that have been measured and no doubt some that have not.[21] It may be these long-term adjustments of the brain tissue that result in the antidepressant action.

A few final comments. These antidepressant drugs are not stimulants and at clinical dose levels have little effect on normal individuals. Animal studies[22] show that long-term administration of an antidepressant increases the sensitivity of the reward systems in the brain. Whether enhancement of reward systems in humans would occur is not known but the mechanisms that have been described for the control of the release and reuptake of noradrenaline may underlie the variability among people in their sensitivity to rewards, as well as set the level of their general affective mood.

Well over half of the prescriptions written for antidepressants are written by nonpsychiatrists. This is unfortunate since they frequently prescribe too little for too short a time to decrease the depression. It is understandable, though, since the tricyclics can cause severe side effects: about one user in 20 will have disorientation, hallucinations, or other anticholinergic effects (see Chapter 18). Large doses (several grams) can be lethal, so quantities prescribed to suicidal patients need to be restricted. A 1980 alert to physicians by the FDA[23] pointed out how dangerous the tricyclics can be when accidentally taken by children: 1000 emergency room visits a year, resulting in 500 hospitalizations and 10 deaths.

There has been some excitement among those working in laboratories and hospitals about a diagnostic laboratory test for primary unipolar depression: the dexamethasone suppression test

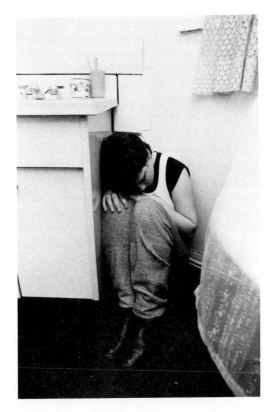

Depression is a serious, debilitating disorder that often responds to antidepressant medication.

(DST). The details need not concern us here but you should know that the test is only about 40% to 60% accurate in identifying those patients who are primary unipolar depressives. However, it eliminates about 90% of those who are not.[24] That is, there are few false positive results but false negative results still exist. So far, this test is of little value in the diagnosis or management of individual patients.

Probably the single most effective treatment for the depressed patient is electroconvulsive therapy (ECT). One report summarized the available good studies and showed that in seven of eight studies ECT was more effective in relieving the symptoms of depression than was placebo. Further, in four studies ECT was more effective than the most effective class of antidepressant drugs, and in three other studies the two treatments were equal. One factor that makes ECT sometimes the clear treatment of choice is its more rapid effect than that found with current antidepressant drugs. Reversal of the depression may not occur for 2 or 3 weeks with drug treatment, but with ECT results sometimes are noticed almost immediately. When there is a possibility of suicide, ECT is thus the obvious choice, and there is no danger in pursuing both drug and ECT treatment simultaneously.[25]

Lithium

In the late 1940s two medical uses were proposed for salts of the element **lithium.** In the United States, lithium chloride, which tastes much like sodium chloride (table salt), was introduced as a salt substitute in heart patients. However, above a certain level lithium is quite toxic and since there was no control over the dose, many users became ill and several died. This scandal was so great in the minds of American physicians that a proposed beneficial use published in 1949 by an Australian, John Cade, produced little interest in this country.

Cade had been experimenting with guinea pigs, examining the effects of lithium on urinary excretion of salts. Since it appeared to have sedative properties in some of the animals, he administered the compound to several disturbed patients. The manic patients all improved, whereas there seemed to be no effect on depressed or schizophrenic patients. This was followed up by several Danish studies in the 1950s and early 1960s, and it became increasingly apparent that the large majority of manic individuals showed dramatic remission of their symptoms after a lag period of a few days when treated with lithium carbonate or other lithium salts.

Three factors slowed the acceptance of lithium in the United States. First, of course, was the salt-substitute poisonings, which gave lithium a bad reputation as a potentially lethal drug. Second, mania was not seen as a major problem in the United States. Remember that manic patients feel energetic and have an unrealistically positive view of their own abilities, and such people are unlikely to seek treatment on their own. Also, patients who became quite manic and lost touch with reality would probably have been called schizophrenic in those days, perhaps at least partly because a treatment existed for schizophrenia. In fact, the antipsychotic drugs can control mania in most cases. The third and possibly most important factor is economic and relates to the way new drugs are introduced in the United States: by companies who hope to make a profit on them. Since lithium is one of the basic chemical elements (number 3 on the periodic chart) and its simple salts had been available for various purposes for many years, it would be impossible for a drug company to receive an exclusive patent to sell lithium. A company generally must go to considerable expense to conduct the research necessary to demonstrate safety and effectiveness to the FDA. If one company had done this, as soon as the drug was approved any other company could also sell lithium, and it would be impossible for the first company to recoup its research investment. Finally, the weight of the academically conducted research and the clinical experience in Europe was such that several companies received approval to sell lithium in 1970.

Treatment with lithium requires 10 to 15 days before symptoms begin to change. Lithium is both safe and toxic. It is safe because the blood level can be monitored routinely and the dose adjusted to ensure therapeutic but not excessive blood levels. It is a toxic agent but may be used with caution with patients with a kidney or cardiovascular disorder. The more minor side effects of gastrointestinal disturbances and tremor do not seem to persist with continued treatment. If excessively high blood levels persist, central nervous system and neuromuscular symptoms appear; these can progress to coma, convulsions, and death if lithium is not stopped and appropriate treatment instituted.

The clinical use and effectiveness of lithium has had some interesting effects in several areas. The mechanism of action is still not clear, but one biochemical effect is that lithium increases the synthesis of serotonin in the brain. Of primary importance in the therapeutic use of lithium is the realization that lithium acts as a mood-normalizing agent in individuals with bipolar manic-depressive illness. Lithium will block both the manic state and the depressed state. Lithium has only moderate effects on unipolar depressions.

These very selective clinical effects of lithium have forced better diagnostic decisions and have given a new basis for belief that unipolar and bipolar mood disorders are not the same illness. This fact is most clearly seen in Table 13-3, which contains the treatment outcome of one study.[26] Either lithium, placebo, or imipramine (a tricyclic) was given to hospitalized patients, who were later discharged and observed for a prolonged period. For patients diagnosed as unipolar, a relapse means an episode of depression, whereas for the bipolar patients relapse can mean either a depressed or a manic period.

The results are relatively clear: lithium is very effective in preventing relapses in biopolar subjects, whereas imipramine treatment showed no clinical improvement compared to placebo. With unipolar subjects imipramine was superior to lithium, but both drugs were superior to placebo treatment. It is of interest to note one major difference between the unipolar and bipolar patients: 55% of next-of-kin relatives of bipolar patients had some type of psychiatric illness, compared to only 28% of the unipolar patients. This suggests that there may be a stronger genetic component in bipolar mood disorders than in unipolar disorders.

THE CONSEQUENCES OF DRUG TREATMENTS FOR MENTAL ILLNESS

There is no question that the use of modern psychopharmaceuticals, which began in the mid-1950s in the United States, has affected the lives of millions of Americans who have been treated with them. But the availability of these effective medications has also brought about revolutionary changes in our society's treatment of and rela-

Table 13-3

Drug treatment 2-year outcome in unipolar and bipolar patients

	Percent of patients with relapses during treatment for	
	First 4 months	Next 20 months
Unipolar subjects		
Lithium	30	41
Imipramine	32	29
Placebo	73	85
Bipolar subjects		
Lithium	22	18
Imipramine	46	67
Placebo	54	67

tionship with our mentally ill citizens. Fig. 13-1 depicts quite graphically what happened to the population of our large mental hospitals over the period from 1946 to 1986.[27] These hospitals had grown larger and larger and held a total of over half a million people in the peak years of the early 1950s. The year in which chlorpromazine was first introduced in the United States, 1955, was the last year in which the population of these hospitals increased. Remember that the antipsychotics do not cure schizophrenia or other forms of psychosis, but they can control the symptoms to a great degree, allowing the patients to leave the hospital, live at home, and often to earn a living. These drugs began the liberation of mental patients from hospitals, where many of them had previously stayed year after year, committed for an indefinite time.

The movement out of mental hospitals was accelerated in the 1960s, with the establishment of federally supported community mental health centers. The idea was to treat mental patients closer to home and in a more natural environment, at lesser expense, and on an outpatient basis. Needless to say, the opportunity for such a program to work was greatly enhanced by the

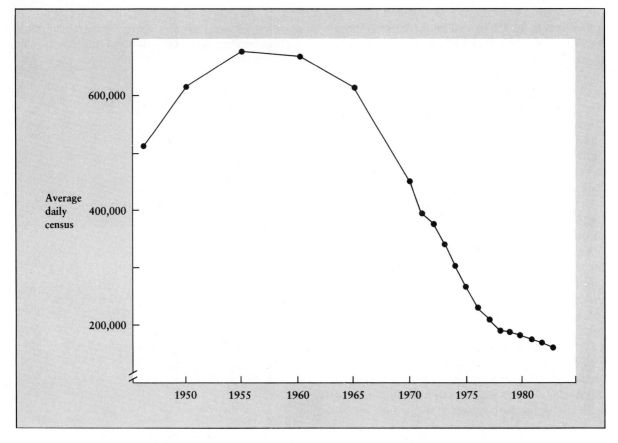

Figure 13-1. Number of patients in nonfederal psychiatric hospitals in the United States.

availability of potent, effective psychopharmaceuticals, especially the antipsychotics.

The mental health professions have been affected by these drugs. It is probably safe to say that the majority of psychiatrists in practice today spend less time doing psychotherapy than did their colleagues in the 1950s. In fact, for many psychiatrists the first issue is to establish an appropriate drug regimen, and only after the initial symptoms are controlled will they engage in much talk therapy. For some psychiatrists the prescription pad has completely taken the place of the couch. This may be sensible, in terms of overall cost effectiveness, but it has certainly altered the doctor/patient relationship.

Concomitant with the liberation of patients from hospitals and their return to the communities came a concern with their civil rights. Indefinite commitment to a hospital has been declared unconstitutional, and all states have developed procedures to protect the rights of individual patients. Hearings are required before a person can be committed for treatment against their will, and it is usually necessary to demonstrate a clear and present danger to the patient's own person or to others. Periodic reviews of the patient's status are called for, and if at any time the immediate danger is not present, the patient must be released. Again, it is not possible to argue that mental patients should not have these rights, but the availability

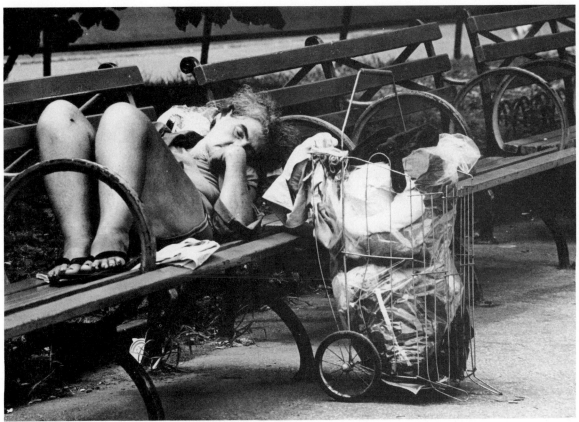

© Joel Gordon 1983

The homeless mentally ill have become a topic of special concern.

of psychoactive medications helps to create an unusual situation. A patient may be quite dangerously psychotic, be admitted for treatment, and after a few weeks on an antipsychotic drug may be sufficiently in control to be allowed to leave the hospital. However, if the patient remains suspicious or simply doesn't like to take the medication, which most don't, he or she will eventually stop taking it and again become psychotic. Or patients may be released to the community, perhaps functioning with medication or perhaps not, too sick to really take care of themselves, but not sick enough to present an immediate danger. The plight of our homeless, rootless, mentally ill citizens has been the subject of magazine and television reports, and we may expect efforts to change the way these people are treated in the future.

Summary

The large number of people who suffer from some sort of mental disorder during their lifetime now find themselves treated with drugs to a greater degree than ever before. Although before the 1950s it was possible to refer to drug treatment for the mentally ill as a "chemical straitjacket," implying nothing more than decreased activity, the introduction of the phenothiazine antipsy-

---

Issue: Catch-22 for the mentally ill

In an article in Newsweek magazine,[28] a 30-year-old x-ray technician named Vickie Wish described the tragedy of her mother's schizophrenia. In her terms, "Hospitals take her in, lock her up, inject her with drugs—and wait the legal amount of involuntary holding time and then send her back out on the streets." Wish described the routine of filing a petition for an involuntary commitment against her own mother, the 72-hour holding period for observation, the court hearing, and the institutionalization. Her mother had had a dozen suicide attempts and a dozen hospitalizations, and sometimes she "escaped." She was once found after 6 weeks, hundreds of miles away, sleeping on a park bench. She weighed 85 pounds and had spent some nights in jail. The mother felt this was all part of her job "for the CIA."

Vickie found it ironic that, in spite of her mother's obvious need for help, because her problem was mental and she didn't want help, there was no way for her to get any except through involuntary commitment.

Three weeks after the mother's last hospitalization, she took an overdose of her medication and died in Vickie's bed, where Vickie found her.

---

chotics resulted in something different: drugs that seemed to act on the psychotic symptoms in a somewhat selective manner. Although the antipsychotic drugs do have side effects associated with them, notably pseudoparkinsonism, there is little doubt of their effectiveness in reducing psychotic behavior. Both the antipsychotic action and the production of pseudoparkinsonism are caused by the action of the drugs at dopamine receptors, which they block.

The antidepressant drugs, which were introduced later in the 1950s, are not as uniformly effective, but they do succeed in reducing the severity of episodes of depression in most individuals. The tricyclics form the most important group of antidepressants. The mechanism by which drugs exert antidepressant action is unknown, but it is important to note that these drugs do not elevate the mood of people who are not depressed.

The single most effective and rapid treatment for severe depression is electroconvulsive shock.

Mania and bipolar affective disorders are treated with lithium salts. This drug is effective for these conditions, and it can be used safely if blood levels are monitored.

The widespread use of these drugs has helped to liberate mental patients from the large mental hospitals and has changed our entire system of mental health care delivery.

REFERENCES

1. Maugh TH: Biochemical markers identify mental states, Science 214:39, October 1981.
2. American Psychiatric Association: Diagnostic and statistical manual of mental disorders, ed 3, revised, Washington DC, 1987.
3. Weiner RD: Electroconvulsive therapy. In Sullivan JL and Sullivan PD, editors: Biomedical psychiatric therapeutics, Boston, 1984, Butterworth.
4. Goldman D: Treatment of psychotic states with chlorpromazine, Journal of the American Medical Association 157:1274-1278, 1955.
5. Cole JO: Phenothiazines. In Simpson LL, editor: Drug treatment of mental disorders, New York, 1976, Raven Press.
6. Freyhan FA: The immediate and long range effects of chlorpromazine on the mental hospital. In Chlorpromazine and mental health, proceedings of a symposium under the auspices of Smith, Kline and French Laboratories, Philadelphia, 1955, Lea & Febiger.
7. Klein DF and Davis JM: Diagnosis and drug treatment of psychiatric disorders, Baltimore, 1969, The Williams and Wilkins Co.
8. Kessler KA and Waletzky JP: Clinical use of the antipsychotics, American Journal of Psychiatry, 138(2):202, February 1981.
9. Veterans Administration: Drug treatment in psychiatry, Washington, DC, 1970, US Goverment Printing Office.
10. Prien RF, Caffey EM, Jr, and Klett CJ: Pharmacotherapy in chronic schizophrenia, Department of Medicine and Surgery, Veterans Administration, May 1973.
11. Prien RF and Klett CJ: An appraisal of the long-term use of tranquilizing medication with hospitalized chronic schizophrenics, Schizophrenia Bulletin No 5, pp 64-73, 1972.
12. Prien RF, Gillis RD, and Caffey EM, Jr: Intermittent pharmocotherapy in chronic schizophrenia, Hospital and Community Psychiatry 24:317-322, 1973.
13. Rivera-Calemlim L and others: Correlation between plasma concentrations of chlorpromazine and clinical response, Communications in Psychopharmacology 2:215, 1978.

14. May PRA: Cost efficiency of treatments for the schizophrenic patient, American Journal of Psychiatry 127:1382-1385, 1971.
15. Bernstein JG: Rational use of antipsychotic drugs. In Bernstein J, editor: Clinical psychopharmacology, ed 2, Littleton, Mass, 1984, John Wright-PSG, Inc.
16. Snyder SH: Dopamine receptors, neuroleptics and schizophrenia, American Journal of Psychiatry, 138(4):460, April 1981.
17. Iversen LL: Dopamine receptors in the brain, Science 188:1084-1089, 1975.
18. Tardive dyskinesia: summary of a task force report of the American Psychiatric Association, Task Force on late neurological effects of antipsychotic drugs, American Journal of Psychiatry, 137(10):1163, October 1980.
19. Tarsy D and Baldessarini RJ: The tardive dyskinesia syndrome. In Klawans HL, editor: Clinical Neuropharmacology, 1, New York, 1976, Raven Press.
20. Schoonover SC: Depression. In Bassuk EL, Schoonover SC, and Gelenberg AJ, editors: The practitioner's guide to psychoactive drugs, ed 2, New York, 1983, Plenum Press.
21. Friedhoff AJ and Schooler NR: Receptor modulation as a treatment strategy, Psychopharmacology Bulletin, 21:43-47, 1985.
22. Fibiger HC and Phillips AG: Increased intracranial self stimulation in rats after long-term administration of desipramine, Science 214:683, November 1981.
23. HHS News P80-56, November 18, 1980.
24. Coppen A and Metcalfe M: The dexamethasone suppression test in depression: a World Health Organization Collaborative study, British Journal of Psychiatry 150:459-462, 1987.
25. Small JG and Small IF: Electroconvulsive therapy update, review, Psychopharmacology Bulletin 17(4):27, 1981.
26. Pokorny AD and Prein RF: Lithium in treatment and prevention of affective disorder, Diseases of the Nervous System 35(7):327-333, 1974.
27. Hospital Statistics 1987, American Hospital Association, Chicago, Ill.
28. Wish VR: Catch-22 for the mentally ill, Newsweek, December 9, 1985.

Chapter 14

Narcotics

OBJECTIVES

After reading this chapter, you should be able to:

Discuss the opium poppy as the original source of narcotic drugs and the history of this important plant substance.

Describe how narcotic addiction has changed over the years up to the present.

Explain how the narcotics work in the nervous system and what their effects are.

List the ways in which narcotic drugs have been used to benefit human health and well-being.

Discuss the dependence characteristics and the toxic properties of the narcotics.

Describe some of the behavioral patterns of narcotic abusers.

And soon they found themselves in the midst of a great meadow of poppies. Now it is well known that when there are many of these flowers together their odor is so powerful that anyone who breathes it falls asleep, and if the sleeper is not carried away from the scent of the flowers he sleeps on and on forever. But Dorothy did not know this, nor could she get away from the bright red flowers that were everywhere about; so presently her eyes grew heavy and she felt she must sit down to rest and to sleep. . . . Her eyes closed in spite of herself and she forgot where she was and fell among the poppies, fast asleep. . . . They carried the sleeping girl to a pretty spot beside the river, far enough from the poppy field to prevent her breathing any more of the poison of the flowers, and here they laid her gently on the soft grass and waited for the fresh breeze to waken her.[1,pp.69,70,72]

From the land of Oz to the streets of Harlem the poppy has caused much grief—and much joy. **Opium** is a truly unique substance. This juice from the plant *Papaver somniferum* has a history of medical use, perhaps 6000 years long. Except for the last century and a half, opium stood alone as the one agent physicians could use and obtain sure results. Compounds containing opium solved several of the recurring problems for medical science wherever used. Opium relieved pain and suffering magnificently. Just as important in the years gone by was its ability to reduce the diarrhea and subsequent dehydration caused by dysentery, which is still a leading cause of death in under-developed countries.

Parallel with the medical use of opium was its use as a deliverer of pleasure and relief from anxiety. Because of these effects, extensive recreational use of opium has also occurred throughout history. And, through all those years, the problem of dependence on opium was experienced by many of its users.

HISTORY

Opium

Early history. The most likely origin of opium is in a hot, dry, Middle East country several millennia ago when some unknown native discovered that for 7 to 10 days of its year-long life *Papaver somniferum* produced a substance that, when eaten, would ease pain and suffering. The opium poppy is an annual plant 3 to 4 feet high with large flowers 4 to 5 inches in diameter. The flowers may be white, pink, red, purple, or violet.

Opium is produced and available for collection for only a few days, between the time the petals drop and before the seed pod matures. Today, as before, to harvest the opium, workers move through the fields toward evening and use a sharp multiclawed tool to make shallow cuts into, but not through, the unripe seed pod. During the night a white substance oozes from the cuts, oxidizes to a red-brown color, and becomes gummy. In the morning the resinous substance is carefully scraped from the pod and collected in small balls. This raw opium forms the basis for the opium medicines used through history and is the substance from which morphine is extracted and then heroin is derived.

The importance and extent of use of the opium poppy in the early Egyptian and Greek cultures are still under debate, but in the Ebers papyrus (circa 1500BC) a remedy is mentioned "to prevent the excessive crying of children." Since a later Egyptian remedy for the same purpose clearly contained opium (as well as fly excrement), many writers report the first specific medical use of opium as dating from the Ebers papyrus.

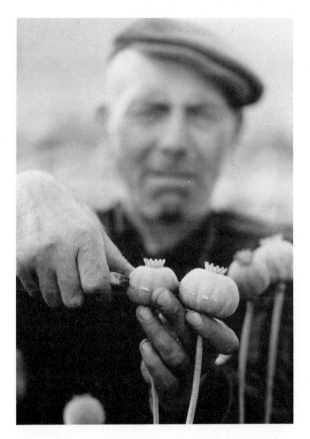

Opium has been extracted from the seed pods of the poppy for thousands of years.

Homer's *Odyssey* (1000BC) contains a passage that some authors believe refers to the use of opium. A party was about to become a real drag because everyone was sad thinking about Ulysses and the deaths of their friends, when:

> Helen, daughter of Zeus, poured into the wine they were drinking a drug, nepenthes, which gave forgetfulness of evil. Those who had drunk of this mixture did not shed a tear the whole day long, even though their mother or father were dead, even though a brother or beloved son had been killed before their eyes. . . .[2,p.6]

The drug could only have been opium.

Opium was important in Greek medicine. Galen, the last of the great Greek physicians, emphasized caution in the use of opium but felt that it was almost a cure-all, since it

> resists poison and venomous bites, cures chronic headache, vertigo, deafness, epilepsy, apoplexy, dimness of sight, loss of voice, asthma, coughs of all kinds, spitting of blood, tightness of breath, colic, the iliac poison, jaundice, hardness of the spleen, stone, urinary complaints, fevers, dropsies, leprosies, the troubles to which women are subject, melancholy and all pestilences.[2,p.111]

Recreational use even then must have been extensive, since Galen commented on the opium cakes and candies that were being sold everywhere in the streets. Although the concepts of addiction and withdrawal had not yet been established, a recent writer suggested that the reports on the behavior and health of the Roman emperor in this period, Marcus Aurelius, clearly indicate that he was addicted to opium and occasionally suffered withdrawal symptoms.[3]

Greek knowledge of opium use in medicine died with the decline of the Roman Empire and thus had little influence on the world's use of opium for the next 1000 years. To the south in North Africa, though, the Arabic world clutched opium (and hashish) to its breast, since the Koran forbade the use of alcohol in any form. Opium and hashish became the primary social drugs wherever the Islam culture moved, and it did move. The Mohammedans were active fighters, explorers, and traders. While Europe rested through the Dark Ages, the Arabian world reached out and made contact with India and China. Opium was one of the products they traded, but they also sold the seeds of the opium poppy, and home cultivation began in these countries. By the tenth century AD, opium was referred to in Chinese medical writings.

During this period when the Arabian civilization flourished, two Arabian physicians made substantial contributions to medicine and to the history of opium. Shortly after 1000AD, Biruni composed a pharmacology book. In his descriptions of opium was what some believe to be the first written description of addiction.[4] In this same period, the best-known Arabian physician, Avicenna, was using opium preparations very effectively and extensively in his medical practice. His writings, along with those of Galen, formed the basis of medical education in Europe as the Renaissance dawned, and thus the glories of opium were advanced. (Strange but true that a physician as knowledgeable as Avicenna, and a believer in the tenets of Islam, should die as a result of drinking too much of a mixture of opium and wine.)

Early in the sixteenth century, European medicine had a phenomenon by the name of Paracelsus. A true iconoclast and Renaissance man, he denounced all the famous medics of history—Hippocrates, Galen, Avicenna—as well as his contemporaries. He apparently was a successful clinician and accomplished some wondrous cures for the day. One of the secrets of Paracelsus was a potion called laudanum. Although it is not clear that his laudanum contained opium, he did use opium very extensively in his treatment of patients. Paracelsus was one of the early Renaissance supporters of opium as a panacea and referred to it as the "stone of immortality."

Because of the increasing awareness of the broad effectiveness of opium as a result of Paracelsus and his followers, a variety of new opium preparations was developed in the sixteenth, seventeenth, and eighteenth centuries. Only two will be mentioned, partly because of their importance in medical history and partly because they are still available today by the same names in many places. The first compound is laudanum, as prepared by Dr. Thomas Sydenham, the father of clinical medicine. (Although the name is the same as Paracelsus's compound, this seems to be the only similarity.) Sydenham's general contributions to English medicine are so great that he has been called the English Hippocrates. He spoke more highly of opium than did Paracelsus, saying that "without opium the healing art would cease to exist." His landanum contained 2 ounces of strained opium, 1 ounce of saffron, and a dram of cinnamon and of cloves dissolved in 1 pint of Canary wine and taken in small quantities.

STIMULANTS

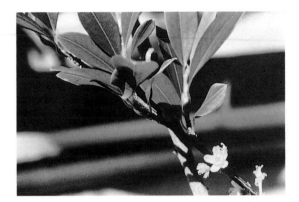

Coca plant

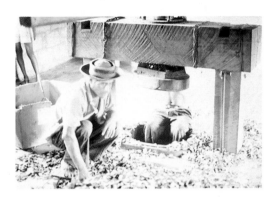

A cocaine lab

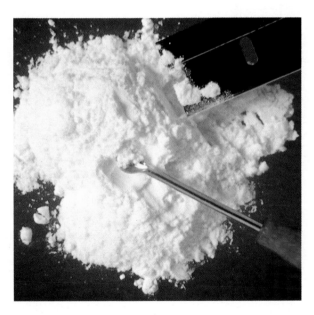

Cocaine

These pages show some of the illegal and prescription drugs discussed
in this text.

DEPRESSANTS

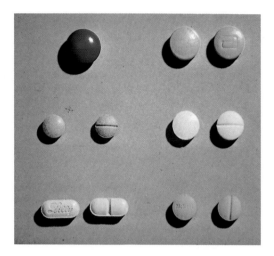

Various barbiturates

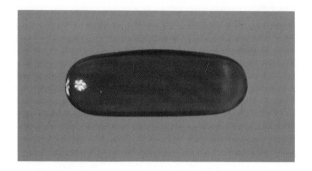

Chloral hydrate

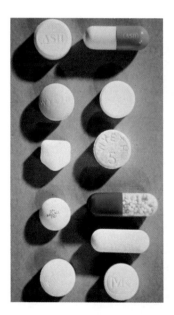

Meprobamates

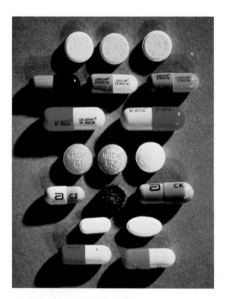

Benzodiazepines, from top to bottom: diazepam, chlordiazepoxide, flurazepam, clonazepam, clorazepate, lorazepam, and oxazepam

NARCOTICS

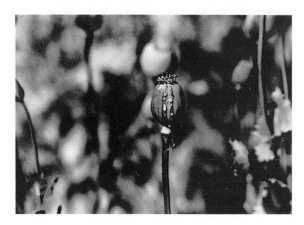

Incised seedpod of the poppy plant

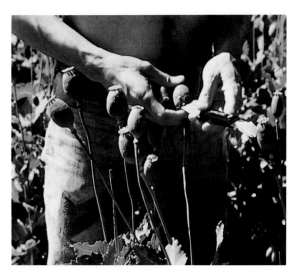

Milky fluid of the seedpods

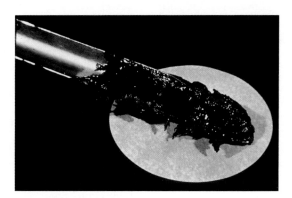

Opium gum

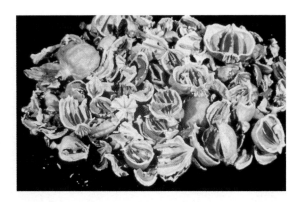

Poppy straw

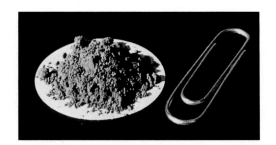

Poppy straw concentrate

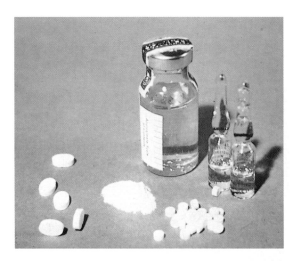

Codeine

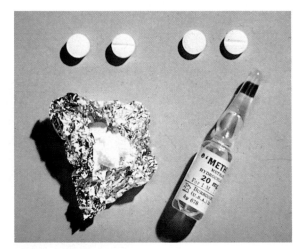

Hydromorphone

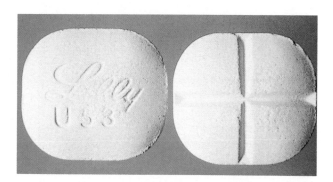

Methadone, a synthetic narcotic

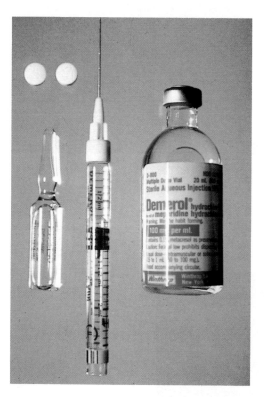

Meperidine (Demerol), a synthetic narcotic analgesic

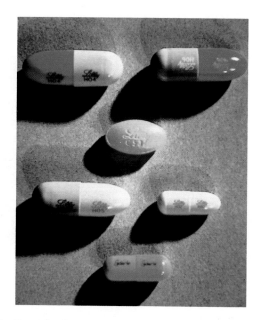

Propoxyphene (Darvon), a synthetic narcotic analgesic

CANNABIS AND ITS EXTRACTS

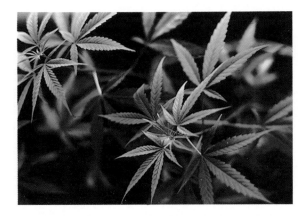

Cannabis plants

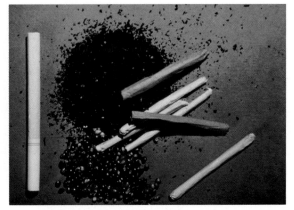

Marijuana cigarettes

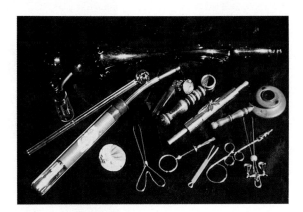

Cannabis paraphernalia

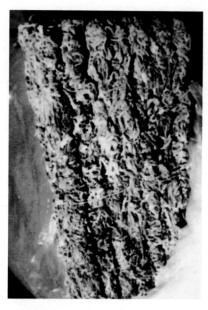

Thai sticks

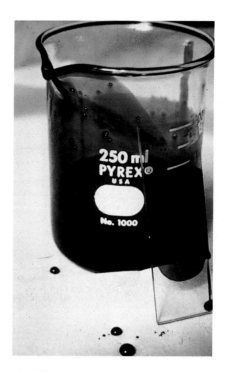

Hashish oil

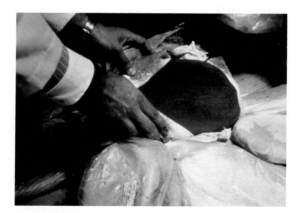

Hashish

PSYCHEDELICS

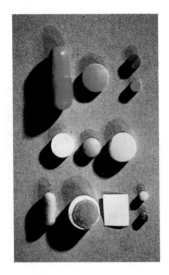

Various forms of psychedelics

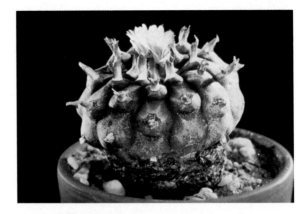

Peyote cactus

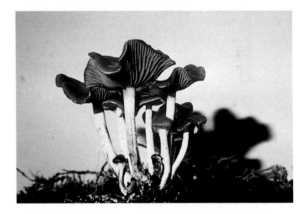

Psilocybe mushroom containing psilocybin, which is chemically related to lysergide (LSD)

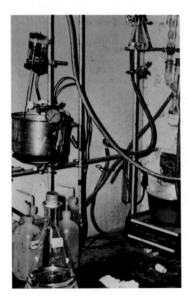

Illegal production of LSD

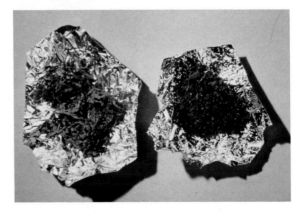

Angel dust: phencyclidine (PCP) on plant material for smoking

Writers and opium: the keys of paradise. In a momentous year for opium, 1805, Thomas De Quincey, a 20-year-old English youth who had run away from home at 17, purchased some laudanum for a toothache and received change for his shilling from the apothecary. His response to this dose was described:

I took it: and in an hour, O heavens! what a revulsion! what a resurrection, from its lowest depths, of the inner spirit! what an apocalypse of the world within me! That my pains had vanished was now a trifle in my eyes; this negative effect was swallowed up in the immensity of those positive effects which had opened before me, in the abyss of divine enjoyment thus suddenly revealed. Here was a panacea . . . for all human woes; here was the secret of happiness, about which philosophers had disputed for so many ages, at once discovered; happiness might now be bought for a penny, and carried in the waistcoat-pocket; portable ecstasies might be had corked up in a pint-bottle; and peace of mind could be sent down by the mail.[5,p.179]

For the rest of his life De Quincey used laudanum, although he possibly was no longer addicted at his death. He did not try to conceal the extent of his addiction. Rather, his writings are replete with insight into the opiate-hazed world, particularly his article "The Confessions of an English Opium-Eater," which was published in 1821 (and in book form in 1823). ("Opium eating" throughout this period was the phrase generally used to refer to laudanum drinking.)

Several other famous English authors were also addicted to laudanum, including Elizabeth Barrett Browning and Samuel Taylor Coleridge. Coleridge's magnificently beautiful "Kubla Khan" was probably conceived and composed in an opium reverie and then written down as best as he could remember it. However, De Quincey is of primary interest here, as Baudelaire will be with hashish. His emphasis was on understanding the effects that opium has on consciousness, experience, and feeling, and as such he provided some of the most vivid accounts of the power of opium.

Opium does not produce new worlds for the user.

If a man, "whose talk is of oxen," should become an opium-eater, the probability is, that (if he is not too dull to dream at all)—he will dream about oxen; whereas, in the case before him [De Quincey], the reader will find that the opium-eater boasteth himself to be a philosopher; and accordingly, that the phantasmagoria of *his* dreams (waking or sleeping, day-dreams or night-dreams) is suitable to one [of] that character. . . .[6,p.156]

Opium does, however, change the way the world is perceived. For example, "an opium eater is too happy to observe the motion of time."[5]

The contrast between the feelings, effects, and experiences that result from alcohol were discussed extensively and sharply contrasted with those accompanying the use of opium:

crude opium . . . is incapable of producing any state of body at all resembling that which is produced by alcohol. . . . It is not in the quantity of its effects merely, but in the quality, that it differs altogether. The pleasure given by wine is always rapidly mounting, and tending to a crisis, after which as rapidly it declines; that from opium, when once generated, is stationary for eight or ten hours. . . . The one is a flickering flame, the other a steady and equable glow. But the main distinction lies in this—that, whereas wine disorders the mental faculties, opium, on the contrary (if taken in a proper manner), introduces amongst them the most exquisite order, legislation, and harmony. Wine robs a man of his self-possession; opium sustains and reinforces it. Wine unsettles the judgment. . . . Opium, on the contrary, communicates serenity and equipoise to all the faculties. . . .[5,pp.180-181]

In spite of all the good things De Quincey said about opium and the effects it had on him, he suffered from its use. For long periods in his life he was unable to write as a result of his addiction. As with most things: "Opium gives and takes away. It defeats the *steady* habit of exertion; but it creates spasms of irregular exertion. It ruins the natural power of life; but it develops preternatural paroxysms of intermitting power."[7,p.424]

Publication of De Quincey's book in 1823 and its first translation into French in 1828 were events that spurred the French Romantic writers into exploration with opium and hashish in the 1840s and later. Baudelaire's famous book *The Artificial Paradises* was composed of two parts, the first being an original account of the effects of hashish and the second his translation of *The Confessions of an English Opium-Eater.* Baudelaire was to repeatedly comment that much of what he wrote at various times about the effects of opium could equally be said about hashish.[8] The only associated American article of note in this period, "An Opium Eater in America,"[9] appeared in an American magazine in 1842.

The Opium Wars.   Although opium and the opium poppy had been introduced to China well before the year 1000, there was only a moderate level of use by a select, elite group. Spreading much more rapidly after its introduction was tobacco smoking. It is not clear when tobacco was introduced to the Chinese, but its use had spread and become so offensive that in 1644 the Emperor forbade tobacco smoking in China. The edict did not last long (as is to be expected), but it was in part responsible for the development of opium smoking.

Up to this period the smoking of tobacco and the eating of opium had existed side by side. The restriction on the use of tobacco and the population's appreciation of the pleasures of smoking led to the subterfuge of combining opium and tobacco for smoking. The amount of tobacco used was gradually reduced and soon omitted altogether. Very rapidly the smoking of opium spread, although opium eating had never been very attractive to most Chinese,[10] perhaps, at least partly, because smoking results in a rapid effect compared to oral use of opium.

In 1729 China's first law against opium smoking mandated that opium shopowners were to be strangled. Once opium for nonmedical purposes was outlawed, it was necessary for the drug to be smuggled in from India, where poppy plantations were abundant. Smuggling opium was so profitable for everyone—the growers, the shippers, and the customs officers—that unofficial rules were gradually developed for the game.[2] The background to the Opium Wars is too lengthy and complex to even attempt to sketch adequately.

However, some points must be made to explain why the British went to war so they could continue pouring opium into China against the wishes of the Chinese national government.

Since before 1557, when the Portuguese were allowed to develop the small trading post of Macao, pressure had been increasing on the Chinese emperors to open the country up to trade with the "barbarians from the West." Not only the Portuguese but the Dutch and the English repeatedly knocked on the closed door of the Chinese. Near the end of the seventeenth century the port of Canton was opened under very strict rules to foreigners. Tea was the major export, and the British shipped out huge amounts. There was little that the Chinese were interested in importing from the "barbarians," but opium could be smuggled so profitably that it soon became the primary import. The profit the British made from selling opium paid for the tea they shipped to England.[11]

In the early nineteenth century the government of India was actually the British East India Company. As such it had a monopoly on opium, which was legal in India. However, smuggling it into China was not. The East India Company auctioned chests of opium cakes to private merchants, who gave the chests to selected British firms, who sold it for a commission to Chinese merchants. In this way the British were able to have the Chinese "smuggle" the opium into China! The number of chests of opium, each with about 120 pounds of smokable opium, that were annually imported to China increased from 200 in 1729 to about 5000 at the century's end to 25,000 chests in 1838.

The following year, 1839, the emperor of China made a fatal mistake—he sent an honest man to Canton to suppress the opium smuggling. Commissioner Lin demanded that the barbarians deliver all their opium supplies to him and subjected the dealers to confinement in their houses. After some haggling, the representative of the British government ordered the merchants to deliver the opium—20,000 chests worth about $6 million—which was then destroyed and everyone set free. Pressures mounted, though, and an incident involving drunken American and British sailors killing a Chinese started the Opium War in 1839. The British army arrived 10 months later, and in 2 years, largely by avoiding land battles and by using the superior artillery of the royal navy ships, won a victory over a country of more than 350 million citizens. As victors, the British were given the island of Hong Kong, broad trading rights, and $6 million to reimburse the merchants whose opium had been destroyed.

Through it all, the smuggling of opium continued. There was another Opium War in the 1850s, but the British imports of illegal opium continued until 1908, when Britain and China agreed to limit imports of opium from India.

The Chinese opium trade posed a great moral dilemma for Britain. The East India Company protested until its end that it was not smuggling opium into China, and technically it was not. From 1870 to 1893 motions in Parliament to end the extremely profitable opium commerce failed to pass but did cause a decline in the opium trade. In 1893 a moral protest against the trade was supported, but not until 1906 did the government support and pass a bill that started the process which ended the opium trade by 1913.[12]

Morphine

In 1805 in London, England, 20-year-old De Quincey eased a toothache and fell into the abyss of divine enjoyment. In Hanover, Germany, another 20-year-old worked on the experiments that were to have great impact on science, medicine, and the pleasure seekers. In 1806, this German youth, Frederich Sertürner, published his report of over 50 experiments, which clearly showed that he had isolated the primary active ingredient in opium. The active agent was 10 times as potent as opium. Sertürner named it **morphium** after Morpheus, the god of dreams. Use of the new agent developed slowly, but by 1831 the implications of his chemical work and the medical value of **morphine** were so overwhelming that this pharmacist's assistant was given the French equivalent of the Nobel Prize. Later work into the mysteries of opium found over 30 different al-

kaloids, with the second most important one being isolated in 1832 and named **codeine,** the Greek word for poppy head.

The availability of a clinically valuable, pure chemical of known potency is always capitalized on in medicine. The major increase in the use of morphine came as a result of two nondrug developments, one technological and one political. The technological development was the perfection of the hypodermic syringe in 1853 by Dr. Alexander Wood. This made it possible to rapidly deliver morphine directly into the blood or tissue rather than the much slower process of eating opium or morphine and waiting for absorption to occur from the gastrointestinal tract. A further advantage of injecting morphine was thought to exist. Originally it was felt that morphine by injection would not be as addicting as the oral use of the drug. This belief was later found to be false.

The political events that sped the drug of sleep and dreams into the veins of people worldwide were the American Civil War (1861 to 1865), the Prussian-Austrian War (1866), and the Franco-Prussian War (1870). Military medicine was, and to some extent still is, characterized by the dictum "first provide relief." Morphine given by injection did work rapidly and well, and it was administered regularly in large doses to many soldiers for the reduction of pain and relief from dysentery. The percentage of returning veterans from these wars were addicted to morphine was high enough that the illness was later called "soldier's disease" or the "army disease."

Heroin

Toward the end of the nineteenth century, a small but important chemical transformation was made to the morphine molecule. In 1874 two acetyl-groups were attached to morphine, yielding **heroin,** which was placed on the market in 1898 by Bayer Laboratories. The chemical change was important because heroin is about three times as potent as morphine. The pharmacology of heroin and morphine is identical except that the two acetyl groups increase the lipid solubility of the molecule, and thus the molecule enters the brain more rapidly. The additional groups are detached, yielding morphine. Therefore, effects of morphine and heroin are identical except that heroin is more potent and acts faster.

The history of heroin provides strong support for those who argue for extended experimental study of new therapeutic agents before they are marketed. Heroin was originally marketed as a nonaddicting substitute for codeine.[13] It seemed to be the perfect drug, more potent yet less harmful. Although not introduced commercially until 1898, heroin had been studied, and many of its pharmacological actions were reported in 1890.[14] By January 1900 a comprehensive review article concluded that tolerance and addiction (habituation) to heroin were only minor problems.

Habituation has been noted in a small percentage . . . of the cases. . . . All observers are agreed, however, that none of the patients suffer in any way from this habituation, and that none of the symptoms which are so characteristic of chronic morphinism have ever been observed. On the other hand, a large number of the reports refer to the fact that the same dose may be used for a long time without any habituation.[15]

The basis for the failure to find addiction and the resulting attitudes probably was the fact that heroin was primarily used as a substitute for codeine, which meant oral doses of 3 to 5 mg used for brief periods of time. Slowly the situation changed, and a 1905 text on *Pharmacology and Therapeutics* took a middle ground on heroin by saying that it "is stated not to give rise to habituation. A more extended knowledge of the drug, however, would seem to indicate that the latter assertion is not entirely correct."[16,p.860] In a few more years everyone knew that heroin was the most addicting of the opiates.

Narcotic Addiction before the Harrison Act

In the second half of the nineteenth century three forms of opiate addiction were developing in the United States. The long-useful oral intake of opium, and now morphine, increased greatly as patent medicines became a standard form of self-medication. After 1850 Chinese laborers were imported in large numbers to the west coast, and they introduced opium smoking to this country. The last form, medically the most dangerous and ultimately the most disruptive socially, was the injection of morphine.

Around the turn of the century the percentage (and perhaps the absolute number) of Americans addicted to one of the opiates was very probably greater than at any other time before or since. Several authorities, both then and more recently, agree that no less than 1% of the population was addicted to opium, although accurate statistics are not available. In spite of the high level of addiction, it was not a major social problem. In this period:

The public then had an altogether different conception of drug addiction from that which prevails today. The habit was not approved, but neither was it regarded as criminal or monstrous. It was usually looked upon as a vice or personal misfortune, or much as alcoholism is viewed today. Narcotics users were pitied rather than loathed as criminals or degenerates—an attitude which still prevails in Europe.[17,p.211]

The opium smoking the Chinese brought to this country never became widely popular, although around the turn of the century about one fourth of the opium imported was smoking opium. Perhaps it was because the smoking itself occupies only about a minute and is then followed by a dreamlike state of reverie that may last 2 or 3 hours—hardly behavior that is conducive to a continuation of daily activities or consonant with the outward, active orientation of most Americans in that period. Another reason why opium smoking did not spread was that it originated with Orientals, who were scorned by whites. Similarly, the opium smoking that did occur among whites was found within the asocial and antisocial elements of this culture. Amusingly, even the underworld has its standards of morality, and opium smokers looked down on those who used their drugs by injection. In a New York opium-smoking den early in this century "one of the smokers discovered a hypodermic user in the bathroom giving himself an injection. He immediately reported to the proprietor that there was a 'God-damned dope fiend in the can.' The offender was promptly ejected."[17]

The growth of the patent medicine industry after the Civil War has been well documented. Everything seemed to be favorable for the industry, and it took advantage of each opportunity. There were few government regulations on the industry, and as a result addicting drugs were an important part of many tonics and remedies, although this fact did not have to be indicated on the label. Since labeling of ingredients was not required, a user who had become aware that he was addicted and who wanted to purchase a cure could be sold a remedy labeled as a cure that contained almost as much of the addicting drug as he had been receiving in the original tonic.

The generally poor level of health care in the country and a large number of maimed and diseased veterans created a need for considerable medical treatment. Patent medicines promised, and in part delivered, the perfect self-medication. They were easily available, not too expensive, socially acceptable, and, miracle of miracles, they did work. The amount of alcohol and/or opiates in many of the nostrums was certain to relieve the user's aches, pains, and anxieties.

Two other points help explain the increase in the sales of patent medicines. One was the lack of sophistication and education of most Americans during this period, and the other was the use of fantastic advertising campaigns. Medicine shows, testimonials, songs, newspaper and magazine ads all said the same thing: "You feel ill! *This* product will cure." People believed and bought!

Gradually some medical concern developed over the number of people who were addicted to opiates, and this concern was a part of the motivation that led to the passage of the 1906 Pure Food and Drugs Act. In 1910 a government expert in this area made clear that this law was only a beginning.

The thoughtful and foremost medical men have been and are cautioning against the free use of morphine and opium, particularly in recurring pain. The amount they are using is decreasing yearly. Notwithstanding this fact, and the fact that legislation, federal, state and territorial, adverse to the indiscriminate use and sale of opium and morphine, their derivatives and preparations, has been enacted during the past few decades, the amount of opium per capita imported and consumed in the United States has doubled during the last forty years. . . . It is well known that there are many factors at work tending to drug enslavement, among them being the host of soothing syrups, medicated soft drinks containing cocaine, asthma remedies, catarrh remedies, consumption remedies, cough and cold remedies, and the more notorious so-called "drug addiction cures." It is often stated that medical men are frequently the chief factors in causing drug addiction.[18,pp.105-106]

Data were presented in this paper that tended to support the belief that medical use of opiates initiated by a physician was one, if not *the*, major cause of addiction in this country at that time. A 1918 government report clearly indicted the physician as the major cause of addiction in addicts of "good social standing."

That physicians widely used opiates as drugs in treatment is understandable in light of articles that had been published, such as one in 1889 titled "Advantages of Substituting the Morphia Habit for the Incurably Alcoholic." The author stated:

In this way I have been able to bring peacefulness and quiet to many disturbed and distracted homes, to keep the head of a family out of the gutter and out of the lock-up, to keep him from scandalous misbehavior and neglect of his affairs, to keep him from the verges and actualities of delirium tremens horrors, and above all, to save him from committing, as I veritably believe, some terrible crime.[19]

Besides all those good things, morphine addiction was cheap: by one estimate it was 10 times as expensive to be an alcoholic—all of 25 cents a day. The article concludes:

I might, had I time and space, enlarge by statistics to prove the law-abiding qualities of opium-eating peoples, but of this any one can perceive somewhat for himself, if he carefully watches and reflects on the quiet, introspective gaze of the morphine habitue, and compares it to the riotous, devil-may-care leer of the drunkard.[19]

This middle history period, 1806 to 1914, is rich in material on the use of opiates that gives background to the thesis that if drugs are widely used, it is because they meet the needs of a culture. An 1880 report called addiction a "vice of middle life."[20] The typical opiate addict of this period was a 30- to 50-year-old white woman who functioned well and was adjusted to her life as a wife and mother. She bought opium or morphine legally at the local store, used it orally, and caused few, if any, social problems. She may have ordered her "family remedy" through the mail from Sears, Roebuck—two ounces of laudanum for 18 cents or 1½ pints for $2.

Do not be misled. There *were* problems associated with addiction during this period. There are always individuals who are unable to control drug intake, whether the drug is used for self-medication or recreation. Because of the high opiate content of patent medicines and the ready availability of addicting drugs for drinking and/or injecting, very high levels of drug were frequently used. As a result, the symptoms of withdrawal were very severe—much worse than today—and there were no medications or treatment programs to reduce the pain or anxiety.

After the Harrison Act

The complex reasons for the passage of the 1914 Harrison Act were discussed in detail in Chapter 3. Remember that this was a fairly simple revenue measure. However, as is true of most laws, it is not the law itself that becomes important in the ensuing years, but the court decisions and enforcement practices that evolve as the law interacts with the people it effects.

Eliminating legal sources

The passing of the Harrison Act in 1914 left the status of the addict almost completely indeterminate. The Act did not make addiction illegal and it neither authorized nor forbade doctors to prescribe drugs regularly for addicts. All that it clearly and unequivocally did require was that whatever drugs addicts obtained were to be secured from physicians registered under the act and that the fact of securing drugs be made a matter of record. While some drug users had obtained supplies from physicians before 1914, it was not necessary for them to do so since drugs were available for purchase in pharmacies and even from mail-order houses.[20,p.5]

In 1915 the United States Supreme Court decided that possession of smuggled opiates was a crime, and thus users not obtaining the drug from a physician became criminals with the stroke of a pen. An addict could still obtain his supply of drugs on a prescription from a physician until this avenue was removed by the 1920 Webb and the 1922 Behrman Supreme Court decisions. Even though the Lindner case in 1925 reversed these earlier decisions and stated that a physician could prescribe drugs to a nonhospitalized addict just to maintain him, the doctors had been harassed and arrested enough. Though it was legal to prescribe drugs to an addict, few physicians would do so. Attempts in the early 1920s to maintain clinics for the treatment of opiate addicts failed for a number of reasons, including poor management and disapproval by law enforcement officials.

The number of oral opiate users began to decline after the Harrison Law was passed, and the primary remaining group were those who injected morphine or heroin. That has stayed true up to the present. By 1920, about the only source of opiates for a nonhospitalized addict was an illegal dealer. The cost through this source was 30 to 50 times the price of the same drug through legitimate sources, which no longer were available to the addict. As a consequence, then, of the 1914 law and the Supreme Court decisions in the early 1920s, the opiate user was forced to either stop using the drug or buy from an illegal dealer. To maintain a supply of the drug in this way was expensive. Many addicts resorted to criminal activity, primarily burglary and other crimes against property, to finance their addiction.[21]

During this period, law enforcement agencies and the popular press brought about a change in the attitudes of society toward the addict. Thus in the 1920s

the addict was no longer seen as a victim of drugs, an unfortunate with no place to turn and deserving of society's sympathy and help. He became instead a base, vile, degenerate who was weak and self-indulgent, who contaminated all he came in contact with and who deserved nothing short of condemnation and society's moral outrage and legal sanction. The law enforcement approach was accepted as the only workable solution to the problem of addiction.[22]

Changing the addict population. The change in the type of addict population in the United States from the 1920s to the 1980s is easier to specify than the number of addicts in this country after 1914. After the Harrison Act, there almost certainly was a decline in the number of addicts using opiates orally and thus a drop in white middle-aged users. One paper comments that between World War I and World War II heroin received little publicity and was primarily used by "people in *the life*—show people, entertainers and musicians; racketeers and gangsters; thieves and pickpockets; prostitutes and pimps."[23] The transition from the 1930s to the 1950s in the United States has been best described by an internationally recognized expert who worked in the area of drug addiction through this period.

If you go back to 1935 the other problems, apart from alcohol, were primarily the opiates and cocaine, usually taken together in the form of the so-called "speed-ball" and then as now . . . drug use was multiple. These individuals that I know used morphine, cocaine, heroin, bromides, phenobarbital or whatever happened to come along but they preferred the opiates and cocaine. The people of those days were really predominately white individuals, they were on the whole members of various criminal trades, pickpockets and so on, and in fact most of them had been involved in these criminal trades either before or after their onset of their career of using drugs. These people more or less disappeared during the Second World War which practically made these drugs unavailable . . . the old fashioned addict, the expert pickpocket, the short change

artist couldn't get drugs. This group was succeeded, after the war was over, by a new kind of opiate taker. These were primarily individuals from the minority groups in the big city slums and in contrast to the older addicts who got good drugs, who knew good stuff when they got it, this new group were getting drugs extremely diluted, full of all kinds of other poisons and were a very different kind of people. They were not expert thieves, in fact very inexpert.[24,p.32]

In the early years after World War II heroin use slowly increased in the lower-class, slum areas of the large cities. Heroin was inexpensive in this period; a dollar would buy enough for a good high for three to six people; $2-a-day habits were real and not uncommon. As the fifties passed by, heroin use spread rapidly. Some authorities believe that it was increasing heroin use as much as anything else that removed the street gangs and their wars from city streets by the end of the decade. As demand increased, so did the price and the amount of adulteration.

The 1960s. A brief summary of heroin use from 1940 to 1970 suggests that all rules changed in November 1961.[23] A critical shortage of heroin developed, prices tripled, and adulteration was carried to new heights. Since this increased profits, the price and adulteration level stayed the same when heroin was again in good supply. This article suggested that it was the large increase in price that disrupted the previous social cohesiveness among addicts, increased considerably the amount of crime, and contributed to the general social disorganization of the ghettos, where most addicts lived.

In the 1960s the use of heroin and other drugs skyrocketed. Flower children, hippies, Tim Leary, and LSD received most of the media attention, but within the central core of the large American cities the number of regular and irregular heroin users increased daily. As you might expect, mainstream U.S.A. gradually became concerned with the heroin problem of the large cities. The increase in crime was the key, since most addicts were black or Latin, and the white majority saw little relevance of the addiction to their own personal, family, and social problems. What the man in the street didn't appreciate was that the young criminal population—both addicted and nonaddicted—was becoming increasingly nonwhite, meaning it wasn't just drugs that were involved. Of more interest perhaps is the report that among youthful offenders in the period from 1968 to 1972 "heroin addicts . . . were found to be older, better educated, and more intelligent than nonaddicts."[25,p.222]

Vietnam. The attitude of the man in the street toward the relevance of addiction to his personal life changed rapidly with the reports that began to filter out of Southeast Asia toward the end of the 1960s. Public anxiety increased dramatically with the possibility that the Vietnam conflict might produce thousands of addicts among the soldiers stationed there.

The Department of Defense established a Task Force on Drug Abuse in 1967; initial reports emphasized concern over the widespread use of marijuana by troops in combat zones as well as in rest and rehabilitation areas. In 1970 public and federal concern began to focus on the problem of heroin addiction among service personnel stationed in Southeast Asia.[26]

Heroin was about 95% pure and almost openly sold in South Vietnam, whereas purity in the United States was about 5% in 1969. Not only was the Southeast Asia heroin undiluted, it was inexpensive. Ten dollars would buy about 250 mg, an amount that would cost over $500 in the United States. The high purity of the heroin made it possible to obtain psychological effects by smoking or sniffing the drug. This fact, coupled with the completely wrong belief that addiction occurs only when the drug is used intravenously, resulted in about 40% of the users sniffing, about half smoking, and only 10% mainlining their heroin.[27]

Some early 1971 reports estimated that 10% to 15% of the American troops in Vietnam were addicted to heroin. As a result of the increased magnitude and visibility of the heroin problem, the U.S. government took several rapid steps in mid-1971. One step was to initiate Operation Golden Flow, a urine testing program for opiates in servicemen ready to leave Vietnam. The testing program, which tested *only* for opiates, was later expanded to include other American personnel.

In October 1971, the Pentagon released figures for the first 3 months of testing, which showed that 5.1% of the 100,000 servicemen tested showed traces of opiates in their urine. The Army had a higher incidence of users (6.4%) than either the Air Force (1.3%) or the Navy (1.7%), and most of the opiate users were concentrated in the lower ranks.

In retrospect the Vietnam drug use situation was "making a mountain out of a molehill," but much was learned. An excellent follow-up study[28] of veterans who returned from Vietnam in September 1971 showed that most of the Vietnam heroin users did *not* continue heroin use in this country. Only 1% to 2% were using narcotics 8 to 12 months after returning from Vietnam and being released from the service, approximately the same percentage of individuals found to be using narcotics when examined for induction into the service.

One of the important things learned from the Southeast Asia caper was that narcotic addiction and compulsive use is *not* inevitable among occasional users. The pattern of drug use in Vietnam also supports the belief that under certain conditions—availability and low cost of the drug, boredom, unhappiness—there is a relatively high percentage of individuals who will use narcotic drugs recreationally.

The 1970s. Since the late 1960s the federal government has made a serious effort to estimate the number of heroin users in the United States. As we learned in Chapter 1, this is an impossible task to perform with much accuracy, since heroin use is conducted in great secrecy and is not uniformly distributed across the country. Nevertheless, several sophisticated statistical techniques have been brought to bear, combining various sources of information. Different groups of researchers have estimated the number of heroin addicts from 1970 to the mid-1980s, and the estimates mostly range between 400,000 and 500,000.[29] Perhaps because of considerable variability in the estimates, no particular trends or patterns can be seen in these data, and one might argue that heroin addiction is a fairly stable problem that hasn't really changed much over this period. This is roughly true if one looks at the addicted population.

Even though the heroin use problem has remained relatively stable over the past 20 years, there have been small "waves" of increased availability of the drug, which probably produces some small effect on use. Some of the recent waves can be followed by looking at Table 14-1, which presents data from the DEA's Domestic Monitor Program.[30] In this program, the DEA makes small retail purchases of heroin in different cities around the country, and then estimates the average price and purity. Looking at Table 14-1, it is possible to see that in the mid-1970s there was a period when purity was relatively high—around 6%, and the price was relatively low. By 1980 the average purity was closer to 4%, and the price was higher. Toward the end of the 1980s it appears that there was another increase in availability, with higher purity and declining prices. Although these general trends are reflective of the nationwide pattern,

you should be aware that the price and purity vary widely from time to time within a year and from location to location. For example, in 1987 several packages of heroin were purchased ranging in purity from 28 to 67%, roughly 10 times the usual concentration.

In 1972, the major source of U.S. heroin was from opium grown in Turkey and converted into heroin in southern French port cities, such as Marseille. This "French connection" accounted for as much as 80% of U.S. heroin before 1973. In 1972, Turkey banned all opium cultivation and production, in return for $35 million the United States provided to make up for the financial losses to farmers and to help them develop new cash crops.[31] This action, combined with a cooperative effort with the French[32] (also partially funded by

Table 14-1		
Estimated average purity and price of heroin in the United States		
Year	**Purity (% heroin)**	**Price (per mg)**
1974	5.8	$1.15
1975	6.1	1.22
1976	6.3	1.30
1977	5.3	1.58
1978	4.4	1.88
1979	3.6	2.25
1980	3.8	2.21
1981	3.9	2.31
1982	5.0	2.13
1983	4.5	2.15
1984	4.7	2.37
1985	5.3	2.30
1986	6.1	2.12
1987	5.9	2.00

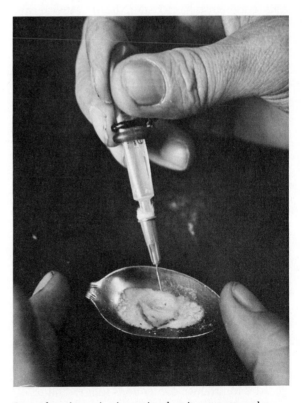

Street heroin varies in purity, but it averages only about 5% heroin.

the United States), did lead to a reduction in the supply of heroin on the streets of New York in 1973.

This relative shortage did not last for long. In Mexico, opium is processed into morphine by a different process, and the resulting pure heroin has a brown color. By 1975 the Drug Enforcement Administration estimated that 80% or more of all U.S. heroin was **Mexican brown.** The supply was plentiful, the price low, and the purity high.[33] Beginning in 1974 the United States began to finance opium eradication programs in Mexico. Although it is a hopeless task to try to eliminate all such production, these monumental and expensive efforts did slow the importation from Mexico to some extent, and the second epidemic of the 1970s began to decline.[34]

At the end of the 1980s, almost half of our heroin supply apparently originated in Southwest Asia (Afghanistan, Pakistan, Iran). Mexico was the next biggest contributor, with the Golden Triangle area of Southeast Asia (Burma, Laos, and Thailand) producing about 14% of the total (Chapter 5). Production of opium and availability of refined heroin from all three of these regions increased during the second half of the 1980s, which is reflected in the increased purity and decreased prices on the streets.

PHARMACOLOGY OF THE NARCOTICS
Chemical Characteristics

Raw opium contains about 10% by weight of morphine and a smaller amount of codeine. The addition of two acetyl groups to the morphine molecule results in diacetylmorphine, otherwise known as heroin (once a brand name owned by Bayer) (Fig. 14-1). The acetyl groups allow heroin to penetrate the blood-brain barrier more readily, and heroin is therefore two to three times more potent than morphine.

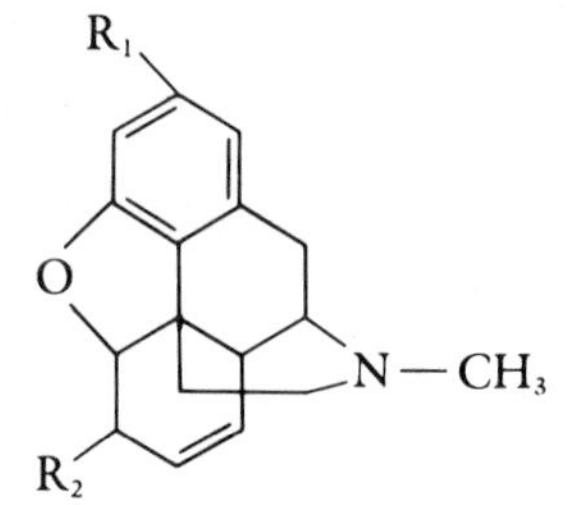

Medicinal chemists have worked hard over the decades to produce compounds that would be effective pain killers, trying to separate the analgesic effect of the narcotics from their dependence-producing effects without success. As a result,

Figure 14-1. Narcotic agents isolated or derived from opium.

there are several synthetic narcotics sold as prescription pain relievers (Table 14-2). Especially interesting among these is fentanyl, which is approximately 100 times as potent as morphine, and sufentanyl, which is even more potent. These are used primarily in conjunction with surgical anesthesia.

In addition to the narcotic analgesics, this search for new compounds led to the discovery of **narcotic antagonists,** drugs that block the action of morphine, heroin, or other narcotics. The administration of a drug such as naloxone or naltrexone can reverse the depressed respiration resulting from a narcotic overdose. If given to an individual who has been taking narcotics and has become physically dependent, these antagonists can precipitate an immediate withdrawal syndrome, as though the previously taken narcotic had been instantly removed from the body.

Mechanism of Action

The 1970s will be long remembered in pharmacology as the decade in which the interaction between the narcotics and the central nervous sys-

Table 14-2

Some prescription narcotic analgesics

Generic name	Trade name(s)	Recommended dose (mg)
Morphine		10-30
Codeine		30-60
Methadone	Dolophine	2.5-10
Meperidine	Demerol	50-150
Oxycodone	Percodan	2.25-4.50
Oxymorphone	Numorphan	1-1.5
Hydrocodone		5-10
Hydromorphone	Dilaudid	1-4
Dihydrocodeine		32
Propoxyphene	Darvon	32-65
Pentazocine	Talwin	30
Fentanyl	Sublimaze	0.05-0.10

tem finally began to be understood. Previous studies had suggested that the opiates act through specific receptors in the brain. One fact pointing to an opiate receptor was the finding that it is only the *l*-form that is effective, i.e., the action of the drug is dependent on the shape of the molecule. As relationships between chemical structures and narcotic activity were studied, the theoretical construct of an opiate receptor seemed more and more real: active morphine-like drugs would fit the receptor and activate it, whereas the narcotic antagonists could act by occupying the receptor sites without activating them, thus preventing access by molecules of the active narcotics.

A pharmacologist at Stanford University, Avram Goldstein, developed the technique by which opiate receptors could be measured using radioactively labeled molecules, but his group was unable to detect the receptors with much accuracy. In 1973, Pert and Snyder at Johns Hopkins University used naloxone with a high degree of radioactive labeling to measure opiate receptors in rat brain tissue.[35] Their technique not only demonstrated that the theoretical opiate receptor was quite real, but allowed the mapping out of the brain areas that contained opiate receptors.

What are opiate receptors doing sitting around in the synapses of the brain? Waiting for someone to extract the juice from a poppy? The distribution of these receptors didn't agree with the distribution of any known neurotransmitter substance, so scientists all over the world went to work looking for a substance in the brain that could serve as the natural activator of these opiate receptors. Groups in England and Sweden each succeeded in 1974: a pair of molecules, leu-enkephalin and met-enkephalin, were isolated from brain extracts. These **enkephalins** acted like morphine and were many times more potent. It was interesting that these enkephalin molecules were from a chemical class known as **peptides,** sequences of amino acids linked together, and it was soon recognized that the same sequence of amino acids occurred in a larger molecule that had been isolated first from the pituitary gland. This led to the discovery of a group of **endorphins** (endogenous morphine-like substances) that are also found in brain tissue and also have potent opiate effects.

These discoveries opened a number of doors for scientists, some of which have helped to answer questions and others of which have led only to more questions. It is now clear that both beta-endorphin and the enkephalins are contained within neurons and released from terminals to act as neurotransmitters or as modulators of neural activity.[36] Beta-endorphin is contained in a relatively small number of long-axon neurons that interconnect the hypothalamus, forebrain limbic structures, the medial thalamus, and the locus ceruleus. Enkephalins are found in a larger number of short-axon neurons within the basal ganglia, hypothalamus, amygdala, substantia nigra, and other areas. Both types of neurons innervate the midbrain central gray, a region known to be involved in pain perception. However, there are many other sites of interaction between these two systems and areas that relate to pain, and pain itself is a complex psychological and neurological phenomenon, so we cannot say that we understand completely how the opiates act to reduce pain.

In addition to the presence of these endogenous opiates in the brain, we know that large amounts of endorphins are released from the pituitary gland in response to stress. Also, the enkephalins are released from the adrenal gland. The functions of these peptides circulating through the blood as hormones are poorly understood at this point. They could perhaps reduce pain by acting in the spinal cord, but they are unlikely to produce direct effects in the brain, because they do not cross the blood-brain barrier. In the late 1970s it was speculated that long-distance runners experience a release of endorphins that may be responsible for the so-called runner's high. Unfortunately, the only evidence in support of this notion was measurements of blood levels of endorphins that seemed to be elevated in some, but not all, runners. These endorphins were presumably from the pituitary and should not be capable of producing a high. It is not known whether exercise alters *brain* levels of these substances.

BENEFICIAL USES
Pain Relief

The major therapeutic indication for morphine and the other narcotics is the reduction of pain. After the administration of an analgesic dose of morphine some patients report that they are still aware of pain, but the pain is no longer aversive. Frequently, though, the pain stimulus is not attended to by the drug user. He is not aware of the pain stimulus until it is pointed out to him, and when made aware of the stimulus, he does not perceive it as aversive. The narcotic agents seem to have their effect in part by diminishing the awareness the individual has of the aversive stimulus and in part on his response to the stimulus. Morphine, then, primarily reduces the emotional response to pain, the suffering, and to some extent also decreases knowledge of the pain stimulus. The effect of narcotics is relatively specific to pain. Fewer effects on mental and motor ability accompany analgesic doses of these agents than with equipotent doses of other analgesic and depressant drugs. Continuous dull pain is relieved more effectively than sharp intermittent pain, but most types of pain are reduced following administration of narcotic agents. Although one of the characteristics of these drugs is their ability to reduce pain without inducing sleep, drowsiness is not uncommon after a therapeutic dose. (In the addicts' vernacular, the patient is "on the nod.") The patient is readily awakened if he sleeps, and dreams during the sleep period are frequent.

Intestinal Disorders

Narcotics have long been valued for their effects on the gastrointestinal system. Not only have they been used to quiet colic, but the only life-saving effect of these drugs is through their ability to counteract diarrhea. In years past and today in many underdeveloped countries, contaminated food or water has resulted in many severe intestinal infections (dysentery). Particularly in the young or the elderly, the diarrhea and resulting dehydration can be a major cause of death.

The narcotic agents decrease the number of peristaltic contractions, which is the type of contraction responsible for moving food through the intestines. At the same time, however, there may be an increase in other gastrointestinal contractions, with the result that there is much activity but little movement of material. Considerable water is absorbed from the intestinal material; this fact, plus the decrease in peristaltic contractions, often results in constipation in patients taking the drugs for pain relief. This side effect has saved many lives of dysentery victims. Although modern synthetic narcotic derivatives are now sold for this purpose, good old-fashioned paregoric, an opium solution, is still available for the symptomatic relief of diarrhea.

Cough Suppressants

The narcotics also have the effect of decreasing activity in what the advertisers refer to as the cough control center in the medulla. Although coughing is often a useful way of clearing unwanted material from the respiratory passages, at times "nonproductive" coughing can itself become a problem. Since the purification from

---

Your turn: people and pain

People hold a variety of personal attitudes about pain and the use of drugs to relieve it. Answer the following questions for yourself:

1. If you were going to the dentist to have a simple cavity filled, would you expect/demand a local anesthetic or other pain reliever, or would you prefer to bear the expected amount of discomfort without drugs if possible?

2. If you broke a leg or were recovering from minor surgery, would you take all available medication to avoid pain, or would you minimize the medication and bear as much pain as possible?

3. If it were necessary for you to receive large doses of a narcotic drug for pain relief for a couple of weeks so that mild physical dependence occurred (some discomfort on ceasing the drug), do you feel that you might have a tendency to seek out more drugs on your own because of the dependence?

4. In cases of postoperative pain, should physicians prescribe an amount of narcotic that is clearly sufficient and allow the patient to reduce the dose at will or should the physician prescribe a minima! amount and allow the patient to ask for more if needed?

After answering these questions for yourself, discuss your answers with a friend or a small group of classmates.

---

opium of codeine, it has been widely used for its *antitussive* properties and is still available in a number of prescription cough remedies. Nonprescription cough remedies contain dextromethorphan, a narcotic analogue that is more selective in its antitussive effects.

CAUSES FOR CONCERN

Dependence Potential

Tolerance. Tolerance develops to most of the effects of the narcotic drugs, although with different effects tolerance may occur at different rates. If the drug is used chronically for pain relief, for example, it will probably be necessary to increase the dose to maintain a constant effect. The

same is true for the euphoria sought by recreational users: repeated use results in a decreased effect that can be overcome by increasing the dose. Cross tolerance exists among all the narcotics, such that tolerance to one reduces the effectiveness of each of the others. Siegel[37] and others have shown that psychological processes can play an important role in the tolerance to narcotics. As a user repeatedly injects the narcotic, the stimuli associated with taking the drug consistently predict various physiological effects (changes in body temperature, intestinal motility, respiration rate, and so on). With repeated experience, the addict's body comes to anticipate those effects and to counteract them. This can be revealed by animal experiments in which, after repeated morphine injections, a placebo injection produces changes in body temperature opposite to those originally produced by morphine. This is analogous to Pavlov's experiments in which a bell repeatedly signaled powdered meat being placed in a dog's mouth: eventually the dog came to anticipate the dry meat powder by salivating in response to the bell. Thus, some of the body's tolerance to narcotics results from conditioned reflex responses to the stimuli associated with taking the drug. To demonstrate how important these conditioned protective reflexes can become, Siegel and his colleagues injected rats with heroin every other day in a particular environment, so that the environment could serve as a predictive signal that heroin effects were about to occur. After 15 such injections, rats were given a much larger dose of heroin, half in the environment previously associated with heroin and half in a different environment. Among the group given the large heroin injection in the different environment, most of the rats died. However, among the group given heroin in the environment that had previously predicted heroin, most of the rats lived.[38] Those rats had presumably been "warned" by the stimulus situation, and conditioned reflexes occurred that counteracted some of the physiological effects of the drug.

Biochemical mechanisms for tolerance have been studied extensively in the norepinephrine-containing cells of the locus ceruleus: activation of opiate receptors normally inhibits the action of an enzyme, adenylate cyclase. After prolonged exposure to opiates, there is an increased level of this enzyme, which tends to counteract its inhibition.[39]

Physical dependence. Concomitant with the development of tolerance is the establishment of physical dependence: in a person who has used the drug chronically and at high doses, as each dose begins to wear off, certain withdrawal symptoms begin to appear. These symptoms and their approximate timing after heroin or methadone are listed in Table 14-3. This list of symptoms might have more personal meaning for you if you compare it to a good case of the "24-hour" or "intestinal" flu: combine nausea and vomiting with diarrhea, aches, and pains and a general sense of misery and you have a pretty good idea of what a moderate case of narcotic withdrawal is like: rarely life-threatening, but most unpleasant. If an individual has been taking a large amount of the narcotic, then these symptoms may be much worse than those caused by "24-hour flu" and last at least twice as long. Note that **methadone,** a longer-lasting synthetic narcotic, produces withdrawal symptoms that are usually less severe and always appear later than with heroin. Cross dependence is seen among the narcotics: no matter which of them was responsible for producing the initial dependence, withdrawal symptoms can be prevented by an appropriate dose of any narcotic. This is the basis for the use of methadone in treating heroin addicts, since substituting legal methadone prevents withdrawal symptoms for as much as a day.

An interesting clue to the biochemical mechanism of withdrawal symptoms has been the finding that *clonidine,* an alpha adrenergic agonist that is used to treat high blood pressure, can diminish the severity of narcotic withdrawal symptoms. Studies on brain tissue reveal that opiate receptors and alpha adrenergic receptors are found together in some brain areas, including the norepinephrine-containing cells of the locus ceruleus. Clonidine and morphine produce identical effects on the enzyme activity and neurophysiology of these cells. In other brain areas, opiate receptors are found that are not associated with alpha adrenergic receptors, which is why clonidine does not produce narcotic-like euphoria and is not a good analgesic.[39]

Psychological dependence. That the opi-

Table 14-3

Sequence of appearance of some of the abstinence syndrome symptoms

Signs	Approximate hours after last dose	
	Heroin and/or morphine	**Methadone**
Craving for drugs, anxiety	6	24
Yawning, perspiration, running nose, teary eyes	14	34 to 48
Increase in above signs plus pupil dilation, goose bumps (pilo-erection), tremors (muscle twitches), hot and cold flashes, aching bones and muscles, loss of appetite	16	48 to 72
Increased intensity of above, plus insomnia; raised blood pressure; increased temperature, pulse rate, respiratory rate and depth; restlessness; nausea	24 to 36	
Increased intensity of above, plus curled-up position, vomiting, diarrhea, weight loss, spontaneous ejaculation or orgasm, hemo-concentration, increased blood sugar	36 to 48	

ates produce psychological dependence is quite clear; in fact, experiments with the opiates were what led to our current understanding of the importance of the reinforcing properties of drugs. Animals allowed to self-administer low doses of morphine or heroin intravenously will learn the required behaviors quickly and perform them for prolonged periods, even if withdrawal symptoms have never been experienced. This is an example of what psychologists refer to as *positive reinforcement:* a behavior is reliably followed by the presentation of a stimulus, leading to an increase in the probability of the behavior and its eventual maintenance at a higher rate than before. Remember that the rapidity with which the reinforcing stimulus follows the behavior is an important factor, which is why fewer experiences are needed with a narcotic injected intravenously than with one taken orally.

Once physical dependence has developed and withdrawal symptoms are experienced, the conditions are set up for another behavioral mechanism, *negative reinforcement.* In this situation, an act (drug taking) is followed by the *removal* of a stimulus (withdrawal symptoms), leading to further strengthening of the habit. In heroin addiction, the rapid and potent euphoric effect resulting from intravenous injection, combined with the appearance of early withdrawal symptoms after only a few hours and their rapid alleviation by another injection, leads to the development of strong psychological dependence. Remember, however, that heroin was prescribed in low doses and taken orally by many patients for several years during which it was believed to be nonaddictive. Although heroin is more potent than morphine and may be slightly more addictive because of its more rapid access to the brain, morphine taken intravenously is clearly more addicting than heroin taken orally.

The needle habit. Each heroin administration is followed by a decrease in discomfort, an increase in pleasure, or both. As a result, the behavior itself of preparing and injecting the drug and the setting in which it occurs acquire pleasurable, positive associations through learning

mechanisms. Because of this conditioning, the *process of using* heroin becomes rewarding as well as the *use* of heroin. One occasional user commented on the ritual of heroin use:

> Once you decide to get off it's very exciting. It really is. Getting some friends together and some money, copping, deciding where you're going to do it, getting the needles out and sterilizing them, cooking up the stuff, tying off, then the whole thing with the needle, booting, and the rush, that's all part of it. . . . Sometimes I think that if I just shot water I'd enjoy it as much.[40]

Perhaps strangely to the reader, that last statement is true for some individuals who label themselves "addicts." Things aren't always what they seem to be. One out of five individuals who apply for treatment in one large city center is clearly not physically dependent: they show *no* response to a narcotic antagonist. Another 15% to 20% show only "a very mild reaction to a large naloxone injection. . . . "[41,p.35] These individuals have been called "needle freaks"—they are psychologically dependent on shooting up and may or may not be physiologically dependent on the drug.

> The heroin addict of today is very different from the addicts we saw ten years ago. We've seen an evolution of drug-taking patterns during the time we've been involved—from the "Aquarian Age junkie," as we call them, through the "Nixon Era junky," the transitional junky, to a new and extremely different group. . . .
>
> This new junkie is not a true heroin addict. There will be needle marks all over him, he may have abscesses, but upon testing you will find that he is not truly addicted.[42]

A research team headed by a psychiatrist, Charles O'Brien, has studied the process of eliminating (extinguishing) the needle habit. A long-acting, experimental narcotic antagonist was administered and the patients allowed to shoot up, using their own equipment and rituals. Since most addicts usually shoot up in a bathroom, the researchers used a special bathroom where the patients could inject their drugs. Under double-blind conditions the users injected saline or a high or low dose of a narcotic. No matter which he used, there was no effect because of the administration of the antagonist. Both objective and subjective measures were used, and "all of the self-injections are rated by the patients as pleasurable at first."[41,p.36] Only after three to five injections were the subjective reports neutral. Continued self-injections under these conditions resulted in the patients reporting they they hated the whole process. Remember always that there is variability in any biological system: one patient continued to report euphoria after each injection for 26 trials, and he regularly showed the pupillary constriction that accompanies the injection of a narcotic! That patient was one of those receiving saline, so it was not a question of the narcotic dose being high or the antagonist dose being low.

Toxicity Potential

Acute toxicity. One specific effect of the narcotics is to depress the respiratory centers in the brain so that respiration slows and becomes shallow. This is perhaps the major side effect of the narcotic agents and one of the most dangerous, since death resulting from respiratory arrest can easily follow an excessive dose of these drugs. The basis for this effect is that the respiratory centers become less responsive to carbon dioxide levels in the blood. It is this effect that keeps heroin/morphine and methadone near the top of the list of mentioned drugs in DAWN coroner's reports. Remember that this respiratory depression is additive with the effects of alcohol or other sedative-hypnotics, and there is evidence that a large fraction of those who die from heroin overdose have elevated blood alcohol concentrations and might better be described as dying from a combination of heroin and alcohol. Narcotic overdose may be diagnosed on the basis of the "narcotic triad": coma, depressed respiration, and pinpoint pupils. Emergency medical treatment calls for the use of naloxone (Narcan), which antagonizes the narcotic effects within a few minutes.

The behavioral consequences of having narcotics in the brain are probably less dangerous. Those who inject heroin may "nod off" into a dream-filled sleep for a few minutes, and opium smokers are famous for their "pipe dreams." It is perhaps not surprising that individuals under the influence of narcotics are likely to be less active and less alert than they otherwise would be. There is a clouding of consciousness that makes mental work more difficult. And narcotics users are not only less likely to be interested in sex, males may even suffer from primary impotence as a direct result of the presence of the drug.

Narcotics also stimulate the brain area controlling nausea and vomiting, which are other frequent side effects. Nausea occurs in about half of ambulatory patients given a 15 mg dose of morphine. Also, nausea and vomiting are a common reaction to heroin injection among street users.

Chronic toxicity. Although early in this century many medical authorities believed that chronic narcotic use weakened the user both mentally and physically, there is no scientific evidence that exposure to narcotic drugs per se causes long-term damage to any tissue or organ system. Many street users of narcotics do suffer from sores and abscesses at injection sites, but these can be attributed to the lack of sterile technique. Also, the practice of sharing the same needle to inject drugs into the veins can result in the spread of such blood-borne diseases as serum hepatitis and AIDS. Again, this is not a result of the drug, but of the technique used to inject it.

Patterns of Abuse

The heroin addict. Only a glimpse of some of the mechanics of a heroin user's life can be presented here. Withdrawal signs may begin about 4 hours after the last use of the drug, but many addicts report that they begin to feel ill only 6 to 8 hours after the last dose. That puts most addicts on a schedule of three to four injections every day. Today's addict is not spending a lot of time nodding off in opium dens as in the good old days. When you have a very important appointment to keep every 6 to 8 hours, every day of the week, every day of the year, you've got to hustle not to miss one of them. Remember, there are no vacations, no weekends off for the regular user, just 1200 to 1400 appointments to keep.

And each one costs money. Heroin is frequently sold on the street in "nickel or dime" bags: $5 or $10 for a small plastic bag containing . . . Good question—what's in the bag? In 1987 the material in a $10 bag might have had 3 to 5 mg or 25 mg. Of course, you may not get any heroin, and you can't complain to the Better Business Bureau. At any rate, your addiction may cost you $20 to $100 a day.

The variability in amount of heroin is a problem because of the possibility of an overdose (OD). Addicts should worry about an OD with each new batch of drug used. A sophisticated user buying from a new or questionable source will initially try a much smaller than normal amount of the powder to evaluate its potency.

Once the user has acquired the drug, he prepares it for injection. Usually, he

mixes the powder with unsterile water, heats the mixture briefly in a spoon or bottle cap with a match or lighter, then draws the heroin into a syringe or eyedropper through cotton, thus filtering out the larger impurities. The heroin is then injected intravenously without any attempt at skin cleansing.[43]

Under these conditions it is not surprising that infections do occur. The preferred equipment today for injection is the eyedropper with a hypodermic needle attached, since the rubber bulb of the dropper is easier to operate than the plunger of a syringe.

The most common form of heroin use by male addicts is to inject the drug intravenously, that is, to "mainline" the drug. A convenient site is the left forearm (for right-handed users), and the frequent use of dirty needles will leave the arm marked with scar tissue. If the larger veins of the arm collapse, then other body areas will be used. Many beginning addicts start by "skin-popping"—subcutaneous injections. "Skin-popping" increases the danger of tetanus but decreases the risk of hepatitis compared to mainlin-

ing. Because of the lack of sterility or even cleanliness, hepatitis, tetanus, and abscesses at the site of injection are not uncommon in street users who inject drugs.

If the addict survives the perils of an overdose, escapes the dangers of contaminated equipment, and avoids being caught, there are still some dangers. Since heroin is a potent analgesic, its regular use *may* conceal the early symptoms of an illness such as pneumonia. The addict's lack of money for, or interest in, food frequently results in malnutrition. With low resistance from malnutrition and the symptoms of illness unnoticed as a result of heroin use, the addict becomes quite susceptible to serious disease.

If all these dangers are overcome, the addict may continue to use opiates to an advanced age. Sometimes, though, the addict who avoids illness, death, or arrest and who does not enter and stay in a rehabilitation program or withdraw himself from the drug may no longer feel the need for the drug and gradually stop using it. The data are still very much debated, but this "maturing out" is probably what happens to a large number of addicts. One authority reports that if an addict lives, he remains addicted for only about 8 or 9 years. This is an average, however, and according to this report the earlier a user starts, the longer he remains addicted, with maturing out generally occurring in the 35- to 45-year age period.[44] Even if he lives, the street life of an addict isn't a rose garden.

The street scene is continually shifting on all illegal drug use, and future trends are difficult to specify with certainty. As a general statement, however, and this is true of all drug use, there is a gradual homogenization of users. Every year, in drug use as in other behaviors, the differences between males and females, blacks and whites become less distinct. In the period from 1969 to 1970 four males entered drug treatment programs for every female. In 1980 the ratio was three to one. Over this same period the proportion of those admitted to treatment programs who were black decreased from 55% to 30%. The proportion who were white increased from 30% to 58%. By 1987 it appeared that blacks and whites each represented about 40% of narcotic users, with hispanics accounting for 11%. These data, of course, also obscure important regional variation, with more hispanic users in Los Angeles and San Antonio, more whites in Minneapolis, Phoenix, Kansas City and Miami, and more blacks in Baltimore, Newark, and Detroit.[45]

Misconceptions and preconceptions. There has been so much written in the popular press about heroin use and heroin users that readers may believe that they know enough about it. This section deals with some of the major misconceptions most people, including many professionals, have about nonmedical use and misuse of narcotics. One of the most common is that mainlining heroin or morphine induces in everyone an intense pleasure unequaled by any other experience. Addicts talk in glowing terms of the "rush" or "kick" they frequently experience.[46] Often it is described as similar to a whole-body orgasm that persists up to 5 or more minutes. Some addicts report that they try with every injection to reexperience the extreme euphoria of the first injection, but they always have a lesser effect. There are studies, however, as well as clinical and street reports, that some people experience only nausea and discomfort following the initial intravenous administration of morphine or heroin.[47] For whatever reasons, some of these users persist and the discomfort decreases, that is, shows tolerance more rapidly than the euphoric effects. Under these conditions the injections soon result primarily in pleasant effects. To maintain these pleasurable feelings, though, the dose level must gradually be increased. There is no resolution of what type of individual—socially, psychologically, or biochemically—readily experiences pleasure in contrast to those whose initial symptoms are unpleasant.[48] It is true, however, that even with the narcotics some addicts must partially learn which experiences are defined as pleasurable. One author has referred to the two "powerfully pleasurable effects"—the initial brief rush and then the longer tranquility—and then commented:

This sequence of events occurs with virtually every nontolerant person, although the first few experiences may be accompanied by vomiting. Even so, the sensations are often pleasurable ("You don't mind vomiting behind smack").[49]

Another misconception has to do with the development of withdrawal symptoms. The addict undergoing withdrawal without medication is always portrayed as being in excruciating pain, truly suffering. It depends. With a large habit, withdrawal without medication is truly hell. The opiate addiction scene is changing too rapidly to be definite about today's user, but most street addicts are described as having "ice cream habits," that is, they use a low daily drug dose.

Perhaps the most common misconception about heroin is that after one shot, you are hooked for life. None of the narcotics, or any other drug, fits into that fantasized category. Becoming addicted takes some time, perhaps a week, and persistence on the part of the beginner. Regular use of the drug seems to be more important in establishing physiological addiction than the size of the dose used. Becoming physiologically addicted is possible on a weekend, but it frequently requires a longer period with three or four injections a day.[40]

There are probably about 500,000 narcotic addicts in the United States. There may be two to three times as many heroin *chippers*—occasional users. Several reports and studies have appeared on the characteristics of these occasional users, but no consistent differences, compared to addicts, have yet been found other than the pattern of use. One review of this topic contains several case histories, and you must appreciate that there are no "typical" chippers, but Arthur D. is representative.

Arthur D. is a forty-year-old white male with a wife and three children who works regularly as a union carpenter. He has no family history of alcoholism or drug dependency.

Drug use began with occasional marijuana use at age sixteen, which became daily use by age eighteen. By nineteen he had stopped his heavy drinking though he continued regular marijuana use, which included

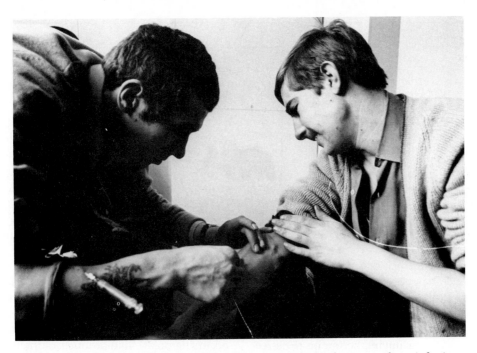

One user helps another "shoot up." Note the apparent lack of concern about infection.

some dealing in marijuana. For about one and a half years from ages twenty to twenty-two he experimented with psychedelics, and for two years from ages twenty-one to twenty-three he used amphetamines with some frequency.

Mr. D. first used heroin at age twenty-four. He used it sporadically for two years, but with growing frequency, until at age twenty-seven he recognized that he had a habit. He was married at age thirty-two to a woman who disapproved of his use of narcotics in particular and of drugs in general. Although his drug use had sharply decreased, it never ceased. For the last ten years his use of heroin has been confined to weekends, with an occasional shot during the week. For the last five years, however, this occasional "extra" shot has virtually ceased. His wife does not use heroin at all but will smoke marijuana with him occasionally. As a result of her disapproval of his drug use and the people with whom he uses drugs, on almost every weekend he will select a time to go to a using friend's home and get high there.[50,p.10]

The 1980s: new users, new drugs. Heroin addiction will continue to appear in various groups in each new generation. In the mid-1980s, low-class junkies were joined by a group of young, wealthy, "respectable" heroin users, both in the United States and Europe. A new, very pure form of heroin called **black tar** appeared on the streets in 1986. As if the variable nature of street heroin coming from different sources around the world weren't confusing enough, the street scene has become further complicated by the presence of various synthetic drugs. Street users have become wise to fentanyl, a potent prescription narcotic available in sterile solution for injection. Illicit chemists have developed derivatives of fentanyl and sold them on the streets as "China White," or "synthetic heroin." The interesting thing about these "designer drugs" is that the chemists are able to vary the molecule to produce drugs that have not yet been listed as controlled substances.

Another synthetic heroin, MPPP, which is a derivative of meperidine (Demerol), has been produced by several illicit laboratories. However, there is substantial danger of trace amounts of the

---

Issue: AIDS and the IV drug user

A new danger for IV drug users came into national prominence in the 1980s: acquired immune deficiency syndrome (AIDS). This disease, which was first described in 1981, kills about half its victims. By the beginning of 1986 more than 16,000 cases had been documented.

The AIDS virus attacks the body's immune system, leaving the victim susceptible to a variety of other infections. The virus does not survive well on its own, however, and must be transmitted through a body fluid such as blood or semen. Because IV drug users often share needles, there is a high risk of AIDS among that group. Certainly this will frighten some individuals away from IV use of heroin or at least make them more careful about sharing needles and perhaps about cleanliness in general.

There is an ironic twist to this problem: because it is primarily a disease associated with male homosexuals and drug addicts, there are some in our society who have a hard time becoming too concerned about it. Are your own attitudes about AIDS influenced by your perception of the type of people likely to contract it?

---

impurity MPTP being included, and this incredibly toxic substance has been responsible for the occurrence of permanent brain damage in several users in the 1980s. MPTP results in destruction of dopamine neurons, leading to a form of Parkinson's disease. Anyone buying heroin on the street these days faces multiple dangers, and the only regulation seems to be that famous old free-market concept, *caveat emptor* (let the buyer beware).

Summary

Opium, from which the narcotic drugs morphine and codeine can be extracted, was used in its raw form for centuries, both medicinally and for pleasure. It had significant influences on medicine, literature, and world politics through the 1800s. The importance of opium has declined with the purification of morphine and the later development of heroin and the synthetic narcotics.

Addiction to narcotics has been recognized for a long time, but no concerted effort to control addiction was tried until the patent medicine era of the late 1800s, combined with opium-smoking by Chinese Americans, led to federal regulations in the early 1900s. The typical narcotic addict changed from a middle-aged, middle-class female using narcotics by mouth to a young, lower-class male using heroin by intravenous injection.

A variety of synthetic narcotics are now available along with the natural products of the opium poppy. These drugs all act at opiate receptors in the brain and in other nervous tissue. These receptors are normally acted upon by the naturally occurring opiate-like products of the nervous system and endocrine glands, endorphins and enkephalins.

The narcotics produce tolerance, physical dependence, and psychological dependence and are considered "model" drugs of addiction. Besides the concern over addiction to these drugs, they are also capable of producing acute poisoning by suppressing the respiration rate. In overdoses, death occurs because breathing ceases.

There is a great variety of behavioral patterns exhibited by current narcotic addicts. In addition to the stereotype of the lower-class addict who avoids painful withdrawal symptoms only by illegal activities, we have occasional users, "chippers," and perhaps an increasing number of young, wealthy heroin users. This variety of behavioral pattern is matched by a variety of heroin with wide ranges of purity coming from all over the world, as well as new "designer drugs," at least one of which has been accompanied by terrible side effects.

REFERENCES

1. Baum LF: The new wizard of Oz, New York, 1944, Grosset & Dunlap, Inc.

2. Scott JM: The white poppy; a history of opium, New York, 1969, Funk & Wagnalls.

3. Africa TW: The opium addiction of Marcus Aurelius, Journal of the History of Ideas 22:97-102, 1961.

4. Hamarneh S: Sources and development of Arabic medical therapy and pharmacology, Sudhoffs Archiv fur Geschichte der Medizin und der Naturwissenschaften 54:34, 1970.

5. De Quincey T: Confessions of an English opium-eater, New York, 1907, E.P. Dutton & Co., Inc.

6. Turk MH: Selections from De Quincey, Boston, 1902, Ginn & Co.

7. De Quincey works, vol 206. Quoted in Lowes JL: The road to Xanadu, Boston, 1927, Houghton Mifflin Co.

8. Mickel EJ: The artificial paradises in French literature, Chapel Hill, NC, 1969, The University of North Carolina.

9. Blair W: An opium-eater in America, The Knickerbocker (New York Monthly Magazine) 20:47-57, 1842.

10. Hahn E: The big smoke, The New Yorker, pp 35-43, February 15, 1969.

11. Kramer JC: Opium rampant: medical use, misuse and abuse in Britain and the West in the 17th and 18th centuries, British Journal of Addiction, p 377, 1979.

12. Edwards G: Opium and after, Lancet 1(8164):351, February 16, 1980.

13. Kramer JC: Heroin in the treatment of morphine addiction, Journal of Psychedelic Drugs 9(3):193-197, 1977.

14. Dott DB and Stockman R: Proceedings of the Royal Society of Edinburgh, p 321, 1890.

15. Manges M: A second report on the therapeutics of heroine, New York Medical Journal 71:51, 82-83, 1900.

16. Wilcox RW: Pharmacology and therapeutics, ed 6, Philadelphia, 1905, P. Blakiston's Son & Co.

17. Lindesmith AR: Addiction and opiates, Chicago, 1968, Aldine Publishing Co.

18. Kebler LF: The present status of drug addiction in the United States. In Transactions of the American Therapeutic Society, Philadelphia, 1910, FA Davis Co.

19. Black JR: Advantages of substituting the morphia habit for the incurably alcoholic, The Cincinnati Lancet—Clinic 22:538-541, 1889.

20. Lindesmith AR: The addict and the law, Bloomington, 1965, Indiana University Press.

21. Markham JM: The American disease, New York Times, sec 7, April 29, 1973.

22. Smith R: Status politics and the image of the addict, Issues in Criminology 2(2):157-175, 1966.

23. Preble E and Casey JJ, Jr: Taking care of business—the heroin user's life on the street, International Journal of the Addictions 4(1):1-24, 1969.

24. Isbell H: Discussion, Symposium on Problems of Drug Dependence, Fourteenth Annual Conference Veterans Administration Cooperative Studies in Psychiatry, Houston, Texas, April 1, 1969, Highlights of the Conference, Veterans Administration, Washington, DC, 1969, US Government Printing Office.

25. Platt JJ and others: Recent trends in the demography of heroin addiction among youthful offenders, The International Journal of the Addictions 11(2):221-236, 1976.

26. Inquiry into alleged drug abuse in the armed services, Report of a special subcommittee of the Committee on Armed Services, House of Representatives, Ninety-second Congress, First Session, April 23, 1971, Washington, DC, 1971, US Government Printing Office.

27. The world heroin problem. Committee Print, House of Representatives, Committee on Foreign Affairs, Ninety-second Congress, First Session, May 27, 1971, Washington, DC, 1971, US Government Printing Office.

28. Robins LN: The Vietnam drug user returns, Special Action Office for Drug Abuse Prevention Monograph, Series A, No 2, May 1974, Contract No HSM-42-72-75.

29. Brodsky MD: History of heroin prevalence estimation techniques. In Self-report methods of estimating drug use, NIDA Research Monograph No 57, Washington, DC, 1985, US Government Printing Office.

30. The supply of illicit drugs to the United States, National Narcotics Intelligence Consumers Committee, Washington, DC, 1988.

31. Thomas H: Turkey agrees to '72 ban on poppies, United Press International, July 1, 1971.

32. Hess JL: U.S. and France sign antidrug accord, New York Times, February 27, 1971, p 3.

33. Mexico, Drug Enforcement 3(1):6-12, Winter, 1975-1976.

34. Riding A: Mexico making headway in war on opium poppies, New York Times, February 24, 1980, p 1.

35. Pert CB and Snyder SH: Properties of opiate-receptor binding in rat brain, Proceedings of the National Academy of Sciences 70:2243-2247, 1973.

36. Feldman RS and Quenzer LF: Fundamentals of Neuropsychopharmacology Sunderland, Mass, 1984, Sinauer.

37. Siegel S: Morphine analgesic tolerance: its situation specificity supports a pavlovian conditioning model, Science 193:323-325, 1976.

38. Siegel S, Hinson RE, Krank MD and others: Heroin "overdose" death: contribution of drug-associated environmental cues, Science 216:436-437, 1982.

39. Aghajanian GK: The neurobiology of opiate withdrawal: receptors, second messengers, and ion channels. Psychiatry Letter 3:57-60, 1985.

40. Powell DH: A pilot study of occasional heroin users, Archives of General Psychiatry 28:586-594, 1973.

41. O'Brien CP: "Needle freaks": psychological dependence on shooting up. In Medical World News, Psychiatry Annual, New York, 1974, McGraw-Hill Book Co.

42. Gay G: Heroin addiction patterns have changed, MD says, Drugs and Drug Abuse Education Newsletter 6:9, 1975.

43. Louria DB, Hensle T, and Rose J: The major medical complications of heroin addiction, Annals of Internal Medicine 67:1-22, 1967.

44. Winick C: Maturing out of narcotic addiction, Bulletin on Narcotics 14(1):1-8, 1962.

45. Data from the Drug Abuse Warning Network (DAWN), DHHS Publication No (ADM) 88-1584, US Government Printing Office, 1988.

46. Mathis JL: Sexual aspects of heroin addiction, Medical Aspects of Human Sexuality 4(9):98-109, 1970.

47. Isbell H and White WM: Clinical characteristics of addictions, The American Journal of Medicine 14:558-565, 1953.

48. Balster RL and Harris LS: Drugs as reinforcers in animals and humans; Symposium, Federation Proceedings 41(2):209-246, 1982.

49. Goldstein A: Heroin addiction and the role of methadone in its treatment, Archives of General Psychiatry 26:291-297, 1972.

50. Hunt CG and Zinberg NE: Heroin use: a new look, Drug Abuse Council, Inc., September 1976.

Chapter 15

Hallucinogens

OBJECTIVES

After reading this chapter, you should be able to:

Explain why psychoactive drugs have played an important role in many of the world's religions.

Describe the history of the discovery and use of LSD.

Identify the psychological similarities among the indole hallucinogens and the current scientific attitude about how they work in the brain.

Describe several psychoactive plants, the chemicals contained in them, the class of hallucinogen to which they belong, and what their psychological effects are.

From the soft, quiet beauty of the sacred *Psilocybe* mushroom to the angry, mottled appearance of the toxic *Amanita,* from the mountains of Mexico to the streets of Anytown, U.S.A., from before history to the end of the twentieth century, man has looked, searched, sought after the perfect aphrodisiac, spiritual experiences, other worlds. The plants have been there to help; it's worth repeating that plants have an adaptive edge if they produce chemicals that alter the biochemistry of animals. If they make us feel sick, we are unlikely to eat them again, and if they kill us, we are certain not to eat them again. But humans long ago learned to "tame" some of these plants, to use them in just the right way and in just the right amount to alter perceptions and emotions without too many unpleasant consequences.

ANIMISM AND RELIGION

Animism, the concept that animals, plants, rocks, and streams derive their special characteristics from some spirit contained within the object, is a common theme in most of the world's religions. Plants that are able to alter man's perception of the world and of himself fit right into such a view. If the plant contains a spirit, then eating the plant transfers that spirit to the person who ate it, and the spirit of the plant may speak to the consumer, make him feel the plant's joy or provide him with special powers or insights.

In primitive societies, certain individuals became specialists in the ways of these plants, learning when to harvest them and how much to use under what circumstances. These traditions were passed down from one generation to another, and colorful stories were used to teach the principles to apprentices. Although our modern term for these individuals is medicine man, because of their knowledge of drug-containing plants, their function in primitive societies had less to do with what we would call medicine today than with what we would now call religion. Thus these plants and their psychoactive effects were probably important reasons for the development of spiritual and religious practices and folklore in many different societies all over the world.[1]

TERMINOLOGY AND TYPES

The issue of what to call this group of drugs is an old one. In 1931, Lewin referred to a class of **phantastica,** drugs that could replace the present world with a world of fantasy. Peyote, psilocybin, and LSD all produce this type of effect. In the 1960s, these drugs were described by enthusiastic users as allowing them to see into their own minds, and the term **psychedelic** (mind vision) was widely used. Because the drugs are capable of producing hallucinations and some altered sense of reality, a state that could be called psychotic, they have been referred to as **psychotomimetic** drugs. Since one thing common to these drugs is some tendency to produce hallucinations, we will refer to them by the name **hallucinogens.**

Although the drugs are all called hallucinogens for our purposes, in fact there are important differences among them. They can be classified according to their chemical structures, known pharmacological properties, how much loss of awareness occurs, and how dangerous they are. The first types we will review are the classical phantastica: they are capable of altering perceptions, while allowing the person to remain in communication with the present world. The individual under the influence of these drugs will often be aware of both the "fantasy" world and the "real" world at the same time, may talk avidly about what is being experienced, and will be able to remember much of it later. These drugs may be seen as having more purely hallucinogenic effects in that they do not produce much acute physiological toxicity, that is, there is relatively little danger of dying from an overdose of LSD, psilocybin, or mescaline.

INDOLE HALLUCINOGENS

The basic structure of the neurotransmitter serotonin is referred to as an **indole** nucleus. Fig. 15-1 illustrates that the hallucinogens LSD and psilocybin also contain this structure. For that reason and the fact that some other chemicals with this structure have similar hallucinogenic effects, we refer to one group of the hallucinogens as the indoles.

d-Lysergic Acid Diethylamide

The most potent and notorious of the hallucinogens and the one that brought these drugs into the public eye in the 1960s, is not found in nature at all. Although there are naturally occurring compounds that resemble the indole *d*-lysergic acid diethylamide (LSD), their identity as hallucinogens was not known until after the discovery of LSD. LSD was originally synthesized from ergot alkaloids extracted from the ergot fungus *Claviceps purpurea*. This mold occasionally grows on grain, especially rye, and eating infected grain results in an illness called **ergotism.**

St. Anthony's fire.   Grain that has been infected with the ergot fungus is readily identified and is usually destroyed. During periods of famine, however, the grain may be used in making bread. In France between 945 AD and 1600 AD there were at least 20 outbreaks of ergotism, the illness that results from eating infected bread. Although the cause of the illness was established before 1700, only symptomatic treatment exists even today. There are two forms of the disease. In one there are tingling sensations in the skin

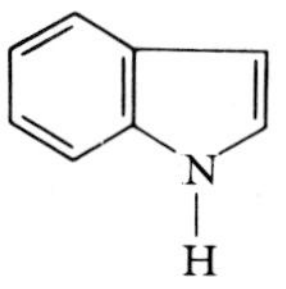

the indole nucleus

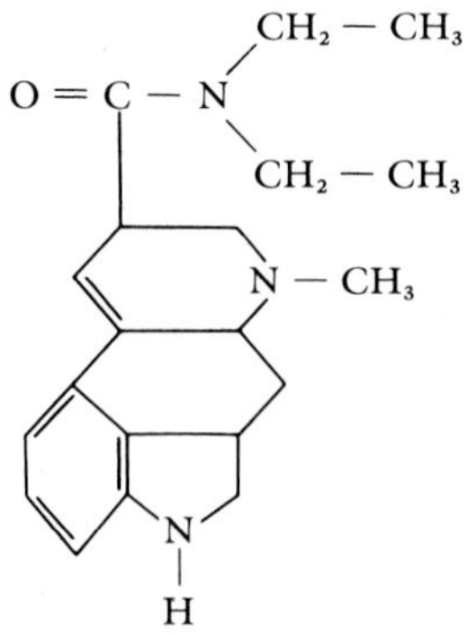

d-lysergic acid diethylamide (LSD) (9, 10-didehydro - *N,N* - diethyl - 6 - methyl - ergoline - 8β - carboxamide).

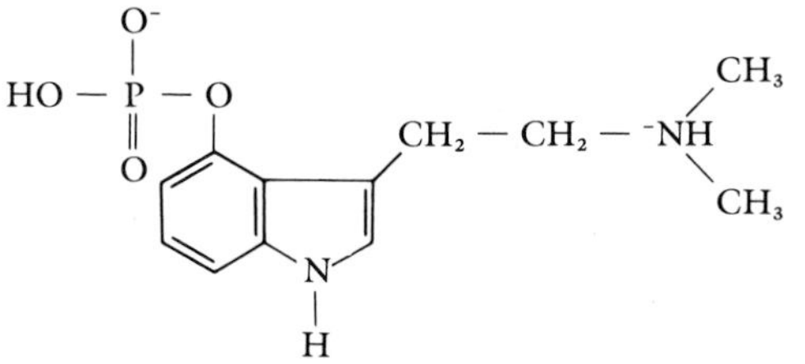

Psilocybin
(3-[2-(dimethylamino)ethyl]-indol-4-ol dihydrogen phosphate ester)

Figure 15-1. Indole hallucinogens.

and muscle spasms that develop into convulsions, insomnia, and various disturbances of consciousness and thinking. In the other form, gangrenous ergotism, the limbs become swollen and inflamed, with the individual experiencing "violent burning pains" before the affected part becomes numb. Sometimes the disease moves rapidly, with less than 24 hours between the first sign and the development of gangrene. Gangrene develops because the ergot causes a contraction of the blood vessels, cutting off blood flow to the extremities.

During the twelfth century ergotism became associated with St. Anthony, although the reason for this is not completely clear. It may be that the hospital for the treatment of ergotism was built near the shrine of St. Anthony because he had suffered from a minor attack of ergotism. Some suggest that the demons he reported battling were the result of the disease.[2] Others believe the illness was called St. Anthony's Fire because those who made the pilgrimage to Egypt, where St. Anthony had lived, were cured. No matter, those who journeyed to Egypt as well as those who entered the hospital did lose their symptoms, probably as a result of a diet that did not include ergot-infected rye.

Two interesting articles in 1976 discussed a possible link between convulsive ergotism and the Salem village witch trials of 1692 in which 20 people were executed. The first article[3] built a very strong case that (1) the original symptoms exhibited by the "possessed" eight girls were similar to those seen in convulsive ergotism and (2) the conditions were right for the growth of the ergot fungus on the rye that was the staple cereal. The second article[4] constructed an equally convincing case that ergotism could *not* have been involved and that the "possession" was psychological in origin. In fact, we will never *know* for sure; there are, however, enough similarities and lingering doubts that ergotism seems to remain a possible basis for the Salem incident.

LSD discovery and early research.   In the Sandoz Laboratories in Basel, Switzerland, in 1938 Dr. Albert Hofmann synthesized *l*ysergsaure*d*iethylamid, the German word from which LSD comes and the equivalent of the English d-lysergic acid diethylamide. Hofmann was working on a series of compounds derived from ergot alkaloids that had as their basic structure lysergic acid. LSD was synthesized because of its chemical similarity to a known stimulant, nikethamide. It was not until 1943, however, that LSD entered the world of biochemical psychiatry when Hofmann recorded in his laboratory notebook:

Last Friday, April 16, 1943, I was forced to stop my work in the laboratory in the middle of the afternoon and to go home, as I was seized by a peculiar restlessness associated with a sensation of mild dizziness. Having reached home, I lay down and sank in a kind of drunkenness which was not unpleasant and which was characterized by extreme activity of imagination. As I lay in a dazed condition with my eyes closed (I experienced daylight as disagreeably bright) there surged upon me an uninterrupted stream of fantastic images of extraordinary plasticity and vividness and accompanied by an intense, kaleidoscope-like play of colors. This condition gradually passed off after about two hours.[5, pp. 184-185]

Hofmann later said, "The first experience was a very weak one, consisting of rather small changes. It had a pleasant, fairy tale-magic theater quality."[6] He was sure that the experience resulted from the accidental absorption, through the skin of his fingers, of the compound with which he was working. The next Monday morning Hofmann prepared what he thought was a very small amount of LSD, 0.25 mg, and made the following record in his notebook:

April 19, 1943: Preparation of an 0.5% aqueous solution of *d*-lysergic acid diethylamide tartrate.

4:20 P.M.: 0.5 cc (0.25 mg LSD) ingested orally. The solution is tasteless.

4:50 P.M.: no trace of any effect.

5:00 P.M.: slight dizziness, unrest, difficulty in concentration, visual disturbances, marked desire to laugh. . . .

At this point the laboratory notes are discontinued:

The last words could only be written with great difficulty. I asked my laboratory assistant to accompany me home as I believed that my condition would be a repetition of the disturbance of the previous Friday. While we were still cycling home, however, it became clear that the symptoms were much stronger than the first time. I had great difficulty in speaking coherently, my field of vision swayed before me, and objects appeared distorted like images in curved mirrors. I had the impression of being unable to move from the spot, although my assistant told me afterwards that we had cycled at a good pace. . . .

Six hours after ingestion of the LSD-25 my condition had already improved considerably. Only the visual disturbances were still pronounced. Everything seemed to

sway and the proportions were distorted like the reflections in the surface of moving water. Moreover, all objects appeared in unpleasant, constantly changing colors, the predominant shades being sickly green and blue. When I closed my eyes, an unending series of colorful, very realistic and fantastic images surged in upon me. A remarkable feature was the manner in which all acoustic perceptions (e.g., the noise of a passing car) were transformed into optical effects, every sound causing a corresponding colored hallucination constantly changing in shape and color like pictures in a kaleidoscope. At about 1 o'clock I fell asleep and awakened the next morning somewhat tired but otherwise feeling perfectly well.[5, pp. 185-186]

The amount Albert Hofmann took orally is five to eight times the normal effective dose, and it was the potency of the drug that attracted attention to it. Mescaline had long been known to cause strange experiences, alter consciousness, and lead to a particularly vivid kaleidoscope of colors, but it takes 4000 times as much mescaline as LSD. LSD is usually active when only 0.05 mg (50 µg) is taken, and in some people a dose of 0.03 mg is effective.

The first report on LSD in the scientific literature came from Zurich in 1947, but it was 1949 before the first North American study on its use in humans appeared. In 1953 Sandoz applied to the Food and Drug Administration to study LSD as an investigational new drug. Between 1953 and 1966 Sandoz distributed large quantities of LSD to qualified scientists throughout the world. Most of this legal LSD was used in biochemical and animal behavior research.

Besides an interest in trying to develop "model psychoses" in animals and humans so that treatments could be developed, the major thrust of LSD research had to do with its alleged ability to access the "subconscious mind." This notion probably derived from the dreamlike quality of the reports of LSD experiences and the long-held psychoanalytic view that dreams represented subconscious thoughts trying to express themselves. Thus LSD was widely used as an adjunct to psychotherapy. When a psychiatrist felt that a patient had reached a roadblock and was unable to dredge up repressed memories and motives, LSD might be used for its psychedelic (mind-viewing) properties. Thus LSD took over as a modern truth serum, replacing sodium pentothal and scopolamine.

Two other potentially therapeutic uses were studied: for various theoretical reasons it was believed that LSD might be a good treatment for alcoholics, and initial reports of its effectiveness were quite positive. Later, it was hoped that LSD would allow terminal cancer patients to achieve a greater understanding of their own mortality. Thus many such patients were allowed to explore their feelings while under the influence of this fantasy-producing agent.

In April 1966, the Sandoz Pharmaceutical Company recalled the LSD it had distributed and withdrew its sponsorship for work with LSD. Large quantities of illegally manufactured LSD of uncertain purity were being used in the street, and Sandoz decided to give the responsibility for the legal distribution of LSD to the federal government.

Scientific study of the hallucinogens declined in the 1970s. The Reverend Walter Clark, a theologian and well-known advocate of controlled research on psychedelic drugs, provided data to support what he wrote in 1975:

Because of bureaucratic restrictions and public fear of the highly publicized dangers of the drugs both real and supposed, responsible investigators have too often retired from the field, despite their interest in the drugs and the conviction of many that these drugs are exceedingly promising tools in mental health and for the study of the human mind and development.[7]

Dr. Clark was partially whistling in the dark, since research with marijuana has the same bureaucratic restrictions and is legally studied by thousands of scientists. More probably, hallucinogenic research had reached a dead end where new ideas were needed and not forthcoming. A 1974 report by an NIMH research task force on hallucinogenic research stated:

Virtually every psychological test has been used to study persons under the influence of LSD or other such

hallucinogens, but the research has contributed little to our understanding of the bizarre and potent effects of this drug.[8]

Partly as a reality-oriented response to this type of evaluation and partly because of the dead ends, the National Institute of Mental Health stopped its in-house LSD research on humans in 1968 and stopped funding university human research on LSD in 1974. The National Cancer Institute and the National Institute on Alcohol Abuse and Alcoholism stopped supporting psychedelic research in 1975 because it was nonproductive.

The unraveling of CIA/army human research programs using hallucinogens began with a June 1975 report of the Rockefeller Commission on the CIA. A 43-year-old biochemist, Frank Olson, had committed suicide on November 28, 1953, less than 2 weeks after CIA agents had secretly slipped LSD into his after-dinner drink. This drug caused a panic reaction in Dr. Olson, and he was taken to New York City for psychiatric treatment. The Olson family had been told only that he had jumped or fallen from his tenth-story hotel room in Manhattan. In 1975 when this was uncovered, President Ford rapidly apologized to the Olson family at the White House and said the incident was "inexcusable and unforgiveable . . . a horrible episode in American history."[9] It was not until October 1976 that enough government red tape was cut to make it possible to award $750,000 to the Olson family.

Awareness of the Olson death started Congress and journalists digging for more, this time into the military as well. The army's interest in, and human experiments on, the use of psychedelics for warfare and for interrogation of prisoners and spies was not hidden. It was open knowledge in the scientific and military communities that such research was conducted at Edgewood Arsenal in Maryland, where Dr. Olson was poisoned, and at several major universities in the United States.

It was easy to see how the military and intelligence agencies got involved in this work. "American military and intelligence officials watched men with glazed eyes pouring out rambling confessions at the Communist purge trials in Eastern Europe after World War II, and for the first time they began to worry about the threat of mind-bending drugs as weapons."[10] They worried enough to repeatedly contact Dr. Hofmann about the feasibility of large scale production of LSD,[11] and the CIA considered buying 10 kg in 1953 for $240,000. We can all be pleased that they decided against the purchase, which would have provided 100 million doses!

As the information kept pouring out of government files in the 1975-1976 period, it became clear that the army-sponsored research on 585 soldiers and 900 civilians between 1956 and 1967 had been very poorly done. The army and some of the university scientists had violated many of the ethical codes established as a result of the Nuremberg war crimes trials after World War II. Three failures were especially blatant: many of the volunteers were not really volunteers, many of the participants could not quit an experiment if they wanted to, and the participants were not told the nature of the experiment.

This horror story could go on almost without end; mention could be made of CIA agents picking up patrons in bars and secretly putting LSD in their drinks or of the administration of LSD to unsuspecting civilians around the world. The inspector general of the army issued a long report that criticized almost every aspect of the army's involvement with human drug research: its conception, its execution, and its productivity.[12] Perhaps a mountain has been made out of this molehill in the passing parade, but at the very least it should all too strikingly bring home the dangers of giving drugs to persons without their knowledge. These drugs can literally be mind-breaking when used incautiously.

Recreational use. The illegal LSD story starts with legal psilocybin, or perhaps at West Point, where Timothy Leary discovered Oriental mysticism.

The story proper starts in the summer of 1960 in Mexico, where for the first time Leary used the magic mushrooms containing psilocybin. As he later said, he realized then that the old Timothy Leary was dead; the "Timothy Leary game" was over. Working at Harvard University, Leary collaborated with Dr. Richard Alpert and discussed the meaning and implication of this new world with Aldous Huxley.

During the 1960-1961 school year Leary and Alpert began a series of experiments on Harvard graduate students using pure psilocybin, which they had obtained through a physician. Leary's original work was apparently done under proper scientific controls and with a physician in attendance because drugs were used. The use of a physician was later eliminated, and then other controls were dropped. In fact, Leary believed strongly that not only the subject should use the drug but also the experimenter, so that he could communicate with the subject. This practice removes the experimenter from the role of an objective observer and can hardly be classified as seriously scientific.

Leary's drug taking in the role of an experimenter and the apparent abandonment of any possible former semblance of a scientific approach were questioned by the Harvard authorities and other scientists. A combination of things not acceptable to the university gradually developed from 1961 to 1963. Some of the major issues were that no doctor was present when drugs were administered, undergraduates were used in drug experiments, and drug sessions were conducted outside the laboratory in Leary's home as well as at other places off campus. As a result of many factors, Alpert and Leary were dismissed from their academic positions in the spring of 1963.[13]

All was reasonably quiet in 1964 and 1965. Alpert, now known as Baba Ram Dass, separated from Leary and lectured on the West Coast, while Leary settled at an estate in Millbrook, New York, which was owned by a wealthy supporter of Leary's beliefs. In 1964 Leary announced that drugs were not necessary to rise above and go beyond one's ego. He reiterated this again in 1966 after he was arrested for possession of marijuana at the Millbrook estate.

Also in 1966 Leary started his religion, the League of Spiritual Discovery, with LSD as the sacrament. The League got off to a slow start, and Leary's home base at Millbrook was under attack around the same time. Concern was that Leary would attract "drug addicts to Millbrook. When their money runs out, they will murder, rob and steal, to secure funds with which to satisfy their craving."[14]

Although he was the guru of the age, Leary's sacrament was already being secularized. Increasing numbers of young people were responding to the motto of the League for Spiritual Discovery, "Turn On, Tune In, and Drop Out." Leary phrased it meaningfully:

Turning on correctly means to understand the many levels that are brought into focus; it takes years of discipline, training, and discipleship. To turn on on a street corner is a waste. To tune in means you must harness rigorously what you are learning. . . .

To drop out is the oldest message that spiritual teachers have passed on. You can get only by giving up.[15]

Noble words, perhaps, but street corner turn-ons were becoming more frequent. A combination of many things increased the use of hallucinogens, and especially LSD, during the early and mid-1960s. LSD's promise of new sensations (which were delivered), of potent aphrodisiac effects (which were not forthcoming),[16] of kinship with a friendly peer group (which occurred) spread the drug rapidly.

In the summer of 1966 delegates to the annual convention of the American Medical Association passed a resolution urging greater controls on hallucinogens. They were a little uptight, as was the nation; in part, the resolution stated that

these drugs can produce uncontrollable violence, overwhelming panic . . . or attempted suicide or homicide, and can result, among the unstable or those with preexisting neurosis or psychosis, in severe illness demanding protracted stays in mental hospitals.[17]

LSD use appears to have reached a peak during 1967 and 1968, after which it tapered off. Several factors probably contributed to this decline, including widely publicized concern over "bad trips," prolonged psychotic reactions, chromo-

some damage, self-injurious behavior, and "flashbacks." In reaction to these concerns, many people began to avoid hallucinogens, whereas others shunned the synthetic LSD for the natural experiences produced by psilocybin or mescaline (actually, into the mid-1970s these natural substances, while in demand, were in short supply, and most street samples of either psilocybin or mescaline contained primarily LSD or PCP).

After a series of arrests on drug charges, Timothy Leary was sent to a minimum security prison in 1969, from which he escaped in 1970. After wandering around the world for a couple of years, he surrendered and was sent back to prison. Before his release in 1976, he stated that he was "totally rehabilitated" and would "never, under any circumstances, advocate the use of LSD or any drug."[18] Touring college campuses on the lecture circuit in the early 1980's, Leary talked about "how to use drugs without abusing them."[19]

LSD pharmacology. LSD is odorless, colorless, tasteless, and one of the most potent psychochemicals known to man. Let's remind ourselves about the pharmacological meaning of potent: it takes little LSD to produce effects. A drug could be highly potent and yet not produce much in the way of effects. For example, LSD has never been definitely linked to even one human overdose death. In rats, reliable behavioral effects can be produced by 0.04 mg/kg, whereas the LD 50 is about 16 mg/kg, 400 times the behaviorally effective dose.

Absorption from the gastrointestinal tract is rapid, and most humans take LSD through the mouth. At all postingestion times, the brain contains less LSD than any of the other organs in the body, so it is not selectively taken up by the brain. Half of the LSD in the blood is metabolized every 3 hours, so blood levels decrease fairly rapidly. LSD is metabolized in the liver and excreted as 2-oxy-lysergic acid diethylamide, which is inactive.

Tolerance develops rapidly, repeated daily doses becoming completely ineffective in 3 to 4 days. Recovery is equally rapid, so weekly use of the same dose of LSD is possible. Cross tolerance has been shown between LSD, mescaline, and psilocybin, and the effects of each can be blocked or reversed with chlorpromazine. Physical dependence or addiction has not been shown to LSD or to any of the hallucinogens.

LSD is a sympathomimetic agent, and the autonomic signs are some of the first to appear after LSD is taken. Typical symptoms are dilated pupils, elevated temperature and blood pressure, and an increase in salivation.

The fact that the indole structure of LSD resembles that of serotonin led first to the idea that LSD works by acting at serotonin receptors. Injections of radioactive LSD into animals demonstrate that serotonin receptors are the primary, but not the only, binding sites for LSD.[20] Electrophysiological recordings from serotonin-containing neurons in the raphe nuclei of rats reveal that LSD injections cause a complete cessation of spontaneous electrical activity at doses comparable to those producing behavioral effects.[21] Thus there is fairly general agreement that many of the primary CNS effects of LSD are by actions on the serotonin systems.

There are, however, several problems with this explanation of LSD effects. A basic problem relates to the fact that mescaline and other catechol hallucinogens, which have been assumed to act on the catecholamines norepinephrine and/or dopamine, have psychological effects that are reported to be similar to those of LSD. Rats trained to press one lever after an injection of LSD and another lever after a saline (placebo) injection will respond on the LSD lever if given other indole or catechol hallucinogens, but not if given PCP, anticholinergics, stimulants, sedatives, or opiates.[22] Thus the highly specific "LSD stimulus" in a rat appears to be similar to the stimuli produced by other indole and catechol hallucinogens. It has been suggested that the catechol hallucinogens are flexible enough to assume a shape that would allow them to fit the "LSD receptor," which could be a serotonin receptor.[23]

Whereas most of the behavioral effects of LSD and the catechol hallucinogens can be blocked by drugs that act as serotonin-receptor antagonists, others cannot. Add to this that there are several subtypes of serotonin receptors, some of which are excitatory and others inhibitory, and that LSD can act as either an agonist or an antagonist at different serotonin receptors, you can begin to see how complicated this issue becomes. At the present time, the best evidence seems to indicate that LSD and other hallucinogens, including mescaline and psilocybin, act by stimulating the "serotonin-2" subtype of receptors.[24] Among a large group of hallucinogenic chemicals, there is a high correlation between their potency in binding to this type of receptor from rat brains and their potency in producing hallucinogenic effects in humans.

The LSD experience. Regardless of the chemical mechanism, most scientists feel that an important effect is the modification of perception, particularly of visual images. Some of the experiences reported, especially after low doses, might best be described as illusions, or perceptual distortions, in which an object that is in fact present is seen in a distorted form (brighter than normal, moving, multiple images of the same object). Siegel,[25] who conducted laboratory research on the visual images reported after the ingestion of various drugs, reported that some images can be seen with eyes open or closed and thus represent hallucinations rather than illusions. One stage of such hallucinogen-induced imagery consists of form-constants: lattices, honeycomb or chessboard designs, cobwebs, tunnel, alley or cone shapes, and spiral figures. These shapes were generally combined with intense colors and brightness. At another stage, complex images, such as landscapes, remembered faces, or objects, may be combined with the form-constants (e.g., a face might be seen "through" a honeycomb lattice or multiple images of the face might appear in a honeycomb configuration). Siegel suggested that the perceptual processing mechanisms may be activated at the same time the sensory inputs are either reduced or impaired, thus allowing vivid perception of images that come from inside, rather than outside, the brain.

Besides changes in visual perception, users also report an altered sense of time, changes in the perception of one's own body (perhaps indicating

Your turn: music and drugs

Although the lyrics of popular songs have often referred to recreational drug or alcohol use, the practice of referring to popular illicit drugs in music first became widespread during the 1960s. Sometimes the references were direct and sometimes hidden as in the Beatles "Lucy in the *Sky* with *Diamonds*."

How many of today's hit records include references to drugs or drug use? One way to find out would be to listen to the lyrics of some appropriate sample, either ten records in a row from a rock radio station or the top ten records in a given week. What proportion of the songs contain explicit comments, either positive or negative, about drugs? Are there some apparently hidden references?

a reduction in somatic sensory input), and some alterations of auditory input. A particularly interesting phenomenon is that of *synesthesia,* a "mixing of senses," in which sounds may appear as visual images, or the visual picture may be altered in rhythm with music.

Altered perception is combined with enhanced emotionality, perhaps related to the arousal of the sympathetic branch of the autonomic nervous system. Thus one might experience the images as exceptionally beautiful or awe inspiring, because of an enhanced tendency to react with intense emotion. Alternatively, an object appearing to break apart or move away from or toward the perceiver might be reacted to with intense sadness or with fear. This fear can result in a pounding heart and rapid, shallow breathing, which further frightens the tripper and may lead to a full-blown panic reaction.

Part of the wonder of these agents is that they do not give repeat performances. Although each trip differs, the general type of experience and the sequence of experiences are reasonably well delineated. When an effective dose is taken orally (30 to 100 μg), the trip will last 6 to 9 hours. It can be greatly attenuated at any time through the administration of chlorpromazine intramuscularly.

The initial effects noticed are autonomic responses that develop gradually over the first 20 minutes. The individual may feel dizzy or hot and cold; his mouth may be dry. These effects diminish and, in addition, are less and less the focus of attention as alteration in sensations, perceptions, and mood begin to develop over the following 30 to 40 minutes. In one study, after the initial autonomic effects, the sequence of events over the next 20 to 50 minutes was mood changes, abnormal body sensation, decrease in sensory impression, abnormal color perception, space and time disorders, and visual hallucinations. One visual effect was described beautifully:

The guide asked me how I felt, and I responded, "Good." As I muttered the word "Good," I could see it form visually in the air. It was pink and fluffy like a cloud. The word looked "Good" in its appearance and so it had to be "Good." The word and the thing I was trying to express were one, and "Good" was floating around in the air.[26]

About 1 hour after taking LSD, the intoxication is in full bloom, but it is not until near the end of the second hour that changes occur in the perception of the self.

Usually these changes center around a depersonalization. The individual may feel that the sensations he experiences are not from his body or that he has no body. Body distortions are common, the sort of thing suggested by the comment of one user: "I felt as if my left big toe were going to vomit!" Not unusual is a loss of self-awareness and loss of control of behavior.

Two frequent types of overall reactions in this stage have been characterized as "expansive" and "constricted." In the expansive reaction (a good trip) the individual may become excited and grandiose and feel that he is uncovering secrets of the universe or profundities previously locked within himself. Feelings of creativity are not uncommon: "If I only had the time, I could write the truly great American novel." The other end of the continuum is the constricted reaction in which the user shows little movement and frequently becomes paranoid and exhibits feelings of persecution. The prototype individual in this situation is huddled in a corner fearful that some harm will come to him or that he is being threatened by some aspect of his hallucinations. As the drug effect diminishes, normal psychological controls of sensations, perceptions, and mood return.

Adverse reactions. The adverse reactions to LSD ingestion have been repeatedly emphasized in the popular, as well as scientific, literature. Since there is no way of knowing how much illegal LSD is being used or how pure the LSD is that people are taking, there is no possibility of determining the true incidence of adverse reactions to LSD. Adverse reactions to the street use of what is thought to be LSD may result from many factors. It is important to always remember that drugs obtained on the street frequently are not what they are claimed to be—in purity, chemical composition, or quantity.

A 1960 study surveyed most of the legal U.S. investigators studying LSD and mescaline effects in humans. Data were collected on 25,000 administrations of the drug to about 5000 individuals. Doses ranged from 25 to 1500 µg of LSD and 200 to 1200 mg of mescaline. In some cases the drug was used in patients undergoing therapy; in other cases the drug was taken in an experimental situation to study the effects of the drug. Only LSD and mescaline used under professional supervision were surveyed. The results are noted in Table 15-1.

A 1964 article, "The LSD Controversy,"[27] stated:

It would seem that the incidence statistics better support a statement that the drug is *exceptionally safe* rather than dangerous. Although no statistics have been compiled for the dangers of psychological therapies, we would not be surprised if the incidence of adverse reactions, such as psychotic or depressive episodes and suicide attempts, were at least as high or higher in any comparable group of psychiatric patients exposed to any active form of therapy.

but then went on to say:

It is also important to distinguish between the proper use of this drug in therapeutic or experimental setting

Table 15-1
Estimated rates of major complications associated with LSD

Groups studied	Number per 1000 persons		
	Attempted suicide	Completed suicide	Psychotic reaction over 48 hours
Subjects in experiments	0	0	0.8
Patients undergoing psychotherapy	1.2	0.4	1.8

and its indiscriminate use and abuse by thrill seekers, "lunatic fringe," and drug addicts. More dangers seem likely for the unstable character who takes the drug for "kicks," curiosity, or to escape reality and responsibility than someone taking the drug for therapeutic reasons under strict medical aegis and supervision.

It is also important to emphasize that a clear distinction must be made between the pure LSD used in the "therapeutic or experimental setting" and the impure drug or combination of drugs most frequently used in the street.

Two types of adverse reactions that may develop during the drug-induced experience are the panic reaction, which is an extreme anxiety attack, usually results from the individual's response to some particular aspects of the experience and is typified in the following case history:

A 21-year-old woman was admitted to the hospital along with her lover. He had had a number of LSD experiences and had convinced her to take it to make her less constrained sexually. About half an hour after ingestion of approximately 200 microgm., she noticed that the bricks in the wall began to go in and out and that light affected her strangely. She became frightened when she realized that she was unable to distinguish her body from the chair she was sitting on or from her lover's body. Her fear became more marked after she thought that she would not get back into herself. At the time of admission she was hyperactive and laughed inappropriately. Stream of talk was illogical and affect labile. Two days later, this reaction had ceased. However, she was still afraid of the drug and convinced that she would not take it again because of her frightening experience.[28]

When an overt psychosis develops, remedial treatment is not usually so rapid, and the next individual to be described was hospitalized for prolonged treatment. Usually such psychosis occurs in individuals with a precarious hold on reality in the nondrug condition. The flood of new experiences and feelings is too much for this type of person to integrate.

A 23-year-old man was admitted to the hospital after he stood uncertain whether to plunge an upraised knife into his friend's back. His wife, an intelligent, non-psychotic but masochistic woman, reported that he had been acting strangely since taking LSD approximately 3 weeks before admission. He was indecisive and often mute and shunned physical contact with her. On admission he was catatonic, mute and echopractic. He appeared to be preoccupied with auditory hallucinations of God's voice and thought he had achieved a condition of "all mind." On transfer to another hospital 1 month after admission, there was minimal improvement.

During his adolescence the patient had alternated between acceptance of and rebellion against his mother's religiosity and warnings of the perils of sex and immorality. He had left college during his 1st year after excessive use of amphetamines. He attended, but did not complete, art school. His marriage of 3 years had been marked by conflict and concern about his masculinity. Increasing puzzlement about the meaning of life, his role in the universe and other cosmic problems led to his ingestion of LSD. Shortly after ingestion he was ecstatic and wrote to a friend, "We have found the peace, which is life's river which flows into the sea of Eternity." Soon afterward, in a brief essay, he showed some awareness of his developing psychosis, writing, "I am misunderstood, I cried, and was handed a complete list of my personality traits, habits, goals, and ideals, etc. I know myself now, I said in relief, and spent the rest of my life in happy cares asylum. AMEN."[28]

One of the frightening and interesting adverse reactions to LSD is the **flashback.** More than any other reaction, the recurrence of symptoms weeks or months after an individual has taken LSD brings up thoughts of brain damage and permanent biochemical changes.

Flashbacks consist of the recurrence of certain aspects of the drug experience after a period of normalcy and in the absence of any drug use. The frequency and duration of these flashbacks are quite variable and seem to be unpredictable. They are most frequent just before going to sleep, while driving, and in periods of psychological stress. It was suggested that flashbacks may be attempts to resolve and master traumatic experiences. They seem to occur primarily in immature individuals and diminish in frequency and intensity with time if the individual stops using psychoactive drugs.

Where do all these reports leave us? Is LSD, or any of the better-known hallucinogens, a dangerous drug? It is clear that some people do show immediate and/or long-lasting negative reactions to a hallucinogenic experience. The evidence strongly suggests that if the individual using the drug has a marginal adjustment in the nondrug condition, there is a higher probability of a bad reaction than if he is reasonably well adjusted. However, considering the fact that even an apparently normal, mentally healthy person can have a bad trip or a prolonged adverse reaction, all these drugs must be approached with extreme caution.

Beliefs about LSD. LSD is truly a legend in its own time. Although there are no data, probably more people have more ideas about what LSD does and does not do than they have about any other drug. Only a few of these beliefs can be mentioned.

Creativity. One of the most widely occurring beliefs is that these hallucinogenic agents increase creativity or release creativity that our inhibitions keep bottled inside us. There have been several experiments that have attempted to study the effects of LSD on creativity, but there is no good evidence that the drug increases it. In one laboratory study using LSD at doses of 0.0025 or 0.01 mg/kg body weight, "the authors concluded that the administration of LSD-25 to a relatively unselected group of people for the purpose of enhancing their creative ability is *not* likely to be successful."[29] An experiment with professional artists under the influence of LSD concluded: "for the creative artist, drugs are likely to produce more negative than positive results."[30]

Therapy. Another common belief is that LSD has therapeutic usefulness, particularly in the treatment of alcoholics, even though reports of results with LSD in alcoholism gradually changed from glowing and enthusiastic to cautious and disappointing. One well-controlled study compared the effectiveness of one dose of either 0.6 mg of LSD or 60 mg of dextroamphetamine in reducing drinking by alcoholics. No additional therapy, physical or psychological, was used. The authors found that "LSD produced slightly better results early, but after six months the results were alike for both treatment groups."[31]

Some investigators reported considerable success with LSD in reducing the pain and depression of patients with terminal cancer. The LSD experiences were part of a several-day program involving extensive verbal interaction between the therapist and patient. Although not successful in every case, the LSD therapy was followed by a reduction in the use of narcotics, "less worry about the future," and "the appearance of a positive mood state." The authors concluded that they have a treatment "which may be highly promising for patients facing fatal illness if implemented in the context of brief, intensive, and highly specialized psychotherapy catalyzed by a psychedelic drug such as LSD." A scientific peer review by NIMH[32,p.8] concluded: "Research on the therapeutic use of LSD has shown that it is not a generally useful therapeutic drug . . . as an adjunct to a routine psychotherapeutic approach . . . [or] as a treatment in and of itself. . . ."

Chromosomes. A credibility gap in the world of drugs developed in 1967 between the press and the public with the publication of a scientific report that LSD caused damage to chromosomes of white blood cells (leukocytes) in vitro. This report was quickly followed by a study showing a higher than normal incidence of chromosomal damage in the white blood cells of LSD users. These data received much attention in the mass media and are thought to be one of the reasons for the decrease in LSD use that has occurred since 1967. Not so widely publicized were the reports that did *not* show any relationship in vitro or in vivo between white blood cell chromosome damage and LSD use.

The popular reports also had a way of neglecting to emphasize (or mention) that the effects were on white blood cells and not on the germ cells, which are the only cells involved in reproduction. A poster distributed by the National Foundation—March of Dimes in this period showed a young man, in front of a possibly pregnant young woman, making the statement: "Give me one good reason why I shouldn't use LSD." The poster replies: "We can give you 46. . . . Broken chromosomes may cause birth defects. LSD can break chromosomes. Need we say more?" They had already said more than most careful scientists would have liked. We can now look back on this period with more detachment. The weight of evidence gathered over the years does *not* support the claim that LSD can cause birth defects or cancer in its human users.

Psilocybin

The magic mushrooms of Mexico have a long history of religious and ceremonial use. These plants, as well as peyote, dropped from western sight (but not from native use) for 300 years. The mushrooms were to be particularly suppressed. The name *teonanacatl* can be translated as "God's flesh" or as "sacred mushroom," and either name was very offensive to the Spanish priests.

It was not until the late 1930s that it was clearly shown that these mushrooms were still being used by natives in southern Mexico and that the first of many species was identified. The real breakthrough came in 1955. During that year a New York-banker-turned-ethnobotanist and his wife established rapport with a native group still using

Your turn: attitudes toward LSD

In light of what you have learned about LSD, it will be interesting for you to see how other people view it, preferably people who have not recently studied the topic. Make up a list of questions covering both knowledge about and attitudes toward LSD. Be sure to include questions about why people took LSD in the 1960s, benefits, risks, and whether its use is still prevalent. Then find time to conduct interviews with several people, asking the questions you have developed. See if you can summarize consistencies in the knowledge and beliefs of these people, comparing the summary with the facts as presented in the text.

mushrooms in religious ceremonies. Gordon Wasson became the first outsider to participate in the ceremony and to eat of the magic mushroom. In language quite unlike a banker you can almost hear Wasson's soul cry out as he tries to describe the experience:

It permits you to travel backwards and forward in time, to enter other planes of existence, even (as the Indians say), to know God. . . .[33]

The mushroom that seems to have the greatest psychoactive effect is *Psilocybe mexicana*. The primary active agent in this mushroom is **psilocybin** which the discoverer of LSD, Albert Hofmann, isolated in 1958 and later synthesized.

The dried mushrooms contain 0.2% to 0.5% of psilocybin. The hallucinogenic effects of psilocybin are quite similar to those of LSD and the catechol hallucinogen mescaline, and cross-tolerance exists among these three agents.[34]

The psychoactive effects are clearly related to the amount used, with up to 4 mg yielding a pleasant experience, relaxation, and some body sensations. Higher doses cause considerable perceptual and body image changes with hallucinations in some individuals. Accompanying these psychic changes are dose-related sympathetic arousal symptoms. There is some evidence that psilocybin

has its central nervous system effects only after it has been changed in the body to psilocin. Psilocin is present in the mushroom only in trace amounts but is about one and one-half times as potent as psilocybin. Perhaps the greater CNS effect of psilocybin is the result of its higher lipid solubility.

One of Leary's followers used psilocybin in the now classic Good Friday study. The Good Friday study was designed to investigate the ability of psilocybin to induce meaningful religious experiences in individuals when the drug is used in a religious setting. Twenty seminarians participated in a double-blind study, with half receiving 30 mg of psilocybin and half placebos, 90 minutes before attending a religious service. Tape recordings of the subjects' experiences were made immediately after the 2½-hour service, which was held in a chapel. Within a week a questionnaire was completed, followed by a similar one 6 months later. The first was directed at determining the magnitude and type of change that occurred during the experiment, and the later one at assessing the durability of the change. Leary later summarized the outcome of the Good Friday study by saying:

the results clearly support the hypothesis that, with adequate preparation and in an environment which is supportive and religiously meaningful, subjects report mystical experiences significantly more than placebo controls.[35]

Given access to some spores of the mushroom and proper growing conditions, it is possible to cultivate psilocybe M. in a closet. As a consequence of illegal production in the United States the use of this mushroom has continued into the 1980s, with sporadic outbursts of availability. Although occasionally a major mushroom producer will be discovered, most of the production seems to be on a local, amateur basis. Young people may obtain a few "shrooms" to consume at a party, usually in small quantities and in combination with alcoholic beverages. Under such circumstances it is difficult to tell how much of an effect is produced by the mushrooms and how much by the social situation and the alcohol.

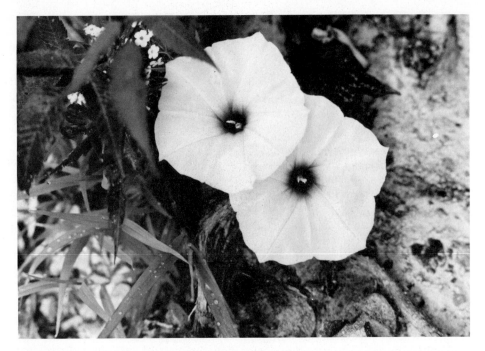

Although morning glory seeds were used as religious plants in Mexico before Columbus, the seeds of most types of morning glories available in the United States have little or no hallucinogenic action.

Morning Glory

Of the psychoactive agents used freely in Mexico in the sixteenth century, **ololiuqui,** seeds of the morning glory plant *Rivea corymbosa,* perhaps had the greatest religious significance.

These seeds tie America to Europe even today, because, when Albert Hofmann analyzed the seeds of the morning glory, he found several active alkaloids as well as *d*-lysergic acid amide. *d*-Lysergic acid amide is about one tenth as active as LSD. The presence of *d*-lysergic acid amide is really quite amazing (to botany majors) because prior to this discovery in 1960, lysergic acid had been found only in much more primitive groups of plants such as the ergot fungus.[36]

A different species of morning glory, *Ipomoea violacea,* seems to be the primary source in the United States of most commercial morning glory seeds containing effective amounts of these alkaloids. Considering the psychoactivity of these seeds, the commercial names seem quite appropriate: Pearly Gates, Flying Saucers, Heavenly Blue!

DMT

Only brief mention will be made of DMT, since it is not widely used in the United States, although it has a long, if not noble, history. In fact, on a worldwide basis, DMT is probably the most important naturally occurring hallucinogenic compound, and it occurs in many plants. Dimethyltryptamine is the active agent in Cohoba snuff, which is used by some South American and Caribbean Indians. It is ineffective when taken orally, unless in the presence of a monoamine oxidase inhibitor, and must be snuffed, smoked, or taken by injection.

The effective intramuscular dose (of the drug, not the snuff, which is not readily available) is about 1 mg/kg of body weight. Since the effect lasts only about an hour, it can be used during lunch; the experience was called a "businessman's trip."[37]

CATECHOL HALLUCINOGENS

This group of drugs, although having psychological effects quite similar to the indole types, is based on a different structure, that of the catechol nucleus. That nucleus forms the basic structure of the catecholamine neurotransmitters, norepinephrine and dopamine. Fig. 15-2 shows this basic structure and the structures of some catechol hallucinogens. Look for the catechol nucleus in each of the hallucinogens, and then compare these structures to the structure of amphetamine and other stimulants shown in Chapter 7.

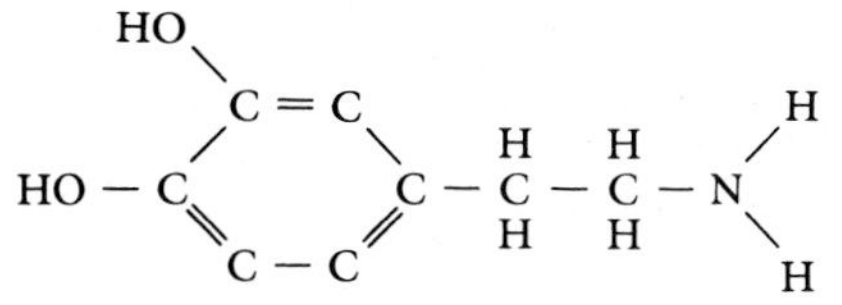

Mescaline

Peyote (from the Aztec *peyotl*) is a small, spineless, carrot-shaped cactus, *Lophophora williamsii* Lemaire, which grows wild in the Rio Grande Valley and southward. It is mostly subterranean, and only the grayish-green pincushion-like top appears above ground. . . .[38]

In pre-Columbian times the Aztec, Huichol, and other Mexican Indians ate the plant ceremonially either in the dried or green state. This produces profound sensory and psychic derangements lasting twenty-four hours, a property which led the natives to value and use it religiously.[39]

Only the part of the cactus that is above ground is easily edible, but the entire plant is psychoactive. This upper portion, or crown, is sliced into disks that dry and are known as "mescal buttons." These slices of the peyote cactus remain psychoactive indefinitely and are the source of the cactus between the yearly harvests. The journey by Indians in November and December to harvest the peyote is an elaborate ceremony, sometimes taking almost a month and a half. When the mescal buttons are to be used, they are soaked in the

The basic catecholamine structure (dopamine)

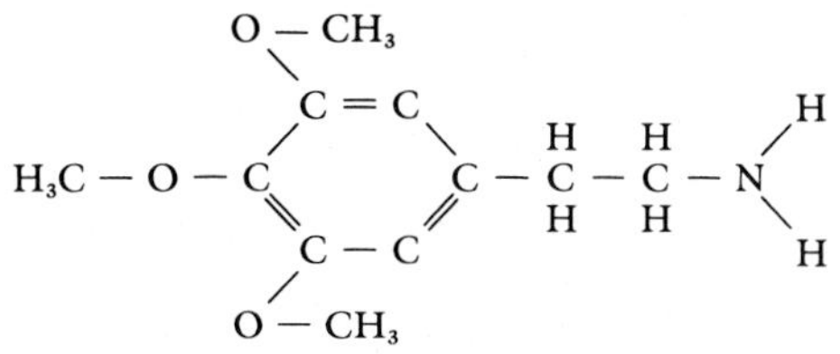

3,4,5 trimethoxyphenylethylamine (mescaline)

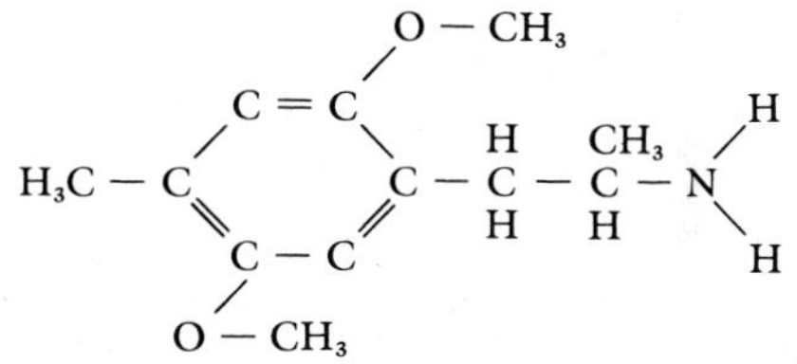

2′,5′ dimethoxy-4′-methylamphetamine (DOM)

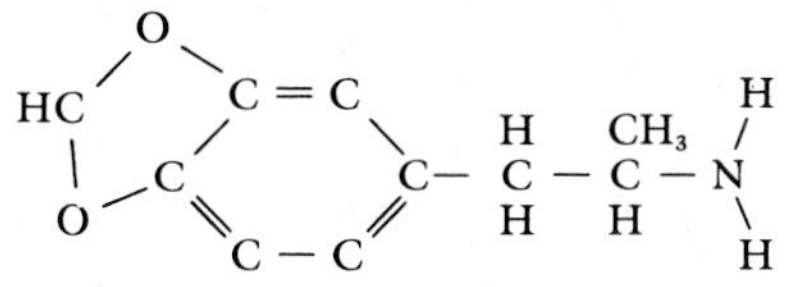

3,4 methylenedioxy amphetamine (MDA)

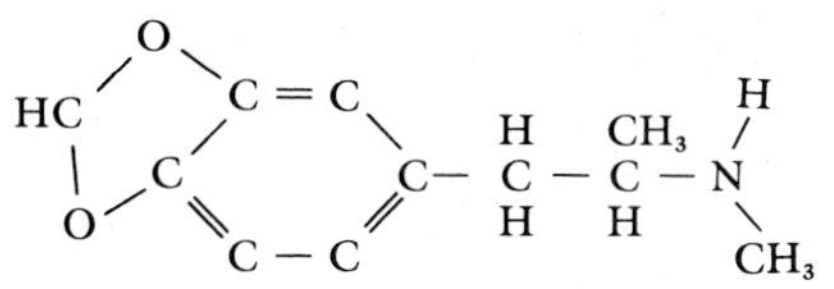

3,4 methylenedioxy methamphetamine (MDMA)

Figure 15-2. Catechol hallucinogens.

mouth until soft, then formed by hand into a bolus and swallowed.

Mescal buttons should not be confused with the mescal beans or with mescal liquor, which is distilled from the fermentation of the agave cactus. Mescal buttons are slices of the peyote cactus and contain **mescaline** as the primary active agent. Mescal beans, however, are dark red seeds from the shrub *Sophora secundiflora*. These seeds, formerly the basis of a vision-seeking cult, contain a highly toxic alkaloid, cytisine, the effects of which somewhat resemble those of nicotine, causing nausea, convulsions, hallucinations, and occasionally death from respiratory failure. The mescal bean has a long history, and there is some evidence that use of the bean diminished and ceased when the safer peyote became available in the southwestern United States. In the transition from a mescal bean to a mescal button cult there appeared, in some tribes, a period in which a mixture of peyote and mescal seeds was concocted and drunk. These factors contributed to considerable confusion in the early (and some recent) literature.[36]

Although there was evidence that the use of peyote had moved north into the United States as early as 1760, it was not until the late nineteenth century that a peyote cult was widely established among the Indians of the plains.

From that time to the present, Indian missionaries have spread the peyote religion to almost a quarter of a million Indians, some as far north as Canada. The development of the present form of this sect has been summarized:

the independent groups of the Peyote Religion have federated into the Native American Church during the 20th century, like the independent congregations of the Jesus Cult federated into the Catholic Church during the 4th century. However, just as not all congregations accepting the basic doctrines of Christianity belonged to the Catholic Church, so not all groups accepting the basic doctrines of Peyotism belong to the Native American Church.[40]

In 1960 peyotism was "the major religious cult of most Indians of the United States between the Rocky Mountains and the Mississippi. . . ."[38]

The **Native American Church** of the United States was first chartered in Oklahoma in 1918 and is an amalgamation of Christianity and traditional beliefs and practices of the Indians. Its basic beliefs are simply stated in the articles of incorporation:

The purpose for which this corporation is formed is to foster and promote religious believers in Almighty God and the customs of the several Tribes of Indians throughout the United States in the worship of a Heavenly Father and to promote morality, sobriety, industry, charity, and right living and cultivate a spirit of self-respect and brotherly love and union among the members of the several Tribes of Indians throughout the United States . . . with and through the sacramental use of peyote.[41]

As in all religions there has developed a whole series of rituals surrounding the use of peyote in religious ceremonies. Peyote is also used in other ways because the Indians attribute spiritual power to the peyote plant. As such, peyote is believed to be helpful, along with prayers and modern medicines, in curing illnesses. It is also worn as an amulet, much as some Christians wear a St. Christopher's medal, to protect the wearer from harm.

Hallucinogenic use. Near the end of the nineteenth century, Heffter isolated several alkaloids from peyote and showed that mescaline was the primary agent only for the visual effect induced by peyote. Spath in 1919 finally synthesized mescaline and most experiments on the psychoactive and/or behavioral effects since then have used synthesized mescaline. There have now been over 30 psychoactive alkaloids identified in peyote, but mescaline does seem to be the agent responsible for the vivid colors and other visual effects. The fact that mescaline is not equivalent to peyote is not always made clear in the literature.[42]

One of the early investigators of the effects of peyote was Dr. Weir Mitchell, who used an extract of peyote and who reported, in part:

The display which for an enchanted two hours followed was such as I find it hopeless to describe in language which shall convey to others the beauty and splendor of what I saw. Stars, delicate floating films of color, then an abrupt rush of countless points of white light swept across the field of view, as if the unseen millions of the Milky Way were to flow in a sparkling river before my eyes . . . zigzag lines of very bright colors . . . the wonderful loveliness of swelling clouds of more vivid colors gone before I could name them.[43,p.34]

Another early experimenter was Havelock Ellis. Interestingly, he took his peyote on Good Friday in 1897, 65 years before the much noted Good Friday experiment with psilocybin. His experience is described in detail in a 1902 article titled "Mescal: A Study of a Divine Plant"[44] in *Popular Science Monthly,* but a brief quotation gives the essence of the experience:

. . . On the whole, if I had to describe the visions in one word, I should say that they were living arabesques. There was generally a certain incomplete tendency to symmetry, the effect being somewhat as if the underlying mechanism consisted of a large number of polished facets acting as mirrors. It constantly happened that the same image was repeated over a large part of the field, though this holds good mainly of the forms, for in the colors there would still remain all sorts of delicious varieties. Thus at a moment when uniformly jewelled flowers seemed to be springing up and extending all over the field of vision, the flowers still showed every variety of delicate tone and tint.

It may well be that not every individual wants every educational opportunity that is offered him. William James, surprisingly, was one who did not. He wrote to his brother Henry: "I ate one but three days ago, was violently sick for twenty-four hours, and had no other symptoms whatever except that and the Katzenjammer the following day. I will take the visions on trust." Even Dr. Weir Mitchell, who had the effect previously recorded, said: "These shows are expensive. . . . The experience, however, was worth one such headache and indigestion but was not worth a second."

Even if you get by without too much nausea and physical discomfort, which the Indians also report, all may not go well. Huxley, whose 1954 *The Doors of Perception*[45] made him a guru in this area, admitted: "Along with the happily transfigured majority of mescaline takers there is a minority that finds in the drug only hell and purgatory." It is reported that natives sometimes wished for "bad trips" when taking this or other plants. By meeting their personal demons, they hoped to conquer them and remove problems from their lives.

Pharmacodynamics of mescaline. Mescaline is readily absorbed if taken orally, but only very poorly passes the blood-brain barrier (which explains the high doses required). There is a maximal concentration of the drug in the brain after 30 to 120 minutes. About half of it is removed from the body in 6 hours, and there is evidence that some mescaline persists in the brain for up to 9 to 10 hours. Similar to the indole hallucinogens, the effects obtained with low doses, about 3 mg/kg, are primarily euphoric, while doses in the range of 5 mg/kg give rise to a full set of hallucinations. Most of the mescaline is excreted unchanged in the urine, and the metabolites identified thus far are not psychoactive.

A dose that is psychoeffective in humans causes pupil dilation, pulse rate and blood pressure increases, and an elevation in body temperature. All of these effects are similar to those induced by LSD, psilocybin, and most other alkaloid hallucinogens. There are other signs of central stimulation, such as EEG arousal, following mescaline intake. In rats the LD 50 is about 370 mg/kg, 10 to 30 times the dose that causes behavioral effects. Death results from convulsions and respiratory arrest. Tolerance develops more slowly to mescaline than to LSD, and there is cross-tolerance between them. As with LSD, mescaline intoxication can be blocked with chlorpromazine.

Although mescaline and the other catechol hallucinogens have a structure that resembles the catecholamine neurotransmitters, it has been proposed that they may in fact operate via the same mechanism as LSD, perhaps mainly via serotonin actions. The fact that the psychological effects of these two chemical classes are so similar in both humans and rats, the pharmacological blockade of most behavioral effects of both by serotonin antagonists and the cross-tolerance among them all suggest a common mechanism, and studies of the structures of catechol hallucinogens indicate certain similarities to the overall LSD structure.[23]

Amphetamine Derivatives

There is a large group of synthetic hallucinogens that are chemically related to amphetamine. However, these drugs have little amphetamine-like stimulant activity. Thanks to certain chemical substitutions on the ring part of the catechol nucleus, these drugs are more mescaline-like (Fig. 15-2).

DOM (STP). DOM is 2,5-dimethoxy-4-methylamphetamine. According to most users, DOM is called STP, and street talk is that the initials stand for serenity, tranquility, and peace. Its actions and effects are highly similar to those of mescaline and LSD, with a total dose of 1 to 3 mg yielding euphoria most often, and 3 to 5 mg a 6- to 8-hour hallucinogenic period. This makes DOM about a hundred times as potent as mescaline but only one thirtieth as potent as LSD.

DOM has a reputation for inducing an extraordinarily long experience, but this seems to be caused by the very large amounts being used. Pills of DOM bought on the street contain about 10 mg—a very big dose. Reports by users had suggested that DOM was unlike other hallucinogens and that its effects were enhanced rather than blocked by chlorpromazine. Controlled laboratory work with normal volunteers, however, has clearly shown that the effects of DOM are similar to those of other hallucinogens and that chlorpromazine does attenuate the DOM experience.[46]

An excellent review from the Haight-Ashbury Clinic contains most of the essential information about the rise and fall of DOM use:

It appears then that DOM produces a higher incidence of acute and chronic toxic reactions than any of the other commonly used hallucinogens. . . . It appears that the effects of DOM are like a combination of amphetamine and LSD with the hallucinogenic effects of the drug very often putting the peripheral amphetamine-like physiological effects out of perspective. . . .[47,p.4]

MDA and others. In addition to DOM, many other amphetamine derivatives have been synthesized and shown to have hallucinogenic properties. Most of these, such as DOET, TMA-2, and the various MDAs, have effects very similar to those of DOM and mescaline, as well as LSD and the indole types. There is some indication that one type of derivative, MDA (Fig. 15-2), has effects that are subjectively somewhat different.[23] MDA, which is somewhat more potent than mescaline, has seen some recreational use through illicit manufacture. Because of the variety of possible hallucinogenic amphetamine derivatives and because most of these chemicals are not specifically listed as controlled substances, illicit drug makers have been drawn to this group of chemicals in the production of various "designer drugs" to be sold on the street as hallucinogens.

MDMA. One of the amphetamine derivatives received special attention in July of 1984 when the DEA proposed scheduling it. MDMA is similar in structure to MDA, but is apparently quite different from the other hallucinogens. Rats trained to discriminate DOM from saline did show some generalization from the DOM stimulus to MDA, but not to MDMA. Furthermore, there is no cross-tolerance between MDA and MDMA.[23] Although there was some use of MDMA on the streets (it was called "ecstasy" or "XTC"), which prompted the DEA to propose scheduling it, what was surprising was that a number of psychiatrists came forth who had been quietly using MDMA, a drug that while not approved by the FDA, was not illegal. These psychiatrists testified against the scheduling of MDMA, insisting that it was not a true hallucinogen and that it had a special ability to promote empathy, thus aiding the psychoanalytic process.[48]

There is some evidence supporting this claim of increased empathy: in a 1987 study 100 people completed detailed questionnaires describing the effects of their previous use of MDMA.[49] While such retrospective reports are less reliable than reports obtained during or immediately after the experience, a remarkably common report (90% of the individuals) was that they experienced a heightened sense of "closeness" with other people. Other common effects were an increased heart rate, dry mouth, grinding of the teeth, profuse sweating, and other autonomic effects. Although several people reported that objects seemed more "luminescent," very few reported actual visual hallucinations.

The bad news is that this otherwise fairly benign drug may cause permanent brain damage. Several laboratories have reported that rats given MDMA injections show a selective destruction of serotonin neurons in their brains. Then a similar effect was reported in monkeys at only two to three times the normal human dose, and this led many observers to conclude that similar brain damage probably would occur in human MDMA users.[50] It should be stressed that this effect is *not* caused by LSD, mescaline, psilocybin, or most other drugs, and that the evidence that MDMA causes damage is strong enough to be taken very seriously.

PCP

In the 1950s, Parke, Davis & Company investigated a series of drugs in the search for an efficient intravenous anesthetic. On the basis of animal studies, they selected 1-(1-phenylcyclohexyl) peperidine hydrochloride (PCP, generic name phencyclidine) for testing in humans. The studies on monkeys had indicated that **PCP** was a good analgesic, but did not produce good muscle relaxation nor did it produce sleep. Instead the animals showed a sort of "dissociation" from what was happening: "During the operation the animal had its eyes open and looked about unconcernedly." In 1958 the first report was published on the use of PCP (brand name Sernyl) for surgical anesthesia in 64 humans.[51] Sernyl produced good analgesia without depressing blood circulation or respiration and did not produce irregularities in heartbeat. Loss of sensation occurred within 2 or 3 minutes of beginning the intravenous infusion, after about 10 mg of the drug had been delivered. They later had no memory for the procedure, did not remember being spoken to, and remembered no pain. Compared to existing anesthetics, which tend to depress both respiration and circulation through general depression of the CNS, this type of "dissociative" anesthetic seemed to be quite safe. However, the psychological reactions to the

drug were unpredictable. During administration of the drug a few patients became very excited and a different anesthetic had to be used. A large number of people were "unmanageable" as they emerged from the anesthetic, exhibiting severely manic behavior. This and later reports indicated that many people given anesthetic doses of Sernyl reported changes in body perception, hallucinations, and in about 15% of the patients, a "prolonged confusional psychosis," lasting 12 to 96 hours after the drug was discontinued. This period of confusion was characterized by feelings of unreality, depersonalization, persecution, depression, and intense anxiety.

News of this new hallucinogen soon reached Dr. Luby, a psychiatrist, who began testing it in both normal and schizophrenic subjects.[52] All the subjects reported changes in perception of their own bodies, with one normal subject saying, "my arm feels like a 20-mile pole with a pin at the end." Another said, "I am a small . . . not human . . . just a block of something in a great big laboratory." There were a number of reports of floating, flying, dizziness, and of alternate contraction and expansion of body size. All subjects also showed some type of thought disorder. Some made up new words, uttered strings of unrelated words, or repeated words or simple phrases over and over. Also, all became increasingly drowsy and apathetic. At times a subject would appear to be asleep but when asked a direct question would respond. When asked, "Can you hear me?" subjects often responded, "No!" The majority became either angry or uncooperative. Many of the normal subjects said they felt as if they were drunk from alcohol. All subjects displayed diminished pain, touch, and position sense, and all showed nystagmus (rapid oscillations of the eyes) and a slapping, ataxic walk. Luby and his colleagues felt that PCP was different from LSD or mescaline in that there were few reports of intense visual experiences and many more reports of body image changes. The disorganized thinking, suspiciousness, and lack of cooperation made the PCP state resemble schizophrenia much more than the LSD state.

Thus by 1960 PCP was well characterized as an excellent anesthetic for monkeys, a relatively safe but troublesome anesthetic for humans, and a hallucinogen different from LSD and mescaline, with profound effects on body perception. Parke, Davis withdrew Sernyl as an investigational drug for humans in 1965 and in 1967 licensed another company to sell Sernylan as an animal anesthetic. It was particularly used with primates, in both research laboratories and zoos. Also, because of its rapid action and wide safety margin, Sernylan was used in syringe bullets to immobilize stray, wild, or dangerous zoo animals. Because of the popular term "tranquilizer gun" for this use, PCP became popularly, and inaccurately, known as an animal "tranquilizer."

Even though Sernyl was never marketed for human use, a related chemical from the same series was marketed as an anesthetic. Ketamine, which has somewhat more depressant activity than PCP and fewer prolonged reactions, is nevertheless quite similar. The 1989 *Physician's Desk Reference* contained the following special note about ketamine:

"Emergence reactions have occurred in approximately 12 percent of patients.

"The psychological manifestations vary in severity between pleasant dream-like states, vivid imagery, hallucinations, and emergence delirium. In some cases these states have been accompanied by confusion, excitement, and irrational behavior which a few patients recall as an unpleasant experience. The duration ordinarily is no more than a few hours; in a few cases, however, recurrences have taken place up to 24 hours postoperatively."[53,p.1558]

In late 1967, workers at the Haight-Ashbury Medical Clinic obtained samples of a substance being distributed as the "Peace Pill." The drug was analyzed, determined to be PCP, and its identity and dangers were publicized in the community in December, 1967. By the next year it was reported that this drug had enjoyed only brief popularity and then disappeared. It appeared briefly in New York in 1968 as "hog" and at other times as "trank." Into the early 1970s, PCP was apparently regarded as pretty much a "garbage" drug by street

people. In the early 1970s, PCP crystals were sometimes sprinkled onto oregano, parsley, or alfalfa and sold to unsuspecting youngsters as marijuana. In this form, it became known as "**angel dust.**" Because PCP can be made inexpensively and relatively easily by amateur chemists, when it is available it usually doesn't cost much. Eventually, the rapid and potent effects of angel dust made it a desired substance in its own right. Joints made with PCP sometimes contained marijuana, sometimes another plant substance, and were known as "killer joints," or "sherms" (because they hit you like a Sherman tank). By the late 1970s, PCP use was the most common cause of drug-induced visits to hospital emergency rooms in many communities, and in some neighborhoods young users could be seen "moonwalking" down the street (taking very high, careful, and slow steps) on any Saturday night.

Some users develop a profound psychological dependence on PCP, in spite of its unpredictability and the behavioral impairment it produces. One user reported:

Immediately after smoking the Dust I started experiencing the effects. All my troubles seemed to go away. I felt a little drunk and had some trouble walking around the apartment. Objects appeared either very far away or very close and I couldn't really judge distance at all. . . . I liked being apart from things, and felt outside my body for most of the trip. That was fun. Before I smoked I had been troubled about some exams coming up and felt I wasn't really prepared. All that anxiety vanished with the Dust . . . I felt at peace. It was a good feeling . . . I want to be there always.[54]

That subject was unusually descriptive about the experience. Most often, PCP users do not say much that makes sense while the drug is having its effects, and later the user doesn't remember much of what happened.

The dependence-producing properties of PCP have also been studied in monkeys, which will learn to respond to produce intravenous injections of the drug.[55] This is in contrast to LSD and other hallucinogens, which will not support animal self-administration and do not produce behavioral dependence in most users.

Because some PCP users have been reported to behave violently, there is a question whether PCP tends to promote violence directly or whether it is a side effect of the suspicion and anesthesia produced by the drug. Most users do not report feeling violent and feel so uncoordinated that they can't imagine "picking a fight." However, police who have tried to arrest PCP users have had trouble subduing them, because many of the commonly used arrest techniques rely on restraining holds that result in pain if the arrestee resists. Since the PCP user is anesthetized, such restraint techniques are less effective.[56] Manual restraint by more than one officer may be required to arrest some PCP users, although one might question how different this is from the problem of arresting a violent drunk who is "feeling no pain."

That PCP users may not feel pain has resulted in some gruesome stories about users biting or cutting off their own fingers and so forth. As with earlier stories about LSD users blinding themselves by staring at the sun, these stories cannot be substantiated and most likely did not really occur. One oft-repeated story probably falls into the category of "police folklore." Every cop knows for a fact the story about the PCP user who was so violent, had such superhuman strength, and was so insensitive to pain that he was shot 28 times (or some similar large number) before he fell. Although everyone knows that this happened, no one can tell you exactly when or where. One might dismiss such folklore as harmless, unless it contributes to events such as the shooting, six times at close range, of an unarmed, naked, 35-year-old biochemist who was trying to climb the street sign outside his laboratory. This story really did happen, on August 4, 1977, during the height of the PCP epidemic. The lethal shots were fired by a Los Angeles policeman. The coroner's office reported that the victim's blood did contain traces of a drug similar to PCP.[57]

The mechanism of PCP's action on the brain was a mystery for several years, since PCP does alter many neurotransmitter systems but did not appear to act directly on any of them. In 1979 it was reported that a specific receptor for PCP was present in the brain, and in 1981 the identity between the receptor and another that had previously been considered a subtype of opiate receptor was reported.[58] The drug cyclazocine, which has some opiate activity and has also been reported to produce hallucinations, binds well to this PCP receptor, but morphine, naloxone, and other opiates do not. Thus the receptor is probably better characterized as being selective for PCP, ketamine, and other similar drugs rather than as a type of opiate receptor. The presence of such a receptor has led to speculation about a possible endogenous substance, facetiously called "angel-dustin," that would normally act on the receptor. It is not far from there to the speculation that excessive amounts of this hypothetical "angel-dustin" in some individuals might be responsible for schizophrenia.

ANTICHOLINERGIC HALLUCINOGENS

The potato family contains all the naturally occurring agents to be discussed here. Three of the genera—*Atropa*, *Hyoscyamus*, and *Mandragora*—have a single species of importance and were primarily restricted to Europe. The fourth genus, *Datura*, is world-wide and has many species containing the active agents.

The family of plants in which all these genera are found is *Solanaceae*, herbs of consolation, and three pharmacologically active alkaloids are responsible for the effects of these plants. **Atropine,** which is *dl*-hyoscyamine, **scopolamine** or *l*-hyoscine, and *l*-hyoscyamine are all potent central and peripheral cholinergic blocking agents. These drugs occupy the acetylcholine receptor site but do not activate it; thus, their effect is primarily to block muscarinic cholinergic neurons, including the parasympathetic system. The structures of the two most widely studied anticholinergic agents, atropine and scopolamine, are shown in Fig. 15-3.

These agents have potent peripheral and central effects, and some of the psychological responses to these drugs are probably a reaction to peripheral

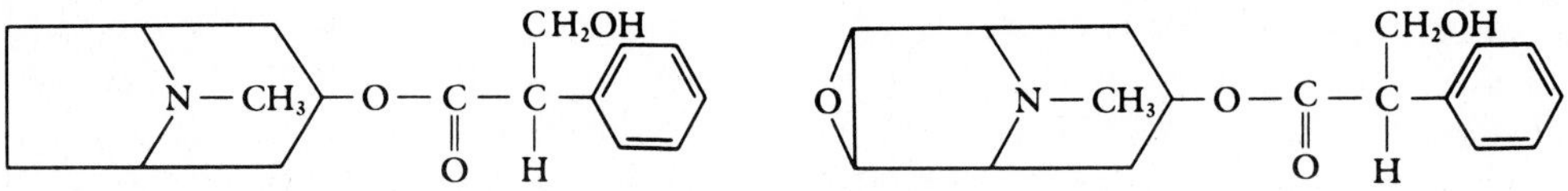

Atropine (*dl*-hyoscyamine)
(1αH,5αH-tropan-3α-ol, [+]-tropate [ester])

Scopolamine (*l*-hyoscine)
(6β,7β-epoxy-1αH,5αH-tropan-3α-ol,[−]-tropate [ester])

Figure 15-3. Naturally occurring anticholinergic hallucinogens.

changes. These alkaloids block the production of mucus in the nose and throat. They also prevent salivation, so the mouth becomes uncommonly dry, and perspiration stops. Temperature may increase to fever levels (109° F has been reported in infants with atropine poisoning), and heart rate may show a 50-beat-per-minute increase with atropine. Even at moderate doses these chemicals cause considerable dilation of the pupils of the eyes with a resulting inability to focus on nearby objects.

With large enough doses, a behavioral pattern develops which resembles that of a toxic psychosis; there is delirium, mental confusion, loss of attention, drowsiness, and loss of memory for recent events. These two characteristics—a clouding of consciousness and no memory for the period of intoxication—plus the absence of vivid sensory effects separate these drugs from the indole and catechol hallucinogens.

Belladonna

The deadly nightshade, *Atropa belladonna,* has as its active ingredient atropine, which was isolated in 1831. The name of the plant reflects two of its major uses in the Middle Ages and before. The genus name reflects its use as a poison. The deadly nightshade was one of the plants used extensively by both professional and amateur poisoners, since 14 of its berries contain enough of the alkaloid to cause death.

Belladonna, the species name, refers to the "beautiful woman," a term that is a result of the use of the extract of this plant to dilate the pupils of the eyes. Interestingly, Roman and Egyptian women knew something that science did not learn until quite recently. In the 1950s it was demon-

strated, by using pairs of photographs identical except for the amount of pupil dilation, that most people judge the girl with the most dilated eyes as the prettiest.

Of more interest here than pretty girls or poisoned men is the sensation of flying reported by witches. The first step toward completing this experiment is to make an ointment. Although there are many recipes, a good one seems to be baby's fat, juice of water parsnip, aconite, cinquefoile, deadly nightshade, and soot.

When the ointment is made, it is rubbed on the body and especially liberally between the legs and on a stick that is to be straddled. This stick served as a phallic symbol during the ceremony of the Sabbat. The Sabbat, or Black Mass, worshipped Satan, and both males and females engaged in a nightlong orgy. Straddling the stick and hopping and shrieking around a circle they felt able "to be carried in the aire, to feasting, singing, dansing, kissing, culling and other acts of venerie, with such youthes as they loue and desire most!"[59,p.81] The feeling of levitation perhaps comes from the irregular heartbeat in conjunction with drowsiness. Some have reported that changes in heart rate coupled with falling asleep sometimes results in a sensation of falling (or flying)[60] but a more likely explanation is simply the power of suggestion.

Other actions were important in causing the effects of the Sabbat. The pounding of the heart would certainly convey excitement, and the excitement might cause sexual arousal. One of the reputations of belladonna was as an aphrodisiac, so it may all fit together. Perhaps the physiological effects of the agents coupled with a good placebo effect was enough for the witches who attended the Sabbat.

Mandrake

The famous **mandrake** plant *(Mandragora offici-narum)* contains all three alkaloids. Although many drugs could be traced to the Bible, it is particularly important to do so with the mandrake because its close association with love and love-making has persisted from Genesis to recent times.

In the time of wheat-harvest Reuben went out and found some mandrakes in the open country and brought them to his mother Leah. Then Rachel asked Leah for some of her son's mandrakes, but Leah said, "Is it so small a thing to have taken away my husband, that you should take my son's mandrakes as well?" But Rachel said, "Very well, let him sleep with you tonight in exchange for your son's mandrakes." So when Jacob came in from the country in the evening, Leah went out to meet him and said, "You are to sleep with me tonight; I have hired you with my son's mandrakes." That night he slept with her. . . .[61,p.33]

The root of the mandrake is forked and, if you have a vivid imagination, resembles a human body. The root contains the psychoactive agents and was endowed with all sorts of magical and medical properties. It was the association with the human form that led Juliet in her farewell to use the phrase: "And shrieks like mandrakes torn out of the earth, That living mortals hearing them run mad."

Henbane

Compared to the deadly nightshade and the mandrake, the *Hyoscyamus niger* has had a most uninteresting life. This is strange, since it is pharmacologically quite active and contains both scopolamine and *l*-hyoscyamine. There are other plants of this genus that contain effective levels of the alkaloids, but it is *Hyoscyamus niger* that appears throughout history as **henbane,** a highly poisonous substance and truly the bane of hens as well as other animals.

Pliny in 60 AD said: "For this is certainly known, that, if one takes it in drink more than four leaves, it will put him beside himself." Hamlet's father must have had more than four leaves because it was henbane that was used to poison him.

Datura

The distribution of the many *Datura* species is worldwide, but they all contain the three alkaloids under discussion—atropine, scopolamine, and hyoscyamine—in varying amounts. Almost as extensive as the distribution are its uses and its history. Some hint of the length of this history is seen in a quote from a 1970 article[62]: "The Chinese valued this drug far back into ancient times. A comparatively recent Chinese medical text, published in 1590, reported that 'when Buddha preaches a sermon, the heavens bedew the petals of this plant with rain drops.'" The text does suggest the importance of the plant, *Datura metel,* by associating it with Buddha, much as tea and Daruma were related in legend.

Halfway around the world 2500 years before the Chinese text, virgins sat in the temple to Apollo in Delphi and, probably under the influence of *Datura,*[62] mumbled sounds that holy men phrased as predictions that always came true. The procedure was straightforward, and:

preliminary to the divine possession, she appears to have chewed leaves of the sacred laurel . . . [prior to speaking] . . . she was supposed to be inspired by a mystic vapour that arose from a fissure in the ground.[63,p.831]

Probably either the plant material eaten was one of the *Datura* species or the burning seeds and leaves of the *Datura* plant formed the mystic vapor she inhaled. It should not go unnoticed, as we search for the beyond within, that engraved on the temple at Delphi were the words, "Know thyself."

Datura was and is part of love potions in India, and the practice of mixing the crushed seeds of *Datura metel* in tobacco and food in Asia persists even today.

The ever-busy chronicler Hernandez mentioned the use of *Datura inoxia* by the Aztecs, and the use of various *Datura* species by Indians of the United States Southwest for magical and religious purposes is well substantiated.[36] One of the interesting uses of *Datura stramonium,* which is native and grows wild in eastern United States, was devised by the Algonquin Indians. They used the plant to solve the problem of the adolescent search for identity.

The youths are confined for long periods, given " . . . no other substance but the infusion or decoction of some poisonous, intoxicating roots . . . " and "they became stark, staring mad, in which raving condition they were kept eighteen or twenty days . . . ". These poor creatures drink so much of that water of Lethe that they perfectly lose the remembrance of all former things, even of their parents, their treasure and their language. When the doctors find that they have drunk sufficiently of the wysoccan . . . they gradually restore them to their senses again. . . . Thus they unlive their former lives and commence men by forgetting that they ever have been boys.[62]

This same plant is now called Jamestown weed, or shortened to jimsonweed, as a result of an incident that happened in the seventeenth century. This was fortunately recorded for history in the famous book *The History and Present State of Virginia*,[64,p.139] published first in 1705 by Robert Beverly.

The *James-Town* Weed (which resembles the Thorny Apple of *Peru*, and I take to be the Plant so call'd) is supposed to be one of the greatest Coolers in the World. This being an early Plant, was gather'd very young for a boil'd Salad, by some of the Soldiers sent thither, to pacifie the Troubles of *Bacon;* and some of them eat plentifully of it, the Effect of which was a very pleasant Comedy; for they turn'd natural Fools upon it for several Days:

Although there has been some recent abuse of jimsonweed, the unpleasant and dangerous side effects of this plant serve to limit its recreational use.

Synthetic Anticholinergics

Anticholinergic drugs were once used to treat Parkinson's disease (before the introduction of L-dopa) and are still widely used to treat the pseudoparkinsonism produced by antipsychotic drugs (Chapter 13). Particularly in older people there is concern about inadvertently producing an "anticholinergic syndrome," characterized by excessive dry mouth, elevated temperature, delusions, and

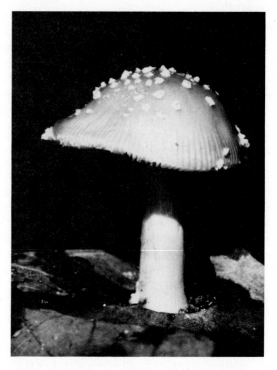

The red- and white-speckled mushroom *Amanita muscaria* played a major role in the early history of Indo-European and Central American religions.

hallucinations. Drugs such as Artane (trihexyphenidyl) and Cogentin (benztropine) have only rarely been abused for their delirium-producing properties.

AMANITA MUSCARIA

If Mexico has magic mushrooms, then Russia and the Scandinavian countries must lay claim to the mushroom that is reusable. The *Amanita muscaria* mushroom is also called "fly agaric," perhaps because it has insecticidal properties! It doesn't kill the flies, but when they suck its juice, it puts them into a stupor for 2 to 3 hours.

The older literature suggests that eating five to ten *Amanita* mushrooms results in severe effects of intoxication such as muscular twitching, leading to twitches of limbs; raving drunkenness with agitation and vivid hallucinations. Later, partial paralysis with sleep and dreams follow for many hours.

Perhaps because the written history on the mushroom is not very old, going back only to about the seventeenth century, and in part because the active chemical constituent still eludes the biochemist, there are many speculations about the role in our history of this red-topped and white-spotted poisonous fungus.

The suggestion has been made that the ambrosia food of the gods—mentioned in the secret rites of the god Dionysius in Greece—was a solution of the *Amanita* mushroom.[65] A really far-out suggestion is that *Amanita muscaria* use formed the basis for the cult that originated about 2000 years ago and today calls itself Christianity.[66] Wasson has proposed that this fungus is the famous unidentified Soma of the Rig Veda poems written about 2000 BC,[65] and most scholars accept this interpretation.

There is no resolution of the role this magic mushroom of the North has played in our past, but its use continues today in several parts of Soviet Russian territory.

Use of the Amanita mushroom by Siberian tribes continues today largely free from social control of any sort. Use of the drug has a Shamanist aspect, and forms the basis for orgiastic communal indulgences. Since the drug can induce murderous rages in addition to more moderate hallucinogenic experiences, serious injuries frequently result.[67]

The mushrooms are expensive; sometimes several reindeer are exchanged for an effective number of the mushrooms. They do have the unique property of being reusable, and during the long winter months they may be worth the price. The mushrooms themselves are not reusable; once eaten, they're gone. But this is a hallucinogen that is excreted unchanged in the urine. When the effect begins to wear off, "midway in the orgy the cry of 'pass the pot' goes out."[68] The active ingredient can be reused four or five times in this way!

For many years the active agent in this mushroom was thought to be *muscarine* (for which the muscarinic cholinergic receptors were named).

Issue: ecstasy and the DEA

In 1985 the DEA temporarily placed the designer drug MDMA, also called Ecstasy, XTC, or Adam, on Schedule I of the list of controlled substances. After the DEA proposed this scheduling, referring to the drug as an hallucinogen, several psychiatrists objected. Many experts, including Lester Grinspoon of Harvard Medical School, apparently felt that MDMA has a low potential for abuse. A New Mexico psychiatrist, Dr. George Greer, had been using MDMA as an adjunct to psychotherapy, in much the way LSD was once used. He reported that it is helpful in improving communication and insight and in decreasing the use of abused substances.[48]

By 1986, scientific evidence was lining up against MDMA. Studies in monkeys and baboons demonstrated that they will self-administer MDMA, indicating its potential for psychological dependence. Most hallucinogens do not reinforce self-administration in such experiments, but amphetamine, cocaine, and heroin do. Also, the first rat experiments had appeared reporting that MDMA caused damage to serotonin systems in the brain. At the end of 1986, the DEA "permanently" placed MDMA on Schedule I.

The legal status of this interesting substance was not yet decided, however. Dr. Grinspoon brought suit in 1987 in the Federal Court of Appeals in Boston. The court eventually ruled against the DEA's procedure for determining "acceptable medical use," and in January of 1988 MDMA was temporarily removed from Schedule I. Six months later, the DEA had redefined its criteria, rereviewed MDMA, and again "permanently" placed it on Schedule I, where it will probably remain.[69]

This substance activates the same type of acetylcholine receptor that is blocked by the anticholinergics. However, pharmacological studies with other cholinergic agonists did not produce similar psychoactive effects. Next, attention focused on *bufotenin*, an indole that is found in high concentrations in the skins of toads. However, the hallucinogenic properties of bufotenin have been in doubt, and *Amanita* species contain only small amounts of it. In the mid-1960s meaningful amounts of two chemicals were found: ibotenic acid and muscimol.

The effects of *Amanita* ingestion are not similar to those of other hallucinogens and that helps to confuse the picture with regard to the mechanism. Ibotenic acid is capable of activating neurons through the excitatory receptors for the neurotransmitter glutamic acid, which is found throughout the CNS. Muscimol can act as an agonist at GABA receptors, which are inhibitory and also found throughout the CNS. Muscimol is more potent than ibotenic acid, and drying of the mushroom, which is usually done by those who use it, promotes the transformation of ibotenic acid to muscimol. Muscimol has been given to humans, resulting in confusion, disorientation in time and place, sensory disturbances, muscle twitching, weariness, fatigue, and sleep.[36]

It should be stressed that, whereas *Amanita muscaria* and other species of related poisonous mushrooms are to be found in North America, they represent a particularly dangerous type of plant to experiment with.

Summary

Hallucinogenic plants and the chemicals they contain have been important to humans for many centuries, not only as medicines, but for spiritual and recreational purposes as well.

LSD, a synthetic hallucinogen, has come to symbolize hallucinogens for most people. This potent agent is capable of altering perceptual processes and enhancing emotionality so that the real world is seen differently and responded to with great emotion. Although LSD does have important physiological effects through the autonomic system, there is a wide range between the psychoactive dose and the estimated lethal dose. Other chemicals that contain the indole nucleus, such as psilocybin (from the Mexican mushroom), may have similar effects.

Mescaline, from peyote cactus, and various synthetic derivatives of amphetamine represent the catechol hallucinogens. Despite differences in chemical structure, most of these drugs have psychological effects quite similar to those of the indole types. MDMA, which is chemically related to the hallucinogenic amphetamine derivatives, is reported to have a different type of psychological effect. MDMA is also the only drug in this group that appears to be capable of producing permanent brain damage in its users.

Angel dust, or PCP, became a national emergency during the late 1970s. Originally developed as an anesthetic, it produces more changes in body perception and fewer visual effects than LSD, and basic thought processes seem to be impaired by this drug. Both PCP and the anticholinergics tend to make the user forget most of what happened under the drug's effect. These anticholinergics are found in many plants throughout the world and have been used not only recreationally, medically, and spiritually, but also as poisons.

There is a vast variety of plants and chemicals that can produce "hallucinogenic" effects, some of which are like LSD or mescaline and others of which could perhaps be called toxic delirium. People will continue to experiment with them, but care is in order, because many of these substances can be dangerous.

REFERENCES

1. Schultes RE and Hofmann A: Plants of the Gods, New York, 1979, McGraw-Hill.
2. Hordern A: Psychopharmacology: some historical considerations. In Joyce CRB, editor: Psychopharmacology: dimensions and perspectives, Philadelphia, 1968, JB Lippincott Co.
3. Caporael LR: Ergotism: the Satan loosed in Salem, Science 192:21-26, 1976.
4. Gottlieb J and Spanos NP: Ergotism and the Salem village witch trials, Science 194:1390-1394, 1976.
5. Hofmann A: Psychotomimetic agents. In Burger A, editor: Drugs affecting the central nervous system, vol 2, New York, 1968, Marcel Dekker, Inc.
6. Horowitz M: Interview with Albert Hofmann, High Times, pp 24-81, July 1976.
7. Clark W: Psychedelic research: obstacles and values, Journal of Humanistic Psychology 15(3):5-17, 1975.
8. Segal J, editor: Research in the service of mental health, research on drug abuse, National Institute on Mental Health, Publication No (ADM) 75-236, US Department of Health, Education, and Welfare, Washington DC, 1975, US Government Printing Office.
9. Johnston L: Ford signs grant of $750,000 in LSD death in CIA test, New York Times, October 14, 1976, p C43.

10. Treaster JB: Mind-drug test a federal project for almost 25 years, New York Times, August 11, 1975, p M42.

11. CIA considered big LSD purchase, Washington Star, August 4, 1975. Knight M: LSD creator says army sought drug, New York Times, August 1, 1975.

12. Taylor JR and Johnson WN: Use of volunteers in chemical agent research, Inspector General Report No DAIGIN 21-75, Washington, DC, March 10, 1976, US Department of Army.

13. Weil AT: The strange case of the Harvard drug scandal, Look, pp 38-48, November 5, 1963.

14. Blumenthal R: Leary drug cult stirs Millbrook, New York Times, June 14, 1967, p 49.

15. Celebration #1, New Yorker 42:43, 1966.

16. Masters REL: Sex ecstasy, and the psychedelic drugs, Playboy 14(11):94-226, 1967.

17. Council on Mental Health and Committee on Alcoholism and Drug Dependence: Dependence on LSD and other hallucinogenic drugs, Journal of the American Medical Association 202:141-144, 1967.

18. Leary, once an LSD advocate, paroled, New York Times, April 21, 1976, p 25.

19. Leary and Liddy, debating specialists, New York Times, September 3, 1981, p B26.

20. Hamon M: Common neurochemical correlates to the action of hallucinogens. In Jacobs BL, editor: Hallucinogens: neurochemical, behavioral and clinical perspectives, New York, 1984, Raven Press.

21. Aghajanian GK: LSD and serotonergic dorsal raphe neurons: intracellular studies in vivo and in vitro. In Jacobs BL, editor: Hallucinogens: neurochemical, behavioral and clinical perspectives, New York, 1984, Raven Press.

22. Appel JB and Rosecrans JA: Behavioral pharmacology of hallucinogens in animals: conditioning studies. In Jacobs BL, editor: Hallucinogens: neurochemical, behavioral and clinical perspectives, New York, 1984, Raven Press.

23. Nichols DE and Glennon RA: Medicinal chemistry and structure-activity relationships of hallucinogens. In Jacobs BL, editor: Hallucinogens: neurochemical, behavioral and clinical perspectives, New York, 1984, Raven Press.

24. Jacobs BL: How hallucinogenic drugs work, American Scientist 75:386-392, 1987.

25. Siegel RK: The natural history of hallucinogens. In Jacobs BL, editor: Hallucinogens: neurochemical, behavioral and clinical perspectives, New York, 1984, Raven Press.

26. Krippner S: Psychedelic experience and the language process, Journal of Psychedelic Drugs 3(1):41-51, 1970.

27. Levine J, and Ludwig AM: The LSD controversy, Comprehensive Psychiatry 5(5):318-319, 1964.

28. Forsch WA, Robbins ES, and Stern M: Untoward reactions to lysergic acid diethylamide (LSD) resulting in hospitalization, New England Journal of Medicine 273:1235-1239, 1965.

29. Zegans LS, Pollard JC, and Brown D: The effects of LSD-25 on creativity and tolerance to regression, Archives of General Psychiatry 16:740-749, 1967.

30. Painting under LSD, Time 94(23):88, December 5, 1969.

31. Hollister LE, Shelton J, and Krieger G: A controlled comparison of lysergic acid diethylamide (LSD) and dextroamphetamine in alcoholics, American Journal of Psychiatry 125:1352-1357, 1969.

32. NIMH research on LSD, Extramural programs fiscal year 1948 to present, prepared September 1, 1975.

33. Crahan ME: God's flesh and other preColumbian phantastica, Bulletin of the Los Angeles County Medical Association 99:17, 1969.

34. Wolbach AB Jr, Isbell H, and Miner EJ: Cross tolerance between mescaline and LSD-25, with a comparison of the mescaline and LSD reactions, Psychopharmacologia 3:1-14, 1962.

35. Leary T: The religious experience: its production and interpretation, Journal of Psychedelic Drugs 1(2):3-23, 1967-1968.

36. Schultes RE and Hofmann A: The Botany and Chemistry of Hallucinogens, Springfield, Ill, 1980, Charles C Thomas.

37. Szara S: DMT (N,N-dimethyltryptamine) and homologues: clinical and pharmacological considerations. In Efron DH, editor: Psychotomimetic drugs, New York, 1970, Raven Press.

38. LaBarre W: Twenty years of peyote studies, Current Anthropology 1(1):45, 1960.

39. LaBarre W: The peyote cult, Hamden, Conn, 1964, The Shoe String Press.

40. Slotkin JS: Religious defenses (the Native American Church), Journal of Psychedelic Drugs 1(2):77-95, 1967-1968.

41. LaBarre W and others: Statement on peyote, Science 114:524, 582-583, 1951.

42. Kapadia GJ and Goyez MBE: Peyote constituents: chemistry, biogenese, and biological effects, Journal of Pharmaceutical Sciences 59:1699-1727, 1970.

43. De Ropp RS: Drugs and the mind, New York, 1957, Grove Press, Inc.

44. Ellis H: Mescal: a study of a divine plant, Popular Science Monthly 61:59, 65, 1902.

45. Huxley A: The doors of perception, New York, 1954, Harper & Row, Publishers.

46. Snyder SH, Faillace L, and Hollister L: 2,5-Dimethoxy-4-methyl-amphetamine (STP): a new hallucinogenic drug, Science 158:669-670, 1967.

47. Smith D and Meyers F: The psychotomimetic amphetamine with special reference to STP (DOM) toxicity. In Smith D, editor: Drug abuse papers, 1969, Section 4, Berkeley, 1969, University of California.

48. MDMA: compound raises medical, legal issues, Brain/Mind Bulletin, April 15, 1985.

49. Peroutka SJ and others: Subjective effects of 3,4-methylenedioxymethamphetamine in recreational users, Neuropsychopharmacology 1:273-277, 1988.

50. Barnes DM: New data intensify the agony over ecstasy, Science 239:864-866, 1988.

51. Greifenstein FE and others: A study of a l-dryl cycle hexyl amine for anesthesia, Anesthesia and Analgesia 37(5): 283-294, 1958.

52. Luby E and others: Study of a new schizophrenomimetic drug—Sernyl, A.M.A. Archives of Neurology and Psychiatry 81:113-119, March 1959.

53. Physician's Desk Reference, ed 43, Oradell, NJ, 1989, Medical Economics Company.

54. Siegel RK: Phencyclidine and ketamine intoxication: A study of four populations of recreational users. In Petersen RC and Stillman RC, editors: Phencyclidine (PCP) abuse: an appraisal, NIDA Research Monograph No 21, Washington, DC, 1978, US Department of Health and Human Services.

55. Balster RL and Chait LD: The behavioral effects of phencyclidine in animals. In Petersen RC and Stillman RC, editors: Phencyclidine (PCP) abuse: an appraisal, NIDA Research Monograph No 21, Washington, DC, 1978, US Department of Health and Human Services.

56. Siegel RK: PCP and violent crime: the people vs peace, Journal of Psychedelic Drugs 12(3-4):317, 1980.

57. Overend W: PCP: death in the "dust," Los Angeles Times, September 26, 1977.

58. Quirion R, Hammer RP, Herkenham M, and others: Phencyclidine (angel dust)/sigma "opiate" receptor: visualization by tritium-sensitive film, Proceedings of the National Academy of Sciences, USA 78:5881-5885, 1981.

59. Briggs KM: Pale Hecate's team, New York, 1962, The Humanities Press.

60. Langdon-Brown W: From witchcraft to chemotherapy, Cambridge, 1941, Cambridge University Press.

61. Gen 30:14-16, The New English Bible, Oxford University Press and Cambridge University Press, 1970.

62. Schultes RE: The plant kingdom and hallucinogens (Part III), Bulletin on Narcotics 22(1):43-46, 1970.

63. Encyclopedia Brittanica, vol 16, 1929.

64. Beverly R: The history and present state of Virginia, 1705, Chapel Hill, NC, 1947, University of North Carolina Press.

65. Graves R: Steps, London, 1958, Cassell & Co.

66. Allegro JM: The sacred mushroom and the cross, New York, 1970, Doubleday & Co, Inc.

67. Wasson RG: Fly agaric and man. In Efron DH, editor: Ethnopharmacologic search for psychoactive drugs, Washington, DC, 1967, National Institute of Mental Health. (See also Wasson RG: Soma, divine mushroom of immortality, New York, 1971, Harcourt, Brace, Jovanovich.)

68. Hallucinogens, Columbia Law Review 68(3):521-560, 1968.

69. Barnes DM: Ecstasy returns to schedule I, Science: 240, 24, 1988.

Chapter 16

Marijuana and Hashish

OBJECTIVES

After reading this chapter, you should be able to:

List the various cannabis species and some of the ways the plant is prepared for use.

Describe the history of cannabis use.

Name those chemicals that are most active in marijuana, and describe the time course of their presence in the body.

Explain the basic physiological and behavioral effects of marijuana, and discuss the current status of medical uses for marijuana.

Identify the issues relating to dependence and toxicity with marijuana.

Marijuana has meant so many things to so many people over the years that it is hard to describe it from a single perspective. We wind up behaving like that famous committee of blind men examining an elephant: the way you describe it depends on where you're standing. The matter of classifying marijuana among the other psychoactive drugs is so complex that we, as with most authors, avoid the issue by setting it off by itself. Marijuana can produce some sedative-like effects, some pain relief, and in large doses produces hallucinogenic effects. Thus many of its users treat it similarly to alcohol; it has been called a narcotic (for both pharmacological, as well as political, reasons); and it is often included among descriptions of hallucinogenic plants. The effects it produces when used as most people use it are, however, sufficiently different from those of other psychoactive drugs to justify its consideration as a unique substance.

CANNABIS
The Plant

Marijuana (or marihuana; either spelling is correct) is a preparation of leafy material from the *Cannabis* plant that is used by smoking. The question is, which *Cannabis* plant, since there is still botanical debate over whether there is one, three, or more species of *Cannabis*. There are many legal

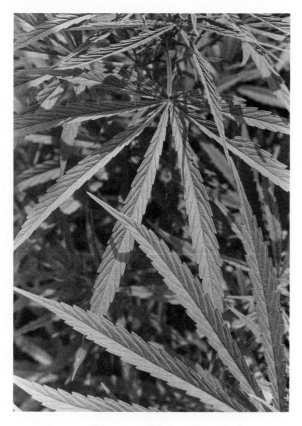

Leaves of the Cannabis (marijuana) plant.

implications over the number of species that are recognized, and the evidence is strong that there are three species of *Cannabis. Cannabis sativa* originated in the Orient but now grows worldwide and primarily has been used for its fibers, from which hemp rope is made. This is the species that grows as a weed in the United States and Canada. *C. indica* is grown for its psychoactive resins and is cultivated in many areas of the world, including selected planters and backyards of the United States. The third species, *C. ruderalis,* grows primarily in Russia and not at all in America. The plant Linnaeus named *C. sativa* in 1753 is what is still known as *C. sativa.*[1]

It was *C. sativa* that George Washington grew at Mount Vernon, most likely not to get high but to make rope. From his fields and many others like it, *C. sativa* spread across the nation, growing spontaneously.

C. sativa that is cultivated for use as hemp grows as a lanky plant up to 18 feet in height. *C. indica* plants cultivated for their psychoactive effects in India are more compact and usually only 2 or 3 feet tall. The psychoactive potency represents an interaction between genetics and environmental conditions. Plants of different species grown under identical conditions produce different amounts of psychoactive material, and the same plants will vary in potency from year to year, depending on the amount of sunshine, warm weather, and moisture.

Preparations from Cannabis

The primary psychoactive agent, Δ-9 tetrahydrocannabinol (THC), is concentrated in the resin of the plant with most of the resin in the flowering tops, less in the leaves, and little in the fibrous stalks. The psychoactive potency of a *Cannabis* preparation depends on the amount of resin present and therefore varies depending on the part of the plant used. We will describe three traditional cannabis preparations from India, each of which corresponds roughly to preparations available currently in the United States. The most potent of these is called *charas* in India, and it consists of pure resin that has been carefully removed from the surface of leaves and stems. **Hashish,** or hasheesh, is a term widely known around the world and in its purest form is pure resin, like charas. It may be less pure, depending on how carefully the resin has been separated from the plant material. Samples of hashish available in the Unted States vary widely in their THC content, averaging about 7% or 8%, and ranging up to about 14% THC. The second most potent preparation is traditionally called *ganja* in India, and it consists of dried plant material, but only from the tops of plants with pistillate flowers (female plants). The male plants are removed from the fields before the female plants can become pollinated and put their energy into seed production; this increases the potency of the female plants. This method of production has become increasingly popular in recent years in the United States for producing high-grade marijuana known as **sinsemilla** (Spanish *sin semilla,* "without seeds"). Sinsemilla samples from the United States also vary widely in THC content, averaging around 4% or 5%, usually not over 7% or 8% maximum, although occasional samples have been reported as high as 10% or 11%. The weakest form in India is *bhang,* which is made by using the entire remainder of the plant after the top leaves have been picked, drying it, and grinding it into a powder. The powder may then be mixed into drinks or candies.[1,p.86] Americans don't usually see this type of preparation, but we may consider it somewhat analogous to low-grade marijuana, which may consist of all the leaves of a plant, perhaps even a cannibis *sativa* plant found growing as a weed. Some of this low-grade domestic marijuana may contain less than 1% THC.

Manually scraping exuded resin off the plant is a tedious process, and a more efficient method of separating the resin from plants has been known for many years. The plants may be boiled in alcohol, then the solids filtered out and the liquid evaporated down to a thick, dark substance once known medically as "red oil of cannabis" and now referred to as *hash oil.* Again, this product varies widely in its potency, but may contain more than 50% THC. Until fairly recently, both medical and psychological effects of cannabis preparations were variable. All the traditional methods could do was produce relatively pure plant resin, but that resin could vary considerably in its THC content.

If we consider only the marijuana available for smoking in the United States, we can see that it may vary widely in potency from a low-grade product containing less than 1% THC to a high-grade sinsemilla containing 8% THC. The usual range of potency for marijuana seems to be 2% to 5%, however. During the 1980s there have been several statements to the effect that the mar-

ijuana available on the streets today is "10 times" more potent than the marijuana of the 1960s, and that all the research showing relatively benign effects of marijuana was based on material containing only 1% to 2% THC. In fact, the entire range of these traditional Indian preparations has been known, and scientific, literary, and medical descriptions of the wide range of effects have been based on this entire range of potencies, for 150 years. It is probably true that U.S. marijuana growers are becoming more sophisticated and producing more sinsemilla, but the overall range of potencies of marijuana available on the streets is still from under 1% to about 8%, with usual samples between 2% and 5%, just as in the early 1970s.[2]

HISTORY
Early History

The earliest reference to *Cannabis* is in a pharmacy book written in 2737 BC by the Chinese emperor Shen Nung. Referring to the euphoriant effects of *Cannabis,* he called it the "Liberator of Sin." There were some medical uses, however, and he recommended it for "female weakness, gout, rheumatism, malaria, beriberi, constipation and absent-mindedness."[3]

Social use of the plant spread to the Moslem world and North Africa by 1000 AD. In this period in the eastern Mediterranean area a legend developed around a religious cult that committed murder for political reasons. The cult was called "hashishiyya," from which our word "**assassin**" developed. In 1299 Marco Polo told the story he had heard of this group and their leader. It was a marvelous tale and had all the ingredients for surviving through the ages: intrigue, murder, sex, the use of drugs, mysterious lands. The story of this group and their activities was told in many ways over the years, and Boccaccio's *Decameron* contained one story based on it. Stories of this cult, combined with the frequent reference to the power and wonderment of hashish in *The Arabian Nights,* were widely circulated in Europe over the years.

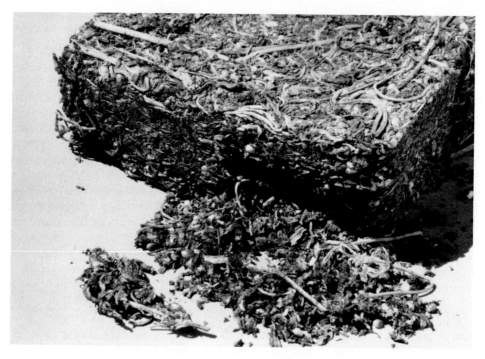

Marijuana is sometimes pressed into a brick weighing about a kilogram (2.2 pounds) for shipping. This may be referred to as a "kilo" or "key."

The Nineteenth Century: Romantic Literature and the New Science of Psychology

At the turn of the nineteenth century, world commerce was expanding. New and exciting reports from the world travelers of the seventeenth and eighteenth centuries introduced new cultures and new ideas to Europe. The Orient and the Middle East had yielded exotic spices, as well as the stimulants coffee and tea. Europe was ready for another new sensation, and she got it. The returning veteran, as usual, gets part of the blame for introducing what Europe was ready to receive.

Napoleon's campaign to Egypt at the beginning of the nineteenth century increased the Romantic's acquaintance with hashish and caused them to associate it with the Near East. . . . Napoleon was forced to give an order forbidding all French soldiers to indulge in hashish. Some of the soldiers brought the habit to

France, however, as did many other Frenchmen who worked for the government or traveled in the Near East.[4,p.63]

By the 1830s and 1840s, everyone who was anyone was using, thinking about using, or decrying the use of mind-tickling agents such as opium and hashish. One of the earliest (1844) popular accounts of the use of hashish is in *The Count of Monte Cristo* by Alexander Dumas. The story includes a reference to the Assassin story and contains statements about the characteristics of the drug that still sound contemporary.

During the 1840s a group of artists and writers gathered monthly at the Hotel Pimodan in Paris' Latin Quarter to use drugs. This group became famous because one of the participants, Gautier, wrote a book, *Le Club de Hachischins,* that described their activities. From this group have come some of the best literary descriptions of hashish intoxication. These French Romantics, like the impressionistic painters of a later period, were searching for new experiences, new sources of creativity from within, new ways of seeing the world outside. A few of the regulars were well-known writers such as Baudelaire, Gautier, and Dumas.

Baudelaire repeatedly used hashish and was an astute observer of the effects in himself and in others. In his book *Artificial Paradises* he echoes what Dumas had written about the kind of effect to expect from hashish:

The intoxication will be nothing but one immense dream, thanks to intensity of color and the rapidity of conceptions; but it will always preserve the particular tonality of the individual. . . . The dream will certainly reflect its dreamer. . . . He is only the same man grown larger . . . sophisticate and ingénu . . . will find nothing miraculous, absolutely nothing but the natural to an extreme.[5]

The extent of Baudelaire's actual experience with hashish is debatable, but he did identify (and exaggerate) three stages of intoxication following oral intake. These are still being rediscovered.

At first, a certain absurd, irresistible hilarity overcomes you. The most ordinary words, the simplest ideas assume a new and bizarre aspect. This mirth is intolerable to you; but it is useless to resist. The demon has invaded you. . . .

It sometimes happens that people completely unsuited for word-play will improvise an endless string of puns and wholly improbable idea relationships fit to outdo the ablest masters of this preposterous craft. But after a few minutes, the relation between ideas becomes so vague, and the thread of your thoughts grows so tenuous, that only your cohorts . . . can understand you.

. . . Next your senses become extraordinarily keen and acute. Your sight is infinite. Your ear can discern the slightest perceptible sound, even through the shrillest of noises.

The strangest ambiguities, the most inexplicable transpositions of ideas take place. In sounds there is color; in colors there is a music. . . . You are sitting and smoking; you believe that you are sitting in your pipe, and that *your pipe* is smoking *you;* you are exhaling *yourself* in bluish clouds.

This fantasy goes on for an eternity. A lucid interval, and a great expenditure of effort, permit you to look at the clock. The eternity turns out to have been only a minute.

The third phase . . . is something beyond description. It is what the Orientals call *kef;* it is complete happiness. There is nothing whirling and tumultuous about it. It is a calm and placid beatitude. Every philosophical problem is resolved. Every difficult question that presents a point of contention for theologians, and brings despair to thoughtful men, becomes clear and transparent. Every contradiction is reconciled. Man has surpassed the gods.[5]

As the end of the nineteenth century approached, the use of the anxiety-relieving drugs increased, but the hashish experience held little interest for the dweller in middle America. Just beginning, however, was the new science of psychology, whose interest was in the workings of the mind. The writings of William James and others introduced the possibility of using psychoactive agents in studying psychological processes. In 1899 one of the psychologists who had been using *Cannabis* in experiments said, "To the psychologist it [*Cannabis*] was as useful as the microscope to the naturalist; it magnifies psychological states and in this way is an aid to its study."[6]

The coming of "marijuana, assassin of youth." During the beginning of the twentieth century, public interest in marijuana and its use was not very widespread. In the early 1920s there were a few references in the mass media to the use of marijuana by Mexican-Americans, but public concern was not aroused. In 1926, however, a series of articles associating marijuana and crime appeared in a New Orleans newspaper. As a result, the public began to take an interest in the drug.

The Commissioner of Narcotics, Harry Anslinger, said that in 1931 the Bureau of Narcotics' file on marijuana was less than 2 inches thick. The same year, the Treasury Department stated:

A great deal of public interest has been aroused by the newspaper articles appearing from time to time on the evils of the abuse of marijuana, or Indian hemp. . . . This publicity tends to magnify the extent of the evil and lends color to an inference that there is an alarming spread of the improper use of the drug, whereas the actual increase in such use may not have been inordinately large.[3,p.130]

Even so, by 1935 there were 36 states with laws regulating the use, sale, and/or possession of marijuana. By the end of 1936 all 48 states had similar laws. The federal worm had also turned. In 1937, at congressional hearings, Anslinger stated that "traffic in marihuana is increasing to such an extent that it has come to be the cause for the greatest national concern."[7] In the 1931-1937 period it is true that the use of marijuana had spread throughout the country, but there is no evidence that there was wide use. The primary motivation for the congressional hearings on marijuana came not because of the use of marijuana as an inebriant or a euphoriant but because of reports by police and in the popular literature stating: "Most crimes of violence . . . are laid to users of marihuana."[8]

When *Scientific American*[9] reported in March 1936 that:

Marijuana produces a wide variety of symptoms in the user, including hilarity, swooning, and sexual excitement. Combined with intoxicants, it often makes the smoker vicious, with a desire to fight and kill.

and *Popular Science Monthly*[10] in May 1936 contained a lengthy article including such statements as:

the Chief of Philadelphia County detectives declared that whenever any particularly horrible crime was committed—and especially one pointing to perversion—his officers searched first in marijuana dens and questioned marijuana smokers for suspects.

it hardly seemed necessary for the reader to be told that marijuana had arrived as "the foremost menace to life, health, and morals in the list of drugs used in America."[10]

The association was repeatedly made in this period between crime, particularly violent and/or perverted crime, and marijuana use. A typical report,[11] cautiously phrased as were all of them, follows:

In Los Angeles, Calif., a youth was walking along a downtown street after inhaling a marijuana cigarette. For many addicts, merely a portion of a "reefer" is enough to induce intoxication. Suddenly, for no reason, he decided that someone had threatened to kill him and

that his life at that very moment was in danger. Wildly he looked about him. The only person in sight was an aged bootblack. Drug-crazed nerve centers conjured the innocent old shoe-shiner into a destroying monster. Mad with fright, the addict hurried to his room and got a gun. He killed the old man, and then, later, babbled his grief over what had been wanton, uncontrolled murder.

"I thought someone was after me," he said. "That's the only reason I did it. I had never seen the old fellow before. Something just told me to kill him!"

That's marijuana!

However, not all articles condemned marijuana as the precipitator of violent crimes. An article in *The Literary Digest* reported that the chief psychiatrist at Bellevue Hospital in New York City had reviewed the cases of over 2200 criminals convicted of felonies. Referring to marijuana he said, "None of the assault cases could be said to have been committed under the drug's influence. Of the sexual crimes, there was none due to marihuana intoxication. . . . It is quite probable that alcohol is more responsible as an agent for crime than is marihuana."[12]

There was very poor documentation of the marijuana-crime relationship, which was stated as proved in the 1930s. A thorough review[13] of Anslinger's writings, including the marijuana and vicious crime cases related throughout this period, concluded that:

In the works of Mr. Anslinger, there are either no references or references to volumes which my assistants and I have checked and which, in our checking, we find to be based upon much hearsay and little or no experimentation. We found a mythology in which later writers cite the authority of earlier writers, who also had little evidence. We have found, by and large, what can most charitably be described as a pyramid of prejudice, with each level of the structure built upon the shaky foundations of earlier distortions.

With such poor evidence supporting the relationship between marijuana use and crime, it seems strange that the true story was never told. There are probably several reasons. One was the Great Depression, which made everyone acutely sensitive to, and wary of, any new and particularly foreign influences. The fact that it was the lower-class Mexican-Americans and Negroes who had initiated use of the drug made the drug doubly dangerous to the white middle class.

Another contributing factor probably was the regular reference in associating marijuana and crime to the murdering cult of Assassins as suggestive of the characteristics of the drug. The 1936 *Popular Science Monthly*[10] reference to the Assassins is the most concise.

The origin of the word "assassin" has two explanations, but either demonstrates the menace of Indian hemp. According to one version, members of a band of Persian terrorists committed their worst atrocities while under the influence of hashish. In the other version, Saracens who opposed the Crusaders were said to employ the services of hashish addicts to secure secret murderers of the leaders of the Crusades. In both versions, the murderers were known as "haschischin," "hash-shash" or "hashishi" and from those terms comes the modern and ominous "assassin."

In none of the original stories and legends where the murders committed by individuals under the influence of hashish; rather, it was part of the reward for carrying out the murders.

No matter. As the thirties rolled on, fear of the marijuana user increased, as did state marijuana-control laws. In the mid-1930s the Narcotics Bureau acted to support federal legislation, and in the spring of 1937 congressional hearings were held.

Passage of the Marijuana Tax Act was a foregone conclusion. There were few witnesses to testify other than law enforcement officers. The bird-seed people had the act modified so they could import sterilized *Cannabis* seed for use in their product. An official of the American Medical Association (AMA) testified on his own behalf, not representing the AMA, against the bill. His reasons for opposing the bill were multiple. Primarily, though, he thought the state antimarijuana laws were adequate and, also, that the social-menace case against marijuana had not been proved at all. The bill was passed in August and became effective on October 1, 1937.

The general characteristics of the law followed the regulation-by-taxation theme of the Harrison Act of 1914. The federal law did not outlaw *Cannabis* or its preparations; it just taxed the grower, distributor, seller, and buyer and made it, administratively, almost impossible to have anything to do with *Cannabis!* In addition, the Bureau of Narcotics prepared a uniform law that many states adopted. The uniform law on marijuana specifically named *C. sativa* as the species of plant whose leafy material is illegal. In recent years there have been some court cases in which the defense has argued that the material confiscated by the police came from *C. indica* and thus was not illegal. In the usual specimens obtained by police and/or presented in court, all distinguishing characters between species are either not present or are obliterated by drying and crushing. Since the cannabinols are generic, present in all species, there is no way of telling what species one has at hand with most confiscated *Cannabis* material. Sometimes the spirit and sometimes the letter of the law wins. Britons are smarter: they refer only to *Cannabis*.

The state laws made possession and use of marijuana illegal per se. In May 1969, 32 years later, the U.S. Supreme Court declared the Marijuana Tax Act unconstitutional and overturned the conviction of Timothy Leary because there was:

in the Federal anti-marijuana law—a section that requires the suspect to pay a tax on the drug, thus incriminating himself, in violation of the Fifth Amendment: and a section that assumes (rather than requiring proof) that a person with foreign-grown marijuana in his possession knows it is smuggled.[14]

After the Marijuana Tax Act

Passage of the Marijuana Tax Act had an amazing effect. Almost immediately there was a sharp reduction in the reports of heinous crimes committed under the influence of marijuana! The price of the merchandise increased rapidly (the war came along, too), so that 5 years after the act the cost of a marijuana cigarette—a reefer—had increased 6 to 12 times and cost about a dollar.

The year after the law was enacted, 1938, Mayor Fiorello LaGuardia of New York City remembered what no one else wanted to recall. What he recalled were two army studies on marijuana use by soldiers in the Panama Canal Zone around 1930. Both reports found marijuana to be innocuous and that its reputation as a troublemaker "was due to its association with alcohol which . . . was always found the prime agent."[15]

Mayor LaGuardia asked the New York Academy of Medicine to study marijuana, its use, its effects, and the necessity for control. The report, issued in 1944, was intensive and extensive and a very good study for its time. The complete report is available[16] and widely discussed, so only a part of the summary is quoted.

It was found that marihuana in an effective dose impairs intellectual functioning in general. . . .

Marihuana does not change the basic personality structure of the individual. It induces a feeling of self-confidence, but this expressed in thought rather than in performance. There is, in fact, evidence of a diminution in physical activity. . . .

Those who have been smoking marihuana for a period of years showed no mental or physical deterioration which may be attributed to the drug.[16,p.408]

This 1944 report, which was completed by a very reputable committee of the New York Academy of Medicine, brought a violent reaction. The AMA stated in a 1945 editorial[17]:

For many years medical scientists have considered cannabis a dangerous drug. Nevertheless, a book called "Marihuana Problems" by New York City Major's Committee on Marihuana submits an analysis of seventeen doctors of tests on 77 prisoners and, on this narrow and thoroughly unscientific foundation, draws sweeping and inadequate conclusions which minimize the harmfulness of marijuana. Already the book has done harm. One investigator has described some tearful parents who brought their 16 year old son to a physician after he had been detected in the act of smoking marihuana. A noticeable mental deterioration had been evident for some time even to their lay minds. The boy said he had read an account of the LaGuardia Committee report and that this was his justification for using marihuana.

As in all such reports and reactions to reports, there is little dispute over the facts, only over the interpretation. Since the LaGuardia Report is in substantial agreement with the Indian Hemp Commission Report of the 1890s, the Panama Canal Zone reports of the 1930s, and the comprehensive reports in the 1970s by the governments of New Zealand, Canada, Great Britain, and the United States, in addition to the 1981 report to the World Health Organization and the 1982 report by the National Academy of Science to the Congress of the United States, it is likely that the conclusions of the LaGuardia Report were and are for the most part valid.

The 1950s and 1960s form a unique period in the history of marijuana. There was a hiatus in scientific research on marijuana and *Cannabis*, but experimentation in the streets increased continually. With the arrival of the "psychedelic sixties,"the popular press could and did emphasize the more sensational hallucinogens. Marijuana, however, was everywhere the action was in the youth culture, but for the most part the major concern was on the more potent agents.

Toward the end of the 1960s, LSD use declined, heroin use increased rapidly in and out of the ghetto, and marijuana use was becoming the initiation rite of the turned-on generation.[18]

PHARMACOLOGY
Cannabinoid Chemicals

The chemistry of *Cannabis* is quite complex, and isolation and extraction of the active ingredient are difficult even today. *Cannabis* is unique among psychoactive plant materials in that it contains no nitrogen and thus is not an alkaloid. This fact was established over 100 years ago by two chemists, the Smith brothers (yes, it's those Smith brothers). Because of its nonnitrogen content, the nineteenth-century chemists who had been so successful in isolating the active agents from other plants were unable to identify the active component of *Cannabis*.

There are over 400 different chemicals in marijuana but only 61 of them are unique to the *Can-*

nabis plant—these are called cannabinoids. One of them, Δ-9-tetrahydrocannibinol (THC), was isolated and synthesized in 1964 and is clearly the most pharmacologically active. Structures of some of these chemicals are shown in Fig. 16-1. 11-Hydroxy-Δ-9-THC is the major active metabolite in the body of THC.

Take special note that the relationship of THC to *Cannabis* is probably more similar to the relationship of mescaline to peyote than of alcohol to beer, wine, or distilled spirits. Alcohol is the *only* behaviorally active agent in alcoholic beverages, but there may be more than one active agent in *Cannabis*.

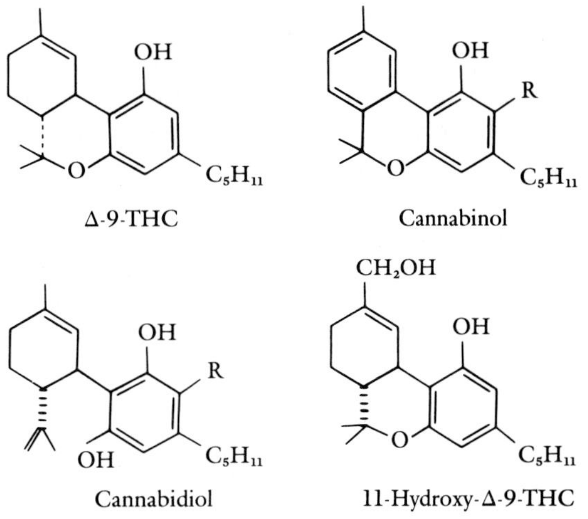

Absorption and Elimination

When smoked, THC is rapidly absorbed into the blood and distributed first to the brain, then redistributed to the rest of the body so that within 30 minutes much is gone from the blood. The psychological and cardiovascular effects occur together, usually within 5 to 10 minutes. The THC remaining in blood has a half-life of about 19 hours but metabolites (of which there are at least 45), primarily 11-hydroxy-THC, are formed in the liver and have a half-life of 50 hours. Complete elimination of one dose of THC and its metabolites may take 30 days. After 1 week 25% to 30% of the THC and its metabolites may remain in the body. THC taken orally is slowly absorbed and the liver transforms it to 11-hydroxy-THC, so little THC reaches the brain after oral ingestion.

The high lipid solubility of THC means that it (and its metabolites) is selectively taken up and stored in fatty tissue to be released slowly. Excretion is primarily through the feces. All of this has two important implications: (1) there is no easy way to monitor (in urine or blood) THC/metabolite levels and relate them to behavioral and/or physiological effects, as can be done with alcohol and (2) the long-lasting, steady, low concentration of THC/metabolites on the brain and other organs may have effects not yet thought of.

With the advent of isolated THC, dose-response relationships could be determined, and the dif-

Figure 16-1. Cannabinoid structures.

ferential response to oral and inhalation modes of intake evaluated.

Threshold doses of 2 mg. smoked and 5 mg. orally produced mild euphoria; 7 mg. smoked and 17 mg. orally, some perceptual and time sense changes occurred; and at 15 mg. smoked and 25 mg. orally, subjects reported marked changes in body image, perceptual distortions, delusions and hallucinations.[19]

Oral intake is more frequently followed by nausea, physical discomfort, and hangover, and the dose level cannot be titrated as accurately as is possible when smoking. There may be other differences in effects between comparable oral and smoking intake, although this has not been studied extensively.

A reminder: *Cannabis* is a drug that has primarily been used in two dosage forms of very different potency. Hashish and *Cannabis* extracts that give rise to the experiences reported by Baudelaire and others are potent hallucinogenic agents. The drug delivery system that spread through the country in the 1920s and 1930s was a much less potent form, marijuana. The active ingredient is the same; the amount differs. Both marijuana and hashish are available and used in the United States today, although the great majority of users restrict themselves to marijuana.

Mechanism of Action

Scientists have been searching for years for a key to help them unlock the mystery of marijuana's action on the nervous system. Of course, the identification and purification of Δ-9 THC was a necessary step. THC has effects on the electrical properties of nerve membranes, alters turnover rates of serotonin and dopamine,[20] and has effects on prostaglandin synthesis[21] to name a few of its effects. Whether any of these is the *basic* effect or whether all are secondary to some other direct action is still not known. An additional problem may be, which of THC's actions are we seeking a mechanism for? The sedative effect may be through a different mechanism from the analgesic and/or the hallucinogenic effects. What appears to be a significant breakthrough was made by researchers at the National Institute of Mental Health laboratories in 1988. They developed a technique to identify and measure highly specific and selective binding sites for THC and related compounds in rat brains.[22] This may be the key to unlock the mystery of THC's action in the brain.

Physiological Effects

Thus far the study of the effects of THC on the physiology of the body has done little more than quantify earlier reports in which resin extracts were used. The established physiological effects of *Cannabis* are dose related, for the most part minor, of indeterminate importance for the psychological effects, and of unknown toxicological significance. For many years there has been substantial agreement on the short-term physiological effects of *Cannabis*.

Physiological changes accompanying marijuana use at typical levels of American social usage are relatively few. One of the most consistent is an increase in pulse rate. Another is reddening of the eyes at the time of use. Dryness of the mouth and throat are uniformly reported. Although enlargement of the pupils was an earlier impression, more careful study had indicated that this does not occur. Blood pressure effects have been inconsistent.

Except for bronchodilation, acute exposure to marijuana has little effect on breathing as measured by conventional pulmonary tests. Heavy marijuana smoking over a much longer period could lead to clinically significant and less readily reversible impairment of pulmonary function.[p.59] The smoking of marijuana causes changes in the heart and circulation that are characteristic of stress. But there is no evidence to indicate that it exerts a permanently deleterious effect on the normal cardiovascular system . . . Marijuana increases the work of the heart, usually by increasing heart rate, and in some persons by increasing blood pressure. This increase in workload poses a threat to patients with hypertension, cerebrovascular disease, and coronary atherosclerosis.[23]

Behavioral Effects

Almost all writers emphasize that a new user has to learn how to smoke marijuana. The first step involves deeply inhaling the smoke and holding it in the lungs for 20 to 40 seconds. Then the user has to learn to identify and control the effects, and, finally, he has to learn to label the effects as pleasant. Because of this learning process, most first-time users do not achieve the euphoric "stoned" or "high" condition of the repeater.

The effects accompanying marijuana smoking by the experienced user are relatively well established.

A cannabis "high" typically involves several phases. The initial effects are often somewhat stimulating and, in some individuals, may elicit mild tension or anxiety which usually is replaced by a pleasant feeling of well-being. The later effects usually tend to make the user introspective and tranquil. Rapid mood changes often occur. A period of enormous hilarity may be followed by a contemplative silence.[17,p.174]

One investigator had experienced marijuana smokers indicate how frequently their marijuana intoxication included each of 206 effects listed on a sheet. Although there are great difficulties in looking for generalizations among idiosyncratic responses, the investigator was able to summarize 124 common subjective effects.

Sense perception is often improved, both in intensity and in scope. Imagery is usually stronger but well controlled, although people often care less about controlling their actions. Great changes in perception of space and time are common, as are changes in psychological processes such as understanding, memory, emotion, and sense of identity. . . .

To the extent that the described effects are delusory or inaccurate, the delusions and inaccuracy are widely shared. It is interesting, too, that nearly all the common effects seem either emotionally pleasing or cognitively interesting, and it is easy to see why marijuana users find the effects desirable regardless of what happens to their external behavior.[24]

The subjective effects of smoking marijuana—the high—are quite difficult to study. First, since tolerance does develop, experienced smokers should show *less* effect than beginning smokers. But almost everyone suggests that you have to learn to use marijuana, and you have to learn to appreciate the psychological effects that occur. This would mean that experienced smokers should show *more* effect than beginning smokers. In addition to these factors, or maybe as part of them, there is much learning and association of the high with the smell, feel, taste, and rituals of using marijuana. This would suggest that an experienced user would report *more* effect from a placebo cigarette than would a beginning user. The placebo cigarette would elicit the feelings associated with (conditioned to) the use of marijuana, and there should be more of these associations in the experienced user. It might also be expected that frequent marijuana users would be *less* sensitive than infrequent users to THC itself, since more of their expectations are involved in the factors related to smoking marijuana. Tables 16-1 and 16-2 speak to these issues.

Placebo cigarettes were made for these studies by extracting the THC and other cannabinols from marijuana with alcohol. The marijuana contained 0.9% THC, and the cigarettes were made so that they contained 9 mg THC, of which about 5 mg would be delivered to the user. This was midrange potency compared to what was being sold

Table 16-1		
Reports of intoxication and measured physiologic changes from experienced users smoking marijuana and placebo cigarettes (n = 100)		
	Number of subjects reporting	
Intoxication level (0 sober, 100 maximum)	**Marijuana**	**Placebo**
0-19	15	35
20-39	11	28
40-59	20	21
60-79	32	12
80-100	22	4
Average	61	34
Average physiological change (pre- to post-smoking)	**Marijuana***	**Placebo†**
Pulse rate (beats/minutes)	+24.00	−4.00
Salivary flow (cc/5 minutes)	−1.60	+0.80
Redness of eye (0-4 scale)	+1.92	+0.04

*All significant, p < 0.05.
†None significant.

on the streets of San Francisco where these double-blind studies were done.[25]

Table 16-1 shows very nicely that, although experienced users report more intoxication from using a THC-containing marijuana cigarette, there is a moderate level of intoxication reported after the use of a similar smelling, tasting, and feeling cigarette without THC. This should not be too surprising, since some experienced users report that they can turn themselves on just by thinking about it. It may be possible to fool the psyche, but not the soma. The physiological changes from use of the active cigarette are what you would expect: increase in heart rate, drying of mouth, reddening of eyes. These changes do not occur with the placebo.

The interaction of learning (reverse tolerance?)

and of tolerance are clear in Table 16-2. Frequent users report less effect when using an active cigarette but more effect to the placebo. Infrequent users do not get as high a high from using the placebo but do report more effect from using the THC-containing cigarette. The same type of response shows up in part B of Table 16-2, but of most interest is the finding that frequent users respond much less to the oral THC than do the infrequent users. This is probably a combination of pharmacodynamic tolerance and absence of the usual associations with getting high. (If I don't see, smell, and feel these things, then I can't be intoxicated.) Even though the subjective effects vary with expectancy and other factors, the physiological effects follow the physiology, and the frequent users show smaller physiological changes to the oral THC than infrequent users.

At the level of social intoxication there is a dose-related impairment in scores of psychomotor and cognitive tests with "moderate impairment . . . during the period of peak intoxication."[19] In laboratory studies naive users report fewer subjective effects but show greater decrement in test performance.[26]

One of the consistent alterations in function is on short-term memory, that is, tasks such as learning and remembering new information or remembering and following a sequence of directions. In everyday use while intoxicated, the marijuana user is unable to easily recall information he just learned seconds or minutes before. This memory lapse affects the general thread of conversation among a group of users, as Baudelaire noted. On this issue one of the truly grand old men of the study of drug effects, A. Wikler, commented:

> The drunkard staggers—
>   only when he walks,
> The pothead forgets—
>   only when he talks.

This impairment of short-term memory is probably the basis for the changes in time sense frequently reported. The user feels that more time has passed than actually has. Such overestimation of the passage of time is the most commonly re-

---

Table 16-2

Reports of intoxication and measured physiological changes in frequent and infrequent marijuana users

	Infrequent users (less than 2 cigarettes a month)	Frequent users (more than 7 cigarettes a month)
Reported level of intoxication after using (averages, range 0-100)		
A. Marijuana cigarette	67	52
Placebo cigarette	22	48
B. Marijuana cigarette	62	56
Oral extract (25 mg THC)	72	32
Placebo cigarette	26	51
Placebo oral extract	2	5
Physiological changes		
Pulse-rate (beats/minute)	+31.0*	+17.0
Salivary flow (cc/5 minutes)	−1.8*	−0.9
Redness of eye (0-4 scale)	+2.1	+1.5

*Significant differences, $p < 0.05$, between infrequent and frequent users.

ported psychological effect of marijuana smoking and has been validated in many experiments.

One particularly important finding is that while reaction time is not greatly affected, if affected at all, there is a great impairment in the ability to engage in *tracking behavior*. Tracking behavior requires sustained attention and this ability is decreased considerably by marijuana. Loss of concentration is perhaps also demonstrated by the finding that the quality of interpersonal communication (the richness of the language and attention to feedback from the other person) goes down under the influence of marijuana.

MEDICAL USES OF CANNABIS

Since *Cannabis* never attained the medical status of opium, its medical report is spotted, but the first report of medical use was by Shen Nung in 2737 BC. Some 2900 years after the Shen Nung report, another Chinese physician, Hoa-tho (200 AD) recommended *Cannabis* resin mixed with wine as a surgical anesthetic. Although *Cannabis* preparations were used extensively in medicine in India and after about 900 AD in the Near East, there was almost nothing about it in European medicine until the 1800s.

Early reports in European medical journals, such as de Sacy's 1809 article titled "Intoxicating Preparations made with Cannabis," awakened more interest in the writers and artists of the period than in medical men. In 1839, however, a lengthy article, "On the Preparations of the Indian Hemp, or Gunjah," was published by a British physician working in India[27]. He reviewed the use of *Cannabis* in Indian medicine and reported on his own work with animals, which suggested that *Cannabis* preparations were quite safe. Having shown *Cannabis* to be nontoxic, he used it clinically and found it to be an effective anticonvulsant and muscle relaxant, as well as a valuable drug for the relief of the pain of rheumatism.

This article by W.B. O'Shaughnessy started the up-and-down history of the medical use of *Cannabis* in Europe and the United States. In 1860 the Ohio State Medical Society's Committee on *C. indica* reported its successful use in the treatment of stomach pain, chronic cough, and gonorrhea. One physcian felt he had to "assign to the Indian hemp a place among the so-called hypnotic medicines next to opium. . . ."[28] By the 1890s a medical text included the statement: "Cannabis is very valuable for the relief of pain, particularly that depending on nerve disturbances. . . ."[3]

One of the difficulties that has always plagued the scientific, medical, and social use of *Cannabis* is the variability of the product. An 1898 brochure reviewed the assay and standardization techniques used with many of the common plant drugs and stated: "In Cannabis Indica we have a drug of great importance and one which all of materia medica is undoubtedly the most variable."[29] Four years later Parke, Davis & Company,[30] using new standardization procedures, claimed that "each lot sent out upon the market by us is of full potency and to be relied upon." They listed a variety of *Cannabis* products available for medical use, including "a Chocolate Coated Tablet Extract Indian Cannabis ¼ grain"!

Passage of the 1937 law resulted in all 28 of the legal *Cannabis* preparations being withdrawn from the market, and in 1941 *Cannabis* was dropped from *The National Formulary* and *The U.S. Pharmacopeia*. Note well that the decline in the medical use of *Cannabis* occurred long before 1937 and that the law did not eliminate an actively used therapeutic agent. Four factors, however, certainly contributed to the declining prescription rate of this plant. One was the development of new and better drugs for most illnesses. Second was the variability of the available medicinal preparations of *Cannabis*, which was repeatedly mentioned in the 1937 hearings.[31] Third, *Cannabis* is very insoluble in water and thus not amenable to injectable preparations. Last, taken orally it has an unusually long (1-hour to 2-hour) latency to onset of action.

With the recent renewed interest in marijuana as a social drug has come some reevaluation and rethinking of the implications of some of the older therapeutic reports. Scientists are looking again at some of the most interesting reported therapeutic effects of *Cannabis*. One is its anticonvulsant activity. A 1949 report [32] found it effective in some cases where phenytoin (Dilantin), the anticonvulsant of choice both then and now, was ineffective. The fact that both Queen Victoria's physician and Sir William Osler, as well as others, found *Cannabis* to be very effective against tension headaches and/or migraine has caused some interest.[33]

A 1972 report showed that marijuana smoking was effective in reducing the fluid pressure of the eye in a glaucoma patient.[34] That report became a cause célèbre in 1975 when a glaucoma patient was arrested for growing marijuana plants on his back porch for medical purposes. This man 15 months later (1) had the charges against him dropped, (2) had his physician certify that the only way for him to prevent blindness was to smoke five joints a day, and (3) had these marijuana joints legally supplied to him by the United States government.[35] A second possible important medical use was reported in 1975. Medication containing THC, the active ingredient in marijuana, was the only kind that was effective in reducing the severe nausea caused by certain drugs used to treat cancer. A 1982 report from the National Academy of Sciences stated that:

> Cannabis and its derivatives have shown promise in the treatment of a variety of disorders. The evidence is most impressive in glaucoma...; in asthma ...; and in the nausea and vomiting of cancer chemotherapy ... [and] might also be useful in seizures, spasticity, and other nervous system disorders. . . .[23,p.150]

On the other hand, Dr. Nahas, a medical researcher and prominent foe of marijuana, feels that:

> For each of these uses, there are other modern drugs with greater bioavailability, specificity, and effectiveness . . . Reproducible absorption, consistent and predictable pharmacological effects may not be achieved. . . . .It appears that it will not become a useful therapeutic agent.[36]

In 1985 the FDA licensed a small drug company, Unimed, Inc., to begin producing a capsule containing THC for sale to cancer chemotherapy patients who are experiencing nausea. It will be interesting to see how many people will use **Marinol,** as the drug is named, and how well it will work, given concerns about slow absorption and variability.[37] The National Organization for the Reform of Marijuana Laws (NORML) wants marijuana cigarettes themselves approved, under the theory that the dose can be better controlled and smoking is therefore safer. Their position received some support from the DEA's chief administrative law judge in 1988, who recommended that the DEA move marijuana from Schedule I to Schedule II so physicians could use it to treat the nausea produced by cancer chemotherapy and also to relieve suffering in cases of multiple sclerosis. He called natural marijuana "one of the safest therapeutically active substances known to man."[38] Needless to say, the DEA as a whole was not ready to take this step.

CAUSES FOR CONCERN
Dependence Potential

For years there was debate over whether tolerance developed to the effects of THC and/or marijuana. Whereas animal studies repeatedly demonstrated tolerance to the behavioral disruption produced by large doses of marijuana, the experiences of human marijuana smokers seemed to indicate that experienced users could get high more readily than inexperienced users, possibly implying reverse tolerance, or sensitization to the drug. We now know that learning plays an important role in the psychological reaction, particularly to low doses of marijuana. That, combined with the fact that THC may build up in the tissues of chronic users, might account for any increased reaction. However, a number of human studies have now demonstrated clear evidence of tolerance to some of the physiological effects of THC (see Table 16-2). If high levels of marijuana are used regularly over a sustained period of time, tolerance will be obvious.

Physical dependence has been demonstrated in laboratory experiments with humans given large doses of THC every 4 hours for 10 to 20 days. Beginning several hours after the last oral dose, subjects showed irritability, restlessness, nausea, and vomiting. These symptoms peaked at 8 hours, and declined over the next 3 days. Sleep disturbances and loss of appetite were also reported.[39] Such withdrawal symptoms are virtually never reported outside the research laboratory. It is of interest that in animal studies, the withdrawal symptoms resemble those of opiate withdrawal to some extent and may have some mechanisms in common.

The strength of a drug's tendency to produce behavioral dependence can be estimated by looking at how many of its users develop patterns of daily, repeated use. With a highly addicting practice like cigarette smoking, the majority of users are daily users of multiple doses. With alcohol and many other drugs, most users avoid such a pattern, but a few develop strong dependence. The marijuana pattern seems to be more similar to that of alcohol use than of cigarette smoking or heroin injection. As David E. Smith of the Haight-Ashbury Medical Center said in 1982: "Regular heavy users who smoke more than 10 joints a day may be rare, but they do exist."[40]

The picture that emerges is that addiction, in the sense of a constant craving, high-frequency use, the buildup of tolerance, and possible withdrawal symptoms is not an issue for the majority of marijuana users who engage in occasional smoking of one or two marijuana cigarettes. However, a small fraction of marijuana users do become dependent on daily use of marijuana. This probably has a lot to do with psychosocial variables and is not seen by most researchers as an inevitable consequence of exposure to marijuana.

Toxicity Potential

The acute physiological effect of marijuana, primarily an increase in heart rate, has not been thought to be a threat to health. However, as the marijuana-using population ages there is concern that individuals with high blood pressure, heart disease, or hardening of the arteries might be harmed by smoking marijuana.[23] The lethal dose of THC has not been extensively studied in animals, and no human deaths have been reported from the use of *Cannabis*. There is general concensus that the lethal dose/effective dose (LD/ED) ratio is much higher for *Cannabis* than it is for alcohol.

Behaviorally, the intoxication produced by marijuana does present some danger, especially if the user is driving. Early experiments using weak marijuana and simple reaction-time driving tests found small effects that experienced users seemed to be able to overcome (behavioral tolerance). However, there have now been a large number of studies using more complex and realistic driving tests that show definite impairments with marijuana. In either computer-controlled driving simulators or in actual driving tests on a closed course, these impairments were found to be dose related. The ability to maintain concentration, correct for wind gusts, and maintain a steady speed were all impaired, as was judgment. A telephone survey of nearly 6000 teenagers found that those who reported driving six or more times per month after smoking marijuana were 2.4 times more likely to be involved in traffic accidents than those who did not drive after smoking marijuana. Studies based on measurements of drugs in the blood of drivers involved in accidents also indicate a role for marijuana in causing accidents.[41]

The other major behavioral problem associated with acute marijuana intoxication is the panic reaction. Much like many of the bad trips with hallucinogens, the reaction is usually fear of loss of control and fear that things will not return to normal. Even our old friend Baudelaire understood this and advised his readers to surround themselves with friends and a pleasant environment before using hashish. Although many people do seek emergency medical treatment for marijuana-induced panic and are sometimes given sedatives or tranquilizers, the best treatment is probably "talking down," or reminding the person of who and where they are, that their reaction is temporary, and that everything will be all right.

Since a large number of Americans are and have been using marijuana chronically, there has been a great deal of concern about the possible long-term effects of chronic marijuana use. There are a couple of physiological concerns that merit attention. One is the effect on lung function and the concern about lung cancer. Experiments have shown that chronic, daily smoking of marijuana does impair air flow in and out of the lungs.[42] It is hard to tell yet whether years of such an effect would result in permanent, major obstructive lung disease in the same way that smoking tobacco cigarettes does. Also, there is no direct evidence linking marijuana smoking to lung cancer in humans. Remember that it took many years of cigarette smoking by millions of Americans before the links with lung cancer and other lung diseases were shown. Marijuana smoke has been compared with tobacco smoke.[23] Whereas some of the constituents differ (there is no nicotine in marijuana smoke and no THC in tobacco), many of the dangerous components are found in both. Total tar levels, carbon monoxide, hydrogen cyanide, and nitrosamines are found in similar amounts (except for tobacco-specific nitrosamines, which are carcinogens). Another potent carcinogen, *benzopyrene,* is found in greater amounts in marijuana than in tobacco. Everyone suspects that marijuana smoking will eventually be shown to cause cancer, but how much of a problem this will be compared to tobacco is hard to say. On the one hand, few marijuana smokers smoke 20 marijuana cigarettes every day, but tobacco smokers regularly smoke this much. On the other hand, the marijuana cigarette is not filtered and the user generally gets as much concentrated smoke as possible as far down in the lungs as possible and holds it there. So, while some of us wait and see when the data will come out, others are participating in the experiment.

The other area of concern seems to be reproductive effects in both males and females. Heavy marijuana smoking can decrease testosterone levels in males, although the levels are still within

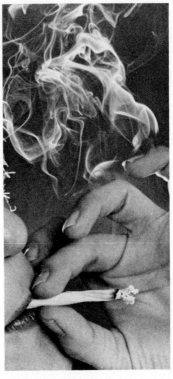

© Joel Gordon 1980

Some of the concerns about marijuana use come from the fact that it is often smoked, and the smoke is likely to have adverse effects on the lungs.

the normal range and the significance of those decreases is not known. There have been reports of diminished sperm counts or abnormal sperm structure in heavy marijuana users, but again the clinical significance of these reports is not clear.[43] A number of studies have reported either lower birth weight or shorter length at birth for infants whose mothers smoked marijuana during pregnancy.[44] Although these effects are small and inconsistent from one study to the next, it is of course wise to avoid use of all drugs during pregnancy.

There have also been reports that marijuana smoking impairs some measures of the functioning of the immune system.[45] Animal studies have found that THC injections can reduce immunity to infection, but at doses well above those obtainable by smoking marijuana. Some human studies of marijuana smokers have suggested reduced immunity, but most have not. If the effect were real, it could result in marijuana smokers being more susceptible to infections, cancer and other diseases, such as genital herpes. A 1984 review pointed out that large-scale epidemiological studies have not been done and small but meaningful effects might be difficult to detect, since most marijuana smokers are young and presumably in good overall health.[41]

Since 1971, when some psychiatric case reports were published identifying an **amotivational syndrome** in marijuana smokers, there has been concern about the effect of regular marijuana use on behavior and motivation. A number of experiments and correlational studies have been aimed at answering this question. One thing to remember is the long half-life of marijuana in the body, so that a daily smoker may in fact be chronically intoxicated and exhibit behavioral or motivational impairments even before his daily dose. There does seem to be evidence for this diminished motivation, impaired ability to learn, and school and family problems in some adolescents who are chronic heavy marijuana smokers. If they stop smoking and remain in counseling, the condition improves.[40] This probably implies a constant state of intoxication rather than some long-lasting change in brain function or personality.

The connection between marijuana use and insanity was one of the main arguments for outlawing the drug in the 1930s, and the notion still remains that marijuana can cause a type of psychosis. There have been reports of psychotic "breakdowns" occurring with rare frequency after marijuana has been smoked, but the causal relationship is in question. The psychotic episodes are generally self-limiting and seem to occur in individuals with a history of psychiatric problems.[41] Smoking a single "joint" will not cause an otherwise healthy person to "go crazy," but perhaps someone who is on the edge of a breakdown could be pushed over the edge by a panic reaction after smoking marijuana.

For about 20 years it has been speculated that amotivational or prolonged psychotic reactions could reflect an underlying damage to brain tissue produced by marijuana. For example, a 1972 report from England indicated that two individuals who demonstrated cerebral atrophy had a history of smoking marijuana. They also, of course, had a history of many other things, but it was suggested that the brain damage may have been caused by the marijuana. Several experiments have since been done, and all fail to find a relationship between marijuana smoking and cerebral atrophy.[45] There have been other incomplete or poorly controlled reports of potential brain damage from animal research, and it has been possible to dismiss most of them as inconclusive. However, two experiments on rats, one appearing in 1987 and the other in 1988, give stronger evidence that THC causes permanent changes in the structure of neurons in the hippocampus. One of the reports related these changes to a persistent deficit in the rats' performance on a radial arm maze. The doses used were in the range of what a very heavy marijuana smoker might obtain, and the treatment was given to the rats everyday for 90 days. Although it is not clear what the implications might be for human beings smoking less heavily and only occasionally, these are clear effects that should lead to cautious concern.

One thing should be said about research on the adverse consequences of marijuana. There is probably no area of science in which emotion has played such an obvious and influential role. Scientists on both sides have become "crusaders" for their cause. Some individuals seem to think it is their professional duty to seek out and publicize every potential evil associated with marijuana, even if the scientific evidence is not as strong as it should be. Others seem to automatically question the negative reports and look for ways to discredit them. We can predict that the emotion, the premature announcement of new scary findings, the repeating of long-discredited stories, and the conflicting reports will continue.

MARIJUANA AND AMERICAN SOCIETY

Remember that our patterns of drug use are but one facet of our evolving society. Our drug use affects and is affected by other social trends in our life. You should at least make note of a couple of important themes for the 1980s, and we'll see how they relate to marijuana use. One trend is the increased emphasis on physical health. Jogging, working out, dieting, drinking less alcohol and caffeine, and smoking less are all reflections of our national concern over shaping up. The health trend obviously works against marijuana use: how many people who won't smoke tobacco will feel good about inhaling marijuana smoke? Second, the 1980s saw a move toward social and political conservatism that would also tend to work against such counterculture behavior as marijuana smoking. And of course, we remember that drug use tends to be faddish. If marijuana was the fashionable drug of the 1970s, then it can't be the fashionable drug of the 1980s. Cocaine apparently had that role.

Data from the yearly survey of high school seniors bears out our idea that marijuana use is down. After peaking in 1978-79, the number of high school seniors who have ever smoked marijuana dropped from just over 60% to under 50% in 1988.[46] Even more dramatic was the drop in daily use, which went from 11% in 1978 to 3% in 1988, and seems to be on a downward course. This goes along with a steady increase in the belief among these students that "people risk harming themselves if they smoke marijuana regularly." Whereas just over one third of the high school seniors agreed with that statement in 1978, three-fourths agreed in 1988.

Although all signs point to decreased use of marijuana in the near future, it is still remarkable how many people have used and continue to use a substance that shouldn't exist at all in our society, according to the Controlled Substances Act and the DEA. That a large fraction of the society continues to violate the laws regarding marijuana is a matter for concern. It is easy to look back and

wish that the 1937 Marijuana Tax Act had never happened. Marijuana use was spreading slowly across the United States and with any luck it might have become acculturated. Society would have adapted to marijuana and adapted marijuana to society. Soon it would have become part of society: perhaps most people would never have used it regularly; of those who did use it most would have known how to use it; some, of course, would have abused it. It has happened before with coffee, tea, tobacco, and alcohol.

The 1937 law prevented all that. It didn't affect most of us a great deal until the 1960s, when a large number of young people began experimenting with drugs. Marijuana, more than anything else, convinced many young people that the government had been lying to them about drugs. They had been told that marijuana would make them insane, enslave them in drug addiction, and lead to violence and perverted sexual acts. Their experience told them that marijuana was pretty innocuous compared to those stories, and it became an important symbol: smoking marijuana struck a blow for truth and freedom. The problem was that laws existed that allowed young people to be sent to jail for 20 years for striking this blow and that didn't sit well with some people. Voice was given to the millions of marijuana users in 1970 when a young Washington lawyer estab-

---

Your turn: use of and attitudes toward marijuana

Marijuana is not a topic that is discussed as much as it was a few years ago. Unless you belong to a group of people that regularly smokes marijuana, you may not know how your friends feel about the topic. Get together with a small group of your friends and discuss how many have ever smoked marijuana, how they feel about people using marijuana, and how prevalent they think marijuana smoking is among people of their age and status. You might, as a group, come up with a short questionnaire to administer to a larger group to see if your estimates are correct.

lished the National Organization for the Reform of Marijuana Laws (NORML) with a grant from the Playboy Foundation. As the founder of NORML put it: "The only people working for reform then were freaks who wanted to turn on the world, an approach that was obviously doomed to failure. I wanted an effective, middle-class approach, not pro-grass but antijail. . . ."[47]

Also, in 1970 the Comprehensive Drug Abuse Prevention and Control Act of 1970 established a Commission on Marijuana and Drug Abuse. Its 1972 report recommended some legislative changes:

> The Commission recommended that federal and state laws be changed so that private possession of small amounts of marihuana for personal use, and casual distribution of small amounts without monetary profit, would no longer be offenses, though marihuana possessed in public would remain contraband. Cultivation, distribution for profit, and possession with intent to sell would remain felonies. Criminal penalties would be retained for disorderly conduct associated with marihuana intoxication and driving under the influence of marihuana, and a plea of marihuana intoxication would not be a defense to any criminal act committed under its influence.[48]

The year 1972 was a turning point in the fight to decriminalize marijuana. In June the American Medical Association came out in favor of dropping penalties for possession of "insignificant amounts" of marijuana and noted that "there is no evidence supporting the idea that marijuana leads to violence, aggressive behavior, or crime."[49] In August the American Bar Association called for the reduction of criminal penalties for possession, and a year later the organization recommended decriminalization. Both traditional liberals and conservatives could support the idea, not to declare marijuana legal, but to make possession of marijuana a civil offense, punishable only by a fine. A week before Christmas in 1972 the best known and most literate of American conservatives, William F. Buckley, proclaimed in favor of the decriminalization of marijuana saying:

> It isn't silly to say that the user should not be molested, even though the pusher should be put in jail. It was so, mostly, under prohibition, when the speakeasy operators were prosecuted, not so the patrons. Thus it is, by and large, in the case of prostitution; and even with gambling; and most explicitly with pornography, the Supreme Court having ruled that you can't molest the owner, even though you can go after the peddler.[50]

In October, 1973, Oregon abolished criminal penalties for marijuana use, substituting civil fines of up to $100. Marijuana offenders are given citations that are processed like traffic tickets. Did marijuana use increase in Oregon as a result of the decriminalization? Yes. By leaps and bounds? No. From the fall of 1974, a year after decriminalization, to the fall of 1977, the percentage of adults over 18 who had "ever used" marijuana went from 19% to 25%. "Current users" went from 9% to 10% over the same period. Please remember that marijuana use was increasing toward its 1978-79 peak all over the country at the same time.

Nine other states made possession of a small amount of marijuana only a civil offense: Alaska, Maine, Colorado, California, Ohio, Minnesota, Mississippi, New York, and North Carolina. One consequence of changing marijuana possession from a felony to a misdemeanor is that it saves money on court costs, juries, and jails. It has been estimated that the state of California enjoyed an average annual savings of over $95 million between 1976 and 1985 as a result of its citation plan for marijuana possession.[51]

At the federal level, action picked up in 1977. In January, "Rosalynn Carter joined her husband, the President, in calling for the decriminalization of marijuana . . ." and revealed that their oldest son had been discharged from the navy for smoking marijuana. Bills to decriminalize marijuana possession were introduced into both houses of Congress, and in August President Carter sent a message to Congress in which he asked them to abolish all federal criminal penalties for the possession of small amounts of marijuana.

President Carter's adviser on drug issues told a

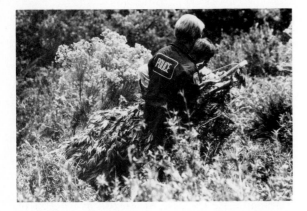

Marijuana crops are being confiscated in the United States, as well as in Mexico and other countries.

congressional committee that the administration "will continue to discourage marijuana use, but we feel criminal penalties that brand otherwise law-abiding people for life are neither effective nor an appropriate deterrent."[52]

If the truth were known, in the late 1970s defacto decriminalization had already occurred in many areas of the country. Law enforcement agencies in many of the larger cities of the United States had stopped arresting marijuana users and did not search out those with small amounts for personal use.

When the Reagan administration came into office in 1980, any hope of federal decriminalization was gone, replaced by a "get tough" (and spend money) attitude toward all illegal drugs. Marijuana is no exception. In addition to increased efforts to intercept marijuana shipments coming from abroad, a nationwide effort was launched in 1985 to combat cultivation of marijuana plants. Over 100 million plants were tugged out of the ground in 1987 by joint state, local, and federal law-enforcement teams.[53] Add to that the "zero-tolerance" seizures of boats, cars, and planes containing even traces of marijuana and the 1988 legislation putting extra pressure on the user (e.g., 10,000 dollar fines at the federal level; Chapter 3), and we can see that the pendulum has definitely swung back.

Issue: should marijuana be decriminalized?

In a 1983 issue of *National Review*, two conservative authors presented their arguments, pro and con, on the issue of decriminalization. Richard Vigilante sought to prove that marijuana is more dangerous than was assumed by Richard Cowan in his 1972 article favoring decriminalization. Reviewing evidence obtained since 1982, he concluded that marijuana is addictive, that it helps users to begin a life of drug abuse that may include heroin or other drugs, that it can cause health problems for its users, that it impairs driving ability, and that it produces an amotivational syndrome.

In reply, Mr. Cowan asserted that he never thought that marijuana was harmless, only that the laws against marijuana were more harmful than marijuana itself. He quibbles with Mr. Vigilante's definition of the term addiction, says that just because heroin users once used pot doesn't mean the use of marijuana led to heroin use. Since heroin users have virtually all used alcohol, too, the type of association is the same. Mr. Cowan minimizes the potential health threats and then decries the government interference with medical research. The result of our laws, he says, is to make marijuana more available to a 16-year-old student who should not have it than to a 60-year-old glaucoma or cancer patient who might benefit from it.

Summary

As with other psychoactive plants, *Cannabis* has a rich history relating both to its medicinal use and to its recreational uses. It became famous as the "Assassin of Youth" in the 1930s and was outlawed in 1937.

Cannabis contains many active chemicals, but the most active is Δ-9 THC. This substance is absorbed rapidly and well by smoking, but slowly and incompletely when taken by mouth. It has a long half life of elimination, and its metabolites may be found for up to a month. Its mechanism of action is not known but selective THC receptors have been found in rat brains.

Marijuana causes an increase in the heart rate and reddening of the eyes as its main physiological effects. Psychologically, it has some properties of sedatives, produces some analgesia, and at high doses may produce hallucinations. In recreational use, some of its most important behavioral effects probably relate to its impairment of memory.

Marijuana has been tested in the treatment of glaucoma and for reducing nausea in patients undergoing cancer chemotherapy, and a legal form of THC is available by prescription.

Tolerance can occur to many of marijuana's effects, and withdrawal symptoms have been demonstrated under laboratory conditions. Although strong behavioral dependence is not common, it does occur in some individuals.

Although many concerns have been raised about the potential toxicity of marijuana, it is clear that over the short run it is much less toxic than alcohol. Marijuana can impair driving, and there is evidence that smoking marijuana leads to an increased frequency of accidents. Most experts agree that chronic smoking of marijuana impairs lung function somewhat and probably increases the risk of lung cancer. Other possible deleterious effects of long-term exposure are less clear. Certainly marijuana use should be avoided during pregnancy, and there is concern about the limited psychosocial development of adolescents who engage in daily, heavy use of marijuana. Long-standing concerns about marijuana-induced brain damage have received support from recent animal studies.

Although possession and use of a small amount of marijuana is not treated as the same type of offense as it was in the 1960s, for most users there is no legal supply for marijuana. The latest federal enforcement push is to combat the cultivation of marijuana within the United States, and to punish users with fines and forefeitures.

REFERENCES

1. Schultes RE and Hofmann A: The botany and chemistry of hallucinogens, Springfield, Ill, 1980, Charles C Thomas.
2. Mijuriya TH and Aldrich MR: Cannabis 1988: old drug, new dangers—the potency question, Journal of Psychoactive Drugs 20:47-55, 1988.
3. Snyder SH: What we have forgotten about pot, New York Times Magazine, pp. 27, 121, 124, 130, December 13, 1970.
4. Mickel EJ: The artificial paradises in French literature, Chapel Hill, NC, 1969, University of North Carolina Press.
5. Baudelaire CP: Artificial paradises; on hashish and wine as means of expanding individuality, translated by Ellen Fox, New York, 1971, Herder & Herder.
6. Unpublished material in the Archives of the American Psychological Association, Department of Psychology, University of Akron, Akron, Ohio.
7. Taxation of marihuana, hearings before the Committee on Ways and Means, House of Representatives, Seventy-fifth Congress, First Session, on HR 6385, April 27-30 and May 4, 1937, Washington, DC, US Government Printing Office.
8. Parry A: The menace of marihuana, American Mercury 36:487-488, 1935.
9. Marihuana menaces youth, Scientific American 154:151, 1936.
10. Wolf W: Uncle Sam fights a new drug menace . . . marijuana, Popular Science Monthly 128:14-119, 1936.
11. Anslinger HJ and Cooper CR: Marijuana: assassin of youth, American Magazine 124:19, 153, 1937.
12. Facts and fancies about marihuana, Literary Digest 122:7-8, 1936.
13. Whitlock L: Review: marijuana, Crime and Delinquency Literature 2(3):367, 1970.
14. Fort J: Pot: a rational approach, Playboy, pp 131, 154, October 1969.
15. The marihuana bugaboo, Military Surgeon 93:95, 1943.
16. Mayor LaGuardia's Committee on Marijuana. In Solomon D, editor: the marihuana papers, New York, 1966, The New American Library.
17. Marijuana problems, Journal of American Medical Association 127:1129, 1945.
18. Kaufman J, Allen JR, and West LJ: Runaways, hippies, and marihuana, American Journal of Psychiatry 126:717-720, 1969.
19. Marihuana and health, Department of Health, Education, and Welfare, Washington DC, 1971, US Government Printing Office.
20. Hamon M: Common neurochemical correlates to the action of hallucinogens. In Jacobs BL, editor: Hallucinogens: neurochemical, behavioral, and clinical perspectives, New York, 1984, Raven Press.
21. Prostaglandins and cannabis. XIV. Tolerance to the stimulatory actions of cannabinoids on arachidonate metabolism, Journal of Pharmacology and Experimental Therapeutics 235:87, 1985.
22. Herkenham M and others: Localization of cannabinoid receptors in brain, Society for Neuroscience Abstracts 14:104, 1988.
23. Marijuana and health, Institute of Medicine, National Academy of Sciences, Washington, DC, 1982, National Academy Press.
24. Tart CT: Marijuana intoxication: common experiences, Nature 226:701-704, 1970.

25. Jones RT: Tetrahydrocannabinol and the marijuana-induced social "high," or the effects of the mind on marijuana. In Singer AJ, editor: Marijuana: chemistry, pharmacology, and patterns of social use, Annals of the New York Academy of Sciences 191:155-165, 1971.

26. Rafaelsen OJ: Cannabis and alcohol: effects on simulated car driving, Science 179:920-923, 1973.

27. O'Shaughnessy WB: On the preparations of the Indian hemp, or gunja, Trans Med m Phys Soc, Bengal, pp. 71-102, 1838-1840; pp 421-461, 1842.

28. Mikuriya TH: Marijuana in medicine: past, present and future, California Medicine 110:34-40, 1969.

29. Standardization of drug extracts, promotional brochure, Detroit, 1898, Parke, Davis & Co.

30. Letter to EP Delabarre, 9 Arlington Ave, Providence, RI, from Parke, Davis & Co, Manufacturing Department, Main Laboratories, Detroit, Superintendent's Office, Control Department, March 10, 1902.

31. Taxation of marijuana, House of Representatives, Committee on Ways and Means, Washington, DC, 1937.

32. Davis JP and Ramsey HH: Antiepileptic action of marihuana-active substances, Federation Proceedings 8:284-285, 1949.

33. Lieberman DM and Lieberman BW: Marihuana—a medical review, New England Journal of Medicine 284:88-91, 1971.

34. Marijuana smoking said to have power to deter glaucoma, New York Times, July 28, 1972.

35. Medical therapy, legalization issues debated at Marijuana Reform Conference, National Drug Reporter 7(1):3-5, 1977.

36. Nahas GG: The medical use of cannabis. In Nahas, GG, editor: Marijuana in science and medicine, New York, 1984, Raven Press.

37. Rhein R: Here comes prescription pot, Business Week, June 24, 1985, p. 104.

38. Conlan MF: Top drug cop weighs use of marijuana as an Rx drug, Drug Topics, December 12, 1988.

39. Jones RT and Benowitz N: The 30-day trip—clinical studies of cannabis tolerance and dependence. In Braude MC and Szara S, editors: Pharmacology of marijuana, New York, 1976, Raven Press.

40. Smith DE and Seymour RB: Clinical perspectives on the toxicology of marijuana: 1967-1981. In Marijuana and youth: clinical observations on motivation and learning, Washington, DC, 1982, US Department of Health and Human Services, US Government Printing Office.

41. Petersen RC: Marijuana overview. In Glantz MD, editor: Correlates and consequences of marijuana use, NIDA Research Issues, No 34, Washington, DC, 1984, US Department of Health and Human Services, US Government Printing Office.

42. Tashkin DP, Calvarese BM, Simmons MS, and others: Respiratory status of seventy-four habitual marijuana smokers, Chest 78:699-706, 1980.

43. Nahas GG: Toxicology and pharmacology. In Nahas GG, editor: Marijuana in science and medicine, New York, 1984, Raven Press.

44. Tennes K and others: Marijuana: prenatal and postnatal exposure in the human. In Pinkert TM, editor: Consequences of maternal drug abuse, NIDA Research Monograph No 59, Washington, DC, 1985, US Government Printing Office.

45. Hollister LE: Health aspects of cannabis, Pharmacological Reviews, 38:1-20, 1986.

46. Johnston LD and others: University of Michigan press release on 1988 National High School Senior Survey, February 28, 1989.

47. Anderson P: The pot lobby, New York Times Magazine, pp 8-9, January 21, 1973.

48. Farnsworth DL: Summary of the Report of the National Commission on Marihuana and Drug Abuse, Tracks, No 9, pp 1-2, 1972.

49. The AMA and pot, Stash Capsules 4(4), August 1972.

50. Buckley WF, Jr: Pot, legalization of, conservative division, New York Times, December 18, 1972.

51. Aldrich MR and Mikuriya T: Savings in California marijuana law enforcement costs attributable to the Moscone Act of 1976—a summary, Journal of Psychoactive Drugs 20:75-81, 1988.

52. Carter seeks end of marijuana curb; cocaine examined, New York Times, March 15, 1977, p. 30.

53. 1987 Domestic cannabis eradication/suppression program final report, Drug Enforcement Administration, US Department of Justice, 1987.

Chapter 17

Drug Education and Prevention

OBJECTIVES

After reading this chapter, you should be able to:

Distinguish between the goals of drug education and drug abuse prevention.

Describe several approaches to drug abuse prevention that have been used in public school settings and how effective each approach has been.

Explain how approaches involving peers, families, and other community agencies can be used to strengthen school-based approaches.

Explain why smoking prevention has been studied more than prevention of other drug use and what some of the latest approaches are.

Discuss a rational approach to prevention programs in your own community.

Why can't we *do* something to keep young people from ruining their lives with drugs? As our society seeks to prevent drug abuse by limiting the availability of such drugs as heroin and cocaine, we are forced to recognize several other facts. First, as long as there is a sizable market for these substances there will be people to supply them. Thus, only if we can teach people not to want the drugs can we attack the source of the problem. Second, these substances will never disappear entirely, so we should try to teach people to live in a world that includes them. Third, our society has accepted the continued existence of tobacco and alcohol, yet some people are harmed by them. Can we teach people to coexist with both legal and illegal substances and to live in such a way that their lives and health are not impaired by them?

DEFINING GOALS AND EVALUATING OUTCOMES

Think about the process you are engaged in while reading and studying from this book. It is aimed at teaching its readers about drugs: their effects, how they are used, and how they relate to society. The goal of the authors is **education.** A person who understands all this information about all these drugs will perhaps be better prepared to make decisions about personal drug use, more able to understand drug use by others, and better prepared to participate in social decisions about drug use and abuse. We would hope that a person who knew all this would be in a position to act more rationally regarding drugs, neither glorifying one and expecting miraculous changes from using it nor condemning it as the essence of evil. For example, the chapter on alcohol, while pointing out the dangers of its use and the problems it can cause, did not attempt to influence the readers to avoid all alcohol use. In a purely educational program, the primary goal is not to alter a person's drug-taking behavior. Our success would be measured by how much a person knew about alcohol or tobacco or marijuana, not by whether a reader of this book is convinced never to drink or smoke.

On the other hand, there exists an old tradition, going back to the "demon rum" programs of the late 1800s, of presenting negative information about alcohol or drugs in the public schools, with the clear goal of influencing behavior. Some of these early programs presented information that was so clearly one sided that they could have been classified as propaganda, rather than education. We would not measure the success of such a program by how much objective information the students gained about the pharmacology of the narcotics, for example. A more appropriate index might be how many of the students did subsequently experiment with the drugs against which the program was aimed. Until the early 1970s, it was simply assumed that these programs would have the desired effect and few attempts were made to evaluate them.

STAGES OF PREVENTION

The goals and methods of a prevention program also depend on the drug-using status of those served by the program. The programs designed to prevent young people from smoking may be different from those used to prevent relapse in smokers who have quit, for example. Borrowing an idea developed in the mental health field, drug-abuse

prevention theorists have discussed three levels or stages of prevention: **Primary** prevention begins before drug use has occurred and includes the education and information programs we usually think of when we discuss prevention. In one of the most widely cited schemes, **secondary** and **tertiary** prevention is described as occurring during early and later stages of drug abuse. These levels of prevention employ approaches such as crisis intervention, referral for treatment, and institutionalization that could be viewed as representing treatment as much as prevention programs. For that reason we have elected to present a similar scheme, but with different definitions for the stages (Table 17-1).

Primary prevention programs are those aimed mainly at young people who have not yet tried the substances in question, or who may have tried tobacco or alcohol a few times. As discussed in the previous section, such programs may encourage complete abstinence from specific drugs or may have the broader goal of teaching people how to view drugs and the potential influences of drugs on their lives, emotions, and social relationships. Because those programs are presented to people with little personal experience with drugs, it might be expected that they would be especially effective. On the other hand, there is the danger of introducing large numbers of children to information about a number of drugs that they might otherwise never have heard of, thus arousing their curiosity about them.

Secondary prevention programs could be thought of as designed for people who have tried the drug in question or a variety of other substances. The goals of such programs are usually the prevention of the use of other, more dangerous substances or preventing the development of more dangerous forms of use of the substances they are already experimenting with. We might describe the clientele here as more "sophisticated" substance users who have not suffered seriously from their drug experiences and who are not obvious candidates for treatment. Most college students would fall into this category, and programs aimed at encouraging responsible use of alcohol among

Table 17-1		
Stages of prevention		
Stage	Clientele	Example
Primary	Young, little or no experience with psychoactive substances	School-based smoking prevention programs
Secondary	Experienced with some psychoactive substances, not in need of treatment	College-based programs in responsible alcohol use
Tertiary	Post-treatment	Relapse prevention

college students are a good example of this stage of prevention.

For alcoholics or cocaine or heroin addicts, treatment programs are the first order of priority. However, once a person has been treated or has stopped the substance use without assistance, we enter another stage of prevention. *Tertiary* prevention is used in our scheme to characterize relapse prevention, or follow-up programs. Since they occur following treatment, these programs are discussed in Chapter 18.

PREVENTION PROGRAMS IN THE SCHOOLS

The Knowledge-Attitudes-Behavior Model

After the increase in the use of illicit drugs by young people in the 1960s, there was a general sense that we were not doing an adequate job of drug education, and most school systems increased their efforts. However, there was a great deal of confusion over the methods to be used. Traditional antidrug programs had relied heavily on representatives of the local police who came in and told a few horror stories, described the legal trouble due anyone who became involved with drugs, and sometimes showed what the drugs looked like or demonstrated the smell of burning marijuana, so that the kids would know what to avoid. Sometimes, especially in larger cities, a former addict would come in and describe how easy it was to get "hooked," the horrible life of the junkie, and the horror of withdrawal symptoms. The 1960s saw more of that, plus the production of a large number of scary antidrug films. There was also the awareness that teachers and counselors knew little about these substances, and many of them attended courses taught by experts in the field. Some of the experts were enforcement-oriented and presented the traditional scare-tactics information, while others were pharmacologists who presented the "dry facts" about the classification and effects of various drugs. Much of this factual information also found its way into the classrooms of the 1960s. It was later pointed out that the programs of this era were based on an assumed model: providing information about drugs would increase the students' **knowledge** of drugs and their effects, this increased knowledge would lead to changes in **attitudes** about drug use, and these changed attitudes would be reflected in decreased drug-using **behavior.**[1]

In the early 1970s this model began to be questioned. A 1971 study indicated that those students with more knowledge about drugs tended to have a more positive attitude toward drug use.[2] Of course, it may have been that prodrug students were more interested in learning about drugs, so this was not an actual assessment of the value of drug education programs. A 1973 report by the same group indicated that four different types of drug education programs were equally effective in producing increased knowledge about drugs and equally ineffective in altering attitudes or behavior.[3] Nationwide, drug use had increased even with the increased emphasis on drug education. There began to be concern about the possibility that drug education may even have contributed to increased drug use. After all, before the 1960s use of marijuana or LSD was rare among school-aged youngsters. Most of them didn't know much about these things, had given them little thought, and had probably never considered using them.

Telling them over and over not to use drugs was a bit like telling a young boy not to put beans in his nose.[4] He probably hadn't thought of it before, and your warning gives him the idea. At least one study in 1972 found that junior high school students who were exposed to a "fact-oriented" course actually increased their experimentation with drugs.[5] These concerns led the federal government in 1973 to stop supporting the production of drug abuse films and educational materials until they could determine what kinds of approaches would be effective.

At this point it was clear that the question of effectiveness depended greatly on the goals of the program. Do we want all students *never to experiment with* cigarettes, alcohol, marijuana, or other drugs? Or do we want students to be prepared to *make rational decisions about drugs?* For example, a 1976 report indicated that students in drug education programs did increase their use of drugs over the 2 years following the program, but were less likely to show drastic escalation of the amount or type of drug use over that period, when compared with a control group.[6] Perhaps by giving the students information about drugs we make them more likely to try them, but we also make them more aware of the dangers of excessive use.

Affective Education

Values clarification.   The next stage of drug education made the assumption that what was lacking in drug-using adolescents was not factual information about drugs, but rather the ability to make appropriate decisions based on that information.[7] Educators had been talking about education as including both a "cognitive domain" and an "affective domain." It was proposed that drug use should not be "flagged" for the students by having special curricula designed just for drugs, but that instead emphasis be placed on teaching generic decision-making skills. Teaching students to analyze and clarify their own values in life, teaching them self-esteem and interpersonal skills, and teaching them how to attain their social and personal goals without drugs or alcohol would

---

> **Examples of values clarification strategies**
>
> **Problem solving**
>
>   Kindergarten and first grade: Children are read a short story, "Amy and the Surprise." The children then discuss Amy's choices, learning that for every problem situation there may be many possible solutions.
>
>   Senior high: Students perform a play titled "Alien Invasion." The students then respond to the proposal that aliens have consumed all drugs on the planet, OTC, prescription, and illegal. We have a chance to start over. Which drugs should we keep?
>
> **Coping skills**
>
>   Kindergarten and first grade: The puppet "Froggy" helps students explore the concept that there are certain feelings associated with stressful situations. They learn where these feelings come from and how to express them.
>
>   Senior high: Students listen to songs about friendship, then discuss the qualities they consider important in a friend.
>
> **Self-concept**
>
>   Kindergarten and first grade: A puzzle, "One of the Bunch," is used to explore the experience of being included and accepted by a group.
>
>   Senior high: Students spin a "feel wheel" and disclose how they feel about the situation described on the wheel. A small group discussion focuses on different reactions to the same situation and how feelings can influence behavior.

A few examples from "Here's Looking At You, Two" Comprehensive Health Education Foundation, Seattle, Washington, supported by NIAAA and NIDA.

make them better able to make decisions that would minimize the negative consequences of drug use. It should be pointed out that groups of parents or other citizens who are concerned about drug abuse have great difficulty understanding and accepting these approaches, because they do not take a direct antidrug approach and the purpose of **values clarification** training is not immediately clear. Examples of values clarification strategies are in the box above.

Alternatives to drugs.   Along with values clarification, another aspect of affective education

Table 17-2		
Examples of some suggested alternatives to drug use		
Level of experience	Motives	Possible alternatives
Physical	Relaxation	Relaxation exercises
	Increased energy	Athletics, dancing
Sensory	Stimulation	Sky-diving
	Magnify senses	Sensory awareness training
Interpersonal	Gain acceptance	Instruction in social customs
Spiritual/ mystical	Develop spiritual insight	Study of religions

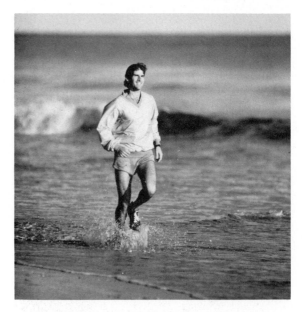

A nondrug high: the adrenaline is flowing, and a sense of well-being is likely to follow.

involved the teaching of **alternatives** to drug use (Table 17-2). Under the assumption that students might take drugs for the experience, for the altered states of consciousness that a drug might produce, students are taught so-called natural highs, or altered states, that can be produced through relaxation exercises, meditation, vigorous exercise, or an exciting sport. Students are encouraged to try these things and to focus on the psychological changes that occur. These alternatives should be discussed with some degree of sensitivity to the audience; for example, it would make little sense to suggest to many inner-city 13-year-olds that such activities as scuba diving or snow skiing would be good alternatives to drugs.

Personal and social skills.   Several studies have indicated that adolescents who smoke, drink, or use marijuana also get lower grades and are less involved in organized sports or school clubs. One view of this is that students may take up substance use in response to personal or social failure. Therefore teaching students how to communicate with others and giving them success experiences has been another component of affective education approaches. For example, one exercise that has been used is having the students operate a school store. This is done as a group effort with frequent meetings of the group. The involved students are expected to develop a sense of social and personal competence without using drugs. Another approach has been to have older students tutor younger students, which is again designed to give the older students a sense of competence. An experiment carried out between 1978 and 1983 in Napa, California combined these approaches with a drug education course, small group discussions led by teachers, and classroom management techniques designed to teach discipline, communication skills, and to enhance the students' self-concepts.[8] Although a small effect on alcohol, marijuana, and cigarette use was found among the girls, the effects were gone by the 1-year follow-up.

"Just Say NO!"

A 1984 review[9] of prevention studies concluded that "(1) most substance abuse prevention programs have not contained adequate evaluation

---

Your turn: alternatives to drugs

As one part of many drug education programs, students are taught that they can produce natural highs, that is, altered states of consciousness similar to those produced by drugs, but without using drugs.

One such alternative that is often mentioned in these programs is skydiving. Obviously an activity of that sort has all the glamour, danger, and excitement most of us would want. Maybe if the kids could do this whenever they wanted, they wouldn't want to try cocaine or marijuana.

But let's examine this as an alternative for a bunch of junior high school kids. First, there's the matter of cost and availability. How realistic is it to think that most of these kids would have any access at all to skydiving? Second, there's the issue of convenience. Even if you were a little rich kid with your own airplane, parachute, and pilot, it's unlikely that you'd be able to go skydiving every afternoon after school. Drugs or alcohol may not provide the best highs in the world, but often they are easy to get and use compared to some of these other activities.

OK, so maybe skydiving isn't a *practical* alternative to drugs for a lot of people. Still, it seems more wholesome and desirable. Let's become social philosophers and ask ourselves why the image of a person skydiving is more positive than the image of a person snorting cocaine. After all, skydiving doesn't make any obvious contributions to society. Let one of your authors play devil's advocate and propose that skydiving is not preferable to taking cocaine. Either way, the person is engaged in dangerous, expensive, self-indulgent activity. Contrast skydiving with cocaine, and see if you can answer for yourself why skydiving has a more positive image than cocaine use. You may have to talk about this with several people before you get a consistent feeling for why our society respects one of these activities so much more than the other. Skiing? Rock-climbing, anyone?

ious interpersonal pressures to begin using drugs; and (4) few studies have demonstrated any degree of success in terms of actual substance abuse prevention." This last point is not entirely a criticism of the programs themselves, but reflects the difficulty of demonstrating statistically significant changes in behavior over some period of time following the programs.

In response to the third point, that affective education approaches have been too general and experiential, the latest efforts at preventing drug use focus on teaching students to recognize peer pressure to use drugs and also teaching specific ways to respond to such pressures without using drugs. This is sometimes referred to as "psychological inoculation." In addition to the focus on substance use, "refusal skills" and "pressure resistance" strategies are taught in a broader context of self-assertion and social skills training. As an example, in the first successful application of this technique a film was made with young actors acting out situations in which one person was being pressured to smoke cigarettes. The film then demonstrated effective ways of responding to the pressure gracefully without smoking. After the film, students discuss alternative strategies and practice the coping techniques. This approach has been demonstrated to be successful in reducing cigarette smoking in adolescent populations. The approach has been adapted for use with groups of various ages and for a wider variety of drugs and other behaviors, and students are taught from kindergarten on to "Just Say No" when someone is trying to get them to do something they know is wrong.

Drug-Free Schools

In 1986, under the direction of Secretary of Education William J. Bennett (later to become the Unites States' first modern drug "czar," Chapter 3), the federal government launched a massive program to support "drug-free schools and communities." Among other things, the government provided millions of dollars worth of direct aid to local school districts to implement or enhance

components; (2) increased knowledge has virtually no impact on substance abuse or on intentions to smoke, drink, or use drugs; (3) affective education approaches appear to be experiential in their orientation and to place too little emphasis on the acquisition of skills necessary to increase personal and social competence, particularly those skills needed to enable students to resist the var-

drug prevention activities. Along with this, Mr. Bennett produced a small book called "What Works: Schools Without Drugs,"[10] which made specific recommendations for schools to follow. This book did not recommend a specific curriculum, and in fact its most significant feature was the emphasis on factors other than curriculum, such as school policies on drug and alcohol use. There are suggestions for policies regarding locker searches, suspension, and expulsion of students. The purpose is not so much to take a punitive approach to alcohol or drug use as to point out through example and through official policy that the school and community are opposed to drug use and to alcohol use by minors. Following this general lead, for example, many schools have adopted "tobacco-free" policies stating that not only the students, but also teachers and other staff people are not to use tobacco products at school or on school-sponsored trips or activities.

In addition to setting policy, according to this approach the curriculum should include teaching about the laws against drugs as well as about the school policies. In other words, as opposed to the 1970s values clarification approach of teaching students how to make responsible decisions for themselves, this approach wants to make it clear to the students that the society at large, the community in which they live, and the school in which they study have already made the decision not to condone drug use or underage alcohol use. This seems to be part of a more general educational trend away from "value-free" schools toward the teaching of values that are generally accepted in our society.

PEERS, PARENTS, AND THE COMMUNITY

Our nation's public schools clearly represent the most convenient conduit for attempts to achieve widespread social changes among young people and that is why most efforts at drug abuse prevention have been carried out there. However, there has also been a recognition that peers, parents, and the community at large also exert powerful social influences on young people. Because these groups are less accessible than the schools there have been fewer prevention programs based on using their influences. Nevertheless, important efforts have been made in all these areas.

Peer Programs

Most such programs have taken place in the school setting, but some have used youth-oriented community service programs (such as YMCA, YWCA, recreation centers) or have focused on "street" youth by employing them in group community service projects. The content of peer programs runs the gamut from specific drug information to generic, affective training involving social skills and so on.[11]

Positive **peer influence** approaches start with the assumption that the opinions of an adolescent's peers represent significant influences on the adolescent's behavior. Often employing an adult group facilitator/coordinator, the emphasis is on open discussion among a group of children or adolescents. These discussions may focus on drugs, with the peer group discussing dangers and alternatives or may simply have the more general goal of building positive group cohesiveness, a sense of belonging, and communication skills.

Peer tutors have been employed in many of the school-based programs. Usually, an older student teaches younger students, either about drugs and other health information or about more general academic subjects. The biggest impact seems to be on the tutor rather than on the younger students.

Peer counselors receive training from adults in listening, how to avoid making judgments, maintaining confidentiality, and how to be supportive of others. Then they make themselves available to their peers to discuss their problems. There must be adult supervision and discussion sessions with the peer counselors, who also are taught to refer serious problems to a professional. For these counselors to be accepted by their peers they should not simply be selected from among

The head of the class.

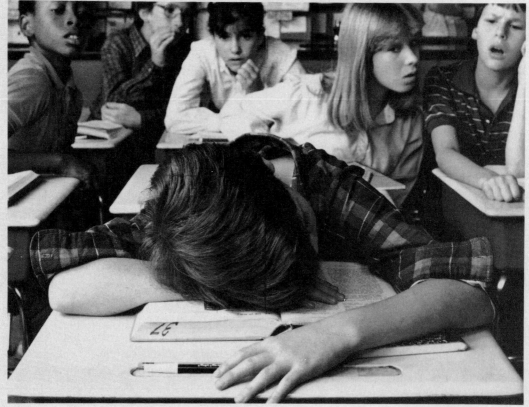

There are two kinds of heads.
The ones that wind up excelling in school.
And the ones that smoke pot and do drugs.
Which head you turn out to be is up to you.
You can resist an offer of drugs.
Just say no.
You'd be surprised how well it works.

Just say no.

 Send for a free booklet, *Peer Pressure: It's Okay To Say No.* Write: Say No To Drugs, P.O. Box 1635, Rockville, Maryland 20850.

A great deal of donated advertising has supported the nationwide "Just Say No" program devised by NIDA.

the brightest and most successful, but perhaps on the basis of surveys among the group. As with peer tutors, the counselors seem to derive more from these programs than the counseled.

Peer participation programs often focus on groups of youth in high-risk areas. The idea here is that young people participate in making important decisions and in doing significant work, either as "peers" with cooperating adults or in programs managed almost entirely by the youths themselves. Sometimes participants are paid for community service work, in other cases they engage in money-making businesses, and sometimes they provide youth-oriented information services. These groups almost never focus on drug use in any significant way; rather, the idea is to help people become participating members of society.

The benefits of all these peer approaches are measurable in terms of acquired skills, improved academic success, higher self-esteem, and a more positive attitude toward peers and school. As to whether they alter drug use significantly, the data either are not available or are inconclusive for the most part.

Parent Programs

The various programs that have worked with parents have been described as taking at least one of four approaches.[12] Most of the programs include more than one of these approaches.

Informational programs provide parents with basic information about alcohol and drugs. Although the parents often want to know simply what to look for, how to tell if their child is using drugs, and what the consequences of drug abuse are, the best programs provide additional information. One important piece of information is the actual extent of use of various types of drugs among young people. Another goal may be to

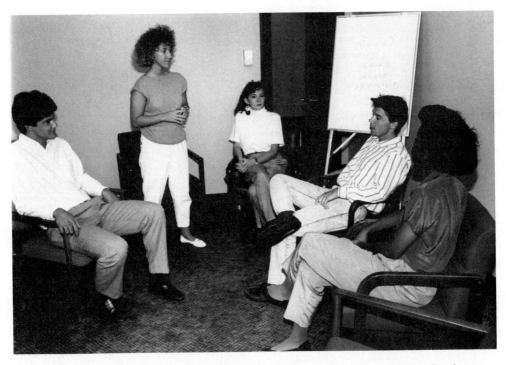

Education and prevention don't happen only in the classroom. Peer counseling has been widely adopted as a means for helping teens to cope with all their problems.

make parents aware of their own alcohol and drug use, to gain a broader perspective of the issue. A basic rationale is that well-informed parents will be able to teach appropriate attitudes about drugs from an early age, as well as being better able to recognize potential problems relating to drug or alcohol use.

Parenting skills may be taught through practical training programs. Communicating with children, decision-making skills, how to set goals and limits, and when and how to say "no" to your child may be learned in the abstract and then practiced in role-playing exercises. Since one risk factor for adolescent drug and alcohol use is poor family relationships, improving family interaction and strengthening communication may help to prevent alcohol and drug abuse.

Parent support groups can be important adjuncts to skills training or in planning community efforts. Groups of parents meet regularly to discuss problem solving, parenting skills, their perceptions of the problem, actions to be taken, and so on.

Family interaction approaches call for families to work as a unit to examine, discuss, and confront issues relating to alcohol and drug use. Other exercises may include more general problem solving or responding to emergencies. Not only do these programs attempt to improve family communication, the parents are placed in the roles of teacher of drug facts and coordinator of family action, thus strengthening their knowledge and skills.

One group that began in Florida and has become active nationwide is PRIDE (Parent Resources and Information on Drug Education). They sponsor speakers, provide information about the dangers of drugs, and provide an opportunity for communication among groups of concerned parents across the United States.

Community Programs

There are two basic reasons for trying to organize prevention programs at the community level. The first is that a coordinated approach employing schools, parent and peer groups, civic organizations, police, newspapers, radio, and television can have a much greater impact than an isolated program that occurs only in the school, for example. Another reason is that drug abuse prevention and drug education are controversial and emotional topics. Parents may question the need for or the methods used in drug education programs in the schools. Jealousies and mistrust about approaches may separate schools, police, church, and parent groups. A program that starts by involving all these groups in the planning stages is more likely to receive widespread community support.

Community-based programs can bring other resources to bear. For example, working with the city council and/or local businesses, alcohol-free parties can be held, recreational facilities developed, and field trips arranged so that when the school-based program talks about alternatives, the alternatives are real. The public media can be enlisted not only to publicize public meetings and programs, but to present drug and alcohol-related information that reinforces what is learned in the other programs. Specific problems, such as driving while intoxicated, can be addressed publicly and attacked from several directions, for example, publicity, education, police practices, parent awareness, vendor awareness.

A number of organized community programs have been attempted.[13] Probably none has ever met all its goals, and each community of necessity comes up with a different program. Under the circumstances, it is impossible to evaluate the general approach, but the assumption is that, if prevention programs are to be done, the broader the bases of support and involvement, the more effective they are likely to be.

SMOKING PREVENTION AS A MODEL

Some of the most sophisticated prevention research in recent years has focused directly on cigarette smoking in adolescents. This problem has two major advantages over other types of drug use as far as prevention research is concerned.

First, a large enough fraction of adolescents do smoke cigarettes so that measurable behavior change is possible in a group of subjects of reasonable size. In contrast, one would have to perform an intervention with tens of thousands of people before significant alterations in the proportion of heroin users would be statistically evident. Second, the health consequences of smoking are so clear with respect to cancer and heart disease that funding is available from federal sources in relatively greater amounts than might be the case for some other substances. Other minor benefits are encountered when doing smoking prevention: there is little or no controversy about the negative health consequences, so that educational programs can present a strong message without being accused of bias. This is much less true with respect to marijuana or alcohol, for example. Also, unlike the situation with alcohol, there is a fairly good consensus over goals: we'd like to prevent adolescents from becoming smokers at all. And there is a relatively simple verification available for self-reported use of tobacco, since saliva samples can be measured for cotinine, a nicotine metabolite.

Virtually all the various approaches to drug abuse prevention have been tried with smoking behavior; in fact, Evans' 1976 smoking prevention paper introduced the use of the psychological inoculation approach based on the **social influence model**.[14] Out of all this research, certain consistencies appear. The most important of these is that it does not seem possible to design and present smoking prevention programs that will be effective in reducing the number of adolescents who begin smoking. Some practical lessons about the components of those programs have also emerged.[15] For example, presenting information about the delayed consequences of smoking (possible lung cancer many years later) is deemed to be relatively ineffective. Information about the immediate physiological effects (increased heart rate, shortness of breath) is included instead. Most other informational aspects are minimized, but one piece of information has been found to be useful. Adolescents tend to overestimate the proportion of their peers who smoke, and presenting factual information about the smoking practices of adolescents reduces the "everybody is doing it" attitude. Films or videotapes demonstrating the kinds of social pressures that peers might use to encourage smoking and some examples of appropriate responses are supplemented with role-playing exercises. It has been found that having each student make a public commitment that he or she will not become a smoker is beneficial. Thus a combination of certain types of basic information along with social and personal skills training has been consistently found to reduce initiation to smoking.

Possible improvements to those approaches are offered by the **cognitive developmental** approach to smoking behavior. McCarthy[16] has criticized the social influence/social skills training model for assuming that all students should be taught social skills or refusal skills without regard to whether they need such training. The model "is that of a defenseless teenager who, for lack of general social skills or refusal skills, passively accedes to social pressures to smoke. . . ." Glynn, Leventhal, and Hirschman[17] have proposed an alternative model in which the individual makes active, conscious decisions about smoking as part of a process of defining himself or herself as a person experimenting with smoking, becoming a smoker, or as a confirmed smoker. The decision-making processes and thus the appropriate prevention strategy might be different at each of these "stages of cognitive development" as a smoker. Furthermore, smokers who begin smoking very young behave differently than smokers who begin as older adolescents (those who start young show more unanimity in selecting the most popular brand).[16] Given what is known about cognitive and social development, perhaps programs should be tailored for the age group being targeted and for various stages in the development of smoking behavior. This model would not replace the social influence methods, which have been shown to be effective, but would modify them to take into account individual differences in smoking-related attitudes and behavior.

Prevention in the Workplace

As a part of the federal government's efforts to reduce the demand for drugs, the Reagan and Bush administrations have encouraged private employers, especially those who do business with the government, to adopt policies to prevent drug use by their employees. In an increasing number of cases, these policies include the possibility of random urine screens. In 1989, rules went into effect requiring all companies and organizations who obtain grants or contracts from the federal government to adopt a "drug-free workplace" plan. The exact nature of the plan is up to the company, but guidelines have been produced by the Department of Labor. Modelled after the Education Department's 1986 book, the Labor Department's is called "What Works: Workplaces Without Drugs."[8] At a minimum they expect employers to state clearly that drug use on the job is unacceptable and to notify employees of the consequences of violating company policy regarding drug use. The ultimate goal is not to catch drug users and fire them, but to prevent drug use by making it clear that it is not condoned.

WHAT SHOULD WE BE DOING?

By now you have picked up some ideas for things to do, as well as some things to avoid doing. But the answer as to what needs to be done in a particular situation depends on the motivations for doing it. Most states require drug and alcohol abuse prevention education as part of a health curriculum, for example. If that is the primary motive for doing something and if there doesn't seem to be a particular problem with substance abuse in the schools, then the best thing would probably be to adopt one of the many modern curricula that have been developed for this purpose, make sure the teachers and other participants are properly trained in it, and go ahead. In selecting among the curricula, a sensible, balanced approach that combines some factual information with social skills training, perhaps integrated into the more general themes of health, personal values, and decision making, would be appropri-

---

Issue: smokeless tobacco—a new prevention problem

Boys all over the country have been putting "just a pinch" of tobacco in their mouths, and the American Cancer Society has become concerned. The interesting thing about this in terms of prevention is that a large number of these boys first use chewing tobacco at the age of 11 or younger. This means that any programs aimed at primary prevention will have to be done in grade schools. Another interesting aspect is that the problem is almost exclusively confined to boys. This may say something about the social function served by chewing tobacco, and studying that function might help in developing new approaches to prevention.

The National Cancer Institute is funding research to develop prevention programs, because evidence to date indicates that the use of oral smokeless tobacco products may increase the risk of oral cancer fivefold. Given the number of boys who are developing this habit, this could represent a serious public health problem several years in the future.

---

ate. Above all, avoid sensational scare stories, "preachy" approaches from the teacher to the student, and avoid having untrained personnel develop their own curricula. Another good thing to avoid is the inadvertent demonstration of how to do things you don't want them to do, that is, don't show them how they shouldn't put beans in their noses!

If, on the other hand, there is a public outcry about the "epidemic" of drugs and alcohol abuse in the community, speakers have come around inflaming passions, and there is a widespread fervor to "do something about it," this represents both a danger and an opportunity. The danger is that this passionate group might attack and undermine efforts already being made in the schools, substituting scary, preachy, negative approaches that may have negative consequences. The opportunity arises if this energy can be organized into a community planning effort, out of which could develop cooperation, increased parent understanding, a focus on family communication, interest in the lives of the community's young people, and increased recreational and creative opportunities.

The key to making this happen is convincing the aroused citizenry of the possibly negative consequences of doing what seems obvious and selling them on the idea of studying what needs to be done. A good place to start might be by writing to the National Institute on Drug Abuse, 5600 Fishers Lane, Rockville, MD 20857, and to the National Institute on Alcohol Abuse and Alcoholism, at the same address. These two government agencies regularly produce updated materials for groups interested in developing drug and alcohol abuse prevention programs. For example, in 1984 NIAAA published *Prevention plus: involving schools, parents and the community in alcohol and drug education,* a 324-page book with detailed examples and resource materials.[11,12]

Summary

The apparent goal of most drug education programs has not been just to impart drug information, but to impart only the type of information that was expected to create negative attitudes toward drug use and therefore to reduce drug-taking behavior. In other words, the goal has usually been prevention of drug abuse rather than an increase in knowledge for its own sake. Judged by whether such programs do in fact reduce drug use, most of the research indicates that they are failures. This caused many people in the 1970s to question the presumed model (the knowledge-attitudes-behavior model).

The 1970s saw the widespread use of various affective education approaches: teaching students to clarify their own values, teaching alternatives to drug use, and teaching students personal and social skills so that they would not need drugs as a substitute for success. These programs have been called generic, in that they cover various health-related behaviors or focus on developing values and social skills without even mentioning drugs or alcohol. Evaluations of these types of programs also have not revealed dramatic successes in preventing drug use.

Recent programs have made an effort to teach specific skills that can help a young person resist peer pressure to engage in substance use. Learning to recognize peer pressure and teaching ways to minimize it or to refuse drugs have been shown to be very effective in reducing the number of new cigarette smokers, but clear demonstrations have not been produced for other types of substance use. In addition, school policies and penalties for violating drug and alcohol policies are seen as supporting the messages heard in the classroom, and are an important part of the federal government's "drug-free schools" model.

Other, less widely used, approaches focus on organized peer groups both in and outside the school setting or involve training parents to be in charge of drug education, values clarification, and learning responsibility within the family setting. Still other approaches try to involve as much of the community as possible, obtaining cooperation from police, schools, civic groups, local media, parent groups, and other interested parties. The federal government also has been encouraging private companies to adopt "drug-free workplace" policies in an effort to prevent drug use on the job. It seems clear that these approaches should have impact, but evaluating them has been difficult.

No program at all is probably preferable to some of the approaches that have been taken. But by avoiding certain approaches and using those that seem to have worked in the past, programs that have drug abuse prevention as a goal can be educational and have beneficial effects on the lives of those involved in them.

REFERENCES

1. Goodstadt MS: Alcohol and drug education: models and outcomes, Health Education Monographs, 6:263-278, 1978.
2. Swisher JD and others: Drug education: pushing or preventing? Peabody Journal of Education 49:68-75, 1971.
3. Swisher JD, Warner RW Jr, Spence CC, and others: A comparison of four approaches to drug abuse prevention at the college level, Journal of College Student Personnel 14:231-235, 1973.

4. How U.S. is smashing "hard drug" rings: interview with John R. Bartels, Jr, Administrator of Drug Enforcement, Department of Justice, US News and World Report, April 1, 1974, pp 38-41.

5. Drug education is linked to use, New York Times, December 3, 1972.

6. Blum RH, Blum E, and Garfield E: Drug education: results and recommendations, Lexington, Mass, 1976, DC Heath & Co.

7. Swisher JD: Prevention issues. In DuPont RI, Goldstein A, and O'Donnell J, editors: Handbook on drug abuse, Washington, DC, 1979, NIDA, US Government Printing Office.

8. Schaps E, Moskowitz J, Malvin J, and others: The Napa drug abuse prevention project: research findings, Washington, DC, 1984, DHHS Publication No (ADM)84-1339, US Government Printing Office.

9. Prevention research. In Drug abuse and drug abuse research, Washington, DC, 1984, DHHS Publication No (ADM)85-1372, US Government Printing Office.

10. What works: schools without drugs, US Department of Education, Washington, DC, 1987.

11. Resnik HS and Gibbs J: Types of peer program approaches. In Gardner SE, editor: Adolescent peer pressure: theory, correlates, and program implications for drug abuse prevention, Washington, DC, 1981, DHHS Publication No (ADM)81-1152, US Government Printing Office.

12. Parent education. In Prevention plus: involving schools, parents, and the community in alcohol and drug education, Washington, DC, 1984, DHHS Publication No (ADM)84-1256, US Government Printing Office.

13. Community approaches. In Prevention plus: involving schools, parents, and the community in alcohol and drug education, Washington, DC, 1984, DHHS Publication No (ADM)84-1256, US Government Printing Office.

14. Evans RI: Smoking in children: developing a social psychological strategy of deterrence, Preventive Medicine, 5:122-127, 1976.

15. Flay BR: What we know about the social influences approach to smoking prevention: review and recommendations. In Bell CS and Battjes R, editors: Prevention research: deterring drug abuse among children and adolescents, Washington, DC, 1985, NIDA Research Monograph 63, DHHS Publication No (ADM)85-1334, US Government Printing Office.

16. McCarthy WJ: The cognitive developmental model and other alternatives to the social skills deficit model of smoking onset. In Bell CS and Battjes R, editors: Prevention research: deterring drug abuse among children and adolescents, Washington, DC, 1985, NIDA Research Monograph 63, DHHS Publication No (ADM)85-1334, US Government Printing Office.

17. Glynn K, Leventhal H, and Hirschman R: A cognitive developmental approach to smoking prevention. In Bell CS and Battjes R, editors: Prevention research: deterring drug abuse among children and adolescents, Washington, DC, 1985, NIDA Research Monograph 63, DHHS Publication No (ADM)85-1334, US Government Printing Office.

18. What works: workplaces without drugs, US Department of Labor, Washington, DC, 1989.

Chapter 18

Substance Abuse Treatment

OBJECTIVES

After reading this chapter, you should be able to:

Describe some of the history, current approaches, and controversies involved in the treatment of alcoholism and narcotic addiction.

List the major characteristics that define typical therapeutic community and outpatient drug-free programs and explain the differences between these approaches.

Discuss approaches that are being used in the treatment of cocaine dependence.

Every year hundreds of thousands of Americans undergo treatment for alcohol abuse, heroin addiction, or abuse of other substances. The word "treatment" conjures up an image of hospitals, nurses, and physicians, but traditional medical approaches form only a small part of the overall treatment picture. As we shall see, the variety of treatment approaches reflects a variety of substance abuse problems, as well as a variety of theories about substance abuse.

DEFINING GOALS AND EVALUATING OUTCOMES

The particular theoretical view one has of alcoholism, narcotic addiction, or substance abuse in general influences not only the treatment approaches one is likely to take, but even the goals of treatment. For example, if one accepts the predominant view of alcoholism as a disease, particularly as a disease with an inherited component, then the only acceptable treatment goal is total **abstinence** from alcohol. Other experts view alcoholism from a psychosocial perspective, and many of these people believe that a possible beneficial outcome of treatment would be controlled social drinking. Likewise, if one views narcotic addiction as inherently evil, undermining the physical and mental health of its victims (a common view until fairly recently), then abstinence from narcotics would be the only acceptable goal. Americans seem to have come around to accepting addiction to the legal narcotic methadone as preferable to heroin addiction, so the goal has changed from eliminating narcotic use to eliminating heroin use. Similarly with cigarette smoking, some programs have focused on cutting down smoking or switching to lower tar and nicotine cigarettes, whereas most programs aim for complete abstinence.

When measuring the success of programs, the goal of total abstinence has certain advantages. First of all, it may be possible to use objective indicators of abstinence. If blood, urine, or saliva tests reveal traces of the substance or its metabolites, then the goal of abstinence has not been met. If the goal is to reduce or control use of a substance, such objective indicators may be useless, and often one has to rely on self-reports by the client as to how much of the substance is being used. Another practical difficulty that arises in evaluating programs whose goals are reduced or controlled use is defining controlled use. This has been a particular argument in alcoholism treatment programs. For example, one controversial **controlled drinking** study considered its graduates to be "functioning well" if they drank less than four drinks per day—an amount that seems too high to abstinence-oriented theorists. This can lead to great confusion when a treatment program claims as successes individuals whom others would see as failures.

A further area of confusion and controversy in both selecting and evaluating treatment programs arises when the subject population is not carefully defined. We should always avoid lumping all "drug users" into the same category. There was a period in the late 1960s and early 1970s when thousands of high-school age youngsters were caught smoking marijuana and, as an alternative to jail, sent to be "rehabilitated" in programs designed for heroin addicts. That was probably a poor use of treatment facilities. Regarding evaluation, the issue of who was being treated has caused the most controversy in the area of alcohol abuse. Some experiments that have claimed to demonstrate controlled drinking by alcoholics have been criticized because the subjects were not "real" alcoholics. One gets the impression at times that this argument can't be won: since to some people alcoholics can never drink socially, if they do learn this trick they really must not have been alcoholics!

TREATING ALCOHOLISM

As we saw in Chapter 9, excessive alcohol consumption is an age-old human problem, and one that exacts enormous costs from contemporary society, both in dollars and in wasted human potential. Where do we place the blame for this difficulty? If we believe that the fault is a moral defect in the alcoholic, then we might "treat" the problem by using the same sort of approach we use with other social transgressions, such as stealing. Historically, these have consisted of social ostracism, imprisonment, or other forms of punishment. If we believe that the fault lies with alcohol itself ("demon rum"), then our treatment consists of attempts to control the availability of alcohol. If we believe that alcoholism is a disease, then we seek medical treatment.

Historically, all these ideas and all these approaches have coexisted. For example, at the turn of the century it was common to view drunkards as social outcasts and to throw them in jail. At the same time the temperance movement was rapidly gaining ground in its rush toward the eventual prohibition of alcohol. Meanwhile, some physicians were advocating the use of morphine or other drugs as preferable substitutes for alcohol.

Alcoholics Anonymous

The formation of **Alcoholics Anonymous** (AA) in 1935 can now be seen as an important milestone in treatment. This group, which has total abstinence as a goal, has given support to the disease model of alcoholism. One of the basic tenets of this group is that the alcoholic is biologically different from the nonalcoholic person and therefore can never safely drink any alcohol at all. Central to this disease model is the idea that the disease takes away the person's control of his own drinking behavior, and therefore removes the blame for the problem. AA members are quick to point out that removing blame for the disease does not remove responsibility for dealing with it. By analogy, we would not blame diabetics for being diabetic, but we do expect diabetics to control their diets, take their medication, and so on. Thus the alcoholic is seen as having the responsibility for managing the "disease" on a day-by-day basis, but need not feel guilty about being different. The major approach used by AA has been group support and a "buddy system." The members of AA help each other through difficult periods and encourage each other in their sobriety.

Although AA has been described as a loose affiliation of local groups, each with its own character, they have in common adherence to a 12-step program of recovery from alcoholism (see boxed item).

Everyone agrees that AA has been helpful for many people and, since it has reached more individuals than any other approach, has undoubtedly helped more people than any other method. Nevertheless, formal evaluations of the success of AA have been few and have not been very positive. For example, studies of court-ordered referrals to AA or to other types of interventions have not shown AA to be more effective. However, AA was developed by and for people who have made a personal decision to stop drinking and who want to affiliate with others who have made that decision and may not be the most appropriate treatment approach for individuals who are coerced into treatment as an alternative to jail. More appropriate (and more difficult and expensive) evaluations of AA should be done to determine which types of alcoholics are most likely to benefit from this organization's program.[1]

Medical Approaches

One of the most influential contributors to the disease concept of alcoholism is E.M. Jellinek, who portrayed alcoholism as a progressive disease

---

The twelve steps of Alcoholics Anonymous
1. We admitted we were powerless over alcohol—that our lives had become unmanageable.
2. Came to believe that a Power greater than ourselves could restore us to sanity.
3. Made a decision to turn our will and our lives over to the care of God *as we understood Him.*
4. Made a searching and fearless moral inventory of ourselves.
5. Admitted to God, to ourselves, and to another human being the exact nature of our wrongs.
6. Were entirely ready to have God remove all these defects of character.
7. Humbly asked Him to remove our shortcomings.
8. Made a list of all persons we had harmed and became willing to make amends to them all.
9. Made direct amends to such people wherever possible, except when to do so would injure them or others.
10. Continued to take moral inventory and when we were wrong promptly admitted it.
11. Sought through prayer and meditation to improve our conscious contact with God *as we understood Him,* praying only for knowledge of His will for us and the power to carry that out.
12. Having had a spiritual awakening as a result of these steps, we tried to carry this message to alcoholics, and to practice these principles in all our affairs.

---

leading characteristically through several stages.[2] In the final and most severe stage, which he called gamma alcoholism, the individual has suffered liver and nervous system damage and has a profound physical dependence so that dangerous withdrawal symptoms appear when alcohol intake is stopped. More recent studies have discounted the notion that all, or even most, alcoholics go through such a consistent set of stages. However, there are a large number of alcoholics who come into treatment with liver and nervous system damage and who will suffer withdrawal symptoms. In fact, thousands of people die each year under these circumstances. In such severe cases it is clear that medical intervention is called for.

Detoxification. The first problem is to get the individual over the immediate crises. There is some danger of death from respiratory depression at first. Clearing the stomach and supporting respiration will hopefully get the individual through this first threat. The next hurdle is to allow the alcohol to clear the system **(detoxification),** while preventing convulsions and delirium tremens because of withdrawal. Intravenous administration of diazepam or another benzodiazepine sedative is an accepted method for controlling these potentially dangerous symptoms.

Treatment. Regardless of which approach is taken to try to alter drinking behavior, the next stage of medical treatment is based on the fact that many alcoholics are malnourished and that at least some of the alcohol-related brain damage may be a result of a vitamin (thiamine) deficiency. Thus an important part of treating chronic alcoholics is providing a nutritious diet supplemented by extra vitamins. There may be other physical problems associated with liver occlusion and altered blood circulation, and these also require symptomatic medical treatment.

Aftercare. Once an individual has been "dried out" and received the primary treatment, it may be appropriate to provide some long-term medical support. A common approach, which may actually be considered part of the treatment itself, is the prescribing of *disulfiram* (Antabuse). Alcohol is normally metabolized in the liver through two enzymatic steps. Disulfiram inhibits the enzyme aldehyde dehydrogenase, the second of these steps. Alcohol is then converted into acetaldehyde, but further conversion is prevented and acetaldehyde builds up in the system. High levels of acetaldehyde usually produce a severe reaction: headache, nausea, vomiting, throbbing of the head and neck, breathing difficulties, and a host of other unpleasant symptoms. Therefore, a person taking disulfiram can't take a drink without becoming ill, and this threat may be sufficient to help many people avoid the impulse to drink. It takes 2 or 3 days after a person stops taking disulfiram before a drink can be taken safely, so a person on this treatment must make a decision

to stop taking disulfiram for that length of time if he or she wants to drink.

Disulfiram treatment has been employed in the court-ordered treatment programs, but there is considerable doubt as to its long-term usefulness when employed in that way. If disulfiram does help, it is by helping those who want to avoid drinking by making it impossible for them to give in to a momentary impulse or to social pressure.

Behavioral Approaches

Aversion therapy is based on the use of Pavlovian conditioning to associate unpleasant events (painful electric shocks or nausea) with the sight, smell and taste of alcoholic beverages. Several of the early experiments attempted to make alcohol aversive by allowing the patients to smell and then taste a drink, immediately after which they would receive an electric shock. Reviews of controlled studies based on this approach reveal that it has not been terribly effective. If instead of electric shocks a drug is given that produces prolonged nausea and vomiting, the aversion appears to be more powerful. A report comparing aversion therapy using an emetic drug with electric shock aversion found that the chemical aversion produced greater improvement in the patients 6 months after treatment.[3] Although chemical aversion treatments may be somewhat effective, they have been shown to work only in patients with a good prognosis (married, employed, and highly motivated).

A more widely used behavioral approach involves **teaching coping skills.** Some of the same behaviors that are taught in prevention programs are used, such as recognizing peer pressure and practicing ways to deal with it. In addition, therapists often get the patients to pay special attention to high-risk situations and teach alternative behaviors that can be used to get through those difficult times. For example, if the individual is used to having a drink or two before dinner it may be suggested that an alternative nonalcoholic drink be substituted, or that the person assist with the dinner preparations, or even that the dinner hour be moved up so that the difficult time gap doesn't exist. The idea is to help the client to manage his or her behavior to decrease the probabilitiy of drinking. Some studies have reported positive results from such treatment approaches, whereas others have not.

Some behavior-management approaches have accepted **controlled drinking** as a desirable outcome and have attempted to teach methods that will limit alcohol intake.[4] Such strategies as switching to drinks with lower alcohol content, keeping track of each drink taken, or even learning to recognize a target blood alcohol level have been tried. A number of such experiments have reported success in producing a higher percentage of improved patients (both abstaining and "controlled") than with traditional abstinence-oriented approaches. However, there is enormous controversy about both the success and the desirability of controlled-drinking approaches.

Is Controlled Drinking a Realistic Goal?

The notion that alcoholism is a disease that produces a loss of control over drinking seems to be inconsistent with AA's belief that alcoholics do have the responsibility to decide to remain sober.[5] This apparent dilemma is resolved by the commonly used phrase, "one drink is too much and a thousand not enough." In other words, the belief is that the alcoholic does have control over that first drink and can choose not to take it, but once alcohol has entered his system he is helpless and his drinking is out of control. This seems to be descriptive of binge drinking, in which a problem drinker may not drink at all for days or weeks and then really "tie one on." But does this notion of loss of control have any further merit? Does it describe the behavior of all alcoholics all the time? A number of experimental studies have been done with hospitalized alcoholics, and virtually all of them report that alcoholics do not differ fundamentally in the types of events that control drinking, although they do drink more than control subjects. Other descriptive studies of the drinking patterns of large numbers of active alcoholics

show a great variety of patterns. Some may drink in this binge fashion, whereas others may have extended periods of what can be described only as controlled drinking. Also, a surprisingly large number of alcoholics who have been through abstention-oriented treatment programs are found on later follow-ups to be drinking, but in a controlled manner.[6]

Just about everyone can agree that anyone who has drinking problems would be best advised to stop drinking and to abstain completely. But there are arguments against having abstention as the only treatment goal. First, problem drinkers may be reluctant to enter treatment if they are required to accept the label of "alcoholic" and the goal of total abstinence. Second, about two thirds of adult Americans are drinkers (and even more among urban, college-educated adults). Thus, assuming that the alcoholic has been part of a social group that accepts or even expects drinking, we are in a sense trying to promote a "deviant" behavior. Third, if abstention has been tried several times with no success, why not try controlled drinking as a treatment goal? Those opposed to such approaches believe that they are doomed to failure, because of the nature of the "disease" of alcoholism. The apparent successes can be argued away either by agreeing that alcoholics may appear to be under control for a few weeks or months or by saying that the controlled drinking successes were not really alcoholics when they entered treatment. These experts are concerned that even discussing the possibility might just encourage alcoholics to drink. After all, they've probably been telling themselves and others for years that they could "handle it." Do we really need scientists providing support for such self-delusion?

A 1976 Rand Corporation report added fuel to this controversy. This study, funded by the National Institute on Alcohol Abuse and Alcoholism (NIAAA), examined treatment effectiveness in eight large treatment centers. After establishing clearly that the alcoholics in these programs were seriously impaired (they drank nine times more than the average person), they found that about

70% of them were improved 18 months after treatment. The controversial conclusion was:

It is important to stress that the improved clients include only a relatively small number who are long-term abstainers. . . . The majority of improved clients are either drinking moderate amounts of alcohol—but at levels far below what could be described as alcoholic drinking—or engaging in alternating periods of drinking and abstention.[7,p.v]

It is important to remember that these programs had abstention as their primary goal, yet controlled drinking seemed to have been the result for a large number of the clients. This report came under immediate and highly emotional attack, as did the Rand Corporation itself and the NIAAA for funding such a study.

The traditional view was vindicated to some extent by the 4-year follow-up of these clients. Of those who had been drinking without symptoms at 18 months, 41% had relapsed by the 4-year follow-up, compared to 30% of those who had been abstaining at 18 months.[8] This was widely hailed as indicating that abstention was a more desirable treatment outcome than controlled drinking. However, we should not ignore the fact that the *majority* of those who were drinking in a controlled fashion at 18 months did not relapse and were found to be either controlled drinkers or abstainers at 4 years. At this point it seems reasonable to conclude that abstention is the preferred goal and the one adopted by the vast majority of programs, but that controlled drinking is a realistic option for many alcoholics.

Brief mention must be made of a specific experiment that has generated controversy far beyond its significance. In 1973, and in a 1976 follow-up report, Mark and Linda Sobell described an experiment comparing "individualized behavior therapy" with a traditional abstinence-oriented treatment.[9] The behavior therapy consisted of training individuals to become "social drinkers" by allowing them to drink in certain limited ways. If the clients exceeded various limits, they received electric shocks. While most clients in both groups had subsequent problems, the So-

bells claimed significantly fewer "failures" in the trained social drinkers than in the abstinence group. In 1982, another group of researchers reexamined these data and contacted a number of the subjects. They published a damaging article implying major weaknesses in the original subject selection and assignment to groups, as well as weaknesses in the follow-up efforts.[10] This generated investigations, more reports, and a seemingly endless series of articles and letters to journal editors, from both defenders and detractors.[11,12] Those opposed to controlled drinking experiments see this controversy as a severe blow to that approach in general. The believers in controlled drinking, while supporting the general conclusion of the Sobells' original reports, also pointed out that even without this experiment there is a large body of evidence supporting the viability of controlled drinking as a treatment goal.

Although research continues on disulfiram, controlled drinking, and other approaches, the mainstay of alcoholism treatment in the United States is and has been a 4 to 6 week visit to one of the growing number of residential (inpatient) treatment facilities. Most of these programs adopt the AA model of alcoholism as a disease, and use individual counseling, group counseling, and family therapy approaches to help the alcoholic "work the steps" (the 12 steps of AA). Because health insurance companies have been willing to pay for such treatment, these residential facilities have become a growth industry during the 1980s.

Is Alcoholism Treatment Effective?

Are the insurance companies getting anything for their money when they pay for someone to go to treatment? The answers to these questions about alcoholism treatment aren't necessarily simple, but we can start by saying a qualified yes. If an individual receives the diagnosis of alcoholism (or alcohol dependence disorder, see Chapters 2 and 9), the prognosis is not good. Most such individuals can be expected to drink again, drink heavily, and have further alcohol-related problems. It is the consensus of many studies that those who enter treatment do better than those who do not. Thus, statistically, alcoholism treatment is effective. However, the same studies show over and over that most of the people who go through treatment will drink again, with typical first-year relapse rates running about 65% to 75%.[13] Therefore it may seem that treatment is not effective for most of the individuals. A further complication has been hinted at: how do we define relapse? If the goal is 100% abstinence, then even one drink at any time after treatment would be considered a relapse and therefore a treatment failure. It is quite possible for someone to go through a treatment program, spend a couple of months going to AA meetings and not drinking, think they have the problem licked, try drinking again, drink too much for a month or two, and then go back to AA and quit drinking. Neither recovery nor relapse should be viewed as a permanent condition.

Many studies over the years have examined the characteristics of the treatment programs and the characteristics of the clients to determine if one type of treatment is better than another, which clients do better than others, and whether certain types of clients do better in certain types of programs. Because of the difficulties in measuring relapse and other indicators of success, this type of research is difficult to do, and individual reports may often be criticized on procedural grounds. But several large-scale studies agree that differences among treatment approaches are less important in predicting success than differences among the clients when they enter treatment. Those clients who have jobs, stable family relationships, minimal psychopathology, no history of past treatment failures, and minimal involvement with other drugs tend to do better than the clients with no jobs, no meaningful relationhips, and so on. What is surprising, and somewhat frustrating, is that the type of treatment program seems to make little or no difference: residential vs. outpatient, shorter vs. longer, intensity of therapy, and theoretical approach are all factors that have not consistently influenced outcome.[14] This seems to imply that insurance companies could save money by providing for shorter term, less intense, outpatient

treatment and still have about the same success rate. However, we are unsure enough about such a conclusion that most companies are continuing to pay for residential treatment while awaiting the outcome of further research.

Occupational alcoholism programs. A new trend that has developed since the late 1960s may solve some of the problems found in most treatment programs: motivation of the individual and maintenance of the family and work support systems.[15] It has been estimated that 6% of the work force in this country engages in destructive drinking, and losses of productivity in illness, accidents, and personal problems amount to billions of dollars each year. With the encouragement of the federal government, many large corporations have organized treatment programs for their alcoholic and potentially alcoholic employees. The federal government has done the same thing for military and civilian employees. Most of the programs—military, government, and industry—are based on the same principles as those listed here[16]:

1. The company makes it plain that it considers alcoholism a disease and will treat alcoholics just as it does employees with any other illness.
2. Supervisors are told to report poor job performance, often the first indicator of alcoholism, to trained counselors in medical or personnel units.
3. If the problem is diagnosed as alcoholism, the employee is given the choice of entering a treatment program or losing his job for poor performance.
4. A worker who enters treatment gets sick leave and medical benefits.
5. Medical records of alcoholism are kept confidential.

The term "employee assistance program" (EAP) is often used for such an approach.

These programs seem to be no more effective than voluntary programs outside the vocational setting. But they are a boon for industry: a program in the Oldsmobile Division of General Motors found that among the participants there was an 82% drop in job-related accidents, a 56% drop in leaves of absence, and a 30% decrease in sickness and accident benefits paid. GM expects to save $3 to $10 for every dollar they invest in the program. Even a city can make money by providing alcoholism treatment. A cost-benefit analysis showed that one state would recover $1.98 for every dollar invested in alcoholism treatment.[17]

For both alcohol and drug treatment this approach seems to be the rising star—great hopes exist, but there is no evidence that the big problem of motivation is solved, in spite of how logical it seems.

> The biggest difficulty in the treatment of an alcoholic is motivating him to seek help. For this purpose . . . no one is in a better position than his employer, who has the power—through the threat of firing or demotion—to intervene in a worker's life, as well as the right to do so once the problem begins to interfere with his work. Neither logic nor tears has the same effect on a problem drinker as the fear of losing what may be his last link to respectability—his job.[18]

TREATMENT OF NARCOTIC ADDICTS
History

Dependence on opium, and later on morphine and heroin, is also a very old problem with a long history of varied treatments. A 1902 medical book on the subject of morphinism described a variety of approaches to treatment, mainly concerned with reducing the morphine intake either slowly or more rapidly (over a few days' time) and dealing with the withdrawal symptoms.[19] The danger of relapse was recognized, with the author recommending cold showers, travel abroad, or a temporary change of lifestyle, such as going west to work on a cattle ranch or in a mine. A few years later, the accepted medical "cure" involved the use of high doses of belladonna or some other anticholinergic to maintain a state of delirium for several days, after which the patient was felt to be cured of the addiction![20,p.249]

After the Harrison Act was passed in 1914, narcotics became less freely available and somewhat more expensive, even through legal sources. This had the purpose of preventing further addictions, but not all those already addicted could afford frequent visits to a private physician. Cities around the country established public narcotic clinics to help these people. Most of the clinics gradually "detoxified" their clients, but in some cases (such as chronic pain conditions) the clients were considered incurable and were offered "social adjustment" treatment, which meant continued maintenance on a narcotic.[20,p.254] After the passage of alcohol prohibition and the establishment of a Bureau of Narcotics, these clinics were all closed down because of pressure from federal agents, and by 1925 there was no longer a legal source of treatment that included providing narcotics for maintenance.

Federal prisons became choked with narcotic addicts by 1930. That and the repeal of prohibition led to the reorganization of the Bureau of Narcotics under Harry Anslinger and the establishment of two federal treatment facilities, one in Lexington, Kentucky and the other in Fort Worth, Texas. The center at Lexington was the first and the more important and served as a combination prison farm, treatment center, and research center where the medical and psychological staff searched for a cure for narcotic addiction. The treatment consisted of gradual withdrawal using morphine, followed by a stay of up to a year, during which the clients would work on the farm and take advantage of the recreational facilities, all the while undergoing psychotherapy and participating in various tests and experiments. The relapse rate following this type of treatment appeared to be above 80% and never got much better than that.[20,p.258] This was the major approach to treating narcotic addicts into the 1960s, at least partly because Anslinger remained adamantly opposed throughout his career, which ended in 1962, to any outpatient treatment program that included giving narcotics to clients.

Current Medical Approaches

Narcotic antagonists. Research at Lexington revealed some interesting properties of drugs

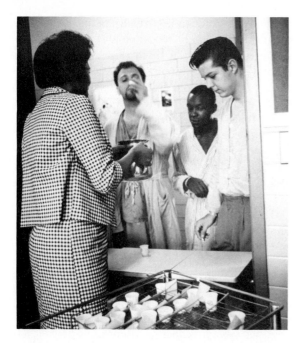

Methadone maintenance programs require the clients to show up each day to receive the methadone. This makes it easier to keep track of the clients and to counsel them on a regular basis.

such as nalorphine, naloxone, and cyclazocine. When given to addicts who had been taking morphine, these drugs percipitated a withdrawal syndrome immediately. And, while taking these drugs, the effects of morphine, heroin, and other narcotics were blocked. Could these narcotic antagonists be a cure for addiction? If an addict were first withdrawn from the narcotic and then given the antagonist on a chronic basis, relapse should not be a problem. If a person did try taking heroin, it would have no effect. While there would be no negative consequence, other than the waste of money, eventually the addict would learn to stop taking heroin, thus curing the addiction. The problem is, of course, that the addict must be highly motivated to take the antagonist. Some of the antagonists, particularly cyclazocine, produce unpleasant side effects. Naloxone, which produces fairly pure antagonism with few side effects, is a short-acting drug that must be taken several times

a day to maintain constant antagonism. With all these difficulties, reports on the effectiveness of narcotic antagonist treatment have not been very promising. More recent experiments have used naltrexone, a long-acting antagonist that was released for marketing as a prescription drug under the brand name Trexan in 1985. A 50-mg tablet can antagonize the effects of a large dose of heroin for 24 hours and a smaller dose for 2 days or more, and it may therefore be given as infrequently as three times a week.[21] Although it is clear that naltrexone therapy is not for everyone, it may be that some highly motivated clients who tend to relapse impulsively may buy themselves some time with it. Also, a court-ordered client could be mandated to come to a clinic three or four times a week and take naltrexone. At least for the duration of the treatment, the client would not be able to become readdicted to heroin or other narcotics. We can expect to see this antagonist receive continued but fairly restricted use. An interesting problem arises if a patient on naltrexone is involved in an accident and requires some pain relief. Current practice would be to give high doses of hydromorphone (Dilaudid) to overcome the antagonism. This should, of course, be done only in a hospital and with extreme caution.

Methadone maintenance.   Methadone (Dolophine) is a synthetic narcotic analgesic developed in Germany during World War II and found to be a substitute for the then-unavailable opium-based agents. It is quite effective when taken orally, and it has a long duration of action. The long duration means not only that it needs to be taken less frequently to prevent withdrawal syptoms, but because the drug leaves the body slowly the withdrawal symptoms are less severe. Although long approved as a narcotic analgesic, it has gained fame as a drug useful in treatment programs for heroin addicts.

The initial study in this area was started in 1964 by Dole and Nyswander, a husband-wife team in New York City. In their initial work heroin addicts were given 20 to 30 mg of methadone orally every day; this was gradually increased over 4 to 6 weeks to 80 to 120 mg given orally once a day.

The theory behind the use of methadone to help rehabilitate addicts is that the long-lasting effects of methadone prevent withdrawal symptoms and block the pleasurable effects of opiates. It disrupts the

pattern of swinging between the states of heroin intoxication and the withdrawal syndrome. "These are three states in the heroin addict's life," says Dr. Dole. "He's either 'straight' (feeling normal), 'high,' or 'sick.' He wakes up sick, takes a shot, and gets high. That lasts a couple of hours, maybe, until he begins coming off the high, and then he'll take another shot if he can get it. He spends very little time being straight, so he usually is not able to hold a job or live normally; he's pretty much a lost soul."[22]

The initial report of the effectiveness of this treatment program on 750 criminal addicts was spectacular.

A four year trial of methadone blockade treatment has shown 94% success in ending the criminal activity of former heroin addicts. The majority of these patients are now productively employed, living as responsible citizens, and supporting families. The results show unequivocally that criminal addicts can be rehabilitated by a well-supervised maintenance program.[23]

Methadone programs expanded rapidly after these reports. Why did we so readily accept the switching of addicts from one narcotic to another? Could we really condone having government-supported narcotic addicts walking around the streets? It may be that programs of this type would not have been possible if Harry Anslinger had not retired in 1962, but one of his major concerns could be avoided. Because methadone can be effective if taken only once or twice a day, the addicts could be required to come to the clinic and take the drug under supervision. Thus addicts were not being supplied with drugs that they could take out on the streets and sell or give to others. Also, there was some confusion over whether methadone was acting purely as a narcotic or whether it had some antagonist properties as well. Note that it was indicated that methadone treatment tended to block the pleasurable effects of heroin and that the program was referred to as

methadone "blockade" treatment by its proponents. This apparent blockade was probably a result of the buildup to high doses of methadone employed in the initial studies. The addicts became tolerant to greater levels of narcotic, and the rather small amount of heroin available in most street "bags" at that time had little effect in a person with such a tolerance. It may be seen as ironic that we were treating narcotic addiction by creating an even greater level of tolerance. Current programs use lower doses, usually under 100 mg per day.

The ethics and morality of the methadone approach were raised early. The heart of the matter was approached in 1969:

although there is no question that methadone maintenance treatment is an effective way of reducing the criminalistic activities of drug addicts, it is a question who is being treated: society or the drug takers . . . each physician who prescribes methadone to a narcotic addict has this moral question to answer: Is he maintaining the patient on drugs for the good of society or for the good of his individual patient? Is he encouraging a kind of "cop out" by reinforcing the hopeless feeling of drug addicts when he wonders whether he can renounce drug use?[24]

Remember too that the 1960s were a time when the majority of addicts were black and there was simultaneously a focus on racial awareness. The idea that large numbers of people might be expected to spend the rest of their lives dependent on a substance, becoming passive supplicants who report to a clinic twice daily for counseling, appeared to some minority leaders to be a frightening experiment in social control.

Despite these concerns, methadone maintenance became widely accepted as the most effective approach to heroin addiction, and by the late 1970s between 75,000 and 100,000 people were enrolled in such programs. There is some division over the primary reason for the effectiveness of methadone. Early workers emphasized the chemical aspects of the program: preventing withdrawal symptoms and craving and blocking the pleasurable effects of heroin. Others see the need for daily appearances at the clinic and the opportunities for frequent counseling as the major reasons for success, with the methadone merely providing a reason for such tight control. In support of this was an early study that indicated that the dose of methadone was not a significant factor. However, more recent studies have indicated that doses of 80 mg per day or more are more effective than doses of 50 mg per day or less.[25]

Even though methadone maintenance is accepted to some extent, it is tightly controlled by the DEA and FDA. Methadone is a regular prescription drug available in both injectable and oral forms for pain relief. But maintenance of addicts has now been formally defined in federal law, and only oral methadone is considered "safe and effective" for this use by the FDA. And this use is not available to every physician, because the FDA still classifies methadone maintenance as investigational, allowing its use only under approved protocols and by approved clinics.[26,pp.263-264] The average American physician is still prohibited from providing any narcotic to an addict for the purpose of maintaining the addiction. The effectiveness of methadone treatment can be measured in several ways. A 1983 review of about 2500 clients in the NIDA-sponsored Treatment Outcome Prospective Study (TOPS) supports the previous reports of positive effects: heroin use declines dramatically, drug-related problems drop, indicators of depression are cut in half during treatment compared to pretreatment levels, commission of nondrug–defined crimes is reduced significantly, and permanent employment is increased slightly.[27]

Why don't all heroin addicts simply come in and sign up for free methadone instead of taking heroin? If their drug-taking behavior were motivated only by the "need" for a narcotic, this would make sense. But let's not forget why most of these people use heroin in the first place: to be part of a subculture, to make a statement about their relationship to the dominant society, or for the experience. And let's not forget that the major reason for continuing to use heroin is probably the positive reinforcement produced by the rapid rise in

blood levels of heroin immediately after an intravenous injection (the "rush"). Slow-acting oral methadone doesn't produce that effect.

Heroin/morphine maintenance.   If we are now willing to supply addicts with narcotics, and if addicts want heroin, why don't we just supply them with heroin and clean syringes and let them inject it intravenously? There are some obvious inconveniences compared to methadone, including the need to administer the drug several times a day, and the use of the needles for intravenous injection. Also, there's the aspect of heroin use mentioned by Dole and Nyswander that the intravenous heroin user spends a lot of time reacting to the last shot or worrying about the next one, with relatively brief periods (only a few hours at a time) of feeling "straight." Oral methadone produces less "up and down" in the blood level of the narcotic and may be more conducive to work, school, or other productive activities. But the major impediment to such an approach is probably the long history Americans have of viewing heroin as an evil substance rather than seeing it as just another narcotic.

Actually, the public clinics that existed in several cities around 1920 can give us some idea of the utility of providing the addict's "drug of choice," which was usually morphine, but was in some cases heroin or codeine. Although Harry Anslinger said many times in later years that these clinics did not work and were hotbeds of criminal activity, a 1974 in-depth review of the clinic in Shreveport, Louisiana gave a more positive assessment.[28] Most of the clients of that program were employed, most were middle-aged, and most had become addicted as a result of medical treatment. The clinic apparently provided an important service for those individuals and has been viewed as a model of what "might have been." Of course, that clinic refused admission to people suspected of being criminals and encouraged "bums" or "loafers" to leave town rather than offering them treatment. The addicts it did serve could in no way be seen as representative of today's addict population.

A great deal has been said about the British

system, in which addicts may register and receive heroin for purposes of maintenance of their addiction. Actually, over the years there really hasn't been a system at all. It's simply the case that Britain never took the step of outlawing the medical use of heroin nor of outlawing the prescribing of narcotics to addicts by physicians. Thus until 1968 there was no program: British heroin addicts simply obtained a prescription from their physician just as they would for any other drug. Some Americans, noting that there were few narcotic addicts in Britain before the 1960s, had suggested that the major cause of our much greater narcotic addiction problem lay in our attempts to control it![29] We'll never know the answer to that one: even though America and England seem quite similar in many ways, they are far from the same society, either now or in the 1920s.

The British were not immune to the social change of the 1960s, and one reflection of that change was that some British youth began to experiment with drugs. Individuals who went to their physicians for heroin and who had developed the addiction recreationally were reported to the Home Office as "nontherapeutic" heroin addicts. The number of such addicts increased from 47 in 1959 to 222 in 1963.[26,p.107] That may not seem like many, but the increase gave support to those who wanted tighter controls. Noting that a few physicians were writing prescriptions for large amounts of heroin, it was concluded that not every physician should be trusted completely where narcotics addicts were concerned. By 1968 the new system was in place: British physicians could still prescribe any medication, including heroin, to nonaddicts. But addicts now had to register as such and could receive heroin or cocaine only from specially licensed physicians in "drug-dependence clinics," which were established in several areas. During the 1970s these clinics dispensed less and less heroin and more and more counseling and oral methadone. By 1978 only 9% of the clinic clients were receiving heroin, either alone or in combination with other drugs.[26,p.199] During the 1970s narcotic addiction continued to increase in Britain, an illicit market for heroin developed, and crime rates increased.

Your turn: where to go for help

You may be interested to know the types of treatment facilities available in your own community. The easiest way to get a start on this is to look in the Yellow Pages under "Drug Abuse and Addiction." There you should find several programs and hospitals advertising their services, even in a small community. In large cities, there will be a long list. Try to guess whether each of these offers a medical approach (e.g., methadone), residential, or outpatient drug-free programs. If you want a more definitive listing of all the programs in your area, write to your state Health Department and ask for a list. The NIDA publishes an up-to-date directory of treatment programs all over the country. You can request a copy by writing to NIDA, 5600 Fishers Lane, Rockville, MD 20857.

If you're confused by all this and want some advice on where to start, we recommend starting with your local community mental health center. These centers are publicly supported and are staffed by professionals, whereas many treatment centers are profit-making corporations employing mainly nonprofessional staff. That doesn't mean that such a program might not be best in a given circumstance, but if so it is probable that the mental health center staff will be able to recommend a good one. It is quite common for individuals to seek treatment first within their own community, from the mental health center or a related program, later to enter a residential facility, and then to be released back to the care of the mental health center. After several such cases the mental health center people get a good idea of how the various residential programs operate and which are the most successful. Another good place to start might be with your school or employer, if they offer counseling services of this type.

A helpful book, "The 100 Best Treatment Centers for Alcoholism and Drug Abuse" (Linda Sunshine and John Wright, Avon Books, New York, 1988) not only describes what those authors believe to be 100 good centers, but also tells in more general terms what to look for and what to avoid in selecting a residential treatment facility.

However, the British still have a much smaller heroin problem than the United States: with a total population about one fourth that of the United States, Britain probably has less than one thirtieth the number of heroin addicts.[26,p.20]

TREATMENT APPROACHES APPLICABLE TO VARIOUS SUBSTANCES

Residential Therapeutic Communities

Synanon. In 1958 Charles Dederick, a recovering alcoholic, felt that an organization such as AA should be able to help narcotic addicts who wanted to be rehabilitated. From quite meager beginnings Synanon grew by the 1970s into a large and apparently successful rehabilitation program and philosophy. The Synanon concepts and practices are extensive, but a few points seem crucial. One is the belief that a narcotic addict is never cured (as AA believes an alcoholic is never cured). Thus he should continue forever to live in the Synanon center or, after being clearly stabilized as a former addict, move into nearby living quarters and stay affiliated and involved with the Synanon program. A second premise of this organization is that the addict must really want to be helped to discontinue drug use. To assure this motivation, there is an open-door policy: a member is free to leave at any time. An important practice is the use of former addicts as staff, with professionals being involved only for emergency medical service. A former addict has several advantages, first that he has "been there" and second, that he has beaten addiction. Thus new members have someone to relate to who understands their problems. The former addict also has the advantage of knowing the tricks of the trade. As a result, he is able to recognize these tricks and demonstrate that they will not be effective at Synanon.

The residents at Synanon are kept busy working. Because of a belief that addicts have difficulty in expressing emotions and in identifying others' emotions, Dederick established the use of "seminars," or group encounters, several times a week. These encounters are often psychologically quite violent. The positive view of them is that they help the addict learn to stop using destructive guards to protect himself and teach him to see himself and others more clearly. A less charitable view is that these sessions serve to threaten or cajole the new members into accepting life at Synanon.

Early reports of Synanon's high rate of success should be examined carefully. The program was

not research oriented, and Dederick pointed out that thousands had left the program.[30] Most of those returned to addiction, but no precise records were kept of the quitters. Thus the high rates of nonaddiction related only to those who stayed with the program.

As the use of many drugs increased in the 1960s, Synanon grew rapidly and began to include a much greater variety of members. For example, youngsters who were caught smoking marijuana were sometimes sent by their families to be rehabilitated at Synanon. Arrestees, whether for marijuana, LSD, amphetamine or other drug use, sometimes volunteered to go to Synanon at the urging of their attorneys to avoid a jail sentence. The businesses Synanon started to provide employment for the residents became large and profitable, and Synanon became a major property holder.[31] In the early 1980s newspaper reports implying that Dederick had himself profited greatly from this "cult" led to threats and to violent encounters between Synanon members and outsiders who began to fear their numbers, wealth, and unanimity. Synanon is still there and still important, but its halo has become tarnished.

Other therapeutic communities. Other residential treatment communities were established in the 1960s, including Daytop Village, Phoenix House, Odyssey House, and Gateway Foundation. Because of the reported successes of such programs (although again such reports were not based on scientific evaluations), their number grew through the 1970s and early 1980s. There are now hundreds of residential facilities across the country, serving narcotic addicts, alcoholics, and abusers of other substances. The one major diference between these therapeutic communities and Synanon is the goal of returning their clients to society. Most of their staff usually consists of recovering alcoholics or former addicts or abusers of other drugs, and there is still a focus on group encounter sessions and on keeping the clients busy. Relatively high success rates reported for these therapeutic communities are again based on those who stick with the program for the full course of the treatment, which may be anywhere from several weeks to several months. The pro-

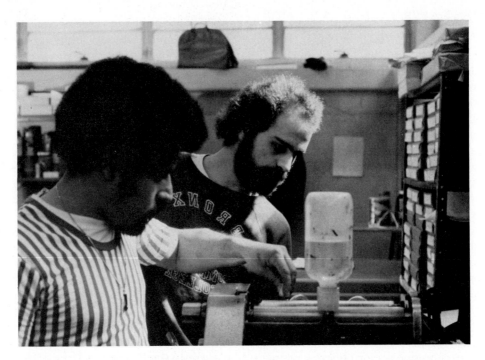

Vocational rehabilitation is an important part of some residential treatment programs.

grams rarely abandon their clients to the outside world, since most have some kind of ongoing follow-up, such as regular group sessions of the program's "graduates." Some therapeutic communities that deal mainly with alcoholics may encourage AA membership as a form of long-term follow-up.

The NIDA-financed Drug Abuse Reporting Program (DARP) has followed the success of a large number of clients admitted to drug abuse treatment programs during the years 1969-1973. In a 1982 follow-up over 4000 of the original sample were contacted and interviewed about their drug use.[32] These and the previous years' data indicate that therapeutic communities do reduce drug use relative to untreated clients or to those who are detoxified and then released. For example, narcotic addicts who had been treated with either methadone maintenance or a therapeutic community approach had about a 20% chance of engaging in daily narcotic use during the last follow-

up year, compared to about 30% from the untreated or detoxified groups. If clients had been treated for less than 90 days in the therapeutic community their outcome measures were not more positive than untreated groups, thus indicating that the length of treatment is an important variable. Other variables among therapeutic communities, such as treatment philosophy or types of services available in the program, did not influence the outcome.

Outpatient Drug-Free Programs

These programs grew from two major sources. In the 1960s, because of a large number of panic reactions to LSD and other illicit drugs, "crisis clinics" were set up in most large communities. These provided alternatives to the emergency room for a person who was frightened and needed someone to talk to until the drug wore off. These facilities ranged from telephone hot lines to emergency-room associated clinics with medical support available to "crash pads" where people could come to sleep off a drug's effects and receive some nonjudgmental advice and counseling. Another major source of outpatient services has been the community mental health centers that have been established all over the nation since the early 1960s. Of the 2000 outpatient services surveyed by NIDA in 1979, about one third were free-standing help centers, another third were affiliated with community mental health centers, and the rest were associated with hospitals, correctional facilities, employers, or other agencies.[33,p.55]

Because of the large number of such programs and their ready availability, they constitute the most popular form of drug abuse treatment, chosen by more than half of all clients. Services range from drop-in "rap" centers to more formal psychotherapy, group counseling, vocational counseling, or other professional services. In contrast to therapeutic communities, the counselors in these programs are more likely to be professional psychologists, social workers, or trained vocational rehabilitation counselors. Also, in contrast to therapeutic communities, clients are less likely to be heroin addicts, and more likely to be marijuana or multiple drug abusers. Perhaps because contacting one of these programs does not seem to be as big a step as entering a residential center, outpatient programs may be more likely to contact drug users earlier in their drug-abuse career, which may help their success rates.

The 1982 follow-up report on the DARP project reported significant positive long-term results from outpatient drug-free programs of about the same magnitude as for methadone maintenance and therapeutic community approaches.[32] Again, the length of treatment was important, but the particular philosophy or type of service offered did not seem to be critical.

The Treatment Outcome Prospective Study (TOPS), which is examining data from a group of clients admitted during 1979-1981, has reported some preliminary findings relative to outpatient drug-free programs. The few heroin addicts who were in outpatient drug-free programs were more likely to use heroin during treatment than were clients in methadone programs, but the use of nonnarcotic drugs seemed to be less in the drug-free program.[34,p.57]

COCAINE TREATMENT

The 1980s saw an enormous increase in the number of people seeking treatment for cocaine dependence. In 1984, 25% of those entering treatment in Denver and almost half those entering treatment in Newark reported cocaine as a major drug problem for them.[35] With all the previous experience we have had in treating drug abuse, how are we reacting to this new challenge? You should be able to predict that some of these people are entering residential programs, but most are being treated on an outpatient basis.

Cocaine overdose is potentially lethal, and medical treatments are being developed to deal with the acute emergencies resulting from excessive cocaine use.[36] Beta-adrenergic blocking drugs, such as propranolol, can be used to treat the rapid, irregular heart rate and high blood pressure. Psychotic symptoms can be controlled with haloperidol (Haldol). If seizures occur, they can be controlled with intravenous diazepam (Valium).

During the withdrawal phase, patients usually become depressed and feel lethargic and irritable. Antidepressant drugs have been shown to be helpful,[37] and are becoming more widely used. One experiment reported that bromocriptine, a dopamine agonist, relieves cocaine withdrawal symptoms without itself being addicting.[38] That treatment has not received much notice, perhaps because of the availability of clonidine, a drug which has been reported to reduce drug craving in heroin addicts, cocaine addicts, and cigarette smokers. The purpose of using a drug to reduce cravings is to prevent the high dropout rate typically seen in the first few days and weeks of cocaine treatment.

After the initial detoxification period, treatment is designed to prevent any attempts to try cocaine use again. Mandatory urine screening at 3-day intervals has been suggested as a useful monitoring device. Group therapy, support groups (groups calling themselves Cocaine Anonymous are available in many areas), and individual psychotherapy, job, and family counseling are all important components of current cocaine treatment programs. Promotion of exercise and general health consciousness fit in with current American trends and are felt to help reduce the "hunger" for cocaine.

Since many cocaine users are middle- or upper-class individuals with both money and status, a behavioral management technique known as "contingency contracting" has been successfully employed.[36] In this approach, an individual who is highly motivated to stop cocaine, but who fears impulsive use, may sign a contract agreeing that using cocaine (as determined by a urine test) will result in the loss of something of great significance (an automobile, a professional license, a large cash deposit) or an automatic notification of an employer. While such contracts must be established with care, if one is freely entered into and if the contingency is sufficiently important, it can be an important aid to behavioral management.

Although still experimental in nature and not yet widely adopted by treatment centers, a promising approach to cocaine addicts focuses on the conditioned stimuli in the addict's environment that become associated with the use of cocaine. For example, seeing a white powder of any kind, or seeing a large amount of cash, may be so strongly conditioned to cocaine use that these stimuli elicit conditioned cravings, withdrawal symptoms, or excitement.[39] By monitoring the client's emotional and physiological responses while discussing such stimuli or while actually presenting stimuli, it is possible to determine which stimuli elicit the strongest emotional responses and are therefore most likely to lead to relapse. The therapists then use "systematic desensitization," a form of extinction procedure, to reduce these conditioned responses. The clients are induced to relax, then to talk about these situations or to step-by-step imagine the sight of drugs, getting ready to use the drug, and so on,

---

Issue: is methadone maintenance forever?

In a NIDA Treatment Research Monograph on the state of the art in treating narcotic addiction, Dr. Richard Resnick, of the New York Medical College, reviewed various approaches to "detoxifying" patients from methadone, ranging from prolonged, slow reduction of the dose to abrupt termination or even to administration of an antagonist to produce immediate withdrawal symptoms and get them over with, which some addicts apparently prefer.[25,27] The assumption behind many of the studies cited by Dr. Resnick is that the goal of a methadone program should be to use the methadone and counseling for as long as is necessary to "treat" the individual so that he or she can then achieve the desired goal of continued abstinence from all narcotics.

Dr. Robert Newman, of Beth Israel Medical Center (also in New York), pointed out that, while detoxification is a valuable service desired by many addicts, many others do not want to be withdrawn. Dr. Newman believes, as do others, that some addicts are using narcotics as a form of self-medication for emotional problems that they have no other way to treat. If these patients receive both objective and subjective benefit from continued methadone maintenance, then it is probably wrong to continually pressure them into attempting detoxification and prolonged abstinence.

---

all the time remaining calm and relaxed. It is hoped that by breaking the emotional reactions to these conditioned stimuli they will no longer elicit cravings and lead to relapse.

As with other drugs, treatment is probably more effective than no treatment, but the failure rate is still high. It will be several years before the effectiveness of different approaches to cocaine dependence can be evaluated.

Summary

The goals, methods, and evaluation of a treatment program for any type of substance abuse depend to some extent on the view one has of that substance and of those who abuse it. This is true whether we are talking about alcohol, heroin, or marijuana users.

These varying views and approaches are quite evident when one looks at the history and current practices of treating alcoholism. Various medical and behavioral approaches have been tried with varying degrees of success. One major and continuing controversy is whether every alcoholic should be treated with total abstinence as the only goal or whether efforts to teach controlled drinking to alcoholics are also worthwhile.

The treatment of narcotic addicts has also employed various medical and behavioral approaches. Again, the goals of treatment have not always been uniform, with many programs seeking total abstinence from all narcotics, and others accepting medically prescribed and therefore controlled use of various narcotics to maintain an addict.

Aside from these specialized programs for alcohol or narcotics, most substance-abuse programs fit into one of two general models: the residential therapeutic community, usually staffed by former substance abusers or the outpatient drug-free programs, which are often associated with community mental health centers and employ trained counselors, psychologists, or social workers.

Because of a large increase in the number of people seeking treatment for cocaine dependence in the 1980s, both old and new approaches are being applied to this problem. There are some promising medical treatments that may help to alleviate the prolonged depression and irritability that occur after cocaine withdrawal. Nevertheless, as with all other drug treatment programs, although they are no doubt better than no treatment at all, the odds for long-term success are not great for any individual client.

REFERENCES

1. Glaser FB and Ogborne AC: What we would most like to know: does AA really work? British Journal of Addiction 77:123-129, 1982.
2. Jellinek EM: The disease concept of alcoholism, New Brunswick, NJ, 1960, Hillhouse Press.
3. Cannon DS, Baker TB, and Wehl CK: Emetic and electric shock alcohol aversion therapy: six- and twelve-month follow-up, Journal of Consulting and Clinical Psychology 49:360-368, 1981.
4. Heather N and Robertson I: Controlled drinking, London, 1981, Methuen & Co.
5. Finagarette H: Alcoholism—neither sin nor disease, The Center Magazine, March/April, 1985, pp 55-63. Reprinted in Annual editions: drugs, society and behavior 86/87, Guilford, Conn, 1986, Dushkin.
6. Pomerleau O, Pertschuk M, and Stinnet J: A critical examination of some current assumptions in the treatment of alcoholism, Journal of Studies on Alcohol 37:849-867, 1976.
7. Armor DJ, Polich JM, and Stambul HB: Alcoholism and treatment, NIAAA Publication R-1739, Washington, DC, 1976, US Government Printing Office.
8. Polich JM, Armor DJ, and Braiker HB: The course of alcoholism: four years after treatment, New York, 1981, John S Wiley and Sons.
9. Sobell MB and Sobell LC: Second-year treatment outcome of alcoholics treated by individualized behavior therapy: results, Behavior Research and Therapy 14:195-215, 1976.
10. Pendery ML, Maltzman IM, and West LJ: Controlled drinking by alcoholics? New findings and a re-evaluation of a major affirmative study, Science 271:169-175, 1982.
11. Marlatt GA: Controlled drinking: the controversy rages on, American Psychologist 40:374-375, 1985.
12. Wallace J: The alcoholism controversy revisited, American Psychologist 41:479-480, 1986.
13. Sixth special report on alcohol and health: DHHS Publication No (ADM) 87-1519, US Department of Health and Human Services, Rockville, MD, 1987.
14. Holden, C: Is alcoholism treatment effective? Science 236:20-22, 1987.
15. Rachin RL, editor: Job-based programs for alcohol and drug problems, Journal of Drug Issues 2:1, 1981.
16. How business grapples with problem of the drinking worker, U.S. News and World Report, p 76, June 15, 1974.
17. Rundell OH and Paredes A: Benefit—cost methodology in the evaluation of therapeutic services for alcoholism, Alcoholism: Clinical and Experimental Research 3(4): 324-333, 1979.
18. Holden C: Alcoholism: on-the-job-referrals mean early detection, treatment, Science 179:363, 1973.
19. Crothers TD: Morphinism and narcomanias from other drugs, reprinted edition, New York, 1981, Arno Press.
20. Latimer D and Goldberg J: Flowers in the blood: the story of opium, New York, 1981, Franklin Watts.
21. Krill-Smith S: Naltrexone treatment. In Patterns and trends in drug abuse: a national and international perspective, Washington DC, 1985, NIDA Publication, US Government Printing Office.

22. Methadone maintenance: how much, for whom, for how long? Medical World News pp 53-63, March 17, 1972.

23. Dole VP, Nyswander ME, and Warner A: Successful treatment of 750 criminal addicts, Journal of the American Medical Association 206:2708-2714, 1968.

24. Myerson DJ: Methadone treatment of addicts, New England Journal of Medicine 281:390-391, 1969.

25. Hargreaves WA: Methadone dosage and duration for maintenance treatment. In Cooper JR et al, editors: Research on the treatment of narcotic addiction: state of the art, DHHS Publication (ADM)83-1281, Washington, DC, 1983, US Government Printing Office.

26. Trebach AS: The heroin solution, New Haven, 1982, Yale University Press.

27. Hubbard RL, Allison M, Bray RM and others: An overview of client characteristics, treatment services, and during-treatment outcomes for outpatient methadone clinics in the treatment outcomes prospective study (TOPS). In Cooper JR et al, editors: Research on the treatment of narcotic addiction: state of the art, Washington, DC, 1983, DHHS Publication No (ADM)83-1281, US Government Printing Office.

28. Waldorf D, Orlich M, and Reinerman C: Morphine maintenance: the Shreveport clinic 1919-1923, Washington DC, 1974, The Drug Abuse Council, Inc.

29. Lindesmith, AR: The addict and the law, Bloomington, Ind, 1965, Indiana University Press.

30. Brecher EM: Licit and illicit drugs, Chapter 12, Boston, 1972, Little, Brown & Co.

31. Lindsey R: Synanon's founder tells how his group changed, New York Times p D12, December 22, 1980.

32. Simpson DD and Sells SB: Evaluation of drug abuse treatment effectiveness: summary of the DARP follow-up research, Washington, DC, 1982, DHHS Publication No (ADM)82-1194, US Government Printing Office.

33. Allison M, Hubbard RL, and Rachal JV: Treatment process in methadone, residential, and outpatient drug free programs, Washington, DC, 1985, DHHS Publication No (ADM) 85-1388, US Government Printing Office.

34. Craddock SG, Bray RM, and Hubbard RL: drug use before and during treatment: 1979-1981 TOPS Admission Cohorts, DHHS Publication (ADM) 85-1387, Washington, DC 1985, US Government Printing Office.

35. Patterns and trends in drug abuse: a national and international perspective, Washington, DC, 1985, NIDA Publication, US Government Printing Office.

36. Treatment of cocaine abuse, NIDA Notes, p 10, December, 1985.

37. Barnes, DM: Breaking the cycle of addiction, Science 241:1029-1030, 1988.

38. Kicking cocaine: experimental therapies ease withdrawal, American Health, p 10, April, 1986.

39. Classically conditioned responses in opioid and cocaine dependence: a role in relapse? In Ray BA, editor, Learning factors in substance abuse, NIDA Research monograph 84. DHHS Publication No (ADM)88-1576, Washington, DC, 1988, US Government Printing Office.

Chapter 19

Drugs and Athletics

OBJECTIVES

After reading this chapter, you should be able to:

Understand the historical development of the use of performance-enhancing drugs by athletes, and of attempts to regulate drug use by athletes.

Be familiar with major concepts and terms such as ergogenic aids and anabolic and androgenic steroids, and understand the importance of psychological factors such as the masking of fatigue in evaluating the performance-enhancing properties of drugs.

Understand what experimental research as well as the experience of athletes tells us about the effects of stimulant drugs on performance, as well as the side effects and dangers of stimulant drug use.

Understand what experimental research and experience tell us about the effects of anabolic steroids on muscular development and strength, as well as the side effects and dangers of anabolic steroids.

Why so much concern over drug use by athletes? Why not focus on drug use by clarinet players or muffler repairmen? There are several answers to this question, and together they demonstrate that there are special reasons to be concerned about drug use in sports. First, there are many athletes who become famous, and through their fame and the fact that they portray youth, strength, and health, they are often seen as role models for young people. When well-known athletes are reported to be using cocaine or some other illicit substance, there is concern that impressionable young people will see drug use in a more positive light. After all, haven't corporate sponsors paid famous athletes to endorse their products, from shoes to breakfast cereal, based on this presumed influence over young consumers? Second, some of the drugs used by athletes are intended to give the user an advantage over the competition, an advantage that is clearly viewed as being unfair. This is inconsistent with our tradition of fair play in sports, and widespread "cheating" of any kind tends to diminish a sport and to diminish public interest in it. Professional wrestling, which is widely viewed as being "rigged" or "staged," is enjoyed more as a form of comic entertainment than as an athletic contest. Most professional and amateur sportspeople guard their honor carefully, and the use of performance-enhancing drugs is seen as a threat to that honor. Third, there is a concern that both the famous and the not-so-famous athletes who use drugs are endangering their health and perhaps their lives for the sake of a temporary burst of power or speed. To the extent that there are real risks associated with the use of these drugs, athletes should be aware of those risks. Since these drugs are often obtained illicitly, we can assume that the providers of the drugs do not present a balanced cost-vs-benefit analysis to the potential user, but instead probably maximize any possible benefit and minimize the dangers.

HISTORICAL USE OF DRUGS IN ATHLETICS

Although we tend to think of drug use by athletes as a recent phenomenon, the use of chemicals to enhance performance may be as old as sport itself. As with many early drugs, some of these concoctions seemed to make sense at the time, but probably had only placebo value. We no longer think that the powdered hooves of an ass will make our feet fly as fast as that animal's, but perhaps it was a belief in that powder that helped the ancient Egyptian competitor's self-confidence. Also, if the other guys are all using it, why take chances?

The early Greek olympians did use various herbs and mushrooms that may have had some pharmacological actions as stimulants, and early Aztec athletes used a cactus-based stimulant resembling strychnine. Since the earliest athletic competitions probably developed in tribal societies as a means of training and preparation for war or for hunting, and since various psychoactive plants were used by tribal peoples during battles or hunts, it is not surprising that the drugs were also used in "sports" from the earliest times.

During the 1800s and early 1900s three types of stimulants were reported to be in use by athletes. Strychnine, which became famous as a rat poison, can at low doses act as a central nervous system stimulant. However, if the dose is too high, seizure activity will be produced in the brain. The resulting convulsions may paralyze respiration, leading to death. At least some boxers were re-

ported to have used strychnine tablets. This may have made them more aggressive and kept them from tiring very quickly, but it was a dangerous way to do it. We'll never know how many of those rugged heroes were killed in this way, but there must have been a few. Thomas Hicks won the marathon in the 1904 St. Louis Olympics, then collapsed and had to be revived. His race was partly fueled by a mixture of brandy and strychnine.[1,p.5] Although the availability of amphetamines later made such dangerous drugs as strychnine less attractive, there is some evidence that occasional use of strychnine continued at the level of world competition into the 1960s. Cocaine was also available in the 1800s, at first in the form of Mariani's Coca Wine (used by the French cycling team), which was referred to in some advertisements as "wine for athletes."[2,p.33] When pure cocaine became available it was quickly adopted into sports. Also, while many athletes used coffee as a mild stimulant, some added pure caffeine to their coffee or took caffeine tablets. There are numerous reports of the suspected "doping" of swimmers, cyclists, boxers, runners, and other athletes during this period. Then, as now, some of the suspicions were raised by the losers who may or may not have had any evidence of doping. Our use of the word "dope" for illicit drugs is derived from a Dutch word used in South Africa to refer to a cheap brandy, which was sometimes given to racing dogs or horses to slow them down. From this came the idea of "doping" horses and then people, more often in an effort to improve rather than impair performance. Dogs and horses received all the substances used by humans, including coca wine and cocaine, prior to the days of dope testing.

It isn't clear when athletes first started using amphetamines for their stimulant effects, but it was probably not long after the drugs were introduced in the 1930s. Amphetamines were widely used throughout the world during World War II, and in the 1940s and 50s there were reports of the use of these "pep pills" by professional soccer players in England and Italy. Boxers and cyclists also relied on this new synthetic energy source. More potent than caffeine, longer-lasting than co-

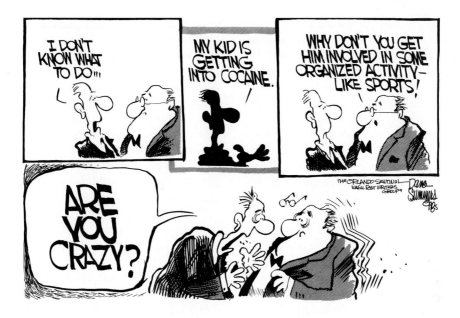

caine, and safer than strychnine, it seemed to be the ideal **ergogenic** (energy-producing) drug for both training and competition. In 1952 the presence of syringes and broken ampules in the speed skating locker room at the Oslo Winter Olympics was an indication of amphetamine's presence in international competition. There were other reports from the 1952 summer games in Helsinki and the 1956 Melbourne Olympics. Unfortunately, several deaths during this period were attributed to overdoses of amphetamines and/or other drugs. By the time of the 1960 Rome games, amphetamine use had spread around the world and to most sports. On opening day a Danish cyclist died during time trials. An autopsy revealed that his death due to "sunstroke" was aided by the presence of amphetamine, which reduces blood flow to the skin, making it more difficult for the body to cool itself. Three other cyclists collapsed that day, and two were hospitalized.[1,p.6] This and other examples of amphetamine abuse led to investigations and to antidoping laws in France and Belgium. Other nations, including the United States, seemed less concerned. Some sports, especially cycling, began to test competi-

tors for drugs on a sporadic basis. Throughout the 1960s there were instances of athletes refusing to submit to tests or failing tests and being disqualified. These early testing efforts were not enough to prevent the death of cyclist Tommy Simpson, an ex-world champion, who died during the 1967 Tour de France. His death was seen on television, and weeks later it was reported that his body contained two different types of amphetamine, and that drugs had been found in his luggage. This led in 1968 to the establishment by the International Olympic Committee of rules requiring the disqualification of any competitor who refuses to take a drug test or who is found guilty of using banned drugs. Beginning with fewer than 700 urine tests at the 1968 Mexico City Olympics, each subsequent international competition has had more testing, more disqualifications, and more controversy.

Most Americans did not seem to be too concerned about drug use by athletes until reports surfaced in the late 1960s and early 1970s that professional football players were using amphetamines during games. Prior to that time, people might not have been very concerned about it even if they had known. You should remember from Chapter 7 that amphetamine underwent a major status change in the United States during the 1960s. For years an increasing number of Americans had used amphetamines to keep them awake, provide extra energy, or to lose weight. They were seen by most people as legal, harmless, "pep pills." It was in that context that the team physicians for professional football teams ordered large quantities of the drugs as a routine part of their supplies, and trainers dispensed them liberally. By the end of the 1960s amphetamine was widely considered to be a drug of abuse and a dangerous drug that could lead to violent behavior. In this context, revelations that many professionals were playing "high" made for sensational headlines. Several National Football League (NFL) players sued their teams for injuries received while playing under the influence of drugs, and the NFL officially banned amphetamine use in 1971. Although the drugs were no longer condoned by the league, the NFL did little at that time to enforce the ban, except to request copies of each team's orders for medical supplies. Athletes who wanted amphetamines still obtained and used them, often through a legal prescription.

During and after World War II it was found that malnourished people could gain weight and build themselves up more rapidly if they were given the male hormone testosterone. Although it is easy for an American to be biased about such things, it does appear that the Soviets were the first to put this hormone to use on a wide scale to build up their athletes. An American team physician at the 1956 Olympics reported that the Soviet athletes were using straight testosterone, sometimes in excessive doses and with unfortunate side effects. Testosterone not only helps both men and women become more muscular, its masculinizing effects on women and enlargement of the prostate gland in men are definite drawbacks. The American physician came back to the United States and helped to develop and test the more selective **anabolic** steroids, which were quickly adopted by American weightlifters and bodybuilders. American and British athletes in such events as discus and shotput were the first to acknowl-

edge publicly that they had used steroids, and there was evidence that steroid use was widespread during the 1960s in most track and field events. These drugs were not officially banned nor were they tested for in international competition until the early 1970s, mainly because a sensitive urine test was not available until then. Of the 2000 urine samples taken during the 1976 Olympics, fewer than 300 were tested for the presence of steroids, and eight of those were positive.[1,p.13] The first international athletes to be found guilty of taking steroids were a Bulgarian discus thrower, a Romanian shotputter, a Polish female discus thrower, and weightlifters from several countries. By that time, the situation appeared to be that individual Western athletes may have chosen to use steroids, but some of the East European countries seemed to have adopted their use almost as a matter of official policy. When the East German swimming coach was asked during the 1976 Olympics why so many of their women swimmers had deep voices, the answer was, "we have come here to swim, not sing."[3,p.19]

During the 1980s, public revelations of drug use by athletes became commonplace, and cocaine was often mentioned. Professional basketball, baseball, and football players in the United States were being sent into treatment centers for cocaine dependence, and several either dropped out or were kicked out of professional sports. Most amateur and professional sports organizations adopted longer and more complicated lists of banned substances, as well as rules providing for more and more participants to be tested. For example, the U.S. National Collegiate Athletic Association adopted in 1986 a list of over 3000 brand name drugs containing banned substances.[4] All participants are to be tested during the championship contest and after all postseason football games. In many events around the world, all contestants must now be subjected to urine tests as a matter of routine.

At the end of the 1980s, some were beginning to question the wisdom of trying to test every athlete for everything. In spite of the enormous expense to which sports organizations have gone, the use of steroids, stimulants, and other perfor-

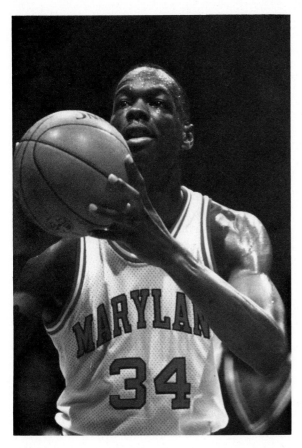

University of Maryland basketball star Len Bias died of heart failure after using cocaine.

Your turn: winning

Imagine that you have gone out for the track team. You compete in the 3000 meter races and have been training hard for the past 2 years. It seems as though you have worked as hard as you could every day, yet it's clear that your times have gotten as fast as they're going to get. The conference championships are tomorrow. Your parents have traveled 300 miles to see you run, and lots of your friends will be there cheering you on. You know your own times, and you know the competition, and, although you expect a close race for the top three spots, you figure to come in fourth. You yourself have never used any type of stimulant drug, but you have heard rumors that several of the fastest runners take amphetamines before the race, and you suspect that it is true. Your conference has not yet adopted a drug-screening program for track, however, so there's no way to know for sure.

Under these circumstances, what would you do if:

1. A guy that you don't know very well but who you heard is a drug dealer offers you some "speed" just for the race?
2. A friend of yours has some prescription diet pills that contain amphetamine, and the friend offers you one?
3. You are offered some cocaine to snort right before the race?
4. You are offered an OTC asthma pill that contains ephedrine?
5. You are offered coffee or tea?

Or would you rather not take artificial stimulants at all, come in fourth, and know you did your best and ran a clean race?

---

mance-enhancing substances seems to some to be as great as ever. At a 1989 meeting on drug use sponsored by the international governing body for track,[5] that organization's medical chairman said, "You start to approach a limit that society has the right to say, 'stop'." He was talking not about drug use but about expensive and intrusive drug testing.

STIMULANTS AS PERFORMANCE-ENHANCERS

The first question to be answered about the use of a drug to increase energy or otherwise enhance athletic performance is: does it work? We might not worry so much about unfair competition if we

didn't feel that the use of a drug would in fact help the person using it. There is another reason why it would be nice if these drugs were ineffective: if we could prove that, then we could presumably convince young people not to take the risk of using drugs because there would be no gain to be had. It is worthwhile pointing out that experiments can never prove that a drug has no effect—you may have done a hundred experiments and not used the right dose or the right test (peak output? endurance? accuracy?). The possibility always exists that someone could come along later with the right combination to demonstrate a beneficial effect. Therefore, be wary when someone tries to use scientific evidence to argue that some drug "doesn't work," "has no effect," "is not toxic," or is otherwise inactive.

We've had a pretty good idea of the effectiveness of amphetamine since 1959, when Smith and Beecher published the results of a double-blind study comparing amphetamine and placebo in runners, swimmers, and weight throwers.[6] Their conclusion was that most of the athletes performed better under amphetamine, but the improvement was small (a few percentage points' improvement). There have been several studies that reported no differences or very small differences in performance, and some medical experts in the 1960s wanted to argue that amphetamines were essentially ineffective and there was no reason for people to use them. An excellent 1981 review of the existing literature put it all into perspective.[7] Pointing out that it had been taking athletes an average of about 7 years for each 1% improvement in the world record speed for the mile run, if amphetamine produces even a 1% improvement it could make an important difference at that level of competition. Their conclusion: "There is an amphetamine margin. It is usually small, amounting to a few percent under most circumstances. But even when that tiny, it can surely spell the difference between a gold medal and sixth place."

Whether amphetamine or other stimulants increase the physical ability (provide "pep," or energy) or act through a psychological mechanism only is an interesting question that cannot be answered at this point. Surely a person who feels more confident may train harder, compete with a winning attitude, try harder, and keep trying longer. With amphetamine, improvements have been seen both in events requiring brief, explosive power (shotput) and in events requiring endurance, such as distance running. In laboratory studies, increases have been found in isometric strength and in work output during endurance testing on a bicycle ergometer (the subjects rode longer under amphetamine conditions). This endurance improvement may be due to the masking of fatigue effects, allowing a person to compete to utter exhaustion (resulting in the deaths of several cyclists, for example).

Caffeine has also been shown to improve endurance performance under laboratory conditions. In one experiment, 330 mg of caffeine (approximately equivalent to three cups of brewed coffee) increased the length of a bicycle ergometer "ride" by almost 20%. In another experiment, when subjects rode for 2 hours, their total energy output was 7% higher after 500 mg caffeine than in the control condition.[8]

We are not aware of any controlled laboratory or field experiments testing the performance-enhancing capabilities of cocaine, but there are certainly athletes who believe in its power, and since its stimulant properties are generally similar to those of amphetamine we can assume that it would be effective under some circumstances. Given cocaine's shorter duration of action, it would not be expected to improve endurance over a several-hour period as well as either amphetamine or caffeine.

With all these and several other CNS stimulants banned by most sports associations, some athletes have continued to use them during training, to allow them to run or ride or swim harder. They then do not use the drug for several days before the competition or during the competition, hoping that traces of the substance will not appear in the urine test. This might make sense, but no one knows the effect of training under one drug condition and competing under another condition. Also, it is possibly during training that overexertion under the influence of a fatigue-masking drug might be most dangerous, leading to muscle injury, a fall or other accident, or, expecially under hot conditions, to the dangerous condition of exhaustion referred to as "sunstroke."

Athletes and others who use amphetamines or cocaine regularly run the risk of developing a dependence on the drug, of developing paranoid or violent behavior patterns, and of suffering from the loss of energy and psychological depression that occur as the drugs wear off (Chapter 7).

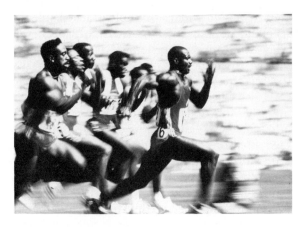

Canadian Olympian Ben Johnson lost his gold medal after testing positive for steroid use.

STEROIDS

The male sex hormone **testosterone** has two major types of effect on the developing human male. **Androgenic** effects refer to the masculinizing actions: initial growth of the penis and other male sex glands, deepening of the voice, and increased facial hair are examples.This steroid hormone also has **anabolic** effects (promoting constructive metabolism; building tissue). These include increased muscle mass, increases in the size of various internal organs, control of the distribution of body fat, increased protein synthesis, and increased calcium in the bones. Beginning in the 1950s, drug companies synthesized various steroids that have less of the androgenic effects and more of the anabolic effects than testosterone. These are referred to as "anabolic steroids," although none of them is entirely without some masculinizing effect.

Whether or not these drugs are effective in improving athletic performance has been controversial: for many years the medical position was that they are not, whereas the lore around the locker room was that they would make anyone bigger, stronger, and more masculine-looking. A lot of people must have had more faith in the locker-room lore than in the "official" word. The 1989 Physician's Desk Reference contains the following statement in bold-face type: "**Anabolic Steroids Have Not Been Shown To Enhance Athletic Ability.**" Try telling that to Ben Johnson, the disqualified winner of the 1988 Olympic Gold Medal in the 100-meter run, or to the people who ran against him.

There is no doubt that testosterone has a tremendous effect on muscle mass and strength during puberty, and experiments on castrated animals can clearly show the muscle-developing ability of the synthetic anabolics.[9] What is not so clear is the effect of adding additional anabolic stimulation to adult males who already have high circulating levels of testosterone. Laboratory research on healthy males who are engaged in weight training and are maintained on a proper diet has often found small increases in lean muscle mass, and sometimes also small increases in muscular strength. There is no evidence for an overall increase in aerobic capacity or endurance in those studies. However, it may never be possible to conduct experiments demonstrating the effectiveness of the high doses used by some athletes. Many athletes report that they take 10 or more times the recommended therapeutic doses of anabolic steroids.[10] In addition, it is common practice for athletes to take more than one steroid at a time (both an oral and an injectable form, for example). This practice is known as "stacking." To expose research subjects to such massive doses would clearly be unethical.

Another impediment to doing careful research on this topic is that these steroids do produce detectable psychological effects. When double-blind experiments have been attempted, the subjects almost always know when they are on steroids, thus destroying the blind control.[11] This is important, because steroid users report that they feel they can lift more or work harder when they are on the steroids. This may be due to central nervous system effects of the steroids leading to a stimulant-like feeling of energy and loss of fatigue, or to increased aggressiveness expressed as more aggressive training, or there could be a good dose of placebo effect operating, enhanced by the clear sensation that the drug is doing something, because you can "feel" it. Some of the scientists

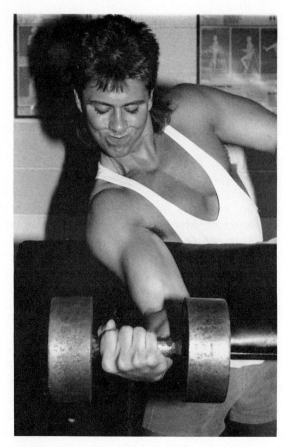

Young body builders who use steroids run many health risks.

studying steroid hormones believe that their main effects are psychological, combined with a "bloating" effect on the muscle, in which the muscle retains more fluids, is larger and weighs more, but has no more physical strength.[1,p.49]

The reported psychological effects, including a stimulant-like "high" and increased aggressiveness, might be beneficial for increasing the amount of work done during training and for increasing the intensity of effort during competition. However, there are also concerns that these psychological effects might produce great problems, especially at high doses. One concern that has

been expressed is that a psychological dependence seems to develop in some users, who feel well when they are on the steroids, but become depressed when they are off. Since many users take the drugs in cycles, this up-and-down mood swing may also interfere with social relationships and other life functions. There has been a great deal of discussion about "roid rage," a kind of manic rage that has been reported by some steroid users.[12] We should be careful on the basis of uncontrolled retrospective reports to attribute instances of violence to a drug, especially when the perpetrator of a violent crime may be looking for an excuse.[13] However, there are a sufficient number of reports of violent feelings and actions among steroid users for us to be concerned and to await further research.

There are also many concerns about the effects of steroid use on the body. In young users who have not attained their full height, these steroids may cause premature closing of the growth plates of the long bones, thus limiting their adult height. For all users, the risk of peliosis hepatitis (bloody cysts in the liver) and the changes in blood lipids possibly leading to atherosclerosis, high blood pressure, and heart disease are potentially serious concerns. Acne and baldness are reported, as is atrophy of the testes and the development of feminine breasts in men.

There are special considerations when females use these anabolic steroids. Because females usually have only trace amounts of testosterone produced by the adrenals, the addition of even relatively small doses of anabolic steroids can have dramatic effects, in terms of both muscle growth and masculinization. Some of the side effects are reversible, such as mild acne, decreased breast size, and fluid retention. The enlargement of the clitoris may be reversible if steroid use is stopped soon after it is noticed. Other effects, such as increased facial hair and deepening of the voice, may be irreversible.[11]

As we found in Chapter 2, when a drug produces dependence, violent crime, and toxic side effects, society may feel justified in trying to place special restrictions on the drug's availability. In 1988, congressional hearings were held on the notion of placing anabolic steroids on the list of controlled substances. Evidence was presented that a large black market has developed for these drugs, amounting to perhaps $100 million dollars per year. In addition, there is concern that adolescent boys, many of whom are not athletic at all, have begun to use steroids in the belief that they will quickly become more muscular and "macho" looking.[14] Although no decision was made on this issue in 1988, prominent sports physicians will probably keep up the pressure for controlled substance scheduling.[15]

OTHER HORMONAL MANIPULATIONS

While the anabolic steroids have been in wide use, other treatments have been experimented with on a more limited basis. Female sex hormones have been used to feminize males so that they can compete in women's events. The woman's gold medal sprinter in the 1964 Olympics was shown by chromosome testing to be a male; she/he had to return the medal! Steroid receptor blocking drugs have probably been used to delay puberty in female gymnasts. In women, puberty shifts the center of gravity lower in the body and changes body proportions in ways that adversely affect ability. Smaller women appear to be more graceful, spin faster on the uneven bars, and generally have the advantage, which is why top female gymnasts are usually in their teens. However, the Soviets have been suspected of tampering with nature: their top three international gymnasts in 1978 were all 17 or 18 years old, but their heights and weights were: 53 inches, 63 pounds, 60 inches, 90 pounds; and 57 inches, 79 pounds.

We have certainly not seen the end of growth-promoting hormonal treatments. Human growth hormone, which is released from the pituitary gland, can potentially increase the height and weight of an individual to gigantic proportions, especially if administered during childhood and adolescence. In fact, in rare instances the excessive production of this hormone creates giants well over 7 feet tall. These giants usually have died at an early age because their internal organs continue to grow. However, administration of a few doses of this hormone at the right time might produce a more controlled increase in body size. Likewise, the growth hormone-releasing hormone, and some of the cellular intermediary hormones by which growth hormone exerts its effects might prove useful. It is not currently possible to test for the presence of these substances, and in spite of the possible dangers the lure of an otherwise capable basketball player growing a couple of inches taller or of a football player being 30 pounds heavier will no doubt cause many young athletes to experiment with these substances when they become more available.[11]

Summary

Although drugs and other performance-enhancing techniques have been used by athletes throughout history, within the past two decades there has been a great deal of publicity and concern over what appears to be massive use of several types of ergogenic drugs.

The use of CNS stimulant drugs appears to have increased and spread throughout most sports with the use of amphetamines during the 1950s and 1960s. Amphetamine and caffeine have both been shown to increase work output and to mask the effects of fatigue, and those substances as well as cocaine are still being used by athletes. Athletes who are likely to be urine tested during competition may use the drugs only for training.

Anabolic steroids are capable of increasing muscle mass and probably strength, although it has been difficult to separate the psychological stimulant-like effect of these drugs from the physical effects on the muscles themselves. These steroids may also produce a variety of dangerous and sometimes irreversible side effects.

The future of this area promises to be a frustrating one, with technological advances in growth-promoting hormones, a strong motivation for young athletes to experiment with them, continued difficulty in doing appropriate and ethical controlled research, increasingly expensive testing procedures to detect more and more new substances, and increasingly sophisticated ways of cheating without getting caught.

REFERENCES

1. Donohue, T., and Johnson, N.: Foul play: drug abuse in sports, Oxford, Basil Blackwell, 1986.
2. Asken, M.J.: Dying to win: the athlete's guide to safe and unsafe drugs in sports, Washington, D.C., Acropolis, 1988.
3. Goldman, B.: Death in the locker room, South Bend, Indiana, Icarus Press, 1984.
4. National Collegiate Athletic Association: NCAA banned drugs reference list, NCAA, Mission, Kansas, 1986.
5. News report from Monte Carlo, Monaco, June 6, 1989.
6. Smith, G.M., and Beecher, H.K.: Amphetamine sulfate and athletic performance, Journal of the American Medical Association 170:542-557, 1959.
7. Laties, V.G., and Weiss, B.: The amphetamine margin in sports, Federation Proceedings, 40:2689-2692, 1981.
8. Noble, B.J.: Physiology of exercise and sport, St. Louis, Times Mirror Mosby, 1986.
9. Williams, M.H.: Ergogenic aids in sports, Champaign, Illinois, Human Kinetics Publishers, 1983.
10. Marshall, E.: The drug of champions, Science 242:183-184, 1988.
11. Taylor W.N.: Hormonal manipulation: a new era of monstrous athletes, Jefferson, N.C., McFarland & Co., 1985.
12. Pope, H.G., and Katz, D.L.: Affective and psychotic symptoms associated with anabolic steroid use, American Journal of Psychiatry 145:487-490, 1988.
13. Lubell, A.: Does steroid abuse cause—or excuse—violence? Physician and Sportsmedicine 17:176-185, 1989.
14. Toufexis, A.: Shortcut to the Rambo look, Time, January 30, 1989, p.78.
15. Taylor, W.N.: Synthetic anabolic-androgenic steroids: a plea of controlled substance status, Physician and Sportsmedicine 15:140-149, 1987.

Chapter 20

A Rational Look at Drug Use

OBJECTIVES

After reading this chapter, you should be able to:

Discuss drug effects and the safety of drugs from the perspective of society at large.

Describe how changes in society have changed our drug-using habits.

Describe the factors that go into labeling a particular type of drug use as drug abuse.

Give some examples of the functions of psychoactive drugs in meeting social needs.

Explain why drug abuse is a social, legal, and political issue much more than it is a medical issue.

In our search to understand drugs and society, we've been almost everywhere–from the Andes to Vienna, from Turkey to the suburbs, from the laboratory to the streets of every city. To what end? Why? For one reason, to know that the drug situation is not new; we have been where we are now many times before. At the same time, we have never been where we are now, never in 4000 years.

How are we the same and how are we different from earlier periods of high drug use? What general principles can be derived about the use of psychoactive drugs? Not concepts about specific drugs in specific societies, but broad principles about the interactions that occur repeatedly among drugs, individuals, and society. Three of these principles are so pervasive and fundamental that they have appeared repeatedly in the preceding chapters. Remember them well.

Basic to any understanding of the problems in the area of drug use, misuse, and abuse is the realization that drug taking is behavior. As such it follows the same rules and can be understood and modified to the same extent as any other kind of behavior. People don't take drugs for the hell of it; they use drugs because they provide an increase in satisfaction or a reduction in discomfort.

Drug use does not occur in isolation; it occurs in

and is understandable only within a context. Drug use is not foreign to the American heritage or the present social milieu. The drug problem is not a tumor that can be plucked from the bosom of society. Drug use and abuse are an integral part of the fabric of our evolving social philosophy. To change patterns of drug use requires changing the social context.

It is not true that the drug problem is a war to be won or lost. Most past and present thinking has been based on the idea that *we* are fighting *them*—the enemy, drug abuse. Unfortunately, Pogo was right: We have met the enemy . . . and they is us. There is no war to be won; like death, taxes, and poverty, there will always be drug problems.

A major goal of this chapter is to consider all of the general principles and to draw some conclusions. Of particular importance are the implications of these principles for the present culture. Finally, after reviewing the major themes and considering their implications, a rational view of drug use today in our society seems possible.

THEMES AND PRINCIPLES
Dimensions and Determinants of Drug Effects

What are the determinants of the behavioral effects of a psychoactive drug? They are multiple and range from pharmacological and biochemical factors to the cultural history and social setting of the user. There is no simple answer to the general question, what is *the* behavioral effect of *this* drug? Nevertheless, at the most fundamental level, all drugs used recreationally on a regular basis directly or indirectly either increase pleasure or decrease discomfort. However, individuals and cultures may differ greatly in whether a particular effect is experienced as pleasant or unpleasant.

To find the common physiological threads weaving through the psychoactive drug experiences, only two broad dimensions of brain activity need to be considered for our purposes: level of arousal and information processing. The activity level of the brain is increased by stimulants, such as caffeine, amphetamine, and cocaine, and de-

creased by depressants, including alcohol and barbiturates. The action of these drugs seems primarily to be through their effect on the reticular formation. Some agents, such as LSD, have an alteration of activation level as a secondary rather than a primary effect.

Most of the drugs that have been adopted by western culture are those primarily affecting arousal level. Perhaps stimulation or depression, and thus a loss of inhibitions, has been compatible with our aggressively achieving but tightly moral society. Caffeine, amphetamine, and cocaine may make us achieve more or may only make us feel that we are achieving more. Alcohol provides us with an excuse to "let down our hair" and do a few things we otherwise wouldn't do. Whether speeded up or slowed down, the user is still focused on the outside "real world."

The distortion-of-information-processing dimension results from one of two types of actions on the nervous system. The distortion can result from alterations of the primary or secondary sensory input pathways, or it can result from impaired retrieval and processing of memories. The hallucinogens, LSD, mescaline, and hashish have their primary effect on the information-processing systems. Images, colors—all experiences—are partly unreal when hallucinogenic drugs are employed. Only at the extremes of the arousal dimension—high activation or extreme depression—does distortion of information processing become an important feature of drugs that primarily influence level of arousal.

Drugs that alter information processing have traditionally been foreign to western civilization. There are probably many reasons for this fact, but one of them certainly has to be that by providing "multiple realities," hallucinogens would impair the single focus that is essential for rapid scientific and technological progress. Yet, after a period of flirtation both with the individual consciousness (as opposed to social consciousness) and with the hallucinogenic drugs, America in the 1980s went right back to achievement orientation and to cocaine (a stimulant) and alcohol as major recreational substances.

Throughout the book it has been demonstrated that to discuss drug use meaningfully it is essential to specify dosage range, mode of administration, frequency of use, and setting in which use occurs. The chewing of coca leaves is a far cry from smoking crack, even though some people simply categorize both as drug misuse. The mild relaxation and euphoria accompanying marijuana smoking have only a tenuous behavioral connection with the very personal hallucinations of hashish.

Expectations are of great importance in determining the effect of an agent, as seen most vividly in work done with placebos. The belief that an authority, the physician, is giving a medicine that will have a specific effect is frequently enough to *in fact* produce the effect, even though an inert agent has been used. The expectations an individual has about various drugs obviously develop from his personal history of experiences and needs that occur in a social context. For this reason it is important that the social context present accurate and credible information about what a drug can and cannot do.

It cannot be emphasized too strongly that the greater the role played by mechanisms of consciousness and the integration of information in producing a drug's effects, the more variable these effects can be. A drug may have very specific biochemical actions and still have quite variable behavioral effects. Such variability results because drugs do not create new patterns of nervous system activity. Rather, they serve only to modify already existing patterns, most of which are the result of an individual's unique personal experiences. That is, these psychoactive drugs act by altering *ongoing information processing* and retrieval of *already stored memories*.

Psychoactive drugs, then, do not add new components to experience, or awareness, or consciousness. They may shape the existing components differently, distort them, mute or intensify them, but the drugs do not take the user beyond himself and his environment. If, in fact, each of us carries some of his own personal heaven or hell, then these agents may make it easier to experience each of these.

In spite of the uniqueness of the drug experience resulting from an interplay of all these factors, generalizations about the effects of these chemicals can be made because of three facts. First, the drugs do have specific biochemical actions (even if they are in part unknown) on areas, functions, or processes of the brain. This means that the range of effects an agent can produce is somewhat restricted. Second, the general culture, as well as the small subgroups in which each of us lives, presents a narrow range of experiences, hopes, and fears. It is from this set of possible experiences that drug effects must be selected. Last, one is taught which drug effects should be sought and emphasized and which are to be minimized. We learn, to some extent, whether the drug-induced effects are to be labeled as desirable or undesirable.

How Safe Are Drugs?

There are at least three ways in which the harmfulness of a drug can be considered. One is the common medical usage referring to the toxic effects and lethality resulting from the use of the drug. Both short-term and long-term toxic effects need to be identified (these may be different). Furthermore, all statements refer only to what is now known. Toxic effects that may appear tomorrow cannot be predicted today. Therefore, medically speaking, the basic rule is to approach all drugs with respect and with caution.

From a medical point of view no drug is safe. With some doses, modes of administration, and frequency of use, all drugs cause toxic effects and even death. It is equally true that at some doses, modes of administration, and frequency of use all drugs are safe. The concern here is whether a drug, *used the way most people use it today,* is physically harmful. From this position, alcohol and marijuana are relatively safe drugs the way most people use them. Nicotine, in contrast, is a very harmful drug, since the usual amount of cigarette smoking does increase mortality rate. (Appreciate, however, that when cigarette smoking began, the lethal effects were much less; people smoked

---

Your turn: social acceptance of drugs

Everyone in our society has been exposed to the idea of drug use, if not directly exposed to each of the drugs. It might be interesting to see how several of your friends react to the idea of someone else using each of several drugs. Try making a chart listing cigarettes, chewing tobacco, alcohol, marijuana, cocaine, heroin, and any other drugs you want. Make some copies and ask several of your friends to put a number from +5 to −5 next to each drug, based on how they would feel about being around someone who was using that drug. Look for consistencies among the group that you ask, and then compare the average ratings with the use data in Chapter 1. Are the more widely used drugs more acceptable to your friends?

---

fewer cigarettes and also did not live long enough for much of the cigarette-induced mortality to appear! If cigarettes appeared today for the first time, it would probably be no more than 5 to 10 years before their contribution to mortality would be identified.)

The regular use of intravenous injections makes any drug dangerous. The possibility of hepatitis, AIDS, general infection, or an overdose clearly labels the usual form of heroin as medically dangerous. The fact that the users of these drugs frequently are also malnourished, with all that implies, only contributes to making the usual use of these agents clearly medically harmful.

Not so easy to categorize as medically safe or dangerous are hallucinogens. In the normal, illegal, street use of these agents there is no way of knowing what drug is actually being used, or the purity of the agent, or the dosage, or whether one or more drugs are contained in the dose as taken. Under these conditions it is not surprising that bad trips, deaths, and long-term psychiatric hospitalizations do occur. Perhaps this situation parallels that seen in the realm of the over-the-counter drugs—safe if used as directed. When purity, dose, and other factors are controlled, hallucinogens have not resulted in a high incidence of adverse

effects. Aspirin is a reasonably safe drug even though about 100 youngsters die annually because of misuse. Oral use of pure hallucinogens is medically more dangerous than oral use of aspirin but not as physically dangerous as regular, moderate cigarette smoking.

An increasing number of individuals are beginning to emphasize other implications of the word "harmful." This position considers the personal-social aspect of a drug's use to be of paramount importance. The question here is, to what extent does use of the drug lead to, or contribute to, a major disruption of the individual's relationship to society? That is, does the use of the drug impair the interaction of the user and the existing culture?

When concern is directed to the degree of drug-induced impairment of the relationship between a user and society, different pictures appear. Nicotine is used regularly without greatly impairing the user's interaction with the world (up to the point where cigarette smoking causes hospitalization or death). Alcohol, however, is not harmless, since at least 10% of those who use it at all use it to an extent that they are unable to function in society. The data are not as well established with respect to marijuana, but many feel that the incidence and extent of social impairment are about the same for users of alcohol and marijuana.

The injected agents and crack also score high as dangerous drugs when impairment of social functioning is considered. Few heroin or intravenous stimulant users or crack smokers manage to maintain a useful relationship with society. It is not easy to categorize the use of hallucinogens, since the data are fragmentary. Users who center their life, for one reason or another, around the use of these drugs become drop-outs and certainly fail to make any contribution to the present society. However, there must also be many occasional and irregular users who do maintain their positions in society, but a percentage division is not possible.

A third possibility is that the use of a drug may also have important interrelations with social trends in the culture. Concern is not with the med-

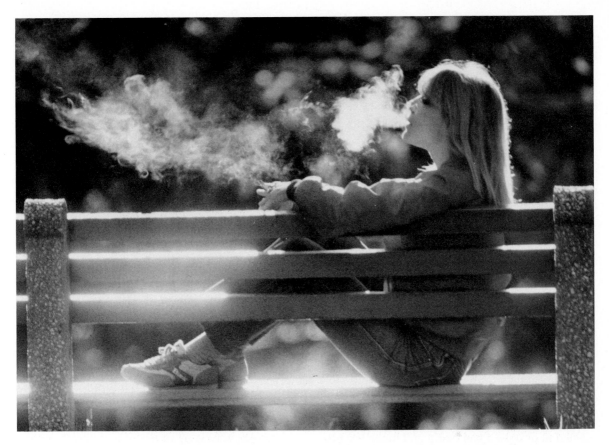

This form of drug use has a number of well-known negative consequences. What personal functions does cigarette smoking serve that make it so hard for us to stop?

ical effects of the drug or with the possible personal consequences of drug use but with the implications that extensive use of the drug may have for the society. Drug consumption by a large number of individuals may be important to the extent that a drug's effects support or oppose certain themes in the culture. That is, does the use of certain drugs fit more compatibly with certain philosophies of life?

Perspective of History

Drug use has affected society, but social changes also affect the use of drugs. One overriding theme has certainly been that the perspective of history

and of other cultures is needed to properly view drug use in America today. Drug use, as with other behaviors, takes place and has meaning only in a context, and the context for all social phenomena must be historical. For example, an important part of the context in which drug use occurs consists of the attitudes held about the drug and the user of the drug. Only by knowing how drugs have been used and viewed in the past can present attitudes toward the use of any drug be fully appreciated.

Throughout history, when a psychoactive drug has been introduced to a culture, its use has spread without stopping. However, until recently, most drugs started in the medicine man's bag of tricks and took years or centuries to disperse. From the chemist's test tube to the hamlets in the hills is now only a matter of weeks or months. Everything moves faster.

The transition from a select group of users of a drug to its acceptance as a critical component of the culture has been seen already with caffeine, nicotine, and distilled spirits. The recent flow of antipsychotic, antianxiety, and antidepressant drugs from the hospital pharmacy to the home medicine cabinet is but a modern version of the spread of a drug. The question still to be answered, of course, is which, if any, of the present illicit drugs will move into the homes of America.

In our society, the spread of a greater and greater number of drugs has been seen. From coffee in the morning through an aspirin during the day to the final nightcap—liquid or pill—we use drugs. Drugs are seen as problem solvers, and for some people they are. They make us feel good, forget the bad; they lift us from the rat race of life to the ecstasy of eternity and remove the boredom of the banal and replace it with the excitement of the ever-new. Drugs are also viewed as causing problems, and for some they do this. They make us ill, kill us, take a bad world and make it worse, and take a bright future and turn in into a dull haze. For most drug users, no matter what drug they use, none of this will happen. Whether legal or illegal, most of us use drugs in such amounts and frequencies that our lives are not seriously altered by our use of drugs. There is, however, the danger of engaging in pharmacological promiscuity and becoming too casual about our use of drugs.

Another principle abstracted from history is that if a psychoactive drug is to be widely used in a society, it must be integrated into and fill some need in that society. Once the agent occupies a niche, it cannot be dislodged except by changing the culture or offering a substitute to meet the same need. For example, in primitive groups the use of psychoactive plants was almost exclusively in a religious or spiritual setting. The active ingredient provided many of the experiences nec-

essary for the participant to maintain the faith that sustained the group structure.

When a particular drug is widely used and used in a particular way, it seems to be a part of the glue that holds a culture together. Whether it is *Datura* in initiation rites or martinis at a business lunch, the drug is a part of and a supporter of that society's prevailing world view. When the drug no longer contributes to and supports the culture, the drug is dropped. More likely, however, the form of the drug use will shift to adjust to the changing culture. In come cases the culture shifts so as to incorporate the use of the drug.

The failure of the Eighteenth Amendment to dislodge alcohol from our society shows clearly that alcohol is firmly entrenched in our culture. It will not be eliminated without an acceptable substitute being offered or a major change occurring in our attitudes about life. The shifting pattern of caffeine use, from the formal and generally less convenient use of coffee to the casual and everywhere available colas, both reflects and supports our changing concepts of work and play. Therefore, the psychoactive drugs a culture selects for regular use and the form of this use can tell much about the culture. Each drug widely used in a particular way is as much of a supporting institution of the society as is its form of government, its churches, and its schools.

There are a number of reasons for the large number of drugs used in our society. Only a few of the more obvious and important will be sketched here. In our generally affluent society each individual learns early that science and technology will supply answers to problems once the problems are identified. Because of the present rate of social and technological change and the great publicity given to even minor discoveries, the expectation of quick solutions to problems is now well ingrained in our culture. Drugs provide these quick solutions. The priming in the medical area was carried out over the first half of this century, so that by the post-World War II period it was easy to believe that drugs would take care of everything, from a cold to cancer.

Throughout the 1950s and 1960s the United

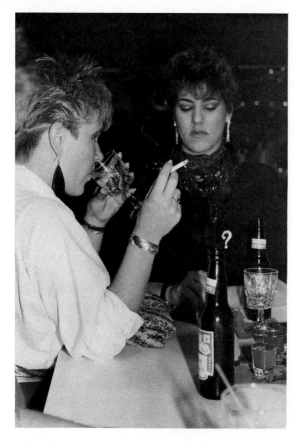

Drug use is a part of our social behavior.

States was flooded with drugs that promised to solve most personal problems. Sniffles? Take a pill. Bad day at school or office? Take two pills. Trouble relating to those around you? Take a tablet. The pressures for increased use of legal drugs to solve problems have been well identified throughout the book, and their effectiveness is clear. The marketplace is replete with exhortations to use this or that drug to remedy a variety of uncomfortable situations. Such advertisements are not false, just misleading. The pill does not cure the cold; it just removes some symptoms! The tablet does not solve the problems you are having with other people, but it does make you less concerned about them.

However, the drugs that were being rapidly de-

veloped and marketed did temporarily solve some major problems for one group of individuals, the physicians. Physicians were confronted with increasing demands on their time, and over half of their patients presented symptoms resulting in large part from nonphysical problems. The drugs of the 1950s and 1960s made it possible for the physician to process a lot of patients and make most of them feel at least temporarily better. Cure, no. Resolution of problems, no. Relief for both the patient and the physician, yes. Little wonder that physicians dispense medication in large amounts.

Another factor that contributes to the increased drug use is simply the availability of more drugs. Not only are there more things to try, but each of the agents offers, and partially delivers, a different effect, and thus different needs of more individuals may be met. Also, an affluent society such as this one may be conducive to increasing drug use. In an economically wealthy society it is possible to drop out and be a reasonably heavy drug user and still survive. This fact may be an important determinant of some individuals' behavior.

Another general cultural trend that seems to interact importantly with the increase in the use of illegal psychoactive drugs is the diminishing importance of the traditional arbiters of public and private behavior. Accepted patterns of behavior are shifting rapidly in many areas of society. The old black-and-white guidelines have been breeched and the social institutions—church, school, family—have not yet found their way out of the gray area where many behaviors "sound wrong, but I guess they are all right."

Closely interwined with the fact that these groups no longer speak with authority on matters of individual behavior is the increase in personal freedom and rights that has accompanied the civil rights and woman's liberation movements. Such an emphasis on personal freedom has already had a major impact on what is moral, legal, and acceptable in the areas of sex and censorship. It seems probable that the expansion of individual rights, that is, the absence of restrictions on behavior that does not immediately and directly harm another person, might soon come to include drug-taking behavior. This thesis has already been repeatedly presented by those advocating reform of the current drug laws. It does appear difficult to justify expanding each indivdual's personal freedom in every area except that of drug use.

In addition to the dissolving traditional moral standards, which in the past have partially countered increased drug use by labeling it as *bad, immoral,* or *sinful,* the shifting patterns of drug use today make it difficult to combine opposition to drug use with already existing prejudices. Identifying the use of alcohol and saloons with the lower class, immigrant Catholic made it easy for the middlle-class, second-generation Protestant to vote for prohibition in the early part of the century. Marijuana prohibition was easy in the 1930s; the drug had an obviously foreign name, it was primarily introduced into this country by Mexicans, and its usage was spread by lower-class blacks. There was little conflict when the heroin problem of the 1950s was considered. The high incidence of use was in the black ghettos, and the drugs were smuggled and sold by a foreign-dominated group, the Mafia. One could nicely compartmentalize the drug, the user, and the seller and be against all three with no problem.

One of the conflicts about drug use during the 1960s and 1970s contrast to previous times, is that things were not so easily compartmentalized. Marijuana and cocaine—"bad" drugs—were being used by white middle-class students and workers— "good" groups. The heroin—bad drug—problem had partly moved to the country club in the suburbs—nice people. No longer was it possible to categorically label those who experiment with drug use as bad, or degenerate, or sick. That began to change again during the 1980s: fewer middle-class kids are trying marijuana and cocaine, and "crack" is fast becoming a problem confined mainly to racial minorities living in urban ghettoes.

Increased pressure for drug use may reflect the fact that the era of instant communication is upon us. The mass media have done an excellent job of spreading the word about the use of drugs, perhaps too good. Perhaps most stories about the use of drugs serve only to increase curiosity about the

drugs and thus increase experimentation. Rarely reaching the level of news is the occasional user of any drug or the socially impaired user whose life *is* drugs. What makes the news is the exciting, the adventurous, the dramatic drug episode. Perhaps, as some have said, it is time for the news media to cool it.

A final aspect of our present society that must be briefly mentioned is the federal government. The national government is playing a pivotal and conflicting role in the expansion of illegal drug use in several ways. It is clear that there is now no consensus at the national level on the medical, personal, or societal meaning of drug use and abuse. Several issues are of concern. Many pronouncements still insist on considering the drug problem as primarily one of law enforcement, when it clearly goes beyond that to become a matter of philosophy. The most basic flaw in the foundation of our federal policy is the emphasis on reactions to problems rather than proposals for the society in which we all live. This is the heart of the issue. It is the sociocultural problems that must be addressed; the questions we ask shape the answers and the actions we take. Rather than devote all our energies and resources to battling the fire that rages around us, we must devote some time and effort to developing a strategy for the future.

A RATIONAL VIEW OF DRUG USE

One of the first steps that must be taken to look rationally at drug use is to clarify terms. The legal aspects of drug usage must be kept separate from the concept of abuse. Only by identifying the different patterns of drug usage do the problems stand out and make it possible to develop solutions.

There are two major ways of looking at patterns of drug use: the legality of the drug use and the psychosocial effects that accompany drug use. These two dimensions are shown in Fig. 20-1. The use-misuse-abuse dimension is clearly a continuum. Most of us use drugs in ways that complement rather than detract from our lives. Some

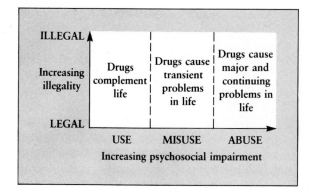

Figure 20-1. Dimensions of drug use.

individuals, however, become so involved in drug use that personal or social problems develop for them. This is drug misuse: using drugs causes significant transient or chronic minor problems for users. Drug abuse, the end of the continuum, occurs when individuals use drugs in such a way that the drugs cause a major and lasting disruption of relationships with society, peers, or themselves. The term *drug abuse* should be restricted to patterns of drug use that impair the individual's ability to function optimally in his personal, social, and vocational life. It complicates rather than clarifies the issues to label a 20-year-old moderate alcohol drinker as a drug abuser, when in fact he is only an illegal drug user. Use of an illegal drug should not automatically be considered drug abuse. Similarly, misuse of a drug, as by overweight, bored, frustrated, depressed suburban housewives who continue to function as adequate wives and mothers, should not be labeled as drug abuse.

The legal-illegal dimension is usually seen as a dichotomy. There are, though, varying degrees of legality or illegality. It may be illegal for a 16-year-old to buy cigarettes from a vending machine, but no one is ever arrested for it. The trend toward the decriminalization of marijuana has added another gray zone: legal to have and use, illegal to sell. The major immediate problem for society is the drug abuser, whether he abuses a legal drug, such as alcohol, or an illegal drug such

as heroin. These abusers are individuals whose life-style is most disruptive and expensive to society.

With terminology clarified, some basic premises should be enunciated. Some are facts, and some are, I believe, reasonable conclusions drawn from the available facts. Some people may feel that the conclusions do not follow from the facts, or that relevant facts were not considered, or that the assumptions made in moving from the facts to the conclusions were wrong. However, I believe these conclusions to be valid and justifiable. The basis for these premises will not be elaborated in detail. Either they appear reasonable enough from the material already presented so that a conceptualization can be suggested, or all the collecting of facts that is possible would have little hope of convincing the reader.

There is an overemphasis on the medical and pharmacological effects of drug use as a basis for making psychosocial and political decisions about drugs. This is everywhere evident; the relative medical safety of marijuana is given as the justification for decriminalization. There is a continuing emphasis on methadone maintenance programs, even though many of the essential psychosocial support systems have been eliminated because of budget cuts. The talk of seriously considering the decriminalization of cocaine was another example of fools and federal officials rushing in where angels fear to tread: the land of inadequate data and misplaced emphasis.

The physical and medical reasons against using some of the presently illegal drugs are valid only for the impure street variety drug. The current, regular intravenous use of heroin, stimulants, or any drug is clearly dangerous and frequently leads to hospitalization and/or death. Used orally and on an occasional basis the potent hallucinogens sometimes result in hospitalization, but with moderate doses of pure drugs there are only infrequent adverse effects. Marijuana, up to now, appears to be as safe (and as dangerous) in moderate social use as alcohol.

Drug-taking behavior seems to belong in the same category of personal freedom as does sexual behavior.

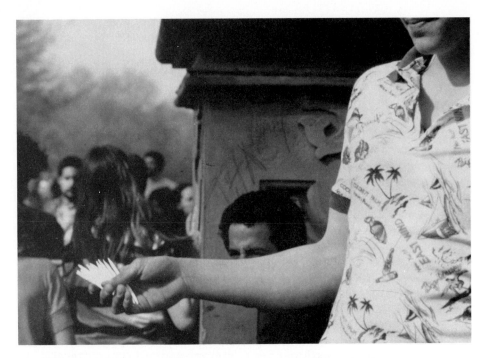

The most serious concern for our society is the use of drugs by the very young.

It is probably easier, though, for nonusers to understand and accept the motivations behind increased individual rather than societal responsibility for one's sexual behavior than to understand or accept personal freedom in drug use. Nevertheless, it seems unlikely that the area of personal rights and freedoms can be increased much further without the right to use certain now-illegal drugs becoming an open question for society and the law.

Among individuals who are satisfactorily intergrated into the present culture, there is a low incidence of use of most illegal drugs. *There is extensive use of a drug only when the drug meets unfilled needs of the individuals in a society.* It seems clear that to diminish drug use or to prevent its further increase, the needs of individuals must be satisfied in a nondrug setting. Society must offer attractive alternatives to a drug-using lifestyle if there is to be a decrease in drug use.

Evidence has been frequently presented that, historically, *drug use has initially altered society and then functioned as one of the stabilizing and supporting forces of the altered culture.* Changing patterns of drug use do change society. Once the change has occurred, the behaviors that develop around the use of the drug oppose additional change. The more unique the drug and the behaviors associated with it use, the more difficult the drug is to assimilate into society, and the greater the change required by society. It is debatable whether the decriminalization of marijuana would greatly alter today's culture. On the other hand, general use of the more potent hallucinogens most likely would result in considerable changes in today's society.

One of the major differences between today and the previous periods is that the stabilizing social institutions have lost some of their stability as well as their influence. *In every previous period of high drug use there have been potent forces countering the extensive use of drugs.* This assured a relatively slow spread of usage and some rational social debate on the meaning of the use of the drug.

There seems little debate over the fact that *for every psychoactive drug in use, legal or illegal, there will be a certain percentage of users who are abusers.* It does not seem possible for a drug to be used without it also being abused by some. This seems a fact of life. As new psychoactive drugs are developed, their abusers will spring up. What is not known is whether each new drug will add to the total number of abusers or whether the number of abusers will remain constant, with only the specific drug being used changing.

One of the amazing things is the almost magical belief many people have that the law and law enforcement are something separate from and independent of society. Failure to appreciate that the law is but one of the reflections of the culture is one of the points of contention in the drug scene today. *Law enforcement works as a social control only when the society wants it to work and that occurs only when the law is in agreement with the major themes and beliefs of the society.* This is the difficulty with considering the drug problem to be a law-enforcement problem. Until a resolution is reached about the role of drug-taking behavior in our culture, the role of law enforcement will be ambiguous.

Another component of this sociocultural, historical approach is that *education can change patterns of behavior,* but *only* if the education is early and is compatible with the life-style and realities of the learner. We must appreciate that the best drug prevention programs may never even mention drugs but instead emphasize life-styles and coping behaviors incompatible with more than occasional drug use. We must appreciate that different ages require different messages, different regions of the country require different approaches, different sociocultural groups require different solutions because they have different problems. Some people "do drugs" because they have too many problems, some because they don't have enough.

The educational problem is not how to prevent illegal drug use and stop drug abuse. No reasonable and informed person believes that either can be done in today's world. What is critical is that we develop strategies, rationales, and actions for min-

---

Issue: law enforcement

For the past several years the DEA has emphasized arrests of large-scale dealers of narcotics and has not put much effort into arresting and charging addicts.

As of 1988, there are plans for a more balanced attack, with increased attention being paid to arresting addicts. The rationale seems to be that the distributors can't be eliminated as long as there is still a market, that is, addicts who are willing to buy.

Is the addict best viewed as a criminal to be arrested, as a victim to be pitied, or as a patient to be treated?

---

imizing the destructive social and personal impact of recreational drug use.

The most serious problem for all of us is the possible increase in drug use by the very young, those 10 to 14 years old. These are beginning critical years in which individual's learn the social skills and personal self-concept that enable them to grow into a socially meaningful and personally rewarding life. It's a hard job to do well. Drugs are so much easier and more fun, for a while at least. Of primary importance is that no actions be taken that increase the availability of drugs for these individuals or increase social sanctions for adolescent recreational drug use.

Beginning use of illegal drugs in the early years of secondary school is a sign of an unhappy, unsuccfessful youth who is midway in the development of a deviant life-style, not the beginning. The evidence is clear from many studies: early drug use results from personality and background factors that results in the rejection of social values and goals. The use of illegal drugs also increases the rate of development of other asocial and antisocial behavior. The prevention of drug use by the young lies in the socialization process and in family relationships.

The basic question in the area of drug use is one of social philosophy: What kind of society do we aspire to, how can we increase the opportunities and specify realistic, socially integrative goals for our citizens to reach out for? The real issues and the hard ones are psychosocial and behavioral and will be solved only from that prespective. The medical problems associated with the illegal use of street drugs can easily be solved if we decide that is what we want to do. Before any actions are taken in prevention, law enforcement, or treatment, we must answer the philosophical questions about our social goals that the drug scene has posed for us.

Summary

The difficulty today in obtaining a clear picture of the changing patterns of drug-taking behavior seems primarily to be a result of viewing drug use as an isolated phenomenon. The facts about the actions and behavioral effects of psychoactive drugs are meaningful only when considered in the context of social history. It is necessary to identify and debate cultural trends that foster and oppose the current increase and diversification of drug-taking behavior if society is to understand and resolve the present crisis in drug use.

Finally, it is important that we address ourselves to the ways in which recreational drug use can remain as punctuation marks on a socially integrated and personally meaningful life, rather than becoming the theme around which our lives are woven. To deal with today's problems of drug use and drug users requires new concepts, new actions, new perspectives. To understand drug use in today's society, it is necessary to look beyond drugs—to look beyond drugs to the broad panorama of our developing social beliefs.

GENERAL REFERENCES

1. Brecher EM: Licit and illicit drugs, Boston 1972 Little Brown & Co.
2. Musto DF: The American disease: origins or narcotic control, New Haven Conn 1973 Yale University Press.
3. Peele S: The meaning of addiction, Lexington Mass 1985, D.C. Health & Co.
4. Thomas E: America's crusade, Time, September 15 1986.

Glossary

abstinence (18) Refraining from the use of a drug or alcohol. Complete abstinence from alcohol means no drinking at all. Abstinence syndrome: withdrawal syndrome.

acetaldehyde (9) The chemical product of the first step in the liver's metabolism of alcohol. It is normally present only in small amounts, as it is rapidly converted to acetic acid.

acute (2) Generally, sharp. In medicine, rapid. Referring to drugs, the short-term effects or effects of a single administration, as opposed to *chronic,* or long-term effects of administration.

ADHD (7) Attention deficit hyperactivity disorder, referring to a learning disability. Terminology of the DSM-III-R.

additive effects (6) When the effects of two different drugs add up to produce a greater effect than either drug alone. As contrasted with *antagonistic* effects in which one drug reduces the effect of another or *synergistic* effects in which one drug greatly amplifies the effect of another.

adenosine (11) A chemical believed to be a neurotransmitter in the CNS, primarily at inhibitory receptors. Caffeine may act by antagonizing the normal action of adenosine on its receptors.

affective disorder (13) A disorder of mood or emotion, in contrast to disorders of thought. Depression, mania, and bipolar (formerly manic-depressive) disorders are examples.

affective education (17) Generally, education that focuses on emotional content or emotional reactions, in contrast to *cognitive* content. In drug education, one example would be learning how to achieve certain "feelings" (of excitement or belonging to a group) without using drugs.

aftercare (18) In drug or alcohol treatment programs, the long-term follow-up or maintenance support that follows a more intense period of treatment.

AIDS (2, 14) Acquired immune deficiency syndrome, a disease in which the body's immune system breaks down, leading eventually to death. Because the disease is spread through the mixing of body fluids, it is more prevalent in intravenous drug users who share needles. The infectious agent is the Human Immunodeficiency Virus (HIV).

alcohol abuse (9) In the DSM-III-R, alcohol abuse is defined as a pattern of pathological alcohol use that causes impairment of social or occupational functioning. Compare to *alcohol dependence.*

alcohol dehydrogenase (9) The enzyme that metabolizes almost all of the alcohol consumed by an individual. It is found primarily in the liver.

alcohol dependence (9) In the DSM-III-R, alcohol dependence is considered a more serious disorder than *alcohol abuse,* in that dependence includes either tolerance or withdrawal symptoms.

alcohol (9) Generally refers to grain alcohol, or ethanol, as opposed to other types of alcohol (for example, wood or isopropyl alcohol), which are too toxic to be drinkable.

alcoholic personality (9) Refers to personality traits, such as immaturity and dependency, that

Numbers in parentheses refer to the chapter in which the term is introduced.

are frequently found in alcoholics in treatment. Many of these consistent traits may be a *result* of years of heavy drinking rather than being a *cause* of alcoholism.

Alcoholics Anonymous (18) A worldwide, loosely organized group of alcoholics who try to help each other to abstain from the use of alcohol.

alcoholism (9) The word has many different definitions, and is, therefore, not a precise term. Definitions may refer to pathological drinking behavior (for example, remaining drunk for 2 days), to impaired functioning (for example, frequently missing work), or to physical dependence. See *alcohol abuse* and *alcohol dependence*.

alternatives (17) (to drugs) Assuming that there are motives for drug use, such as the need to be accepted by a group, many prevention and treatment programs teach alternative methods for satisfying these motives.

Alzheimer's disease (4) A progressive neurological disease that occurs primarily in the elderly. It causes loss of memory and then progressively impairs more aspects of intellectual and social functioning. Large acetylcholine-containing neurons of the brain are damaged in this disease.

Amanita muscaria (15) The fly agaric mushroom, widely used in ancient times for its hallucinogenic properties.

amotivational syndrome (16) A hypothesized loss of motivation that has been attributed to the effects of chronic marijuana use.

anabolic steroids (19) Substances that increase anabolic (constructive) metabolism, one of the functions of male sex hormones. The result is increased muscle mass.

analgesic (12) Pain-relieving. An analgesic drug produces a selective reduction of pain, whereas an *anesthetic* reduces all sensation.

anesthetic (12) Sense deadening. An anesthetic drug reduces all sensation, whereas an *analgesic* reduces pain.

angel dust (15) A street name for phencyclidine (PCP).

animism (15) The belief that objects, plants, and animals contain spirits or souls.

Antabuse (18) Brand name for disulfiram, a drug that interferes with the normal metabolism of alcohol so that a person who drinks alcohol after taking disulfiram will become quite ill. Antabuse interferes with the enzyme aldehyde dehydrogenase so that there is a buildup of acetaldehyde, the first metabolic product of alcohol.

antecedents (1) In the context of Chapter 1, behaviors or individual characteristics that can be measured before drug use and might therefore be somewhat predictive of drug use. These are not necessarily causes of the subsequent drug use.

anticonvulsant (8) A drug that prevents or reduces epileptic seizures.

antidepressant (1, 5, 13) A group of drugs used in treating depressive disorders. The MAO inhibitors and the tricyclics are the major examples.

antihistamine (12) A group of drugs that act by antagonizing the actions of histamine at its receptors. Used in cold and sinus remedies and in OTC sedatives and sleep aids.

antipsychotic (5, 13) A group of drugs that are used to treat psychotic disorders, such as schizophrenia. Also called neuroleptics or major tranquilizers.

antipyretic (12) Fever-reducing. Aspirin is a commonly used antipyretic.

antitussive (14) Cough-reducing. Narcotics have this effect. OTC antitussives generally contain dextromethorphan.

anti-inflammatory (12) Reducing the local heat, swelling, and redness caused by injury or infection. Aspirin has anti-inflammatory properties.

anxiety (13) Describes a number of symptoms that are related to a sense of impending danger. At pathological levels, these symptoms can constitute debilitating disorders.

anxiolytic (8) Term used to describe drugs, such as Valium, used in treatment of anxiety disorders. Literally, anxiety dissolving.

aphrodisiac (8) Any substance that is said to promote sexual desire.

aspirin (12) Originally Bayer's brand name for acetylsalicylic acid, now a generic name for that chemical.

assassin (16) The story is that this term for a hired killer is derived from a hashish-using cult, the hashishiyya.

ataxia (6) Loss of coordinated movement, for example, the staggering gait of someone who has consumed a large amount of alcohol.

attention deficit hyperactivity disorder (7) A learning disability accompanied by hyperactivity. Most common in male children. This DSM-III-R term replaces *hyperkinetic syndrome* and *minimal brain dysfunction* as diagnostic categories.

autonomic nervous system (4) The branch of the peripheral nervous system that regulates the visceral, or automatic functions of the body, such as heart rate and intestinal motility. In contrast to the *somatic,* or voluntary, nervous system.

aversion therapy (18) A form of treatment that attempts to suppress an undesirable behavior by punishing each instance of the behavior. For example, the drinking of alcohol might be punished by electric shocks or by giving a drug that causes nausea.

BAL (9) Blood alcohol level, also called blood alcohol content (BAC). The proportion of blood that consists of alcohol. For example, a person with a BAL of 0.10% has alcohol constituting one tenth of 1% of the blood and is legally intoxicated in all states.

barbiturate (8) A major class of sedative-hypnotic drugs, including amobarbital and sodium pentothal.

basal ganglia (4) A part of the brain containing large numbers of dopamine synapses, it is responsible for maintaining proper muscle tone as a part of the *extrapyramidal motor system.* Damage to the basal ganglia, as in Parkinson's disease, produces muscular rigidity and tremors.

behavioral tolerance (6) Repeated use of a drug may lead to a diminished effect of the drug (tolerance). When the diminished effect occurs because the individual has learned to compensate for the effect of the drug, it is called behavioral tolerance. For example, a novice drinker might be unable to walk with a BAL of 0.20%, whereas someone who has practiced walking while intoxicated would be able to walk fairly well at the same BAL.

behavioral toxicity (2) Refers to the fact that a drug can be toxic because it impairs behavior and amplifies the danger level of many activities. The effect of alcohol on driving is an example.

benzodiazepine (8) The group of drugs that includes Valium (diazepam) and Librium (chlordiazepoxide). They are used as *anxiolytics* or *sedatives,* and some types are used as sleeping pills.

benzoylecgonine (5) A metabolite of cocaine that can be detected in urine samples.

bhang (16) A preparation of cannabis (marijuana) that consists of the whole plant, dried and powdered. The weakest of the commonly used forms in India.

binding (4) The interaction between a molecule and a receptor for that molecule. Although the molecules float onto and off of the receptor, there are chemical and electrical attractions between a specific molecule and its receptor so that there is a much higher probability of the receptor being occupied by its proper molecule than by other molecules.

bioavailability (6) The availability of molecules of a drug at the site of the drug's action in the body. An important concept in comparing different brands of the same generic drug, because one preparation may dissolve better or be absorbed more readily than the other, thus producing greater bioavailability.

bipolar disorder (13) One of the major affective, or emotional, disorders. Periods of mania and periods of depression have occurred in the same individual. Also called *manic-depressive illness.*

blackout (9) A period of time during which a person was behaving, but for which there is no memory. The most common cause of this phenomenon is excessive alcohol consumption, and blackouts are considered to indicate pathological drinking.

blood-brain barrier (6) Refers to the fact that many substances, including drugs, that may circulate freely in the blood do not readily enter the brain tissue. The major structural feature of this barrier is the tightly jointed epithelial cells lining blood capillaries in the brain. Drug molecules cannot pass between the cells but must be able to go through their membranes. Small molecules and molecules that are lipid (fat) soluble cross the barrier easily. Obviously, all psychoactive drugs must be capable of crossing the blood-brain barrier.

brainstem (4) The medulla oblongata, pons, and midbrain. Found between the spinal cord and the forebrain, and generally considered to contain the "oldest" (in an evolutionary sense) and most primitive control centers for such basic functions as breathing, swallowing, and so on.

brand name (5) The name given a drug by a particular manufacturer and licensed only to that manufacturer. For example, Valium is a brand name for diazepam. Other companies may sell diazepam, but Hoffmann-LaRoche, Inc. owns the name Valium.

bright (10) Light-colored, flue-cured tobacco. Compare to *burley*.

British system (18) Generally refers to the fact that heroin addicts in Great Britain may register as addicts and be prescribed legal narcotics, including heroin.

burley (10) Dark-colored, air-cured tobacco. Compare to *bright*.

caffeinism (11) Habitual use of large amounts of caffeine, usually in coffee.

camellia sinensis (11) The plant from which tea is made.

Cannabis (16) *indica, sativa.* The marijuana, or hemp, plant.

carbon monoxide (10) A poisonous gas found in cigarette smoke.

catheter (2) A piece of plastic or rubber tubing that is inserted into a vein or other structure.

central nervous system (4) The brain and spinal cord.

charas (16) A preparation of Cannabis, or marijuana, that is similar to hashish. The most potent form of marijuana commonly used in India.

chemical name (5) For a drug, the name that is descriptive of its chemical structure. As an example, the chemical name sodium chloride is associated with the *generic* name, table salt, of which there may be several *brand* names, such as Morton's.

China white (14) A street name for one of the potent synthetic narcotics.

chipper (14) Refers to an individual who uses heroin occasionally.

chronic (2) Occurring over time. Chronic drug use refers to long-term use, chronic drug effects refer to persistent effects produced by long-term use.

chronic obstructive lung disease (10) Includes emphysema and chronic bronchitis. Cigarette smoking is a major cause of these disorders.

cirrhosis (9) A serious, largely irreversible, and frequently deadly disease of the liver. Usually caused by chronic heavy alcohol use.

coca paste (7) A paste derived from the coca leaf in the process of making cocaine. It is sometimes smoked in South and Central America and Mexico.

coca (7) The plant, Erythroxylon coca, from which cocaine is derived. Also refers to the leaves of this plant.

codeine (14) A narcotic chemical that is present in opium.

coma (6) A state of unconsciousness from which the individual cannot be aroused.

congeners (9) In general, members of the same group. With respect to alcohol, the term refers to other chemicals that are produced in the process of making a particular alcoholic beverage.

controlled drinking (18) The concept that individuals who have been drinking pathologically may be taught to drink in a controlled, nonpathological manner.

controlled substance (3) A term coined for the 1970 federal law that revised previous laws regulating *narcotics and dangerous drugs*. Heroin and cocaine are examples of controlled substances.

crack (5) Street term for a smokable form of cocaine. Also called *rock*.

crank (7) Street name for illicitly manufactured methamphetamine.

crash (7) Originally referred to the rapid emotional descent following a binge of amphetamine use. One symptom is prolonged sleep, and eventually sleeping in general was referred to as crashing.

cumulative effects (6) Drug effects that increase with repeated administrations, usually due to the build up of the drug in the body.

Datura (15) The plant genus that includes many species used for their hallucinogenic properties. These plants contain anticholinergic chemicals.

DAWN (2) The Drug Abuse Warning Network, a federal government system for reporting drug-related medical emergencies and deaths.

DEA (3) The United States Drug Enforcement Administration.

delirium tremens (9) Alcohol withdrawal symptoms, including tremors and hallucinations.

demand reduction (3) Efforts to control drug use by reducing the demand for drugs, as opposed to efforts aimed at reducing the supply of drugs. Demand reduction efforts include education and prevention programs as well as increased punishments for drug users.

depressant (5) Any of a large group of drugs that generally depress the CNS and at high doses induce sleep. Includes alcohol, the barbiturates, and other sedative-hypnotic drugs.

detoxification (18) The process of allowing the body to rid itself of a large amount of alcohol or another drug. Often the first step in a treatment program.

deviance (1) Behavior that is different from established social norms and that social groups take steps to correct.

diagnosis (13) The process of identifying the nature of an illness. A subject of great controversy for mental disorders.

distillation (9) The process by which alcohol is

separated from a weak alcohol solution to form more concentrated distilled spirits. The weak solution is heated and the alcohol vapors are collected and condensed to a liquid form.

dose-response curve (6) A graph showing the relationship between the size of a drug dose and the size of the response (or the proportion of subjects showing that response).

drug disposition tolerance (6) The reduced effect of a drug that may result from more rapid metabolism or excretion of the drug.

drug therapy (1) The use of a drug in an effort to treat an illness.

DSM-III-R (13) The Diagnostic and Statistical Manual, third edition, revised, published by the American Psychiatric Association. It has become a standard for naming and distinguishing among mental disorders.

dysentery (3) A bowel infection that causes severe diarrhea, pain, and fever.

ecstasy (15) Street name for hallucinogen MDMA. Also called "XTC."

ECT (13) Electroconvulsive therapy, or electroconvulsive shock treatment. A procedure in which an electrical current is passed through the head, resulting in an epileptic-like seizure. Although this treatment is now used infrequently, it is still considered to be the most effective and rapid treatment for severe depression.

effective dose (6) The dose of a drug that produces a certain effect in some percentage of the subjects. For example, an ED 50 produces the effect in 50% of the subjects. Note that the dose will depend on the effect that is monitored.

EMIT (5) Enzyme multiplied immunoassay test. The most commonly used urine screening technique for detecting the presence of various drugs.

emphysema (10) A lung disease in which tissue deterioration results in increased air retention and less exchange of gases. The result is difficulty in breathing and shortness of breath. An example of a chronic obstructive lung disease, often caused by smoking.

endorphin (6, 14) An opiate-like chemical that

occurs naturally in the brains of humans and other animals. There are several proper endorphins, and the term is also used generically to refer to both the endorphins and enkephalins.

enkephalin (14) An opiate-like chemical that occurs naturally in the brains of humans and other animals. The enkephalins are smaller molecules than the endorphins.

enzyme (4) A large organic molecule that works to speed up a specific chemical reaction. Enzymes are found in brain cells, where they are needed for most steps in the synthesis of neurotransmitter molecules. They are also found in the liver, where they are needed for the metabolism of many drug molecules.

ephedrine (7,12) A drug derived from the Chinese medicinal herb *ma huang* and used to relieve breathing difficulty in asthma. A sympathomimetic from which amphetamine was derived.

epilepsy (8) A disorder of the nervous system in which recurring periods of abnormal electrical activity in the brain produce temporary malfunction. There may or may not be loss of consciousness or convulsive motor movements.

ergogenic (19) Energy-producing. Refers to drugs or other methods (e.g., blood doping) designed to increase the energy output of an athlete.

ergotism (15) A disease caused by eating grain infected with the ergot fungus. There are both psychological and physical manifestations.

ethical (5) In pharmacy, medicines dispensed only by prescription.

extrapyramidal (4) Refers to a motor control system in the central nervous system that is responsible for maintaining muscle tone and posture. Parkinson's disease causes damage to this system. Antipsychotic drugs also interfere with the extrapyramidal system, often producing symptoms similar to those of Parkinson's disease.

false transmitter (6) One method by which a drug may affect the nervous system. The drug is taken into a neuron and acted on by enzymes to produce a substance resembling the natural neurotransmitter but differing from it functionally: a false transmitter.

FAS (9) Fetal alcohol syndrome.

FDA (3) The United States Food and Drug Administration.

fermentation (9) The process by which sugars are converted into grain alcohol through the action of yeasts.

fetal alcohol syndrome (9) A developmental disorder seen in a fraction of the children born to mothers who drink heavily during pregnancy.

fibrocystic breast disease (11) A benign (noncancerous) but painful disorder characterized by lumps (fibrocysts) in the breasts. There is controversy as to whether caffeine consumption is related to this problem.

flashback (15) An experience reported by some users of LSD in which portions of the LSD experience reoccur at a later time without the use of a drug.

fly agaric mushroom (15) *Amanita muscaria*, a hallucinogenic mushroom that is also considered poisonous.

freebase (7) In general, when a chemical salt is separated into its basic and acidic components, the basic component is referred to as the free base. Most psychoactive drugs are bases that normally exist in a salt form. Specifically, the salt, cocaine hydrochloride, can be chemically extracted to form the cocaine freebase, which is volatile and may therefore be smoked.

functional disorder (13) A mental disorder for which there is no known organic cause. Schizophrenia is a form of psychosis that is considered to be a functional disorder.

ganja (16) A preparation of *Cannabis* (marijuana) in which the most potent parts of the plant are used.

gateway substances (1) Refers to substances such as alcohol, tobacco, and sometimes marijuana that most users of illicit substances will have tried before their first use of cocaine, heroin, or other less widely used illicit drugs.

generic name (5) For drugs, a name which specifies a particular chemical without being chemically descriptive. As an example, the *chemical name,* sodium chloride, is associated with the *generic name,* table salt, of which there may be several *brand names,* such as Morton's.

GRAE (12) Generally recognized as effective, a term defined by the FDA with reference to the ingredients found in OTC drugs (see also GRAS).

GRAHL (12) Generally recognized as honestly labeled (see GRAE and GRAS).

grain neutral spirits (9) Ethyl alcohol distilled to a purity of 190 proof (95%).

grand mal (8) An epileptic seizure that results in convulsive motor movements and loss of consciousness.

GRAS (12) Generally recognized as safe, a term defined by the FDA with reference to food additives and the ingredients found in OTC drugs.

hallucinogen (5) A drug such as LSD or mescaline that produces profound alterations in perception.

hash oil (16) A slang term for oil of cannabis, a liquid extract from the marijuana plant.

hashish (16) A potent preparation of *Cannabis* (marijuana).

henbane (15) A poisonous plant containing anticholinergic chemicals and sometimes used for its hallucinogenic properties. *Hyoscyamus niger.*

heroin (14) Originally Bayer's brand name for diacetylmorphine, a potent narcotic analgesic synthesized from morphine.

HIV (2) Human immunodeficiency virus. The infectious agent responsible for AIDS.

homeostasis (4) A state of physiological balance, maintained by various regulatory mechanisms.

hormones (4) A chemical substance formed in one part of the body that stimulates action in another part of the body.

hyperactive (7) Refers to a disorder characterized by short attention span and a high level of motor activity. The DSM-III-R term is *attention deficit hyperactivity disorder.*

hypnotic (8) Sleep-inducing. For drugs, refers to sleeping preparations.

hypodermic syringe (3) A device to which a hollow needle can be attached so that solutions can be injected through the skin.

hypothalamus (4) A group of nuclei found at the base of the brain, just above the pituitary gland.

immunoassay (5) A method for measuring an organic chemical by inducing an animal to develop an antibody to it, then purifying the antibody and using it to measure the chemical in another tissue sample.

indole (15) A type of chemical structure. The neurotransmitter serotonin and the hallucinogen LSD both contain an indole nucleus.

insomnia (8) Inability to sleep. The most common complaint is difficulty in falling asleep. Often treated with hypnotic drugs.

interferon (12) A chemical produced by the body in response to viral infections. Interferon treatments have been shown to reduce the risk of catching a cold.

intramuscular (6) A type of injection in which the drug is administered into a muscle.

intravenous (6) A type of injection in which the drug is administered into a vein.

kretek (10) A clove cigarette.

laissez faire (2) A doctrine that government should not interfere with business or other activities.

lethal dose (6) The dose of a drug that produces a lethal effect in some percentage of the animals on which it is tested. For example, an LD 50 is the dose that would kill 50% of the animals to which it was given.

leukoplakia (10) A whitening and thickening of the soft tissues of the mouth. The use of chewing tobacco is associated with an increase in leukoplakia, considered to be a "precancerous" tissue change.

limbic system (4) A system of various brain structures that are involved in emotional responses.

lithium (13) A highly reactive metallic element, atomic number 3. Its salts are used in the treatment of mania and bipolar affective disorder.

liver microsomal enzyme (6) An enzyme associated with a particular subcellular component (the microsomal fraction) of liver cells. There are many such enzymes that are important for drug metabolism.

look-alikes (7) Drugs sold legally, usually through the mail, that are made to look like controlled, prescription-only drugs. The most common type contain caffeine and resemble amphetamine capsules or tablets.

ma huang (7) A Chinese herb containing ephedrine, which is a sympathomimetic drug from which amphetamine was derived.

major depression (13) A serious mental disorder characterized by depressed mood. A specific diagnostic term in the DSM-III-R.

malting (9) The process of wetting a grain and allowing it to sprout, to maximize its sugar content prior to fermentation to produce an alcoholic beverage.

mandrake (15) *Mandragora officinarum,* a plant having a branched root that contains anticholinergic chemicals. Now classed among the other anticholinergic hallucinogens, this plant was widely believed to have aphrodisiac properties.

MAO inhibitor (13) A drug that acts by inhibiting the enzyme monoamine oxidase (MAO). Used as an antidepressant.

MDMA (15) Methylenedioxy methamphetamine, a catechol hallucinogen related to MDA. Called "ecstasy" or "XTC " on the street.

medial forebrain bundle (4) A group of neuron fibers that projects from the midbrain to the forebrain, passing near the hypothalamus. Now known to contain several chemically and anatomically distinct pathways, including dopamine and norepinephrine pathways.

medical model (13) With reference to mental disorders, a model that assumes that abnormal behaviors are *symptoms* resulting from a *disease.*

mental illness (13) A term that, to some theorists, implies acceptance of a medical model of mental disorders.

mesolimbic dopamine system (4) A group of dopamine-containing neurons that have their cell bodies in the midbrain and their terminals in the forebrain, on various structures associated with the limbic system. Believed by some theorists to be important in explaining the therapeutic effects of antipsychotic medications.

Also believed by some theorists to be important for many types of behavioral reinforcers.

metabolism (4) (of drugs) The breakdown of drug molecules by enzymes, often in the liver.

methadone maintenance (18) A program for treatment of narcotic addicts in which the synthetic narcotic drug methadone is provided to the addicts in an oral dosage form, so that they may maintain their addiction legally.

Mexican brown (14) A form of heroin that first appeared on American streets in the mid-1970s. Because the heroin is made from the hydrochloride salt of morphine, it is a brown color in its pure form.

moist snuff (10) A type of oral smokeless tobacco that is rapidly increasing in popularity among young American males. A "pinch" of this chopped, moistened, flavored tobacco is held in the mouth, often behind the lower lip.

morphinism (3, 14) An older term used to describe dependence on the use of morphine.

narcolepsy (7) A form of sleep disorder characterized by bouts of muscular weakness and falling asleep involuntarily. The most common treatment employs stimulant drugs such as amphetamine to maintain wakefulness during the day.

narcotic (5) One of a group of drugs similar to morphine, also referred to as opiates, and used medically primarily for their analgesic effects. The Greek root for this word meant numbness, and in early pharmacology writings the term narcotic was used for many psychoactive drugs that were thought to reduce pain or dull the senses. Also, by extrapolation from the Bureau of Narcotics, the term narcotic came in popular use to refer to any illegal drug (now replaced by the term "controlled substance" in legal writings).

narcotic antagonist (14, 18) Any of several drugs that are capable of blocking the effects of narcotic drugs. Used in emergency medicine to treat narcotic overdose, and in some addiction treatment programs to block the effect of any illicit narcotic that might be taken. Nalorphine and naltrexone are examples.

Native American Church (15) A religious organization active among American Indians, in which the hallucinogenic peyote cactus is used in conjunction with Christian religious themes.

NDA (3) In FDA procedures, a New Drug Application. This application, demonstrating both safety and effectiveness of a new drug in both animal and human experiments, must be submitted by a drug company to the FDA before a new drug can be marketed.

neuroleptic (13) Another term for the antipsychotic drugs (also called major tranquilizers).

neurotic (13) A type of mental disorder, mostly now referred to as *anxiety disorders*.

neurotransmitter (4) A chemical that is released by one neuron and that alters the electrical activity in another neuron.

nicotiana (10) Any of several types of tobacco plant, including *N. tobacum* and *N. rustica*.

nicotine (10) The chemical contained in tobacco that is responsible for its psychoactive effects and for tobacco dependence.

nigrostriatal dopamine system (4) A group of dopamine-containing neurons that have their cell bodies in the *substantia nigra* of the midbrain and their terminals in the *corpus striatum* (basal ganglia), which is part of the extrapyramidal motor system. It is this pathway that deteriorates in Parkinson's disease and on which antipsychotic drugs act to produce side effects resembling Parkinson's disease.

nitrosamines, tobacco specific (10) Nitrosamines are a group of organic chemicals, many of which are highly carcinogenic. There are at least four nitrosamines found only in tobacco, and these may account for much of the cancer-causing property of tobacco.

nonspecific effects (6) Effects of a drug which are not changed by changing the chemical makeup of the drug. Also referred to as *placebo* effects.

NORML (16) The National Association for the Reform of Marijuana Laws.

nucleus basalis (4) A group of large cell bodies found just below the basal ganglia and containing acetylcholine. These cells send terminations widely to the cerebral cortex. In Alz-

heimer's disease, there is a loss of these neurons and a reduction in the amount of acetylcholine in the cortex.

opium (14) A sticky substance obtained from the seed pods of the opium poppy and containing the narcotic chemicals morphine and codeine.

organic disorder (13) For mental disorders, those with a known physical cause (e.g., psychosis caused by long-term alcohol use).

OTC (5,12) Over-the-counter drugs (those which can be purchased without a prescription).

papaver somniferum (14) The opium poppy.

paraphernalia (3) In general, the equipment used in some activity. Drug paraphernalia might include such items as syringes, pipes, scales, or mirrors.

parasympathetic (4) The branch of the autonomic nervous system that has acetylcholine as its neurotransmitter and, for example, slows the heart rate and activates the intestine.

Parkinson's disease (4) A disease of the extrapyramidal motor system, specifically involving damage to the nigrostriatal dopamine system. Early symptoms include muscular rigidity, tremors, a shuffling gait, and a masklike face. Occurs primarily in the elderly.

passive smoking (10) Inhalation of cigarette smoke from the air by nonsmokers near someone who is smoking.

patent medicines (3) Proprietary medicines. Originally referred to medicines that were in fact treated as inventions and patented in Great Britain. In America, the term came to refer to medicines sold directly to the public.

PCP (15) Initials for the chemical name 1-(1-phenylcyclohexyl) piperidine. The generic name is phencyclidine. The brand name Sernyl is no longer in use, as PCP is not legally available for human use. A hallucinogen often referred to as Angel Dust.

PDR (5) Physician's Desk Reference, a book listing all prescription drugs and giving prescribing information about each. Updated yearly.

pekoe (11) A grade of tea.

peptide (14) A class of chemicals made up of sequences of amino acids. Enkephalins are small peptides containing only five amino acids, whereas large proteins may contain hundreds.

peyote (15) A hallucinogenic cactus containing the chemical mescaline.

phantastica (15) A term used to describe certain hallucinogens that produce altered perceptions but do not generally impair communication with the real world.

pharmacodynamic tolerance (6) Reduced effectiveness of a drug due to an altered tissue reaction to the drug.

phenothiazine (13) A group of chemicals that includes several antipsychotic medications.

physical dependence (2) Defined by the presence of a consistent set of symptoms when use of a drug is stopped. These withdrawal symptoms imply that homeostatic mechanisms of the body had made adjustments to counteract the drug's effects and without the drug the system is thrown out of balance.

placebo (6) An inactive drug, often used in experiments to control for nonspecific effects of drug administration.

postsynaptic (6) Refers to structures associated with the neural membrane on the receiving side of a synapse.

potency (6) Relates to how little of a drug is required to produce a given effect.

precursor (4) Something that precedes something else. In biochemistry, a precursor molecule may be acted upon by an enzyme and changed into a different molecule. For example, the dietary amino acid tryptophan is the precursor for the neurotransmitter serotonin.

prohibition (9) Refers to the period 1920-1933 during which the sale of alcoholic beverages was prohibited in the United States.

proprietary (5) A medicine that is marketed directly to the public. Also called *OTC, patent,* or *nonprescription* medicines.

prostaglandins (12) Local hormones, some of which are synthesized in response to cell injury and are important for initiating pain signals. Aspirin and similar drugs inhibit the formation of the prostaglandins.

psychedelic (1,15) Another name for hallucinogenic drugs. Has a somewhat positive connotation of mind-viewing or mind-clearing.

psychoactive (1) Used to describe drugs that have their principal effect on the CNS.

psychological dependence (2) A strong tendency to repeat the use of a drug.

psychotic (3) A type of mental disorder characterized by a loss of contact with reality and by deterioration in social and intellecutal functioning.

psychotomimetic (15) Another name for hallucinogenic drugs. Has a negative connotation of mimicking psychosis.

quid (10) A piece of something to be chewed, for example, the wad of chewing tobacco in a person's mouth.

receptors (4) Locations at which neurotransmitters or drugs bind, perhaps triggering a physiological response.

reinforcement (2) The process of strengthening a behavioral tendency by presenting a stimulus contingent on the behavior. For example, the tendency to obtain and take a drug may be strengthened by the stimulus properties of the drug that occur after it is taken, thus leading to psychological dependence.

reuptake (4) One process by which a neurotransmitter chemical may be removed from the synapse. The chemical may be taken back up into the cell from which it was released.

Reye's syndrome (12) A rare brain infection that occurs almost exclusively in children and adolescents. There is some evidence that it is more likely to occur in children who have been given aspirin during a bout of flu or chickenpox.

risk factors (1) Behaviors, attitudes, or situations that correlate with and may indicate the development of a deviance-prone lifestyle that may include drug or alcohol abuse. Examples are early alcohol intoxification, absence from school, and perceived peer approval of drug use.

rock (5) Another name for *crack,* a smokable form of cocaine.

salicylate (12) The class of chemicals that includes aspirin.

schizophrenia (13) A type of psychotic disorder that is chronic and has no known cause.

sedative (8) A drug used to calm a person, reducing stress and excitement.

sinsemilla (16) A process for growing marijuana that is especially potent in its psychological effects due to a high THC content.

sidestream smoke (10) Smoke that comes off a cigarette from the outside rather than being drawn through the cigarette.

smokeless tobacco (10) Includes various forms of chewing tobacco and snuff.

somatic system (4) Part of the nervous system that controls the voluntary, skeletal muscles, for example, the large muscles of the arms and legs.

specific effects (6) Those effects of a drug that depend on the amount and type of chemical contained in the drug.

speed (7) A street term used at one time for cocaine, then for injectable amphetamine, and later for all types of amphetamine. Probably shortened from *speedball.*

stimulant (5) Any of a group of drugs that has the effect of reversing mental and physical fatigue.

street value (5) The theoretical value of an amount of drugs if sold in small quantities on the street.

subcutaneous (6) Under the skin. A form of injection in which the needle penetrates through the skin (about ⅜ inch) but does not enter a muscle or vein.

sulfanilamide (3) A type of antibiotic.

sympathetic (4) Branch of the autonomic nervous system that contains norepinephrine as its neurotransmitter and, for example, increases the heart rate and blood pressure.

sympathomimetic (7) Any drug that stimulates the sympathetic nervous system, for example, amphetamine.

symptom (13) In medicine, some abnormality that indicates a disease. When applied to abnormal behavior, seems to imply a medical model in which some unseen disease causes the abnormal behavior.

synesthesia (15) A phenomenon in which the different senses become mixed, for example, a sound is "seen." May be reported by a person taking hallucinogens.

synthesis (4) Formation of a chemical compound. For example, some neurotransmitter chemicals must be synthesized within the neuron.

tachyphylaxis (7) A rapid form of tolerance in which a second dose of a drug has a smaller effect than a first dose taken only a short time before.

tar (10) With regard to tobacco, a complex mixture of chemicals found in cigarette smoke. After water, gases, and nicotine are removed from the smoke, the remaining residue is considered to be tar.

tardive dyskinesia (13) Movement disorders that appear after several weeks or months of treatment with antipsychotic drugs, which usually become worse if the drug is discontinued.

temperance (9) With reference to alcohol, temperance originally meant moderation, for example, the consumption of beer, which is weaker than spirits. Eventually the temperance movement adopted complete abstinence as their goal and prohibition as the means.

tetahydrocannabinol (16) The most active of the many chemicals found in *Cannabis* (marijuana).

THC (16) Tetrahydrocannabinol.

theobromine (11) A mild stimulant similar to caffeine and found in chocolate.

theophylline (11) A mild stimulant similar to caffeine and found in tea.

tolerance (2, 6) The reduced effectiveness of a drug following repeated administration.

toxic (2) Harmful, destructive, or deadly.

tricyclic (13) Refers to a group of chemicals used in treating depression.

truth serum (13) Refers to the use of drugs to "loosen the tongue," either in association with psychotherapy or interrogation. Although people may speak more freely after some drugs, there is no guarantee of truth.

uptake (4) The process by which a cell expends energy to concentrate certain chemicals within itself. For example, precursor substances which will be synthesized into neurotransmitters must be taken up by the neuron.

values clarification (17) A type of affective education which largely avoids reference to drugs but focuses on helping students to define and defend their own values.

wine cooler (9) A beverage made from mixing wine with a fruit-based soft drink.

withdrawal syndrome (2) The set of symptoms that occur reliably when someone stops taking a drug, also called *abstinence syndrome*.

xanthine (11) The chemical class that includes caffeine, theobromine, and theophylline.

Appendix A

Drug Names

acetaminophen: OTC analgesic, similar to aspirin in its effects.

acetophenazine: *Tindal.* Antipsychotic.

acetylsalicylic acid: aspirin. OTC analgesic.

Adapin: doxepin. Heterocyclic antidepressant.

alprazolam: *Xanax.* Benzodiazepine sedative.

Alurate: aprobarbital. Barbiturate sedative-hypnotic.

Amanita muscaria: Hallucinogenic mushroom.

amitriptyline: *Elavil, Endep.* Heterocyclic antidepressant.

amobarbital: *Amytal.* Barbiturate sedative-hypnotic.

amoxapine: *Asendin.* Heterocyclic antidepressant.

amphetamine: *Benzedrine.* CNS stimulant and sympathomimetic.

Amytal: amobarbital. Barbiturate sedative-hypnotic.

Anavar: oxandrolone. An anabolic steroid.

angel dust: Street name for PCP.

Antabuse: disulfiram. Alters metabolism of alcohol, used to treat alcoholism.

aprobarbital: *Alurate.* Barbiturate sedative-hypnotic.

Artane: trihexyphenidyl. Anticholinergic used to control extrapyramidal symptoms.

Asendin: amoxapine. Heterocyclic antidepressant.

aspirin: acetylsalicylic acid. OTC analgesic.

Ativan: lorazepam. Benzodiazepine sedative.

atropine: Anticholinergic.

Aventyl: nortriptyline. Heterocyclic antidepressant.

belladonna: Poisonous anticholinergic plant.

Benzedrine: amphetamine. CNS stimulant and sympathomimetic. Brand name no longer used.

benzodiazepines: Class of sedative-hypnotics that includes diazepam *(Valium).*

benztropine: *Cogentin.* Anticholinergic used to control extrapyramidal symptoms.

bromide: Group of salts with sedative properties.

butabarbital: *Butisol.* Barbiturate sedative-hypnotic.

Butisol: butabarbital. Barbiturate sedative-hypnotic.

caffeine: Mild stimulant found in coffee and in OTC preparations.

chloral hydrate: *Noctec.* Nonbarbiturate sedative-hypnotic.

chlorazepate: *Tranxene.* Benzodiazepine sedative.

Chlordiazeporide: *Librium.* Benzodiazepine sedative.

chlorpheniramine maleate: OTC antihistamine.

chlorpromazine: *Thorazine.* Antipsychotic.

chlorprothixene: *Taractan.* Antipsychotic.

Brand names in italic

411

Cibalith: lithium citrate. Salt used in treating mania and bipolar affective disorders.

clonidine: *Catapres.* Antihypertensive drug shown to reduce narcotic withdrawal symptoms.

cocaine: CNS stimulant and local anesthetic.

codeine: Narcotic analgesic found in opium.

Cogentin: benztropine. Anticholinergic used to treat extrapyramidal symptoms.

Compazine: prochlorperazine. Antipsychotic.

Cylert: pemoline. Stimulant used in ADD with hyperactivity.

Dalmane: flurazepam. Benzodiazepine hypnotic.

Darvon: propoxyphene. Narcotic analgesic.

Datura: Genus of plants, many of which are anticholinergic.

Demerol: meperidine. Narcotic analgesic.

desipramine: *Norpramine, Pertofrane.* Heterocyclic antidepressant.

Desoxyn: methamphetamine. CNS stimulant and sympathomimetic.

Desyrel: trazodone. Heterocyclic antidepressant.

Dexedrine: dextroamphetamine. CNS stimulant and sympathomimetic.

dextroamphetamine: *Dexedrine.* CNS stimulant and sympathomimetic.

dextromethorphan: OTC cough supressant.

diazepam: *Valium.* Benzodiazepine sedative.

diethylpropion: *Tenuate, Tepanil.* Amphetamine-like appetite supressant.

dihydrocodeine: Narcotic analgesic.

Dilaudid: hydromorphone. Narcotic analgesic.

diphenhydramine: Antihistamine.

disulfiram: *Antabuse.* Alters metabolism of alcohol, used to treat alcoholism.

DMT: Hallucinogen.

Dolophine: methadone. Narcotic analgesic.

DOM: Hallucinogen.

doxepin: *Sinequan, Adapin.* Heterocyclic antidepressant.

dronabinol: *Marinol.* Prescription form of delta-9 tetrahydrocannabinol, used to control nausea in patients undergoing chemotherapy for cancer.

Elavil: amitriptyline. Heterocyclic antidepressant.

Endep: amitriptyline. Heterocyclic antidepressant.

endorphin: Endogenous substance with effects similar to the narcotic analgesics.

enkephalin: Endogenous substance with effects similar to the narcotic analgesics.

ephedrine: Sympathomimetic used in asthma.

Equanil: meprobamate. Nonbarbiturate sedative-hypnotic.

Eskalith: lithium carbonate. Salt used in treating mania and bipolar affective disorders.

fenfluramine: *Pondimin.* Appetite suppressant.

fentanyl: *Sublimaze.* Potent synthetic analgesic.

fluphenazine: *Permitil, Prolixin.* Antipsychotic.

fluoxetine: *Prozac.* Antidepressant medication chemically unrelated to heterocyclics or MAO inhibitors.

flurazepam: *Dalmane.* Benzodiazepine hypnotic.

Halcion: triazolam. Benzodiazepine hypnotic.

Haldol: haloperidol. Antipsychotic.

haloperidol: *Haldol.* Antipsychotic.

henbane: Poisonous anticholinergic plant.

heroin: Narcotic analgesic. Diacetylmorphine.

hydrocodone: Narcotic analgesic.

hydromorphone: *Dilaudid.* Narcotic analgesic.

imipramine: *Tofranil, Janimine.* Heterocyclic antidepressant.

isocarboxazid: *Marplan.* MAO inhibitor used as antidepressant.

Janimine: imipramine. Heterocyclic antidepressant.

Ketalar: ketamine. Dissociative anesthetic.

ketamine: *Ketalar.* Dissociative anesthetic.

laudanum: Tincture (alcohol solution) of opium.

Librium: chlordiazepoxide. Benzodiazepine sedative.

Lithane: lithium carbonate.

lithium carbonate, lithium citrate: Salts used in treating mania and bipolar affective disorders.

Lithobid: lithium carbonate.

lorazepam: *Ativan.* Benzodiazepine sedative.

loxapine: *Loxitane.* Antipsychotic.

Loxitane: loxapine. Antipsychotic.

LSD: Hallucinogen.

Ludiomil: maprotiline. Heterocyclic antidepressant.

Luminal: phenobarbital. Barbiturate sedative hypnotic.

mandrake: Anticholinergic plant.

maprotiline: *Ludiomil.* Heterocyclic antidepressant.

Marinol: dronabinol. Prescription form of delta-9 tetrahydrocannabinol, used to control nausea in patients undergoing chemotherapy for cancer.

Marplan: isocarboxazid. MAO inhibitor used as antidepressant.

Mazanor: mazindol. Appetite suppressant.

mazindol: *Mazanor, Sanorex.* Appetite suppressant.

MDA: Hallucinogen.

MDMA: Hallucinogen.

Mebaral: mephobarbital. Barbiturate sedative hypnotic.

Mellaril: thioridazine. Antipsychotic.

meperidine: *Demerol.* Narcotic analgesic.

mephobarbital: *Mebaral.* Barbiturate sedative-hypnotic.

meprobamate: *Equanil, Miltown.* Nonbarbiturate sedative-hypnotic.

mescaline: Hallucinogen found in peyote cactus.

mesoridazine: *Serentil.* Antipsychotic.

methadone: *Dolophine.* Narcotic analgesic.

methamphetamine: *Desoxyn, Methedrine.* CNS stimulant and sympathomimetic.

methaqualone: *Quaalude, Sopor.* Nonbarbiturate sedative-hypnotic.

methylphenidate: *Ritalin.* Stimulant used in ADD with hyperactivity.

Metrazol: pentylenetetrazol. Convulsant once used in convulsive therapy.

Miltown: meprobamate. Nonbarbiturate sedative-hypnotic.

Moban: molindone. Antipsychotic.

molindone: *Moban.* Antipsychotic.

morphine: Narcotic analgesic.

naloxone: *Narcan.* Narcotic antagonist.

naltrexone: *Trexan.* Narcotic antagonist.

Narcan: naloxone. Narcotic antagonist.

Nardil: phenelzine. MAO inhibitor used as antidepressant.

Navane: thiothixene. Antipsychotic.

Nembutal: pentobarbital. Barbiturate sedative-hypnotic.

Noctec: chloral hydrate. Nonbarbiturate sedative-hypnotic.

Norpramine: desipramine. Heterocyclic antidepressant.

nortriptyline: *Aventyl, Pamelor.* Heterocyclic antidepressant.

Nuomorphan: oxymorphone. Narcotic analgesic.

opium: Narcotic analgesic.

oxandrolone: *Anavar.* An anabolic steroid.

oxazepam: *Serax.* Benzodiazepine sedative.

oxycodone: *Percodan.* Narcotic analgesic.

oxymorphone: *Nuomorphan.* Narcotic analgesic.

Pamelor: nortriptyline. Heterocyclic antidepressant.

paraldehyde: Nonbarbiturate sedative-hypnotic.

paregoric: Tincture (alcohol solution) of opium.

Parnate: tranylcypromine. MAO inhibitor used as antidepressant.

PCP: phencyclidine, "angel dust." Hallucinogen.

pemoline: *Cylert.* Stimulant used in ADD with hyperactivity.

pentazocine: *Talwin.* Narcotic analgesic.

pentobarbital: *Nembutal.* Barbiturate sedative-hypnotic.

pentylenetetrazol: *Metrazol.* Convulsant formerly used in convulsive therapy.

Percodan: oxycodone. Narcotic analgesic.

Permitil: fluphenazine. Antipsychotic.

perphenazine: *Trilafon.* Antipsychotic.

Pertofrane: desipramine. Heterocyclic antidepressant.

peyote: Hallucinogenic cactus containing mescaline.

phencyclidine: PCP, "angel dust." Hallucinogen.

phendimetrazine: Amphetamine-like appetite suppressant.

phenelzine: *Nardil.* MAO inhibitor used as antidepressant.

phenmetrazine: *Preludin.* Amphetamine-like appetite suppressant.

phenobarbital: *Luminal.* Barbiturate sedative-hypnotic.

phentermine: Amphetamine-like appetite suppressant.

phenylpropanolamine: OTC appetite suppressant.

Pondimin: fenfluramine. Appetite suppressant.

Preludin: phenmetrazine. Amphetamine-like appetite suppressant.

prochlorperazine: *Compazine.* Antipsychotic.

Prolixin: fluphenazine. Antipsychotic.

propoxyphene: *Darvon.* Narcotic analgesic.

protriptyline: *Vivactil.* Heterocyclic antidepressant.

Prozac: fluoxetine. Antidepressant medication chemically unrelated to heterocyclics or MAO inhibitors.

pseudoephedrine: OTC sympathomimetic.

psilocybin: Hallucinogen from Mexican mushroom.

Quaalude: methaqualone. Nonbarbiturate sedative-hypnotic.

Restoril: temazepam. Benzodiazepine hypnotic.

Ritalin: methylphenidate. Stimulant used in ADD with hyperactivity.

Sanorex: mazindol. Appetite suppressant.

scopolamine: anticholinergic.

secobarbital: *Seconal.* Barbiturate sedative-hypnotic.

Seconal: secobarbital. Barbiturate sedative-hypnotic.

Serax: oxazepam. Benzodiazepine sedative.

Serentil: mesoridazine. Antipsychotic.

Sernyl: former brand name for PCP.

Sinequan: doxepin. Heterocyclic antidepressant.

Sopor: methaqualone. Nonbarbiturate sedative-hypnotic.

stanozolol: *Winstrol.* An anabolic steroid.

Stelazine: trifluoperazine. Antipsychotic.

Sublimaze: fetanyl. Potent synthetic analgesic.

Talwin: pentazocine. Narcotic analgesic.

Taractan: chlorprothixene. Antipsychotic.

temazepam: *Restoril.* Benzodiazepine hypnotic.

Tenuate: diethylpropion. Amphetamine-like appetite suppressant.

Tepanil: diethylpropion. Amphetamine-like appetite suppressant.

Teslac: testolactone. An anabolic steroid.

testolactone: *Teslac.* An anabolic steroid.

theophylline: Mild stimulant found in tea. Used to treat asthma.

thioridazine: *Mellaril.* Antipsychotic.

thiothixene: *Navane:* Antipsychotic.

Thorazine: chlorpromazine. Antipsychotic.

Tindal: acetophenazine. Antipsychotic.

Tofranil: imipramine. Heterocyclic antidepressant.

Tranxene: chlorazepate. Benzodiazepine sedative.

tranylcypromine: *Parnate.* MAO inhibitor used as antidepressant.

trazodone: *Desyrel.* Heterocyclic antidepressant.

Trexan: naltrexone. Narcotic antagonist.

triazolam: *Halcion.* Benzodiazepine hypnotic.

trifuloperazine: *Stelazine.* Antipsychotic.

triflupromazine: *Vesprin.* Antipsychotic.

trihexyphenidyl: *Artane.* Anticholinergic used to control extrapyramidal symptoms.

Trilafon: perphenazine. Antipsychotic

Valium: diazepam. Benzodiazepine sedative.

Vesprin: triflupromazine. Antipsychotic.

Vivactil: protriptyline. Heterocyclic antidepressant.

Winstrol: stanozolol. An anabolic steroid.

Xanax: alprazolam. Benzodiazepine sedative.

Appendix B

Resources for Information and Assistance

FEDERAL GOVERNMENT AGENCIES

National Clearinghouse for Alcohol and Drug Information
P.O. Box 2345
Rockville, MD 20852
(301) 468-2600

NIDA Cocaine Hotline
1-800-662-HELP

Office on Smoking and Health
5600 Fishers Lane
Rockville, MD 20857
(301) 443-1575

ALCOHOL

Alcohol Research Information Service
1106 E. Oakland
Lansing, MI 48906
(517) 485-9900

Alcoholics Anonymous World Services
P.O. Box 459, Grand Central Station
New York, NY 10163
(212) 686-1100

American Council on Alcoholism
5024 Campbell Blvd. Suite H
Whitemarsh Business Center
Baltimore, MD 21236
(301) 529-9200

American Health and Temperance Society
6830 Eastern Ave., N.W.
Washington, D.C. 20012
(202) 722-6736

BACCHUS of the U.S.
(Boost Alcohol Consciousness Concerning the Health
of University Students)
P.O. Box 10430
Denver, CO 80210
(303) 871-3068

Licensed Beverage Information Council
1250 I St., N.W., Suite 900
Washington, D.C. 20005
(202) 628-3544

MADD (Mothers Against Drunk Driving)
669 Airport Fwy., Suite 310
Hurst, TX 76053
(817) 268-6233

National Alcohol Hotline
1-800-ALCOHOL

National Council on Alcoholism
12 W. 21st St.
New York, NY 10010
(212) 206-6770

National Woman's Christian Temperance Union
1730 Chicago Ave.
Evanston, IL 60201
(312) 864-1396

RID (Remove Intoxicated Drivers)
P.O. Box 520
Schenectedy, NY 12301
(518) 372-0034

SMOKING

ASH (Action on Smoking and Health)
2013 H St., N.W.
Washington, D.C. 20006
(202) 659-4310

Council for Tobacco Research
900 Third Ave.
New York, NY 10022
(212) 421-8885

Smoking Control Advocacy Resource Center
1730 Rhode Island Ave. N.W.
Washington, D.C. 20036
(202) 659-8475

Tobacco Institute
1875 I St., N.W.
Washington, D.C. 20006
(202) 457-4800

DRUGS

Alcohol and Drug Problems Association of North
    America
444 N. Capitol St., N.W., Suite 706
Washington, D.C. 20001
(202) 737-4340

American Council for Drug Education
204 Monroe St., Suite 110
Rockville, MD 20850
(301) 294-0600

Do It Now Foundation
Box 27568
Tempe, AZ 85285
(602)257-0797

Drug Policy Foundation
4801 Massachusetts Ave., N.W., Suite 400
Washington, D.C. 20016-2087

Fair Oaks Hospital
(201) 552-7000
19 Prospect St.
Summit, NJ 07901
Box 100
Summit, NJ 07901
(800) COCAINE

Narcotic Educational Foundation of America
5055 Sunset Blvd.
Los Angeles, CA 90027
(213) 663-5171

National Drug Information Center of Families in Action,
    Inc.
2296 Henderson Mill Rd., Suite 204
Atlanta, GA 30345
(404) 934-6364

National Federation of Parents for a Drug-Free Youth
1423 N. Jefferson
Springfield, MO 65802-1988
(407) 836-3709

NIDA (National Institute on Drug Abuse)
5600 Fishers Lane
Rockville, MD 20857

NORML (National Organization for the Reform of Mar-
    ijuana Laws)
2001 S. St., N.W., Suite 640
Washington, D.C. 20009
(202) 483-5500

PRIDE (Parent Resource Institute for Drug Education)
100 Edgewood Ave., Suite 1002
Atlanta, GA 30303
(800) 241-7946

Credits

Chapter 1   p. 2 (left), Susan Lapides, Joel Gordon; p. 2 (right), Stacy Pick, Stock Boston; p. 3, Michael Hayman, Stock Boston; p. 9, H. Armstrong Roberts; p. 10, Bill Whitehead, Kansas City, KS; p. 17, H. Armstrong Roberts

Chapter 2   p. 22, Fred Mark Tosi, Photo Researchers, Inc.; p. 24, Arthur Sirdofsky, Medichrome/Stock Shop; p. 26, Gerald Thomas, Stock Boston

Chapter 3   p. 39, Mary Evans Picture Library, Photo Researchers, Inc.; p. 41, The Bettmann Archive; p. 47, courtesy Federal Drug Enforcement Administration; p. 52, Mark Perlstein Photography; p. 53, Alon Reininger, Woodfin Camp and Associates; p. 55, Alon Reininger, Woodfin Camp and Associates

Chapter 4   p. 75 (left), Joel Landau, Medichrome/Stock Shop; p. 75, Michael Murphy, Medichrome/Stock Shop

Chapter 5   p. 79, Wolff Communications; p. 80, Wolff Communications; p. 83, Jim Anderson, Woodfin Camp and Associates

Chapter 6   p. 103, Jane Schreibman, Photo Researchers, Inc.

Chapter 7   p. 127, courtesy Drug Enforcement Administration; p. 130, The Bettmann Archives; p. 131 (top), Miami Herald, Black Star; p. 131 (bottom), Andy Levin, Black Star; p. 132, Arthur Tress, Photo Researchers, Inc.; p. 135, Steve Star, Picture Group

Chapter 8   p. 141, Ray Ellis, Photo Researchers, Inc.

Chapter 9   p. 153, Data from Keller, M., and Gurioloi, C.: Statistics on consumption of alcohol and alcoholism, New Brunswick, N.J., 1976, Journal of Studies on Alcohol, Inc.; p. 155, The Bettmann Archives; p. 158,

Data from Beer Marketers INSIGHTS, West Nyack, N.Y., Used by permission; p. 159, Wolff Communications; p. 161, Wolff Communications; p. 163, Blair Seitz, Photo Researchers, Inc.; p. 167, Wolff Communications; p. 172, IHHS facts 1988, Insurance Institute for Highway Safety, Washington, D.C.; p. 173, Reader's Digest $500,000 Don't Drink and Drive College Scholarship Challenge; p. 179, From Streissguth, A.P., et al., Science 209:453-461, 1980; p. 185 (top), Owen Franken, Stock Boston; p. 185 (bottom), Barbara Alper, Stock Boston

Chapter 10   p. 192, FPG International Corp.; p. 195, FPG International Corp.; p. 196, Ciganovic, The Stock Shop; p. 199, Michael Weisbrot, Stock Boston; p. 202, "That's Jake," Tribune Media Services; p. 203, David Garvey, The Stock Shop; p. 205, From The Tobacco Observer, 7(1):1, 1982; p. 206, Photo Researchers, Inc.; p. 208, David York, Medichrome

Chapter 11   p. 217, Data from International Coffee Organization, London; p. 218, Roger Smith, Art Resource, N.Y.; p. 219, Wolff Communications; p. 221, The Bettmann Archives; p. 223, Wolff Communications; p. 224, Data from Consumer Research Magazine, June 1984; p. 225, King Features Syndicate; p. 227, From Physicians Desk Reference for Nonprescription Drugs, 1985

Chapter 12   p. 238, Wolff Communications; p. 250, Wolff Communications

Chapter 13   pp. 254-256, American Psychiatric Association: Diagnostic and Statistical Manual of Mental Disorders, ed. 4, Washington, D.C., 1987; p. 260, Dose ranges from Bernstein, J.G.: Rational use of antipsychotic drugs. In Bernstein J.: Clinical psychopharmacology, ed. 2, Littleton, MA, 1984, John Wright-PSG, Inc.; p. 262, Dose ranges from Schoonover, S.C.: Depression. In Bassuck, E.L., Schoonover, S.C., and

Gelenberg, A.J., editors: The practitioner's guide to psychoactive drugs, ed. 2, New York, 1983, Plenum Press; p. 263, Frances M. Cox, Stock Boston; p. 267, Joel Gordon

Chapter 14 p. 271, Michael Hardy, Woodfin Camp and Associates; p. 281 (left), Data from the Drug Enforcement Administration, 1988; p. 281 (right), Richard Frear, Photo Researchers, Inc.; p. 291, Mary Ellen Mark, Archive Pictures, Inc.

Chapter 15 p. 304, From Cohen, S.L.: Lysergic acid diethylamide: Side effects and complications, Journal of Nervous and Mental Disease 130:30-40, 1960. Copyright © 1982 The Williams & Wilkins Co.; p. 308, Michael O'Brien, Archive Pictures, Inc.; p. 318, Richard Gross, Biological Photography

Chapter 16 p. 324, Jerry Howard, Stock Boston; p. 326, Joyce Photographics, Photo Researchers, Inc.; p. 333, Modified from Jones, R.T.: Tetrahydrocannabinol and the marijuana-induced social "high," or the effects on the mind of marijuana. In Singer, A.J., editor: Marijuana: chemistry, pharmacology, and patterns of social use, Annals of the New York Academy of Sciences 191:144-165, 1971; p. 338, Joel Gordon; p. 342 (left), Frank Oberle, Photographic Resources; p. 342 (right), Vigilante, R., and Cowan, R.C.: Pot-Talk: Is decriminalization advisable? National Review, April 29, 1983. Reprinted in Drugs, society and behavior 86/87, Annual editions, Guilford, Conn, 1986

Chapter 17 p. 348, Modified from Swisher, J.D.: Prevention issues. In Dupont, R.I., et al., editors: Handbook on drug abuse, Washington, D.C., 1979, NIDA, U.S. Government Printing Office; p. 349 (left), Adapted from Cohen, A.Y.: Alternatives to Drug Use: Steps Toward Prevention. U.S. Department of Health, Education and Welfare; p. 349 (right), Janeart Ltd., The Image Bank; p. 352, NIDA; p. 353, Wolff Communications

Chapter 18 p. 367, Robert Goldstein, Photo Researchers, Inc.; p. 372, Doug Magee, Art Resource

Chapter 19 p. 379, Dana Summers Washington Post Writers' Group; p. 381, Focus on Sports; p. 383, Sports Illustrated; p. 384, Wolff Communication

Chapter 20 p. 391, Jim Anderson, Woodfin Camp and Associates; p. 393, Cynthia Dopkin, Photo Researchers, Inc.; p. 396, Jan Halaska, Photo Researchers, Inc.

Index

Italics indicate figures; *t* indicates table.

Checklist for Knowledge of and Interest in Drugs and Drug Use

TO THE INSTRUCTOR

The purpose of this checklist is to secure student appraisal of knowledge and interest in various topics and issues covered by the text. When used at the beginning of the semester, this checklist can help you in planning the organization and emphases of your course. You will notice that there is a degree of correspondence between the items on the checklist and the chapter objectives. The checklist will also provide the student with an orientation to the area of drugs and drug use, giving a brief overview of the topics to be covered.

The answers are coded so that an optical scanner can be used for rapid analysis. If you have access to a test scoring computer that gives you item analyses, you can simply make any arbitrary answer "correct" on your key, ignore the scores, and use the item analysis to get a distribution of responses to each item.

TO THE STUDENT

The results of this questionnaire will not be used for grading purposes. The purpose of this checklist is to allow you to indicate your present knowledge and interest in various areas and issues involved in drugs and drug use. Your replies will be useful in planning the course so that the emphasis and time allotments will best meet the needs and interests of most of the class.

Directions: Read each item carefully. There are no right or wrong answers. Answer each item as honestly as you can. After each item mark a score from 1 to 5 indicating how much you already know about it and another score indicating your interest in the topic. If you are using a computer-scored answer sheet, remember that each odd-numbered answer refers to knowledge and each even-numbered answer refers to interest.

SCORING
Knowledge (Odd-Numbered Items)

1: You have almost no knowledge of this topic.
2: You have a little knowledge of this topic.
3: You know something about this but could profit from learning more.
4: You know almost as much as you want to know about this.

5: You are satisfied that you know enough about this topic.

Interest (Even-Numbered Items)

1: You have no interest in this topic.
2: You have a little interest in this topic.

3: You have some interest and would like to learn more if time were available.
4: You are quite interested and hope that this topic is well covered.
5: This is one of the most interesting topics to you, one that you may even explore beyond what is covered in class.

Drug Use in Society

	KNOWLEDGE		INTEREST	
Historical events that have shaped our society's attitudes about drugs.	(1)	1 2 3 4 5	(2)	1 2 3 4 5
Recent social changes and their relationship to changes in drug use.	(3)	1 2 3 4 5	(4)	1 2 3 4 5
How we gain information about which drugs are being used by how many people.	(5)	1 2 3 4 5	(6)	1 2 3 4 5
What proportion of people report using alcohol, tobacco, marijuana, and cocaine.	(7)	1 2 3 4 5	(8)	1 2 3 4 5
Characteristics of individuals likely to use illicit drugs.	(9)	1 2 3 4 5	(10)	1 2 3 4 5

Social Concerns About Drug Use

The conflict between individual freedom and society's desire to control drugs.	(11)	1 2 3 4 5	(12)	1 2 3 4 5
Relative toxicity of several types of illicit drugs.	(13)	1 2 3 4 5	(14)	1 2 3 4 5
Definition of the term addiction.	(15)	1 2 3 4 5	(16)	1 2 3 4 5
Factors contributing to the addicting potential of drugs.	(17)	1 2 3 4 5	(18)	1 2 3 4 5
Relationship of crime and violence to alcohol and narcotics.	(19)	1 2 3 4 5	(20)	1 2 3 4 5

Regulation of Drug Use

	KNOWLEDGE		INTEREST	
Historical factors leading to the first federal laws regulating drugs.	(21)	1 2 3 4 5	(22)	1 2 3 4 5
How and why federal drug laws have evolved into their current form.	(23)	1 2 3 4 5	(24)	1 2 3 4 5
The process by which a new drug is tested and approved for sale.	(25)	1 2 3 4 5	(26)	1 2 3 4 5
Current laws on controlled substances.	(27)	1 2 3 4 5	(28)	1 2 3 4 5
Current approaches to drug enforcement.	(29)	1 2 3 4 5	(30)	1 2 3 4 5

The Nervous System

How various cells, including nerve cells, communicate by using chemicals.	(31)	1 2 3 4 5	(32)	1 2 3 4 5

How these natural chemicals work to provide meaningful signals in the brain.

(33) 1 2 3 4 5 (34) 1 2 3 4 5

The functions of various major parts of the nervous system.

(35) 1 2 3 4 5 (36) 1 2 3 4 5

The chemical organization found among the pathways of the brain.

(37) 1 2 3 4 5 (38) 1 2 3 4 5

How drugs interact with the brain's chemicals to produce psychoactive effects.

(39) 1 2 3 4 5 (40) 1 2 3 4 5

Chemicals Used as Drugs

KNOWLEDGE *INTEREST*

How legal drugs are marketed and the impact of this industry in the United States.

(41) 1 2 3 4 5 (42) 1 2 3 4 5

The major sources of heroin, cocaine, and marijuana and how they are sold.

(43) 1 2 3 4 5 (44) 1 2 3 4 5

Brand name vs generic name drugs.

(45) 1 2 3 4 5 (46) 1 2 3 4 5

How drugs can be identified.

(47) 1 2 3 4 5 (48) 1 2 3 4 5

Detecting drug use and the controversy over drug screening programs.

(49) 1 2 3 4 5 (50) 1 2 3 4 5

The Actions of Drugs

Placebo effects vs true (specific) drug effects.

(51) 1 2 3 4 5 (52) 1 2 3 4 5

How drug effects change as a function of dose.

(53) 1 2 3 4 5 (54) 1 2 3 4 5

Factors influencing how rapidly a drug acts and for how long.

(55) 1 2 3 4 5 (56) 1 2 3 4 5

Comparing different methods for getting drugs into the body.

(57) 1 2 3 4 5 (58) 1 2 3 4 5

Reasons for developing tolerance to a drug and for withdrawal symptoms.

(59) 1 2 3 4 5 (60) 1 2 3 4 5

Stimulants

KNOWLEDGE *INTEREST*

The origins and early uses of both amphetamine and cocaine.

(61) 1 2 3 4 5 (62) 1 2 3 4 5

The evolution of the stimulants as drugs of abuse.

(63) 1 2 3 4 5 (64) 1 2 3 4 5

The mechanisms by which amphetamine and cocaine act in the brain.

(65) 1 2 3 4 5 (66) 1 2 3 4 5

The medical uses of amphetamine and cocaine.

(67) 1 2 3 4 5 (68) 1 2 3 4 5

Addiction liability and toxicity of amphetamine and cocaine.

(69) 1 2 3 4 5 (70) 1 2 3 4 5

Depressants

The various classes of depressant drugs, for example, barbiturates, Quaalude, Valium.

(71) 1 2 3 4 5 (72) 1 2 3 4 5

	KNOWLEDGE	INTEREST
The mechanisms by which the depressant drugs act in the brain.	(73) 1 2 3 4 5	(74) 1 2 3 4 5
The medical uses of the depressants.	(75) 1 2 3 4 5	(76) 1 2 3 4 5
Addiction liability and toxicity of the depressants.	(77) 1 2 3 4 5	(78) 1 2 3 4 5
Patterns of abuse of depressant drugs.	(79) 1 2 3 4 5	(80) 1 2 3 4 5

Alcohol

	KNOWLEDGE	INTEREST
Production of alcoholic beverages by fermentation and distillation.	(81) 1 2 3 4 5	(82) 1 2 3 4 5
Current trends in sales of beer, wine, and liquor.	(83) 1 2 3 4 5	(84) 1 2 3 4 5
Relationship of blood alcohol level to changes in behavior.	(85) 1 2 3 4 5	(86) 1 2 3 4 5
Medical and social problems associated with alcohol use.	(87) 1 2 3 4 5	(88) 1 2 3 4 5
Problem drinking and alcoholism.	(89) 1 2 3 4 5	(90) 1 2 3 4 5

Tobacco

	KNOWLEDGE	INTEREST
The history of tobacco and its importance to the U.S. economy.	(91) 1 2 3 4 5	(92) 1 2 3 4 5
How cigarettes are made and how they have changed in recent years.	(93) 1 2 3 4 5	(94) 1 2 3 4 5
The health consequences of smoking.	(95) 1 2 3 4 5	(96) 1 2 3 4 5
Smokeless tobacco and clove cigarettes.	(97) 1 2 3 4 5	(98) 1 2 3 4 5
How nicotine acts on the brain and its relationship to tobacco dependence.	(99) 1 2 3 4 5	(100) 1 2 3 4 5

Caffeine

	KNOWLEDGE	INTEREST
Coffee: its history, types, production, and preparation.	(101) 1 2 3 4 5	(102) 1 2 3 4 5
Other sources of caffeine: soft drinks and medications.	(103) 1 2 3 4 5	(104) 1 2 3 4 5
How caffeine acts on the brain and the time course of its action.	(105) 1 2 3 4 5	(106) 1 2 3 4 5
Physiologic and behavioral effects of caffeine.	(107) 1 2 3 4 5	(108) 1 2 3 4 5
Consequences of excessive caffeine use and other health concerns.	(109) 1 2 3 4 5	(110) 1 2 3 4 5

Nonprescription Drugs

	KNOWLEDGE	INTEREST
How the Food and Drug Administration regulates nonprescription products.	(111) 1 2 3 4 5	(112) 1 2 3 4 5
Over-the-counter stimulants, weight-control products, and sedatives.	(113) 1 2 3 4 5	(114) 1 2 3 4 5

Aspirin and other nonprescription pain relievers. (115) 1 2 3 4 5 (116) 1 2 3 4 5
Cold symptoms and how they are treated. (117) 1 2 3 4 5 (118) 1 2 3 4 5
How to select nonprescription drugs by understanding their ingredients. (119) 1 2 3 4 5 (120) 1 2 3 4 5

Drugs for Mental Illness

The symptoms of anxiety disorders, psychoses, and affective disorders. (121) 1 2 3 4 5 (122) 1 2 3 4 5
Drugs used in treating psychoses: how they work and their side effects. (123) 1 2 3 4 5 (124) 1 2 3 4 5
Drugs used in treating depression: types and side effects. (125) 1 2 3 4 5 (126) 1 2 3 4 5
Lithium as a treatment for mania and manic-depressive illness. (127) 1 2 3 4 5 (128) 1 2 3 4 5
Ethics and the social impact of drug treatments for mental disorders. (129) 1 2 3 4 5 (130) 1 2 3 4 5

Narcotics

The opium poppy: its history, its economics, and what it contains. (131) 1 2 3 4 5 (132) 1 2 3 4 5
The evolution of narcotic addiction since the early 1900s. (133) 1 2 3 4 5 (134) 1 2 3 4 5
The mechanism by which narcotics act in the brain. (135) 1 2 3 4 5 (136) 1 2 3 4 5
Medical uses of narcotics. (137) 1 2 3 4 5 (138) 1 2 3 4 5
Dependence liability and toxicity of various narcotics. (139) 1 2 3 4 5 (140) 1 2 3 4 5

Hallucinogens

	KNOWLEDGE	INTEREST

Use of hallucinogens in religious practices. (141) 1 2 3 4 5 (142) 1 2 3 4 5
The history of LSD discovery and use. (143) 1 2 3 4 5 (144) 1 2 3 4 5
Other hallucinogens and their effects, including mescaline, psilocybin, etc. (145) 1 2 3 4 5 (146) 1 2 3 4 5
Various psychoactive plants and the chemicals they contain. (147) 1 2 3 4 5 (148) 1 2 3 4 5
PCP (angel dust, phencyclidine). (149) 1 2 3 4 5 (150) 1 2 3 4 5

Marijuana

Cannabis plants and various preparations from them. (151) 1 2 3 4 5 (152) 1 2 3 4 5
THC as an ingredient of marijuana and how long it stays in the body. (153) 1 2 3 4 5 (154) 1 2 3 4 5

The basic physiologic and behavioral effects of
marijuana.   (155) 1 2 3 4 5   (156) 1 2 3 4 5
Medical uses for marijuana or THC.   (157) 1 2 3 4 5   (158) 1 2 3 4 5
Concerns about dependence and toxicity with
marijuana.   (159) 1 2 3 4 5   (160) 1 2 3 4 5

Education and Prevention

KNOWLEDGE   *INTEREST*

Various possible goals of drug education and drug
abuse prevention programs.   (161) 1 2 3 4 5   (162) 1 2 3 4 5
Drug abuse prevention programs in the public
schools: history and effectiveness.   (163) 1 2 3 4 5   (164) 1 2 3 4 5
Prevention approaches employing peers, families,
and community agencies.   (165) 1 2 3 4 5   (166) 1 2 3 4 5
Smoking prevention programs as an example of
useful approaches.   (167) 1 2 3 4 5   (168) 1 2 3 4 5
How to go about developing a prevention pro-
gram.   (169) 1 2 3 4 5   (170) 1 2 3 4 5

Treatment

Treatment of alcoholism: controversies and cur-
rent approaches.   (171) 1 2 3 4 5   (172) 1 2 3 4 5
Treatment of narcotic addiction.   (173) 1 2 3 4 5   (174) 1 2 3 4 5
Therapeutic community approaches.   (175) 1 2 3 4 5   (176) 1 2 3 4 5
Outpatient approaches to drug abuse treatment. (177) 1 2 3 4 5   (178) 1 2 3 4 5
Current approaches to the treatment of cocaine
dependence.   (179) 1 2 3 4 5   (180) 1 2 3 4 5

Drugs and Athletics

KNOWLEDGE   *INTEREST*

History of the use of drugs to enhance athletic
performance.   (181) 1 2 3 4 5   (182) 1 2 3 4 5
Actions of stimulant drugs in athletes.   (183) 1 2 3 4 5   (184) 1 2 3 4 5
Actions of steroids in athletes.   (185) 1 2 3 4 5   (186) 1 2 3 4 5
Current regulations and drug-testing policies for
athletes.   (187) 1 2 3 4 5   (188) 1 2 3 4 5

Current Issues

Impact of crack cocaine on inner cities.   (189) 1 2 3 4 5   (190) 1 2 3 4 5
Drug-free workplace regulations.   (191) 1 2 3 4 5   (192) 1 2 3 4 5
Recent changes in federal regulations and enforce-
ment efforts.   (193) 1 2 3 4 5   (194) 1 2 3 4 5
(Instructor may add)   (195) 1 2 3 4 5   (196) 1 2 3 4 5

(Instructor may add)

(Instructor may add)

(197) 1 2 3 4 5   (198) 1 2 3 4 5

(199) 1 2 3 4 5   (200) 1 2 3 4 5

Additional Questions

It is sometimes difficult for textbooks and instructors to keep up with the very latest fashions in drug use. However, this class will be more useful if we can address the drugs that some of our students are currently exposed to. That is the purpose of the following question:

What illicit drugs have you been recently hearing about being used at your school or among your friends and acquaintances?

Because some of the talk about drugs is just talk, we'd like to find out about drug use that you yourself have actually seen taking place. We are not trying to identify individuals for the purpose of questioning or prosecuting them, and the answers will be kept anonymous. However, don't answer if you don't want to:

What illicit drugs do you know for a fact are in current use by people you know?